D1093060

Frontal Sinus Surgery

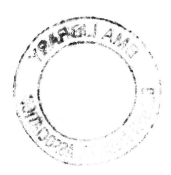

Devyani Lal · Peter H. Hwang

Editors

Frontal Sinus Surgery

A Systematic Approach

Foreword by
Valerie J. Lund, CBE, MB, BS, FRCS, FRCSEd

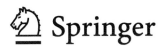

Editors

Devyani Lal, MD, FARS
Professor of Otolaryngology,
Mayo Clinic College of Medicine and
Science,
Associate Dean, Mayo Clinic School of
Continuous Professional Development,
Consultant, Department of
Otolaryngology – Head and Neck
Surgery,
Consultant (Joint),
Department of Neurological Surgery,
Mayo Clinic,
Phoenix, AZ,
USA

Peter H. Hwang, MD, FARS
Professor and Chief,
Division of Rhinology and Endoscopic
Skull Base Surgery,
Department of Otolaryngology – Head
and Neck Surgery,
Stanford University School of Medicine,
Stanford, CA,
USA

ISBN 978-3-319-97021-9   ISBN 978-3-319-97022-6   (eBook)
https://doi.org/10.1007/978-3-319-97022-6

Library of Congress Control Number: 2018965169

This Springer imprint is published by the registered company Springer Nature Switzerland AG
The registered company address is: Gewerbestrasse 11, 6330 Cham, Switzerland

I dedicate this book to my parents, Krishna Murari and Sarita Rani Lal. Their unequivocal love has brought me zest for life, learning and sharing.

This book was only possible with the loving support of my husband, Niresh Pande and my siblings, Ritu and Abhiroop.

Devyani Lal

To my many superb teachers, who have instilled in me a desire to pursue excellence in teaching; and to my students and trainees, who on a daily basis sustain my love for teaching and inspire me to continually sharpen my craft.

Peter H. Hwang

Foreword

Since the inception of endoscopic sinus surgery, it has been widely acknowledged that the frontal sinus provides the greatest challenges to rhinologists. Even prior to endoscopic approaches, the complex outflow anatomy of the frontal sinus and its proximity to the orbit and brain has always made it a potent source of acute and chronic complications which often demanded radical solutions. The proliferation of surgical procedures, devices, and drug delivery systems is indicative of the problems in maintaining mucociliary clearance and patency of the system. For these reasons, it is entirely appropriate for a book such as this to be entirely devoted to this topic, particularly one which adopts a systematic and practical approach.

The editors and senior authors, Dr. Lal and Dr. Hwang, have amassed an impressive array of the "great and the good" to explore all aspects from anatomy, physiology, and pathology through the range of medical management, the many surgical approaches, complications, and associated topics, concluding with a highly instructive step-by-step video demonstrations.

This comprehensive and insightful book is indispensable to all rhinologists at any stage of their careers, but above all, it is a surgeon's book, by surgeons sharing a unique cumulative expertise.

Valerie J. Lund, CBE, MB, BS, FRCS, FRCSEd
Professor of Rhinology, University College London
Honorary Consultant ENT Surgeon
Royal National Throat Nose and Ear Hospital (Royal Free Trust)
Moorfields Eye Hospital
University College Hospital and Imperial College
London, UK

Preface

Frontal sinus surgery is one of the most exacting procedures undertaken by the Otolaryngologist. Surgery in proximity to the eye and brain requires fortitude, and surgery within the convoluted frontal outflow tract requires exquisite delicacy and restraint. Seasoned surgeons approach the frontal sinus with reverence, while learners consider it with trepidation. The editors present a systematic approach to frontal sinus surgery through simplified discussions of critical concepts. A thoughtful, personalized approach optimizes patient outcomes; we therefore discuss all aspects of frontal anatomy, pathology, and surgical approaches. The editors thank the authors of all chapters, each led by global experts on the subject matter. Chapters are richly illustrated with figures and surgical videos, replete with practical pearls and tips. It is the editors' goal to provide this compendium as an aid to the sincere surgeon aspiring to attain expertise in frontal sinus surgery.

Phoenix, AZ, USA   Devyani Lal
Stanford, CA, USA   Peter H. Hwang

Contents

Contributors

Nithin D. Adappa, MD Department of Otorhinolaryngology – Head and Neck Surgery, University of Pennsylvania, Perelman School of Medicine, Philadelphia, PA, USA

Fahad Al-Asousi, MB BCh, BAO, SB-ORL St. Paul's Sinus Centre, St. Paul's Hospital, Department of Otolaryngology – Head and Neck Surgery, Vancouver, BC, Canada

Jeremiah A. Alt, MD, PhD Division of Otolaryngology – Head and Neck Surgery, University of Utah School of Medicine, Salt Lake City, UT, USA

Samantha Anne, MD, MS Pediatric Otolaryngology, Head and Neck Institute, Cleveland Clinic, Cleveland, OH, USA

Rami James N. Aoun, MD, MPH Department of Neurological Surgery, Mayo Clinic, Phoenix, AZ, USA

Pete S. Batra, MD, FACS Department of Otorhinolaryngology – Head and Neck Surgery and Rush Sinus Program, Rush University Medical Center, Chicago, IL, USA

Vidur Bhalla, MD University of Kansas Medical Center, Department of Otolaryngology – Head and Neck Surgery, Kansas City, KS, USA

Benjamin S. Bleier, MD Massachusetts Eye and Ear Infirmary, Harvard Medical School, Department of Otolaryngology, Boston, MA, USA

Christopher D. Brook, MD Boston University Medical Center, Department of Otolaryngology, Boston, MA, USA

Mohamad Raafat Chaaban, MD, MSCR, MBA Department of Otolaryngology, University of Texas Medical Branch, Galveston, TX, USA

Alexander Chiu, MD University of Kansas Medical Center, Department of Otolaryngology – Head and Neck Surgery, Kansas City, KS, USA

Garret W. Choby, MD Division of Rhinology and Endoscopic Skull Base Surgery, Department of Otolaryngology – Head and Neck Surgery, Stanford University School of Medicine, Stanford, CA, USA

Division of Rhinology and Endoscopic Skull Base Surgery, Department of Otorhinolaryngology – Head and Neck Surgery, Mayo Clinic, Rochester, MN, USA

Brian D'Anza, MD Division of Rhinology, Allergy, and Skull Base Surgery, Department of Otolaryngology, University Hospitals – Case Western Reserve University, Cleveland, OH, USA

Anali Dadgostar, MD, MPH, FRCSC St. Paul's Sinus Centre, St. Paul's Hospital, Department of Otolaryngology – Head and Neck Surgery, Vancouver, BC, Canada

John M. DelGaudio, MD Department of Otolaryngology – Head and Neck Surgery, Emory University School of Medicine, Atlanta, GA, USA

Rohit Divekar, MBBS PhD Division of Allergic Diseases, Mayo Clinic, Rochester, MN, USA

D. David Beahm, MD University of Kansas Medical Center, Department of Otolaryngology – Head and Neck Surgery, Kansas City, KS, USA

Jean Anderson Eloy, MD, FACS Department of Otolaryngology – Head and Neck Surgery, Rutgers New Jersey Medical School, Newark, NJ, USA

Center for Skull Base and Pituitary Surgery, Neurological Institute of New Jersey, Rutgers New Jersey Medical School, Newark, NJ, USA

Department of Neurological Surgery, Rutgers New Jersey Medical School, Newark, NJ, USA

Department of Ophthalmology and Visual Science, Rutgers New Jersey Medical School, Newark, NJ, USA

Marco Ferrari, MD Unit of Otorhinolaryngology – Head and Neck Surgery, University of Brescia, Brescia, Italy

Richard J. Harvey, MD, PhD, FRACS Rhinology and Skull Base, Applied Medical Research Centre, UNSW, Sydney, NSW, Australia

Faculty of Medicine and Health Sciences, Macquarie University, Sydney, NSW, Australia

Joseph M. Hoxworth, MD Neuroradiology Division, Department of Radiology, Mayo Clinic, Phoenix, AZ, USA

Mayo Clinic College of Medicine and Sciences, Phoenix, AZ, USA

Peter H. Hwang, MD, FARS Department of Otolaryngology – Head and Neck Surgery, Stanford University School of Medicine, Stanford, CA, USA

Amin R. Javer, MD, FRCSC St. Paul's Sinus Centre, St. Paul's Hospital, Department of Otolaryngology – Head and Neck Surgery, Vancouver, BC, Canada

David W. Kennedy, MD Department of Otorhinolaryngology – Head and Neck Surgery, The University of Pennsylvania, Philadelphia, PA, USA

Suat Kilic, BA Department of Otolaryngology – Head and Neck Surgery, Rutgers New Jersey Medical School, Newark, NJ, USA

Devyani Lal, MD, FARS Department of Otolaryngology – Head and Neck Surgery, Mayo Clinic College of Medicine and Science, Mayo Clinic, Phoenix, AZ, USA

Adrienne M. Laury, MD Otolaryngology, South Texas Veterans Health Care System, San Antonio, TX, USA

Jivianne T. Lee, MD Department of Head and Neck Surgery, University of California Los Angeles David Geffen School of Medicine, Los Angeles, CA, USA

Todd A. Loehrl, MD Department of Otolaryngology, Medical College of Wisconsin, Milwaukee, WI, USA

Division of Surgery, Zablocki VA Medical Center, Milwaukee, WI, USA

Conner J. Massey, MD University of Colorado School of Medicine, Department of Otolaryngology, Aurora, CO, USA

Jose Luis Mattos, MD, MPH Division of Rhinology and Sinus Surgery, Department of Otolaryngology – Head and Neck Surgery, Medical University of South Carolina, Charleston, SC, USA

Ben McArdle, MBBS, FRACS Department of Otolaryngology, Sunshine Coast University Hospital, Birtinya, Qld, Australia

Kevin C. McMains, MD Otolaryngology, South Texas Veterans Health Care System, San Antonio, TX, USA

Lester E. Mertz, MD Division of Rheumatology, Department of Medicine, Mayo Clinic, Scottsdale, AZ, USA

Jayakar V. Nayak, MD, PhD Division of Rhinology and Endoscopic Skull Base Surgery, Department of Otolaryngology – Head and Neck Surgery, Stanford University School of Medicine, Stanford, CA, USA

Piero Nicolai, MD Unit of Otorhinolaryngology – Head and Neck Surgery, University of Brescia, Brescia, Italy

Erin K. O'Brien, MD Department of Otorhinolaryngology, Mayo Clinic Rochester, Rochester, MN, USA

Richard R. Orlandi, MD Division of Otolaryngology – Head and Neck Surgery, University of Utah School of Medicine, Salt Lake City, UT, USA

James N. Palmer, MD Division of Rhinology, Department of Otorhinolaryngology – Head and Neck Surgery, Hospital of the University of Pennsylvania, Philadelphia, PA, USA

Peter Papagiannopoulos, MD Department of Otorhinolaryngology – Head and Neck Surgery and Rush Sinus Program, Rush University Medical Center, Chicago, IL, USA

Arjun K. Parasher, MD Division of Rhinology and Skull Base Surgery, Department of Otolaryngology – Head and Neck Surgery, University of South Florida, Tampa, FL, USA

Department of Health Policy and Management, University of South Florida, Tampa, FL, USA

Chirag Rajan Patel, MD Department of Otolaryngology – Head and Neck Surgery, Loyola University Medical Center, Maywood, IL, USA

Naresh P. Patel Department of Neurological Surgery, Mayo Clinic, Phoenix, AZ, USA

Zara M. Patel, MD Department of Otolaryngology – Head and Neck Surgery, Stanford University School of Medicine, Stanford, CA, USA

David M. Poetker, MD, MA Division of Surgery, Zablocki VA Medical Center, Milwaukee, WI, USA

Department of Otolaryngology, Medical College of Wisconsin, Milwaukee, WI, USA

Alkis James Psaltis, MBBS(hons), PhD, FRACS Department of Otolaryngology Head and Neck Surgery, The University of Adelaide, Adelaide, SA, Australia

Vijay R. Ramakrishnan, MD University of Colorado School of Medicine, Department of Otolaryngology, Aurora, CO, USA

Matthew A. Rank, MD Division of Allergy, Asthma, and Clinical Immunology, Mayo Clinic, Scottsdale, AZ, USA

E. Ritter Sansoni, MD Division of Rhinology and Skull Base Surgery, Department of Otolaryngology – Head and Neck Surgery, St Vincent's Hospital, Sydney, NSW, Australia

Luigi Fabrizio Rodella, MD Section of Anatomy and Physiopathology, University of Brescia, Brescia, Italy

Raymond Sacks, MBBCh, FCS (SA) ORL, FRACS Department of Otolaryngology, Macquarie University, Sydney, NSW, Australia

The University of Sydney, Sydney, NSW, Australia

Alberto Schreiber, MD Unit of Otorhinolaryngology – Head and Neck Surgery, University of Brescia, Brescia, Italy

Theodore A. Schuman, MD Rhinology and Skull Base Surgery, Department of Otolaryngology – Head and Neck Surgery, University of North Carolina at Chapel Hill, Chapel Hill, NC, USA

Joseph S. Schwartz, MD, FRCSC Department of Otolaryngology – Head and Neck Surgery, McGill University, Montreal, QC, Canada

Brent A. Senior, MD Division of Rhinology, Allergy, and Endoscopic Skull Base Surgery, Department of Otolaryngology – Head and Neck Surgery, University of North Carolina at Chapel Hill, Chapel Hill, NC, USA

Dongho Shin, BHSc, MD University of Toronto, Faculty of Medicine, Toronto, ON, Canada

Kristine A. Smith, MD Division of Otolaryngology – Head and Neck Surgery, Department of Surgery, University of Calgary, Calgary, AB, USA

Zachary M. Soler, MD, MSc Division of Rhinology and Sinus Surgery, Department of Otolaryngology – Head and Neck Surgery, Medical University of South Carolina, Charleston, SC, USA

Jessica E. Southwood, MD Department of Otolaryngology, Medical College of Wisconsin, Milwaukee, WI, USA

James A. Stankiewicz, MD Department of Otolaryngology – Head and Neck Surgery, Loyola University Medical Center, Maywood, IL, USA

Janalee K. Stokken, MD Department of Otorhinolaryngology, Mayo Clinic, Rochester, MN, USA

Peter F. Svider, MD Department of Otolaryngology – Head and Neck Surgery, Wayne State University School of Medicine, Detroit, MI, USA

Bobby A. Tajudeen, MD Department of Otorhinolaryngology – Head and Neck Surgery and Rush Sinus Program, Rush University Medical Center, Chicago, IL, USA

Andrew Thamboo, MD, MHSc, FRCSC Department of Otolaryngology – Head and Neck Surgery, Stanford University School of Medicine, Stanford, CA, USA

Aykut A. Unsal, DO Department of Otolaryngology – Head and Neck Surgery, Medical College of Georgia – Augusta University, Augusta, GA, USA

Rickul Varshney, MD, MSc, FRCSC Department of Otolaryngology, McGill University, Montreal, QC, Canada

Ian Witterick, MD, MSc, FRCSC Department of Otolaryngology – Head and Neck Surgery, University of Toronto, Sinai Health System, Toronto, ON, Canada

Bradford A. Woodworth, MD, FACS Department of Otolaryngology, University of Alabama at Birmingham, Gregory Fleming James Cystic Fibrosis Research Center, Birmingham, AL, USA

Alan D. Workman, BA, MD/MTR Department of Otolaryngology, Massachusetts Eye and Ear Infirmary, Boston, MA, USA

Peter-John Wormald, MD, FRACS Department of Otolaryngology Head and Neck Surgery, The University of Adelaide, Adelaide, SA, Australia

Carol H. Yan, MD Department of Otolaryngology – Head and Neck Surgery, Stanford University, Stanford, CA, USA

Shiayin F. Yang, MD Department of Otolaryngology – Head and Neck Surgery, Loyola University Medical Center, Maywood, IL, USA

Evolution and Challenges in Frontal Sinus Surgery

Carol H. Yan and David W. Kennedy

Introduction

The frontal sinuses and their complex anatomy have long challenged surgeons and triggered controversies in their surgical management. The relatively narrow frontal sinus drainage pathway, critical adjacent structures, and high long-term failure rate, combined with relatively difficult angled intranasal access, have created a broad swathe of surgical approaches with initial enthusiasm and subsequent abandonment. More recent attempts at frontal sinus surgery originated in the early eighteenth century with the initial reported cases wrought with morbidity and mortality. Subsequently, a spectrum of frontal sinus surgical techniques evolved. These include external approaches such as the osteoplastic flap, obliteration, cranialization, trephination, and external frontoethmoidectomy. More recently, endoscopic visualization created renewed potential for endonasal techniques, and combined endonasal and external approaches as well as purely endoscopic endonasal approaches have been popularized. The trend of frontal sinus surgery has transitioned from ablative intentions with closure of the frontal ostium, to restorative ones with enlargement of the

frontal outflow tract [1]. In this section, we briefly highlight the advances in techniques and resources that have allowed us to evolve frontal sinus surgery. The overarching goals of surgery include the eradication of disease, the resolution of symptoms, and the restoration of a nasofrontal outflow tract.

Historic Procedures

Early management of frontal sinus surgery from the early eighteenth century to the late twentieth century was predominantly external and focused on obliteration of disease. Some of these procedures still have indications today and will be discussed later in the chapter.

Trephination

The earliest frontal obliteration with a trephine was performed in 1750 by Runge as recorded by Donald [2]. The first published report of frontal sinus surgery with drainage of a mucocele has been credited to Seolberg Wells who conducted a trephine with tube placement [3]. Soon after in 1884, Alexander Ogston described a trephination procedure through the frontal sinus with curettage of mucosa and communication with the ethmoidal sinus for treatment of sinus infection. Luc described a very similar procedure, and in 1896, the Ogston-Luc technique was developed [1, 4]. However, the technique of trephination with frontal mucosal stripping did not gain

C. H. Yan
Department of Otolaryngology – Head and Neck Surgery, Stanford University, Stanford, CA, USA

D. W. Kennedy (✉)
Department of Otorhinolaryngology – Head and Neck Surgery, The University of Pennsylvania, Philadelphia, PA, USA

© Springer Nature Switzerland AG 2019
D. Lal, P. H. Hwang (eds.), *Frontal Sinus Surgery*, https://doi.org/10.1007/978-3-319-97022-6_1

popularity due to a high rate of nasofrontal outflow tract stenosis [5].

Radical Ablation

Frontal sinus obliteration was first introduced as an alternative to the Ogston-Luc procedure. In 1898, Riedel described obliteration of the frontal sinus with complete removal of the anterior table and floor of frontal sinus, stripping of all mucosa, and redraping of forehead skin [4]. This procedure, now known as frontal sinus collapse or the Riedel procedure, was associated with significant cosmetic deformity but improved disease control compared to the Ogston-Luc procedure. In those times, frontal sinusotomies were performed with chisels. Killian modified this technique by preserving a rim of mucosa and bone across the supraorbital ridge in an effort to decrease cosmetic deformity (Fig. 1.1). This technique too, was abandoned due to its high morbidity, post-operative infections, and failure rates [6]. However, frontal sinus collapse still remains a viable option today for some cases of osteomyelitis. In a small frontal sinus with narrow

anterior-posterior (A-P) diameter and with careful drill feathering of the sinus margins, the cosmetic deformity can be minimal. In other cases, a delayed reconstruction can be performed.

External Frontoethmoidectomy

Following disenchantment with disfiguring obliterative procedures, the surgical community explored the option of enlarging the nasofrontal outflow tract through external access to the frontal sinus. Knapp in 1908 entered the frontal sinus via a frontoethmoidectomy through the medial orbital wall. He continued to remove all mucosa of the frontal sinus and also enlarged the frontal outflow tract after addressing the disease. In 1914, Lothrop made the enlargement of the frontal outflow tract a priority and accomplished this via a combined external and intranasal approach to remove the ethmoidal cells, bilateral frontal sinus floors, the superior nasal septum and intersinus septum [7]. Resection of the frontal floor and medial orbital wall caused collapse of orbital soft tissue into the ethmoidal area and subsequent stenosis of the frontal drainage pathway [8]. The

a

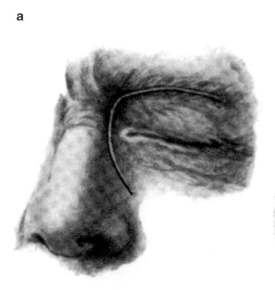

b

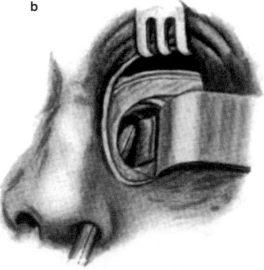

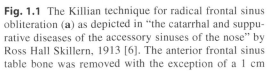

Fig. 1.1 The Killian technique for radical frontal sinus obliteration (**a**) as depicted in "the catarrhal and suppurative diseases of the accessory sinuses of the nose" by Ross Hall Skillern, 1913 [6]. The anterior frontal sinus table bone was removed with the exception of a 1 cm

bar of supraorbital rim to decrease deformity, and a mucosal nasal flap was rotated laterally to cover the frontal recess (**b**). This technique was complicated by high restenosis rates, supraorbital rim necrosis, and mucocele formation

removal of bone without adequate visualization made the procedure dangerous and technically difficult. Its eventual revival and popularization as an intranasal endoscopic operation by Draf was aided by multiple technological advances [9].

Lynch and Howarth in the United States described other modifications of external fronto-ethmoidectomy resulting in improved cosmetic outcome in 1921. This operation was conducted through a medial periorbital incision and pro-ceeded to remove ethmoidal cells as well as a portion of the frontal sinus floor along with a stent placement to ensure adequate drainage. This frontoethmoidectomy technique became known as the Lynch procedure, and its modi-fications have included the addition of a septal flap (Sewall-Boyden) and use of Silastic stents (Neel-Lake) [10, 11]. These additions improved early patency rates up to 85%, but poor long-term results led to its eventual abandonment [10].

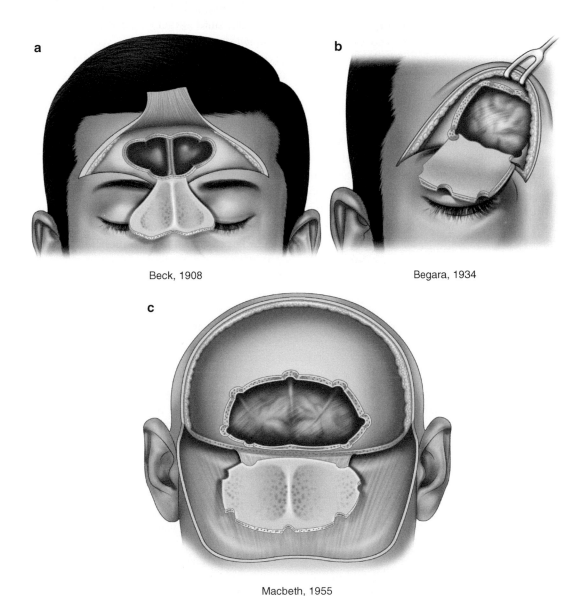

Beck, 1908

Begara, 1934

Macbeth, 1955

Fig. 1.2 Osteoplastic flap techniques as described in J. Dawes in *The Management of Frontal Sinusitis and its Complications*, J. Laryngology and Otology, 1961 [13]. Beck described in 1908 the use of radiographic guidance in his osteoplastic flaps with an incision along the upper margins of the eyebrows (**a**). In 1934, Bergara depicted his flap through the eyebrow incision (**b**) versus Macbeth, who adopted the bicoronal incision for a larger osteoplastic flap (**c**)

Osteoplastic Flaps

Osteoplastic flaps were separately described by Schonborn in 1894 and Brieger in 1895 [12]. Beck in 1908 used radiographic guidance to plan the incision of the flap (Fig. 1.2a). However, technical challenges and concerns of osteomyelitis prevented the flap from gaining popularity until Bergara introduced the eyebrow incision in 1934 (Fig. 1.2b) followed by Macbeth's adoption of the bicoronal incision for a large osteoplastic flap (Fig. 1.2c) [13]. In 1958, Goodale and Montgomery published their series of patients treated with an osteoplastic flap with fat obliteration and reported good success rates. By 1960, the osteoplastic flap, typically with but sometimes without obliteration, became the standard of care. In the 1960s, Becker developed the concept of using a template cut out of the patient's radiographic plate to outline the frontal sinus, allowing for a safer entry into the frontal sinus. The flap avoided significant facial deformity by replacing the bone plate and newer obliteration techniques. However, long-term follow-up demonstrated an increasing failure rate, and even using modern MRI, evaluating for recurrent disease has remained a challenge.

Early Adoption of Endoscopic Techniques

The use of external ablative procedures was limited by recurrent infections and disease due to the closure of the nasofrontal outflow tract, significant scarring and poor cosmetic outcomes. Even with the popular Lynch procedure, over 30% of patients required revision surgery. With these complications, the surgical community became more conservative in use of these approaches. Intranasal approaches were introduced in the beginning of the twentieth century but experienced high morbidity and mortality as the lack of visualization was troublesome.

Early endoscopic techniques were developed by Messerklinger, Wigand, and Draf. The initial work by Messerklinger incorporated the diagnostic use of the endoscope in analyzing mucociliary patterns of the paranasal sinuses. Mucosal apposition in the region of the frontal recess was noted to be the precursor of frontal sinusitis [14]. Wigand described the anatomic landmarks important for identifying the frontal ostium including the anterior ethmoidal artery, middle turbinate, and orbital wall.

In 1985, Kennedy made modifications to the Messerklinger technique and coined the term "functional endoscopic sinus surgery" [15]. Zinreich introduced CT imaging visualization of endoscopic sinus surgery to improve anatomic detail and decrease the very high radiation dose associated with polytomography [16]. Early functional endoscopic surgery also included treatment of mucoceles through marsupialization; approaches that were confronted with significant criticism [17]. Unlike the Lynch procedure, the endoscopic technique focuses on the preservation of as much mucosa as possible within the bony framework of the nasofrontal recess area. Kennedy and colleagues further described the valuable use of endoscopes to visualize the internal lining of the frontal sinus and maintain patency during post-operative surveillance.

Stammberger further popularized the Messerklinger approach, expanded indications for endoscopic disease management and made significant additional contributions to the technique and to the understanding of the regional anatomy [18]. Other early descriptions of endoscopic frontal sinus surgery for chronic sinusitis were described by Schaefer and Close who adopted the combined Messerklinger and Wigand technique along with placement of a Silastic tube if the ostioplasty was less than 6 mm [19]. The authors proposed that patients with frontal sinus ostia less than 4 mm or obstructive hypertrophic mucosa would not be good candidates for endoscopic surgery.

An improved understanding of frontal sinus anatomy facilitated the rapid adoption of endoscopic sinus surgery. Van Alyea's prior work was critical in describing supraorbital ethmoid, agger nasi, intersinus septal cells, and frontal recess cells as potential impediments to drainage of the frontal sinus [20]. The detailed anatomy and technique of removing agger nasi cells in frontal obstruction was further elaborated by Kuhn and colleagues [21].

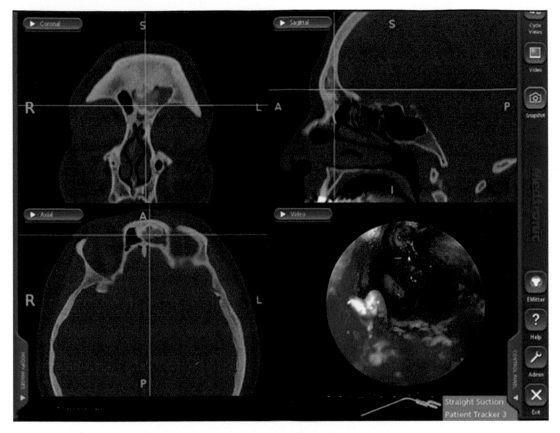

Fig. 1.3 An "outside-in" Draf III procedure being performed for a left-sided frontal osteoma with the help of CT image navigation using the Medtronic fusion navigation system (Minneapolis, MN, USA)

Advent of Modern Endoscopic Frontal Sinus Surgery

Variations of endoscopic frontal sinus surgery were described by Wolfgang Draf in the 1990s as type I, IIa and IIb, and III [9, 22]. Type I involves clearance of the frontal recess with anterior ethmoidectomy but no manipulation of the frontal ostium, type IIa and b involve an extended dissection of the frontal outflow tract with unilateral resection of the frontal sinus floor, while type III involves median drainage and bilateral resection of the frontal floor with removal of the intersinus septum. The Draf III technique, also known as the endoscopic modified Lothrop procedure, was detailed in 1994 in tribute to the original drill out procedure described by Lothrop in 1899 [23]. Close and colleagues warned fellow surgeons that circumferential stripping of frontal recess leads to

stenosis and stressed the importance of radiographic image guidance [23]. Interestingly, both Lothrop and Draf described the procedure to be especially challenging and cautioned against using it as a primary procedure. The availability of high-speed curved drills and image-guided surgery has allowed the Draf III to gain popularity (Fig. 1.3). Promising long-term follow-up data have encouraged expansion of indications for this procedure, most commonly used for chronic frontal sinusitis, for use in surgery for mucoceles and tumors [24]. A meta-analysis reported partial or complete frontal sinus patency to be 95.9% with an overall failure rate (defined as requiring further surgery) to be 13.9% [25]. Subsequently, the re-stenosis rate had been further reduced by the introduction of mucosal grafts or regional mucosal flaps to cover the exposed bone created when the drainage pathway is extended anteriorly and laterally by the drill out.

An important turning point in frontal sinus surgery was the advent of mucosal-sparing techniques. Hilding had previously demonstrated in animals that the removal of mucosa of the maxillary sinus led to accumulation of secretions distally and increased chances of infections [26]. Walsh's Triologic thesis in 1943 suggested that removing diseased frontal sinus mucosa but preserving the frontal outflow tract led to improved outcomes [27]. Multiple studies using animal models demonstrated that a patent, well-mucosalized frontal outflow tract was critical to proper frontal sinus function [28, 47]. Furthermore, the presence of disease in the frontal recess does not mandate revision surgery if the patient is asymptomatic [26, 29]. In a series of 440 subjects who underwent endoscopic sinus surgeries, most of the patients who were noted to have persistent mucosal disease remained asymptomatic [30].

Improvements and Tools in Endoscopic Frontal Sinus Surgery

Improvements in optical aids, instrumentation, and knowledge of pathophysiology have been the critical developments in establishing endoscopic sinus surgery as standard of care for frontal sinus disorders [31].

Frontal Sinus Stents

The use of frontal stents has waxed and waned in the history of frontal sinus surgery. Stents, consisting of a firm rubber tube, were used with Lynch's external frontoethmoidectomy, which employed placement of a firm rubber tube in the nasofrontal tract to maintain patency. However, the stenosis rate remained high at 30%. Neel and colleagues described a modified Lynch (Neel-Lake) operation in 1976 which used silicone (Silastic) rubber sheets to stent the nasofrontal passage with more promising long-term outcomes [11, 32]. In animal studies, stents created from Silastic sheets resulted in improved mucosal regeneration and decreased inflammation [32]. Schaefer and Close used Silastic tubing to stent small endoscopic frontal sinusotomies less than 6 mm [19]. More recently, steroid-eluting bioabsorbable implants placed in the frontal ostioplasty have been shown to be advantageous in several clinical trials. Murr and colleagues performed the original safety and efficacy study for an ethmoid mometasone-eluting implant. In a prospective double-blind, randomized study, they demonstrated decreased inflammation, adhesion, and polyp formation [33]. More recently, a smaller implant placed into the frontal sinus has also been demonstrated to reduce the need for postoperative frontal ostial debridement and to reduce the incidence of stenosis (Propel, Intersect ENT, Menlo Park, CA, USA) (Fig. 1.4c). An office-based corticosteroid-eluting implant (mometasone-furoate impregnated implant, SINUVA, Intersect ENT, Menlo Park, CA, USA) has recently been approved for treatment of recurrent nasal polyps in adult patients who have undergone prior ethmoidectomy.

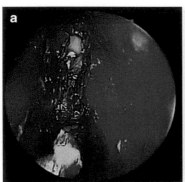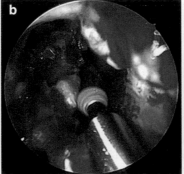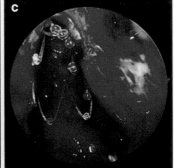

Fig. 1.4 A mucocele of the frontal sinus (**a**) in the process of being opened through a Draf III procedure using a 60,000 rpm high-speed drill, the Medtronic Mini-Midas (Minneapolis, MN, USA) (**b**). A mometasone-eluting stent is placed after completion of the Draf III (Propel, Intersect ENT, Menlo Park, CA, USA) (**c**)

Frontal Sinus Balloon Catheters

Catheter dilation of the paranasal sinuses was inspired by successes in cardiac and vascular procedures. Brown and Bolger performed the first paranasal sinus balloon dilations in 10 patients in 2006 and described a satisfying ease of cannulation while preserving mucosa [34]. Early on, cannulation was performed under fluoroscopic guidance prior to balloon inflation. While studies indicated symptomatic improvement in patients following fluoroscopy-directed balloon dilations, there were concerns regarding patient and physician radiation exposure [35]. Subsequently, light-guided catheters were introduced to utilize transillumination as an alternative method of catheter placement verification. More recently, the addition of image guidance has added additional precision to the catheterization procedure. Balloon catheter dilation can safely be used in the office setting by experienced surgeons for isolated frontal sinus ostium stenosis [36].

There are three current manufactures of frontal sinus balloon devices that have US Food and Drug Administration approval: Acclarent (Irvine, CA, USA), Entellus (Plymouth, MN, USA), and Medtronic (Minneapolis, MN, USA) [37]. Entellus produces XprESS, a device with a malleable tip (Fig. 1.5c), and Path Assist, which acts as a frontal seeker. Working with Fiagon (Berlin, Germany), they have also introduced a computer-assisted image guidance wire, providing accurate tracking of the catheter tip. SpinPlus by Acclarent allows surgeons to navigate multiple frontal sinus ostia by spinning and changing the frontal guidewire trajectory. NuVent, manufactured by Medtronic (Minneapolis, MN, USA), offers surgical navigation with the Medtronic Fusion surgical navigation system (Minneapolis, MN, USA).

Powered Instruments

Powered instrumentation, including microdebriders and drills, have greatly improved the ability to perform mucosa-sparing techniques, particularly in extended frontal dissections. In 1995, Gross and colleagues demonstrated the use of an endonasal soft tissue shaver to perform the Lothrop procedure endonasally without complications [8].

Curved shaver blades and burrs allow for improved visualization and access to the frontal ostia. Microdebriders are available in different sizes and angulations with rotating tips, while various drills can be attached to the microdebrider platform. High-speed drills (60,000 rpm and higher) allow for very fast removal of frontal recess bone but are only available as straight drills (Fig. 1.4b). Angled drill systems running at 12,000 rpm (Diego Elite, Olympus America) and 15,000 rpm (Medtronic Straightshot, Medtronic, Minneapolis, MN, USA) that have built-in suction irrigation systems are available widely. More recently developed, the Medtronic Straightshot M5 Microdebrider functions at 30,000 rpm, allowing for rapid bone removal. Greater mucosal sparing is facilitated through a variety of angled diamond and cutting burrs.

Modern Indications for External Frontal Sinus Surgery

Although endoscopic sinus surgery has become the default approach, there still certain indications that require external frontal sinus surgery. A review of 683 patients with chronic sinusitis showed that external procedures were performed in 5.3% of the cases with the majority being either osteoplastic flaps for neo-osteogenesis of the frontal recess or adjunct trephination [38]. The combination of trephination and endoscopic techniques, known as the "above and below" approach, can be helpful in cases of difficult to reach, laterally based inflammatory and non-inflammatory pathology [39, 40]. Mini-trephinations can also guide us in finding difficult type III or IV frontal cells [41]. The ideal location for trephination has been described as 10 mm from a line passing through the crista galli [42].

There are almost no indications for an external frontoethmoidectomy in today's era. The risk of fibrosis and closure of the frontal ostium with this procedure can result in high rates of recurrent infection and mucocele formation. The Neel-Lake modification of the original Lynch procedure utilizes techniques of mucosa preservation and frontal stenting [11, 32].

In contrast, there is still a role for the osteoplastic flap procedure, such as contemporary indications of tumors, recurring failure from endoscopic approaches for chronic sinusitis,

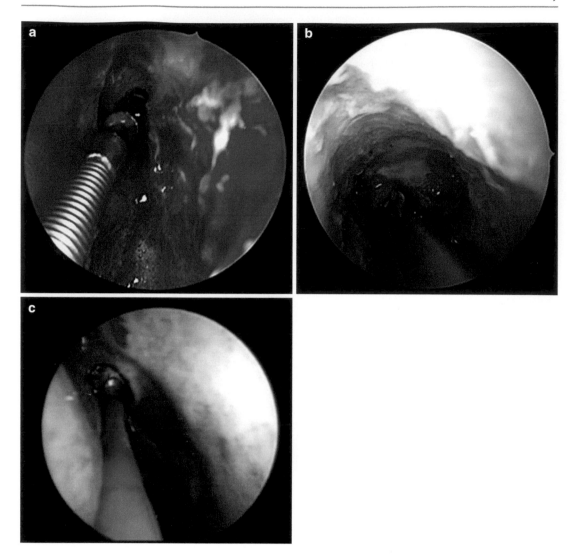

Fig. 1.5 Frontal sinus ostia have been more easily widened with mucosal-sparing techniques due to advancements in frontal sinus instruments including the frontal sinus angled (Hosemann) punch (**a**) and the forward-cutting (cobra) punch (**b**). Frontal sinus balloon catheter dilation (**c**) provides another way of cannulating the frontal ostium while preserving mucosa as shown here with one of the FDA-approved devices XprESS from Entellus (Plymouth, MN, USA)

lesions inaccessible endoscopically, and in some cases of frontal sinus trauma. Osteoplastic flaps today far more likely to be performed in combination with a Draf 3 procedure and without obliteration. This enhances both endoscopic visualization and post surgical radiographic surveillance, although the approach lengthens surgical time. Obliteration techniques are associated with long-term failures. Hardy and Montgomery reported a complication rate of 18% with significant morbidity. Recent studies with longer term follow-up clearly suggest that the failure rate continues to increase significantly over time [43].

New Techniques and Thoughts in Frontal Sinus Surgery

A recurrent challenge for frontal sinus surgery has been narrow frontal ostia and post-operative re-stenosis. While creation of osteoplastic flaps with obliteration is a possible solution, the long-term failure rate and morbidity associated with the procedure prompted the development of advanced endoscopic extended frontal sinusotomy techniques. Woodworth introduced free mucosal grafts to cover the exposed bony surface of the nasofrontal beak following Draf III surgery with promising long-term results, and this has now become standard in our practice [44]. Free septal mucosa grafts are harvested from the anterosuperior septectomy or the posterior third of the inferior turbinate [45]. In Woodworth and colleagues' study, 97% of patients maintained an ostioplasty that was at least 50% of the intraoperative diameter at three years postoperatively. If the septal mucosa is very polypoid, grafts may also be harvested from the nasal floor with minimal or no post-operative morbidity. The graft may be held in place with a mometasone-eluting or a Silastic stent. Mucosal flaps created from the lateral nasal wall can also be rotated to cover the bone exposed during the surgery and have demonstrated significant utility in reducing postoperative crusting.

A long-term study of the Draf III procedure suggested that allergy might be associated with increased re-stenosis rates post-operatively causing some to advocate for primary Draf III procedures in certain patients, particularly those with aspirin-exacerbated respiratory disease (AERD) [24]. On the other hand, Hwang and colleagues have advocated performing only Draf I or total ethmoidectomies in select patients with chronic frontal sinusitis without polyposis to minimize iatrogenic insults to the frontal recess [46].

Summary

Surgical management of frontal sinus disease has shifted dramatically over the last century from external extirpative techniques towards endoscopic surgery that aspires to restore physiological drainage of the frontal outflow tract through mucosal preservation and wide ostioplasties. History cautions us against adopting a one-size fits all approach. Longer term follow up is mandated to evaluate the results of newer techniques. The Draf III procedure does appear to be a very viable approach in long-term management recalcitrant inflammatory disease. The field of frontal sinus surgery continues to evolve rapidly. An adequate A-P diameter was considered paramount for both performing drillout procedures and maintaining long-term patency. However, novel solutions such as the "outside-in" drill out technique now overcome the problems posed by narrow AP width in small frontal sinuses that could not be tackled with the traditional "inside-out" drill out procedure. External approaches, particularly the osteoplastic flap and frontal sinus trephine, still have critical select cases. However, external techniques are now are more likely to be combined with a functional endoscopic approach, thus avoiding extensive mucosal stripping and fat obliteration. New research with longer-term and meticulous follow-up to thoughtfully assess frontal sinus surgery outcomes will guide us in refining and developing indications, techniques and technology.

References

1. Ramadan HH. History of frontal sinus surgery. Arch Otolaryngol Head Neck Surg. 2000;126(1):98–9.
2. Donald P. Surgical management of frontal sinus infections. In: The Sinuses. New York: Raven Press; 1995. p. 201–32.
3. Wells S. Abscess of the frontal sinus. Lancet. 1870;1:694–5.
4. McLaughlin RB. History of surgical approaches to the frontal sinus. Otolaryngol Clin N Am. 2001;34(1):49–58.
5. Coakley C. Frontal sinusitis: diagnosis, treatment, and results. Trans Am Laryngol Rhinol Otol Soc. 1905;11:101.
6. Skillern RH. The catarrhal and suppurative diseases of the accessory sinuses of the nose, vol. 1. Philadelphia and London: J. B. Lippincott Co.; 1913. p. 389.
7. Lothrop HA. XIV. Frontal sinus suppuration: the establishment of permanent nasal drainage; the closure of external fistulae; epidermization of sinus. Ann Surg. 1914;59(6):937–57.
8. Gross WE, Gross CW, Becker D, Moore D, Phillips D. Modified transnasal endoscopic Lothrop procedure as an alternative to frontal sinus obliteration. Otolaryngol Head Neck Surg. 1995;113(4):427–34.
9. Draf W. Endonasal micro-endoscopic frontal sinus surgery: the fulda concept. Oper Tech Otolaryngol Head Neck Surg. 1991;2(4):234–40.
10. Murr AH, Dedo HH. Frontoethmoidectomy with Sewall-Boyden reconstruction: indications, technique, and philosophy. Otolaryngol Clin N Am. 2001;34(1):153–65.
11. Neel HB, McDonald TJ, Facer GW. Modified Lynch procedure for chronic frontal sinus diseases: rationale, technique, and long-term results. Laryngoscope. 1987;97(11):1274–9.
12. Friedman WH. External approaches to the frontal sinuses. In: Diseases of the sinuses: diagnosis and management. 1st ed. PMPH–USA. p. 391–403.
13. Dawes JD. The management of frontal sinusitis and its complications. J Laryngol Otol. 1961;75:297–344.

14. Messerklinger W. On the drainage of the normal frontal sinus of man. Acta Otolaryngol. 1967;63(2):176–81.

15. Kennedy DW, Zinreich SJ, Rosenbaum AE, Johns ME. Functional endoscopic sinus surgery. Theory and diagnostic evaluation. Arch Otolaryngol. 1985;111(9):576–82.

16. Zinreich SJ, Kennedy DW, Rosenbaum AE, Gayler BW, Kumar AJ, Stammberger H. Paranasal sinuses: CT imaging requirements for endoscopic surgery. Radiology. 1987;163(3):769–75.

17. Kennedy DW, Josephson JS, Zinreich SJ, Mattox DE, Goldsmith MM. Endoscopic sinus surgery for mucoceles: a viable alternative. Laryngoscope. 1989;99(9):885–95.

18. Stammberger H. Nasal and paranasal sinus endoscopy. A diagnostic and surgical approach to recurrent sinusitis. Endoscopy. 1986;18(6):213–8.

19. Schaefer SD, Close LG. Endoscopic management of frontal sinus disease. Laryngoscope. 1990;100(2 Pt 1):155–60.

20. Alyea OEV. Frontal cells: an anatomic study of these cells with consideration of their clinical significance. Arch Otolaryngol. 1941;34(1):11–23.

21. Kuhn FA, Bolger WE, Tisdal RG. The agger nasi cell in frontal recess obstruction: an anatomic, radiologic and clinical correlation. Oper Tech Otolaryngol Head Neck Surg. 1991;2(4):226–31.

22. Draf W. Endonasal frontal sinus drainage type I–III according to Draf. In: Kountakis SE, Senior BA, Draf W, editors. The frontal sinus [Internet]. Berlin, Heidelberg: Springer; 2016. p. 337–55. https://doi.org/10.1007/978-3-662-48523-1_25.

23. Close LG, Lee NK, Leach JL, Manning SC. Endoscopic resection of the intranasal frontal sinus floor. Ann Otol Rhinol Laryngol. 1994;103(12):952–8.

24. Georgalas C, Hansen F, Videler WJM, Fokkens WJ. Long terms results of Draf type III (modified endoscopic Lothrop) frontal sinus drainage procedure in 122 patients: a single centre experience. Rhinology. 2011;49(2):195–201.

25. Anderson P, Sindwani R. Safety and efficacy of the endoscopic modified Lothrop procedure: a systematic review and meta-analysis. Laryngoscope. 2009;119(9):1828–33.

26. Jacobs JB. 100 years of frontal sinus surgery. Laryngoscope. 1997;107(11 Pt 2):1–36.

27. Walsh TE. Experimental surgery of the frontal sinus The role of the ostium and nasofrontal duct in postoperative healing. Laryngoscope. 1943;53(2):75–92.

28. Schenck NL. Frontal sinus disease: III. Experimental and clinical factors in failure of the frontal osteoplastic operation. Laryngoscope. 1975;85(1):76–92.

29. Friedman WH, Katsantonis GP. Intranasal and transantral ethmoidectomy: a 20-year experience. Laryngoscope. 1990;100(4):343–8.

30. Wigand ME, Hosemann WG. Endoscopic surgery for frontal sinusitis and its complications. Am J Rhinol. 1991;5(3):85–9.

31. Weber R, Draf W, Kratzsch B, Hosemann W, Schaefer SD. Modern concepts of frontal sinus surgery. Laryngoscope. 2001;111(1):137–46.

32. Neel HB, Whicker JH, Lake CF. Thin rubber sheeting in frontal sinus surgery: animal and clinical studies. Laryngoscope. 1976;86(4):524–36.

33. Murr AH, Smith TL, Hwang PH, Bhattacharyya N, Lanier BJ, Stambaugh JW, et al. Safety and efficacy of a novel bioabsorbable, steroid-eluting sinus stent. Int Forum Allergy Rhinol. 2011;1(1):23–32.

34. Brown CL, Bolger WE. Safety and feasibility of balloon catheter dilation of paranasal sinus ostia: a preliminary investigation. Ann Otol Rhinol Laryngol. 2006;115(4):293–9. discussion 300-301.

35. Bolger WE, Brown CL, Church CA, Goldberg AN, Karanfilov B, Kuhn FA, et al. Safety and outcomes of balloon catheter sinusotomy: a multicenter 24-week analysis in 115 patients. Otolaryngol Head Neck Surg. 2007;137(1):10–20.

36. Luong A, Batra PS, Fakhri S, Citardi MJ. Balloon catheter dilatation for frontal sinus ostium stenosis in the office setting. Am J Rhinol. 2008;22(6):621–4.

37. Sillers MJ, Lay KF. Balloon catheter dilation of the frontal sinus ostium. Otolaryngol Clin N Am. 2016;49(4):965–74.

38. Hahn S, Palmer JN, Purkey MT, Kennedy DW, Chiu AG. Indications for external frontal sinus procedures for inflammatory sinus disease. Am J Rhinol Allergy. 2009;23(3):342–7.

39. Batra PS, Citardi MJ, Lanza DC. Combined endoscopic trephination and endoscopic frontal sinusotomy for management of complex frontal sinus pathology. Am J Rhinol. 2005;19(5):435–41.

40. Patel AB, Cain RB, Lal D. Contemporary applications of frontal sinus trephination: A systematic review of the literature. Laryngoscope. 2015;125(9):2046–53.

41. Seiberling K, Jardeleza C, Wormald P-J. Minitrephination of the frontal sinus: indications and uses in today's era of sinus surgery. Am J Rhinol Allergy. 2009;23(2):229–31.

42. Piltcher OB, Antunes M, Monteiro F, Schweiger C, Schatkin B. Is there a reason for performing frontal sinus trephination at 1 cm from midline? A tomographic study. Braz J Otorhinolaryngol. 2006;72(4):505–7.

43. Hardy JM, Montgomery WW. Osteoplastic frontal sinusotomy: an analysis of 250 operations. Ann Otol Rhinol Laryngol. 1976;85(4 Pt 1):523–32.

44. Illing EA, Cho DY, Riley KO, Woodworth BA. Draf III mucosal graft technique: long-term results. Int Forum Allergy Rhinol. 2016;6(5):514–7.

45. Conger BT, Riley K, Woodworth BA. The Draf III mucosal grafting technique: a prospective study. Otolaryngol Head Neck Surg. 2012;146(4):664–8.

46. Abuzeid WM, Mace JC, Costa ML, Rudmik L, Soler ZM, Kim GS, et al. Outcomes of chronic frontal sinusitis treated with ethmoidectomy: a prospective study. Int Forum Allergy Rhinol. 2016;6(6):597–604.

47. Hilding A. Experimental surgery of the nose and sinuses: II. Gross results following the removal of the intersinus septum and of strips of mucous membrane from the frontal sinus of the dog. Arch Otolaryngol. 1933;17(3):321–27.

Anatomy of the Frontal Sinus and Recess

Alberto Schreiber, Marco Ferrari,
Luigi Fabrizio Rodella, and Piero Nicolai

Introduction

The anatomy of the frontal sinus and frontal recess has garnered considerable interest due to its complexity and exceeding interindividual variability. Since most surgical procedures addressing the frontal sinus are nowadays performed via an endoscopic approach, the surgical anatomy of the frontal recess and surrounding structures should be analyzed in an endoscopic-oriented perspective. On the other hand, anatomy can be difficult to understand in a bidimensional endoscopic view through a narrow corridor without the ability to perceive depth and surrounding structures. The purpose of this chapter is to provide the reader with a multi-perspective view of the frontal recess anatomy so to precisely explain the complex relationship between the uncinate process and surrounding structures, moving from an endoscopic view (both from anterior and posterior perspectives) to gross external anatomy of the lateral nasal wall and frontal sinuses. Step-by-step dissection through such a multi-perspec-tive viewpoint will clarifying the technical surgical concepts that will be discussed in the following chapters. Moreover, detailed multi-planar analysis with high-definition CT images will be utilized to depict the entire three-dimensional architecture of the frontal recess.

Frontal Bone

The frontal bone contributes to make up the bony framework of the face and anterior skull base. It is composed of three portions: squamous, orbital, and nasal. The squamous part is the largest and forms the skeleton of the forehead. As seen from outside, it shows two prominences, called frontal eminences, which correspond to the frontal sinuses. The orbital part forms the orbital roof and, together with ethmoid and sphenoid bones, makes up the anterior skull base. The nasal part is a small portion joining the nasal and maxillary bones.

The frontal sinus is an air space lined by mucoperiosteum that lies within the squamous part of the frontal bone. It shows different grades of pneumatization, ranging from hypoplasia/agenesis to enormous sinuses extending into the nasal part, orbital part, or adjacent bones. On average, the frontal sinus is 24.3 mm in height, 29.0 mm wide (from the midline to the lateral border), and 16.8 mm deep [1].

A. Schreiber · M. Ferrari · P. Nicolai (✉)
Unit of Otorhinolaryngology – Head and Neck Surgery, University of Brescia, Brescia, Italy

L. F. Rodella
Section of Anatomy and Physiopathology, University of Brescia, Brescia, Italy

© Springer Nature Switzerland AG 2019
D. Lal, P. H. Hwang (eds.), *Frontal Sinus Surgery*, https://doi.org/10.1007/978-3-319-97022-6_2

The frontal sinus is connected with the nasal cavity via a drainage pathway passing through anterior ethmoidal complex and the middle meatus.

Middle Meatus

The middle meatus provides ventilation and mucus drainage to the frontal sinus, anterior ethmoidal complex, and the maxillary sinus. The middle meatus is bounded by the middle turbinate medially, and the uncinate process laterally (Fig. 2.1a, b). The ethmoidal bulla lies posterior and superior to the vertical and horizontal portion of the uncinate process, respectively (Fig. 2.2).

The cleft between the free edge of the uncinate process and the ethmoidal bulla is a bidimensional region in the sagittal plane called the hiatus semilunaris. The hiatus semilunaris is the entrance to the ethmoidal infundibulum (Fig. 2.2).

The ethmoidal infundibulum is a three-dimensional space deep and lateral to the uncinate process, anterior and inferior to the ethmoidal bulla, and medial to the orbit and maxillary sinus (Fig. 2.3a).

The physiologic ostium of the maxillary sinus is located lateral to the horizontal portion of the uncinate process. The ethmoidal complex, composed of multiple air spaces, usually drains through several ostia or niches. The most inferior ethmoidal air space usually drains medially into the middle turbinate and is termed the ethmoidal bulla (Fig. 2.4a, b). The cell that lies above the most inferior air space is called "suprabullar cell" and commonly drains anteriorly toward the frontal sinus drainage pathway.

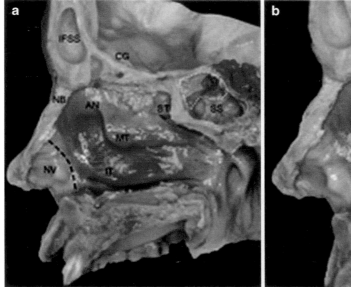
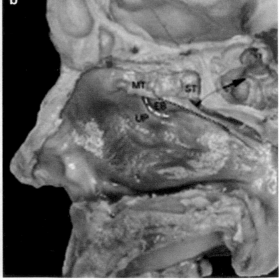

Fig. 2.1 Sagittal paramedian cut of a cadaver head (right side). (**a**) The lateral nasal wall extends from the nasal vestibule (NV) and nasal bone (NB) anteriorly, to the nasopharynx and sphenoid sinus (SS) posteriorly. The nasal floor and olfactory cleft are the caudal and cranial boundaries, respectively. The lateral nasal wall is made up by the inferior turbinate (IT), middle turbinate (MT), superior turbinate (ST), and the area between the limen nasi (black dashed line) and agger nasi (AN), which is called nasal antrum. (**b**) The middle turbinate has been partially removed, leaving the common laminar portion of the middle and superior turbinate to show the middle meatus. The uncinate process (UP) and ethmoidal bulla (EB) lie within the middle meatus and are divided by the hiatus semilunaris (white dashed line). The middle and superior nasal meatus are divided by the basal lamella of the middle turbinate (black dotted line). Black arrow, ventilation pathway of the sphenoid sinus; CG, crista galli; IFSS, interfrontal sinus septum; white dotted line, Onodi's cell (sphenoethmoidal cell)

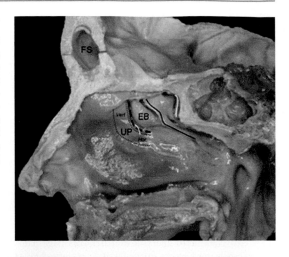

Fig. 2.2 Sagittal paramedian cut of a cadaver head (right side). The uncinate process (UP) and ethmoidal bulla (EB) are the key structures of the middle meatus. The uncinate process has a horizontal (hor) and vertical (vert) portion; black dotted lines show its insertion, anteroinferiorly, and free edge, posterosuperiorly. The hiatus semilunaris (black dashed line) serves as entrance for the ethmoidal infundibulum (white arrow), which is covered by the uncinate process. Black line, basal lamella of the middle turbinate; FS, frontal sinus; white line, basal lamella of the superior turbinate

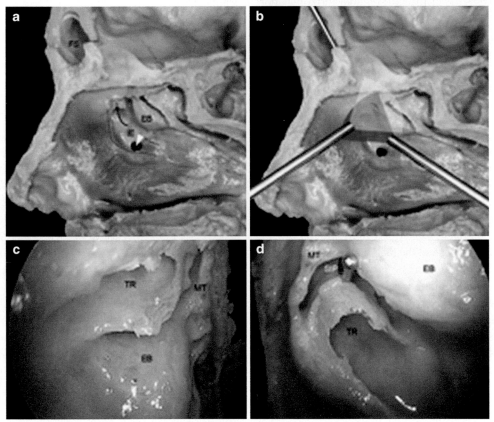

Fig. 2.3 Sagittal paramedian cut (**a, b**) and transnasal endoscopic view (**c, d**) of a cadaver head (right side). (**a**) The horizontal portion of the uncinate process has been removed (black dotted lines) to expose the ethmoidal infundibulum (IE). This space is bounded by insertion of the uncinate process, anteroinferiorly, and ethmoidal bulla (EB), posterosuperiorly. The maxillary ostium (white arrowhead) lies in the infero-posterior portion of the ethmoidal infundibulum. (**b**) Endoscopic fields of view in pictures c (yellow area) and d (red area). (**c**) Endoscopic view through the right nasal fossa. The anterosuperior portion of the ethmoidal infundibulum corresponds to the terminal recess (TR), as shown by the black arrow in picture a. (**d**) Endoscopic view of the ethmoidal infundibulum from the posterior aspect. The lateral insertion of the vertical portion of the uncinate process forms the roof of the terminal recess. The suprainfundibular plate (SIP) is one of the superior insertions of the uncinate process. In this specimen, the frontal sinus drainage pathway runs laterally to the suprainfundibular plate. FS, frontal sinus; MT, middle turbinate

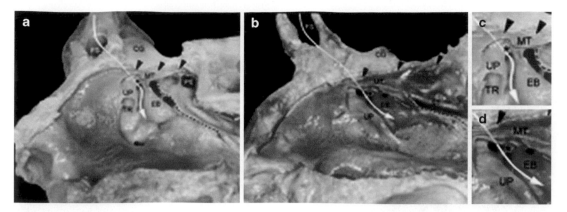

Fig. 2.4 Sagittal paramedian cut of a cadaver head (right side). (**a**) Example of lateral frontal sinus drainage pathway (white arrow), passing between the suprainfundibular plate (black asterisk), medially, and the medial orbital wall, laterally. (**b**) Example of medial frontal sinus drainage pathway (white arrow), passing between the middle turbinate (MT), medially, and suprainfundibular plate, lat-erally. (**c**, **d**) Magnifications of pictures a and b. Black arrowheads, olfactory cleft; black dashed line, basal lamina of the middle turbinate; black dotted line, common laminar portion of middle and superior turbinates; CG, crista galli; EB, ethmoidal bulla; FS, frontal sinus; PE, posterior ethmoidal complex; ST, superior turbinate; TR, terminal recess; UP, uncinate process

Uncinate Process

The uncinate process, which belongs to the eth-moidal bone, affects the framework of the frontal recess due to its several and variable insertions on to the surrounding bony structures. The horizon-tal portion of the uncinate process is attached to the medial maxillary wall, whereas the vertical portion attaches anteriorly to the frontal process of the maxilla and the lacrimal bone. The vertical portion of the uncinate process has lateral, supe-rior, and medial insertions, which are exceed-ingly variable and may resemble a palm tree [2]. Although six types of uncinate process insertions have been traditionally reported [3], a larger number of possible combinations are actually detectable. The specific anatomy of uncinate pro-cess insertions is of paramount importance to understand the relationship between the uncinate process and the frontal sinus drainage pathway [4, 5]. The posterior free edge of the superior por-tion of the uncinate process turns posteriorly, joining the anterior wall of the ethmoidal bulla to form the so-called suprainfundibular plate (Fig. 2.5) [6]. This small bony lamella is the watershed that defines the frontal sinus drainage pathway as medial or lateral to the uncinate pro-cess (Fig. 2.4a–d).

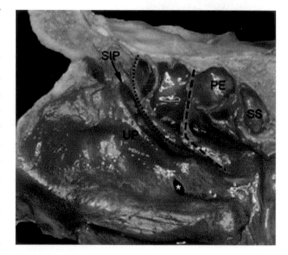

Fig. 2.5 Sagittal paramedian cut of a cadaver head (right side). The suprainfundibular plate is one of the cranial insertions of the uncinate process (UP). It joins the unci-nate process with the anterior wall of the ethmoidal bulla (black dotted line) and is the watershed to classify the frontal sinus drainage pathway as medial or lateral to the uncinate process. Black dashed line, basal lamina of the middle turbinate; PE, posterior ethmoidal complex; SS, sphenoid sinus; white asterisk, accessory ostium of the maxillary sinus

Insertions of the uncinate process vertical portion on the axial and sagittal planes make up, respectively, the horizontal and vertical walls of ethmoidal air spaces located anterior to the fron-

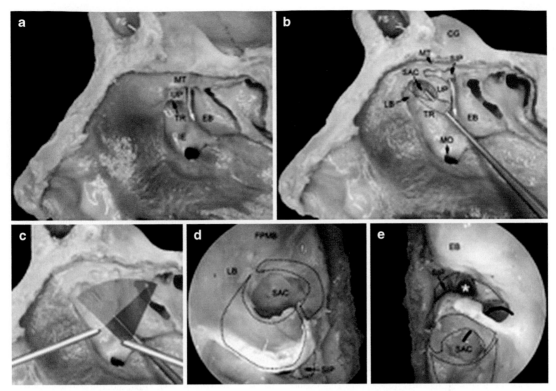

Fig. 2.6 Sagittal paramedian cut (**a–c**) and transnasal endoscopic view (**d, e**) of a cadaver head (right side). (**a, b**) Subtotal removal of the middle turbinate (MT) shows the entirety of the vertical portion of the uncinate process (UP) with several insertions (black dotted lines) onto the surrounding structures. The lowest insertion is the roof of the terminal recess (TR) and the floor of a supra agger cell (SAC), where the ball probe has been placed. The medial wall of the supra agger cell corresponds to an insertion of the uncinate process that reaches the lacrimal bone (LB) and frontal process of the maxillary bone (FPMB).

(**c**) Endoscopic fields of view in pictures d (yellow area) and e (red area). (**d**) Endoscopic view (45° scope) from anterior aspect of the vertical portion of the uncinate process. (**e**) Endoscopic view (45° scope) from posterior aspect of the vertical portion of the uncinate process. The frontal sinus drainage pathway (white asterisk) runs laterally to the suprainfundibular plate (SIP), in front of the ethmoidal bulla (EB). The black line shows the position of the ball probe in picture b. The space between the suprainfundibular plate and middle turbinate ends blindly with a pouch. CG, crista galli; FS, frontal sinus; IE, ethmoidal infundibulum

tal sinus drainage pathway (i.e., terminal recess, lacrimal cell, agger nasi cell, supra agger cell) (Fig. 2.6a–e).

Frontal Recess, Frontal Ostium, and Frontal Infundibulum

In a sagittal view, the frontal recess and the frontal infundibulum are two funnels converging in the frontal ostium (Fig. 2.7a).

The frontal recess is bounded by the frontal process of the maxilla anteriorly, the anterior wall of the bullar complex posteriorly, the medial orbital wall laterally, and the middle turbinate medially

[7]. The frontal recess opens supero-anteriorly into the frontal sinus and infero-posteriorly into the ethmoidal infundibulum (Fig. 2.7a, c). The ethmoidal roof and the lowest axial insertion of the vertical uncinate process are the supero-posterior and infero-anterior boundaries of the frontal recess, respectively. The portion of the medial orbital wall which forms the lateral limit of the frontal recess is made up by the lacrimal bone, anteriorly and inferiorly, and the orbital part of the frontal bone (pars orbitalis ossis frontalis; Fig. 2.8a, b), superiorly. The lamina papyracea lies more posteriorly, lateral to the bullar complex [2]. The cranial spur of the frontal process of the maxillary bone forms the floor of the frontal infundibulum and the

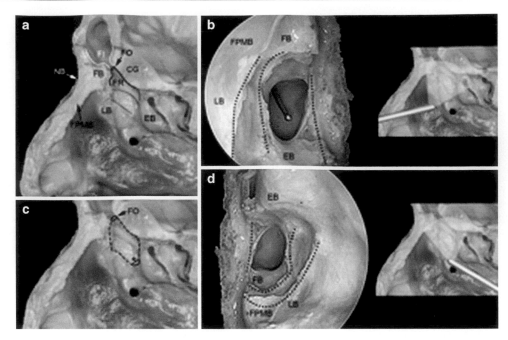

Fig. 2.7 Sagittal paramedian cut (**a**, **c**) and transnasal endoscopic view (**b**, **d**) of a cadaver head (right side). (**a**) Sagittal view of the frontal recess (FR) and frontal infundibulum (FI) that seem like two funnels (black and white lines, respectively) converging in the frontal ostium (FO, black circle). Since the frontal recess has been completely cleared from uncinate process insertions (black dotted line), its boundaries can be identified: the frontal process of the maxillary bone (FPMB) anteriorly; the anterior wall of the ethmoidal bulla (EB) posteriorly; the medial orbital wall laterally; and the middle turbinate (which was entirely removed) medially. (**b**) Endoscopic view (45° scope) of the frontal recess from anterior aspect. A ball probe has been placed into the frontal recess through the frontal infundibulum. The frontal ostium is enclosed between the frontal beak (FB), anteriorly, and the skull base, posteriorly. (**c**) The frontal recess (black dashed line) is opened supero-anteriorly into the frontal sinus via the frontal ostium and infero-posteriorly into the ethmoidal infundibulum through a narrow area between the lowest insertion of the vertical uncinate process and ethmoidal bulla. (**d**) Endoscopic view (45° scope) of the frontal recess from posterior aspect. CG, crista galli; LB, lacrimal bone; NB, nasal bone

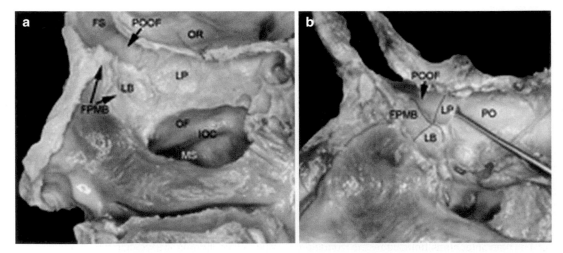

Fig. 2.8 Sagittal paramedian cut of a cadaver head (right side) before (**a**) and after lamina papyracea removal (**b**). The anterior portion of the medial orbital wall is formed by the lacrimal bone (LB), inferiorly, the frontal process of the maxillary bone (FPMB), anteriorly, the pars orbit-alis ossis frontalis (POOF), superiorly, and the lamina papyracea (LP), posteriorly. Black dotted line, sutures between bones; FS, frontal sinus; IOC, infraorbital canal; MS, maxillary sinus; OF, orbital floor; OR, orbital roof; PO, periorbita

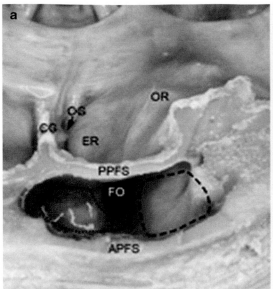 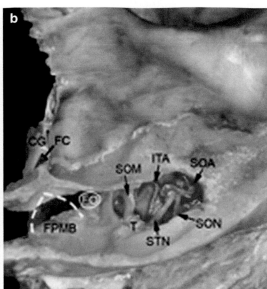

Fig. 2.9 Axial cut of a cadaver head along the frontal bone before (**a**) and after (**b**) removal of the frontal sinus floor on the left side. The frontal sinus floor is made up by the frontal beak (white dashed line) and the frontal process of the maxillary bone (FPMB), medially (black dotted line), and the anteromedial roof of the orbit (black dashed line), laterally to the frontal ostium (FO). APFS, anterior plate of the frontal sinus; CG, crista galli; ER, ethmoidal roof; FC, foramen caecum; ITA, infratrochlear artery; OG, olfactory groove; OR, orbital roof; PPFS, posterior plate of the frontal sinus; SOA, supraorbital artery; SOM, superior oblique muscle; SON, supraorbital nerve; STN, supratrochlear nerve

anteromedial border of the frontal ostium and is defined as the frontal beak (Figs. 2.7a and 2.9a, b). As previously described, the cranial insertions of the uncinate process and the air spaces they bound form the frontal recess (Figs. 2.6b–e and 2.7a–d). All the air spaces contained in the frontal recess and in the surrounding structures can be variably pneumatized resulting in different levels of the frontal sinus drainage pathway complexity.

The frontal infundibulum is the funnel-shaped air space making up the caudal portion of the frontal sinus (Figs. 2.7a and 2.9a, b). The frontal infundibulum narrows down between the orbit laterally, skull base posteriorly, and the frontal beak anteriorly and medially. The same structures can narrow the frontal recess in an "inverted funnel-shaped" manner. Conventionally, the frontal ostium is defined as the narrowest area between the frontal recess and the frontal infundibulum (Fig. 2.7a). The frontal infundibulum forms the frontal sinus floor, which is divided by the frontal ostium in a medial portion (the frontal beak) and a lateral portion (the anteromedial orbital roof) (Fig. 2.9a).

According to the Terracol and Ardouin postnatal development model [8, 9], anterior ethmoidal complex air spaces can be classified in anterior (nasal and orbital) and posterior (bullar) depending on the relationship to the frontal sinus drainage pathway. Anterior air spaces lie anterior to the ethmoidal bulla and posterior to the frontal process of the maxillary bone and can be divided in medial and lateral to the uncinate process. The resulting anteromedial, anterolateral, and posterior air spaces of the anterior ethmoidal complex were called nasal, orbital, and bullar cells, respectively.

Definition of Ethmoidal and Frontoethmoidal Air Spaces

Agger Nasi Cell, Lacrimal Cell, and Terminal Recess

The group of air spaces between the uncinate process, frontal process of the maxilla, and medial orbital wall (orbital cells according to Terracol and Ardouin) may be defined based on

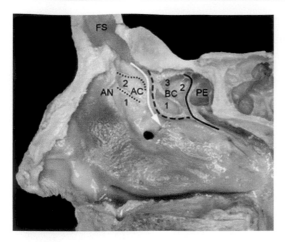

Fig. 2.10 Sagittal paramedian cut of a cadaver head (right side). The agger-bullar classification applied to a cadaver. The agger complex (AC) includes all the air space in front of the frontal sinus drainage pathway (white arrow) and lies postero-lateral to the agger nasi (AN). In this specimen, the agger complex is composed of two air spaces, which are bounded by the insertions of the vertical portion of the uncinate process (black dotted lines). The bullar complex (BC) is enclosed between the anterior wall of the ethmoidal bulla (black dashed lines) and the basal lamella of the middle turbinate (black line). In this specimen, the bullar complex is composed of three air spaces. FS, frontal sinus; PE, posterior ethmoidal complex

their different anteroposterior extension and craniocaudal position. The most caudal air cell in this region is called the lacrimal cell when it lies medial to the lacrimal fossa or agger nasi cell if it extends anteriorly to the agger nasi area. The agger nasi is a bony crest of the frontal process of the maxillary bone that articulates with the middle turbinate (Fig. 2.10). The term terminal recess refers to the last supero-anterior portion of the ethmoidal infundibulum (Fig. 2.3b–d). The terminal recess can be located inferior to the lacrimal/agger nasi cell or can pneumatize into the lacrimal or agger nasi area.

Frontoethmoidal Cells

Air spaces of the anterior ethmoidal complex may extend upward into the frontal sinus, crossing the interface between the frontal, maxillary, and ethmoid bones. Frontoethmoidal cells from the anterolateral air spaces (orbital cells according to Terracol and Ardouin) pass

through the frontal beak and displace the frontal ostium posteriorly and medially. Those arising from the anteromedial air spaces (nasal cells according to Terracol and Ardouin) grow up along the interfrontal sinus septum displacing the frontal ostium laterally. From the bullar complex (bullar cells according to Terracol and Ardouin), frontoethmoidal cells ascend along the skull base, displacing the frontal ostium anteriorly. When these frontoethmoidal cells extend along the orbital roof posterior to the frontal sinus, they pneumatize the posteroinferior portion of the frontal bone and are called supraorbital cells.

Modified Bent and Kuhn Classification and International Frontal Sinus Anatomy Classification

The first anatomical-surgical classification of the frontoethmoidal air spaces was proposed by Bent and Kuhn in 1996 and modified by Wormald in 2005 [10, 11]. The following anatomical structures were defined:

- Agger nasi cell: The most anterior cell that can be seen in a coronal section, anterior to the middle turbinate insertion.

The terms "lacrimal cell" and "terminal recess" were not defined.

- Kuhn's cell: A group of cells lying close to or within the frontal process of the maxillary bone and above the agger nasi cell. They were further classified as follows:
  - Type 1: A single cell not protruding into the frontal sinus
  - Type 2: More than one cell not protruding into the frontal sinus
  - Type 3: At least one cell protruding into the frontal sinus for less than half of its craniocaudal extension
  - Type 4: At least one cell protruding into the frontal sinus for more than half of its craniocaudal extension
- Suprabullar cell: A cell that lies over the most inferior air space pneumatizing the ethmoidal

bulla and not protruding into either the frontal sinus or orbital roof

- Supraorbital ethmoid cell: A suprabullar cell pneumatizing into the orbital roof
- Frontal bulla cell: A suprabullar cell protruding into the frontal sinus
- Interfrontal sinus septal cell: A cell resulting from pneumatization of the interfrontal sinus septum
- Concha bullosa: A cell or recess resulting from pneumatization of the middle turbinate

Recently, a committee of expert endoscopic surgeons formulated the International Frontal Sinus Anatomy Classification by making a number of refinements to the modified Bent and Kuhn classification [12]. Type 1 and 2 Kuhn cells have been grouped under the term "supra agger cell" (Fig. 2.6), and types 3 and 4 under the term "supra agger frontal cell." The frontal bulla cell and interfrontal sinus septal cell have been renamed "supra bulla frontal cell" and "frontal septal cell," respectively. This is detailed in Chap. 4.

According to the Terracol and Ardouin developmental model, supra agger frontal cell, frontal septal cell, and supra bulla frontal cell originate from frontal pneumatization of the orbital, nasal, and bullar cells, respectively.

Agger-Bullar Classification

The agger-bullar classification (ABC) was developed with the intent to synthesize the crucial anatomical information necessary to surgically address the frontal sinus. This summarizes the complex anatomy in a short acronym that is easy to memorize [5].

To apply the ABC, the following 4 steps can be followed (Fig. 2.11a–e):

Step 1. The anterior ethmoidal complex is divided in two compartments. The anterior compartment lies between the frontal process of the maxillary bone and the frontal sinus drainage pathway. The posterior compartment lies between the frontal sinus drainage pathway and the basal lamella of the MT. The anterior compartment is called the "agger complex" (abbreviated as A

complex), and the posterior compartment is called the "bullar complex" (abbreviated as B complex).

Step 2. The number of air spaces is counted for each complex. An air space is defined as a portion of air surrounded by a bony envelope regardless of its shape. Cells, recesses, and irregular air spaces are therefore grouped under the definition of "air space." In this way, it is possible to create an easy-to-remember abbreviation, such as A_xB_y, where x and y are the number of air spaces making up A and B complex, respectively. Finally, if the B complex is composed of four or more air spaces, it is categorized as "large" and represented by an "L" (i.e., A_xB_L).

Step 3. The presence of relevant air spaces is checked as follows:

- Type f air space: An air space protruding into the frontal sinus for less than half of its height; it can be either part of the A or B complex.
- Type F air space: An air space protruding into the frontal sinus for more than half of its height; it can be either part of the A or B complex. For both types, f and F air spaces, the upper surface of the frontal beak is used as the limit to establish the presence or absence of protrusion into the frontal sinus.
- Type R air space: An air space extending from the frontal sinus to the basal lamella of the middle turbinate, without interposed bony lamellas.

If one or more of these spaces was present, the related letter (f, F, or R) is added after the acronym of the related complex (i.e., A_xfB_y). Type R can be added only to B complex (i.e., A_xB_yR).

Step 4. Multiplanar reconstruction is used to detect the path of frontal sinus drainage pathway in relation to the upper insertion of the uncinate process (i.e., the suprainfundibular plate). This spatial relation is classified as medial or lateral, and an "m" or "l" is added before the acronym (i.e., mA_xB_y or lA_xB_y), respectively.

Following the abovementioned simple steps, the surgeon formulates two short acronyms (one per side) summarizing the crucial information required to accomplish the surgical procedure: the position of the frontal sinus drainage pathway

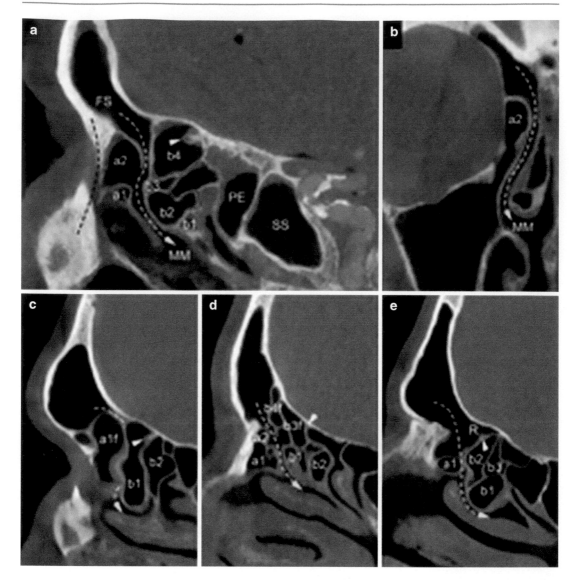

Fig. 2.11 Sagittal (**a**, **c–e**) and coronal (**b**) CT cone-beam images of a cadaver head (**a**, **b**) and live patients (**c–e**). Panel summarizing the main concepts of the agger-bullar classification. (**a**) The agger and bullar complexes have been identified: the agger complex lies between the frontal process of the maxillary bone (black dashed line) and frontal sinus drainage pathway (yellow dashed arrow), and the bullar complex lies between the frontal sinus drainage pathway and basal lamella of the middle turbinate. The former is composed by two air spaces and the latter by four air spaces. (**b**) Coronal reconstruction of the case shown in picture a. The frontal sinus drainage pathway passes medially to the uncinate process (green dotted line). The ABC acronym of this case is mA$_2$B$_4$. (**c**) Sagittal reconstruction of a case with an air space of the agger complex extending into the frontal sinus (a1f), called supra agger frontal cell according to the International Frontal Sinus Anatomy Classification. The ABC acronym of this case is mA$_1$fB$_2$. (**d**) Sagittal reconstruction of a case with two air spaces of the bullar complex extending into the frontal sinus (b3f, b4f), called suprabullar frontal cells according to the International Frontal Sinus Anatomy Classification. The ABC acronym of this case is mA$_2$B$_4$f. (**e**) Sagittal reconstruction of a case with a suprabullar recess (R). The ABC acronym of this case is 1A$_1$B$_3$R

in the frontal recess, the number of anterior and posterior spaces to be marsupialized, and the presence of relevant variants along extent of pneumatization in relationship to the frontal sinus. The ABC is intended to be a practical system for planning frontal sinus surgery.

Frontal Sinus Drainage Pathway

In all endoscopic procedures to the frontal sinus, identification of the frontal sinus drainage pathway is a prerequisite to perform correct and safe surgery. Therefore, the basic information to be preoperatively acquired is the three-dimensional course of the frontal sinus drainage pathway [5].

Although initially called the "nasofrontal duct," the frontal sinus outflow tract is not a linear and cylindrical pathway surrounded by a bony envelope as in a "duct." Conversely, along its course it presents enlargements and narrowings, running tortuously in relation to the shape and pneumatization of FR air spaces. This complexity forces one to infer the course of the frontal sinus drainage pathway through knowledge of spatial relationships with the surrounding spaces. Therefore, the frontal sinus drainage pathway is the result of the competition between the nasal, orbital, and bullar cells (according to Terracol

and Ardouin), in the presence or absence of their extension into the FS (supra agger frontal cell, frontal septal cell, and supra bulla frontal cell, respectively). The general rule is that the predominant pneumatization of the anteromedial (nasal), anterolateral (orbital), and posterior (bullar) air spaces tend to push the frontal sinus drainage pathway in the opposite direction (posterolaterally, posteromedially, and anteriorly, respectively).

Endoscopic Dissection of the Frontal Recess

Classic steps in endoscopic dissection to the frontal recess will be reproduced in a multiperspective view in order to clarify the anatomical structure of the frontal recess. The first step to reach the frontal sinus is the removal of the vertical portion of the uncinate process. This procedure is usually started by placing a cutting retrograde instrument within the ethmoidal infundibulum and removing the intermediate portion of the uncinate process (Fig. 2.12a, b); care should be taken to not damage the orbit and nasolacrimal duct with the instrument that is blindly placed into the ethmoidal infundibulum (Fig. 2.12c). Thereafter, the most cranial

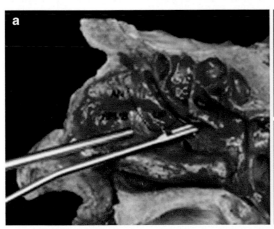
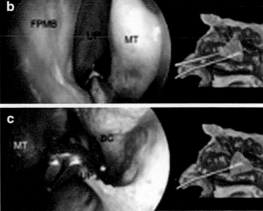

Fig. 2.12 Sagittal paramedian cut (**a**) and transnasal endoscopic view (**b**, from anterior; **c**, from posterior) of a cadaver head (right side). A retrograde cutting instrument is removing the uncinate process (UP) between its horizontal and vertical portions. Attention should be taken to

not damage the lacrimal duct and the periorbita with the tip of the instrument (white asterisk). Black dotted line, vertical portion of the uncinate process; AN, agger nasi; BC, bullar complex; FPMB, frontal process of the maxillary bone; MT, middle turbinate

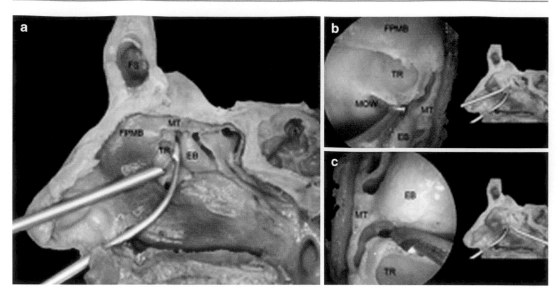

Fig. 2.13 Sagittal paramedian cut (**a**) and transnasal endoscopic view (**b**, from anterior; **c**, from posterior) of a cadaver head (right side). A curved instrument is placed between the terminal recess (TR) and ethmoidal bulla (EB) to probe the drainage pathway of the frontal sinus (FS). FPMB, frontal process of the maxillary bone MOW, medial orbital wall; MT, middle turbinate

portion is removed under guidance of angled scopes by probing the frontal sinus drainage pathway with curved instruments and gently fracturing the uncinate process and its insertions (Fig. 2.13a–c). The frontal sinus drainage pathway always runs along the anterior wall of the ethmoidal bulla and crosses all bony lamellas anterior to the ethmoidal bulla and lateral to the middle turbinate, which are branches of the uncinate process. Once the uncinate process is entirely removed, the frontal ostium can be identified in most of cases and further enlarged by partially removing the frontal beak [13]. A supra agger frontal cell or frontal septal cell be mistaken for the frontal sinus, especially when largely pneumatized into the sinus. Moreover, in the presence of a suprabullar frontal cell, the frontal ostium may not be entirely visible even when the uncinate process is completely removed. In such a scenario, the ethmoidal bulla must be dissected to expose the frontal ostium following the skull base from posterior to anterior. Transillumination and revaluation of preoperative imaging or navigation systems should be considered whenever the frontal recess has an anatomy that is difficult to interpret.

When the ethmoidal bulla is being dissected, there are two critical areas to identify during this maneuver: the medial orbital wall, laterally, and the cribriform plate, medially, which are the points where orbit and skull base can be inadvertently damaged, respectively. When an intact bulla procedure cannot be performed due to frontal recess complexity, the anterior ethmoidal artery should also be additionally identified and preserved during the dissection.

Structures Surrounding the Frontal Sinus and Its Drainage Pathway

Skull Base

The posterior plate of the frontal sinus is the most anterior portion of the anterior skull base and continues infero-posteriorly with the ethmoidal roof medially, and orbital roof laterally (Fig. 2.9a).

Transnasally, the ethmoidal roof is visible when the bullar complex has been entirely removed. It is easily recognized due to its greater thickness compared to the bony lamellae of the bullar complex. The anterior skull base is slightly tilted down from anterior to posterior, and its direction parallels with the hard palate. As seen from above, the ethmoidal roof shows several depressions, called "foveolae," corresponding to the top of air spaces of the bullar complex. Just posterior to the most anterior foveola, the anterior ethmoidal artery runs in a bony canal from lateral to medial and from posterior to anterior (Fig. 2.14a–c) [14]. The anterior ethmoidal artery canal can show dehiscent areas (6–60%) [15, 16] and lie either within (65–86%) [15, 16] or caudal (14–35%) [15, 16] to the ethmoidal roof (even if always connected to the skull base with a bony mesentery). The artery always runs between or within the anterior wall of the ethmoidal complex and the basal lamella of the middle turbinate [15, 16].

The cribriform plate is formed by two thin bony lamellae: the horizontal and vertical lamella. The horizontal lamella is pierced by the olfactory fibers, and the vertical lamella is pierced by the terminal branches of ethmoidal arteries. The horizontal lamella serves as the roof of the olfactory cleft and floor of the olfactory fossa. The vertical lamina is the lateral wall of the olfactory fossa and the highest part of the medial aspect of the frontal recess and bullar complex. The vertical lamella of the cribriform plate is the cranial continuation of the turbinal plate and is the thinnest portion of the anterior skull base that can be easily penetrated (locus minoris resistentiae) (Fig. 2.14c) [17].

The great variability in length and inclination of the vertical lamella, in addition to its frequent asymmetry in the two sides, accounts for surgical risks during endoscopic access to the FS.

Orbit

The anterior portion of the medial orbital wall is formed by the lacrimal bone (LB), inferi-

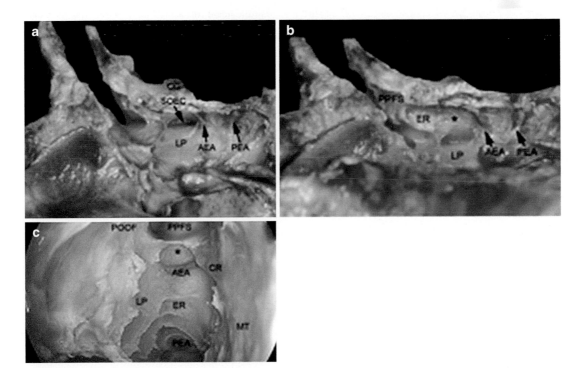

Fig. 2.14 Sagittal paramedian cut (**a**, **b**) and transnasal endoscopic view (**c**) of a cadaver head (right side). The anterior (AEA) and posterior (PEA) ethmoidal arteries run along the ethmoidal roof (ER), from the lamina papyracea (LP) to the vertical lamella of the cribriform plate (CR). The anterior ethmoidal artery is commonly located posterior to the most anterior foveola ethmoidalis (black asterisk). The ethmoidal roof continues anteriorly into the posterior plate of the frontal sinus (PPFS). CG, crista galli; MT, middle turbinate; POOF, pars orbitalis ossis frontalis

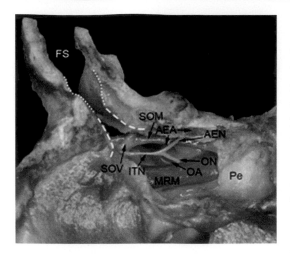

Fig. 2.15 Sagittal paramedian cut of a cadaver head (right side). Medial-to-lateral view of the orbital content after removal of the anterior portion of the medial orbital wall and periorbita (Pe). White dashed line, frontal recess; white dotted line, frontal infundibulum; AEA, anterior ethmoidal artery; AEN, anterior ethmoidal nerve; FS, frontal sinus; ITN, infratrochlear nerve; MRM, medial rectus muscle; ON, ophthalmic nerve; SOM, superior oblique muscle; SOV, superior ophthalmic vein

Summary

The frontal sinus drainage pathway is complex. The final pathway is the result of competing pneumatization between ethmoidal cells and their extension into the frontal sinus. Predominant pneumatization of the anteromedial (nasal), anterolateral (orbital), and posterior (bullar) air spaces tend to push the frontal sinus drainage pathway in the opposite direction (posterolaterally, posteromedially, and anteriorly, respectively) [18]. This chapter provides the reader with a multi-perspective view of the frontal recess anatomy, spanning across endoscopic views to gross anatomy of the lateral nasal wall and frontal sinuses.

References

1. Lang J. Clinical anatomy of the nose, nasal cavity and paranasal sinuses. New York: Thieme Medical Publisher; 1989. p. 62–71.
2. Marquez S, Tessema B, Clement PA, et al. Development of the ethmoid sinus and extramural migration: the anatomical basis of this paranasal sinus. Anat Rec. 2008;291:1535–53.
3. Landsberg R, Friedman M. A computer-assisted anatomical study of the nasofrontal region. Laryngoscope. 2001;111:2125–30.
4. Turgut S, Ercan I, Sayin I, et al. The relationship between frontal sinusitis and localization of the frontal sinus outflow tract: a computer-assisted anatomical and clinical study. Arch Otolaryngol Head Neck Surg. 2005;131:518–22.
5. Pianta L, Ferrari M, Schreiber A, et al. Agger-bullar classification (ABC) of the frontal sinus drainage pathway: validation in a preclinical setting. Int Forum Allergy Rhinol. 2016;6:981–9.
6. Kim KS, Kim HU, Chung IH, et al. Surgical anatomy of the nasofrontal duct: anatomical and computed tomographic analysis. Laryngoscope. 2001;111:603–8.
7. Lund VJ, Stammberger H, Fokkens WJ, et al. European position paper on the anatomical terminology of the internal nose and paranasal sinuses. Rhinology Suppl. 2014;24:1–34.
8. Terrier F, Weber W, Ruefenacht D, et al. Anatomy of the ethmoid: CT, endoscopic, and macroscopic. AJR. 1985;144:493–500.
9. Terracol J, Ardouin P. Anatomie des fosses nasales et des cavités annexes. Paris: Maloine; 1965.
10. Kuhn F. Chronic frontal sinusitis: the endoscopic frontal recess approach. Oper Tech Otolaryngol Head Neck Surg. 1996;7:222–9.

orly, the frontal process of the maxillary bone (FPMB), anteriorly, the pars orbitalis ossis frontalis (POOF), superiorly, and the lamina papyracea (LP), posteriorly (Fig. 2.8b). The lacrimal bone is a thin, delicate bone that separates the frontal recess from the posterior part of the lacrimal fossa. The anterior aspect of the lacrimal fossa is made up by the frontal process of the maxillary bone. The pars orbitalis ossis frontalis is the inferomedial sagittally-oriented extension of the orbital roof. Due to the high variability of uncinate process cranial insertions, air spaces of the agger complex can show different spatial relationships with the lacrimal fossa. The lamina papyracea is made of thin cortical bone with potential dehiscent areas and, together with the periorbita, separates the ethmoidal air spaces from critical neurovascular and muscular structures within the orbit (Fig. 2.15).

The lateral portion of the floor of the frontal sinus is the anteromedial roof of the orbit and separates the content of the sinus from the periorbita and intraorbital structures (Fig. 2.9b).

11. Wormald PJ. Surgery of the frontal recess and frontal sinus. Rhinology. 2005;43:82–5.
12. Wormald PJ, Hoseman W, Callejas C. The international frontal sinus anatomy classification (IFAC) and classification of the extent of endoscopic frontal sinus surgery (EFSS). Int Forum Allergy Rhinol. 2016;6:677–96.
13. Wormald PJ. Endoscopic sinus surgery: anatomy, three-dimensional reconstruction, and surgical technique. 3rd ed. New York: Thieme Medical Publisher; 2012. p. 28–102.
14. Stammberger H, Posawetz W. Functional endoscopic sinus surgery. Concept, indications and results of the Messerklinger technique. Eur Arch Otorhinolaryngol. 1990;247:63–76.
15. Moon HJ, Kim HU, Lee JG, Chung IH, Yoon JH. Surgical anatomy of the anterior ethmoidal canal in ethmoid roof. Laryngoscope. 2001;111:900–4.
16. Simmen D, Raghavan U, Briner HR, Manestar M, Schuknecht B, Groscurth PJNS. The surgeon's view of the anterior ethmoid artery. Clin Otolaryngol. 2006;31:187–91.
17. Kainz J, Stammberger H. The roof of the anterior ethmoid: a locus minoris resistentiae in the skull base. Laryngol Rhinol Otol (Stuttg). 1988;67:142–9. (in German).
18. Ferrari M, Schreiber A, Mattavelli D, Rampinelli V, Buffoli B, Ravanelli M, Bettinsoli M, Rodella LF, Nicolai P. The Terracol and Ardouin developmental model of frontal sinus drainage pathway and surrounding spaces: a radiologic validation. Int Forum Allergy Rhinol. 2018;8(5):624–30.

Radiologic Review for Frontal Sinus Surgery

Joseph M. Hoxworth and Devyani Lal

Introduction

In cases of suspected frontal sinus disease, a detailed clinical examination, even with thorough endoscopic inspection, is often insufficient to evaluate the frontal sinuses. As a result, imaging is critical for the noninvasive assessment of suspected frontal sinus pathology. As is true for all of the paranasal sinuses, computed tomography (CT) is the imaging modality of choice to determine whether the frontal sinuses are diseased and, if so, to assess the severity and identify predisposing conditions. This is achievable because modern multidetector CT is performed using submillimeter isotropic voxels that yield a volumetric imaging dataset suitable for reconstruction in any plane, though standard axial, coronal, and sagittal images are rendered by default for routine diagnostic purposes. Because of exquisite bone detail, the anatomy surrounding the frontal sinus drainage pathway can be accurately defined with CT as a roadmap for the surgeon in terms of preoperative planning, surgical dissection, and intraoperative navigation.

Although noncontrast CT cannot reliably define the soft tissue contents that underlie an opacified sinus, CT can identify features that may merit workup to identify lesions other than routine inflammatory sinus disease. Specifically, bone remodeling, destruction, and expansion must be viewed with suspicion, while abnormal soft tissue extending beyond the confines of the frontal sinuses is an additional "red flag." In cases of suspected sinonasal tumor or sinusitis with orbital and/or intracranial complications, magnetic resonance imaging (MRI) is typically employed because its superior soft tissue contrast leads to improved sensitivity and specificity compared with CT. Based upon greater availability of CT and potential patient contraindications for undergoing MRI, CT can also be acquired with intravenous contrast as an alternative imaging modality, albeit that it is more limited than MRI in discriminating soft tissue pathology.

A radiologic approach to the frontal sinuses can be broadly outlined as:

J. M. Hoxworth (✉)
Neuroradiology Division, Department of Radiology, Mayo Clinic, Phoenix, AZ, USA

Mayo Clinic College of Medicine and Sciences, Phoenix, AZ, USA

D. Lal
Department of Otolaryngology – Head and Neck Surgery, Mayo Clinic College of Medicine and Science, Mayo Clinic, Phoenix, AZ, USA

© Springer Nature Switzerland AG 2019
D. Lal, P. H. Hwang (eds.), *Frontal Sinus Surgery*, https://doi.org/10.1007/978-3-319-97022-6_3

- Definition of anatomy, including relevant anatomic variants
- Characterization of inflammatory sinus disease and any associated complications
- Evaluation of the postoperative diseased frontal sinus
- Assessment of expansile mass-like lesions and sinonasal neoplasms

This chapter will focus on highlighting these key points through an image-based approach.

Definition of Anatomy, Including Relevant Anatomic Variants

Normal frontal sinus anatomy is incredibly variable both in terms of the degree of frontal sinus pneumatization and the presence of numerous air cells that can occur within or adjacent to the frontal sinuses. Although a detailed review of frontal sinus anatomy and physiologic drainage is presented elsewhere in this textbook, a discussion of frontal sinus imaging would be incomplete without a brief treatment of anatomy, as these variants can predispose to disease and potentially contribute to the need for revision endoscopic sinus surgery.

The drainage of the frontal sinus into the nose occurs through a continuous air-filled channel that is a highly variable space based on the ethmoidal air cells. This is termed the frontal recess and is constrained medially by the vertical lamella of the middle turbinate and the lateral lamella of the cribriform plate, while it is bordered laterally by the lacrimal bone and lamina papyracea (Fig. 3.1). As best appreciated in the sagittal plane [1], the frontal recess is bounded anteriorly by the frontal beak and agger nasi (with any associated frontoethmoidal air cells) and posteriorly by additional air cells related to the ethmoidal bulla (bulla ethmoidalis). The frontal recess outflow tract begins at the posteromedial inferior part of the floor of the frontal sinus and then funnels narrower, before widening and opening into the nose, thus forming an hourglass-shaped space. There is no

ductal structure in this recess, and therefore the old terminology of "nasofrontal duct" is erroneous and should not be used. Unlike the maxillary and the sphenoid sinuses, the frontal sinus does not have a true defined frontal ostium. Rather, the narrowest area of the waist of the hourglass-shaped frontal recess is often referred to as the ostium. When viewed in the coronal plane, the frontal recess is bounded medially by the vertical segment of the middle turbinate and laterally by the lamina papyracea. However, within these confines, the attachment of the uncinate process further dictates the pattern of frontal recess drainage (Fig. 3.2). When the uncinate process attaches to the lamina papyracea, frontal sinus drainage is directed medially into the middle meatus. This is the most common pattern of drainage. In contrast, attachment of the uncinate process to the skull base or middle turbinate first channels frontal sinus drainage into the ethmoid infundibulum, ultimately reaching the middle meatus via the hiatus semilunaris. It is important for beginners to be able to clearly distinguish the infundibulum (which lies lateral to the uncinate process, between the uncinate and the orbit) from the middle meatal space which is medial to the uncinate process (lying between the middle turbinate and uncinate).

The size and number of surrounding air cells influence the shape and overall caliber of the frontal recess. Kuhn described these cells in detail and defined the first nomenclature system [2], which was later modified by Wormald [3]. More recently, the nomenclature has been simplified into anterior, posterior, and medial cells in the International Frontal Sinus Anatomy Classification [4].

The most anterior ethmoidal air cell, the agger nasi cell, is positioned above the anterior attachment of the middle turbinate into the lateral nasal wall (Fig. 3.3). Additional air cells arising from the agger nasi region have been previously classified as frontal cells [5]. Type 1 and 2 frontal cells represent either a single cell or a tier of two or more cells above the agger nasi cell, respectively, neither of which extends into the frontal sinus. These are now collectively termed supra agger

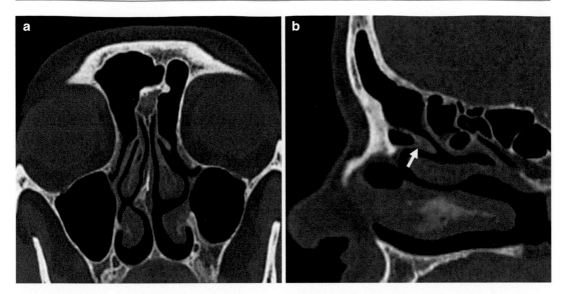

Fig. 3.1 Frontal recess. (**a**) Oblique coronal and (**b**) sagittal CT acquired along the axis of the funnel-shaped frontal recess (blue shading) depicts its close relationship to surrounding structures, including the anterior skull base and lamina papyracea. Note the anterior insertion of the uncinate process (arrow) onto the agger nasi cell

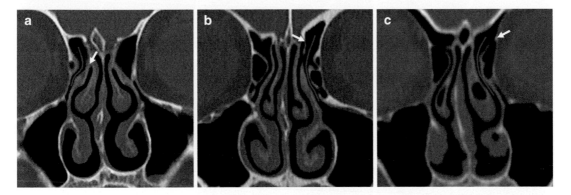

Fig. 3.2 Variation in attachment of the uncinate process. Coronal sinus CT illustrates that the uncinate process (arrow) can attach to the (**a**) middle turbinate, (**b**) skull base, or (**c**) lamina papyracea, and this impacts the direction of frontal recess drainage (blue line). For uncinate attachment to the skull base and middle turbinate, drainage occurs laterally into the ethmoidal infundibulum, while it is directed medially into the middle meatus when the uncinate is attached to the lamina papyracea

cells. A large cell extending from above the agger nasi into the frontal sinus represents a type 3 frontal cell, while a type 4 frontal cell is isolated within the frontal sinus sharing a wall with the inner table and/or floor of the frontal sinus. Given their pneumatization into the frontal sinus, the cells that have historically been designated as types 3 and 4 are now known as supra agger frontal cells. The variable size is recognized on a continuum with larger cells potentially necessitating an extended frontal or combined external/endoscopic approach.

An air cell with a superior attachment to the anterior skull base is commonly identified above the ethmoidal bulla (Fig. 3.4). Whether or not the anterior wall of this air cell extends into the frontal sinus determines if it is termed a supra bulla cell or supra bulla frontal cell. These air cells were previ-

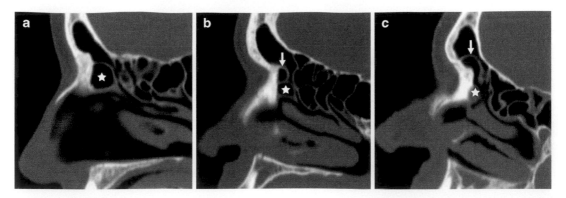

Fig. 3.3 Anterior cells as demonstrated by sagittal CT. (**a**) Note the location of the agger nasi cell posterior (star) to the frontal process of the maxilla. (**b**) Supra agger cell (arrow) is identified above the agger nasi cell (star) and posterior to the frontal beak without extension into the frontal sinus. (**c**) Supra agger frontal cell (arrow) is recognized by its position superior to the agger nasi cell (star) and its extension above the frontal beak to enter the frontal sinus

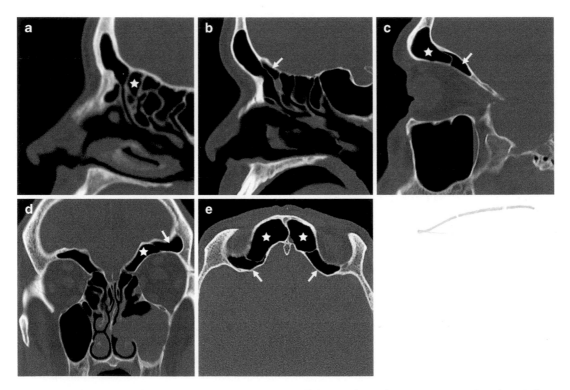

Fig. 3.4 Posterior cells. (**a**) On sagittal CT, a supra bulla cell (star) is located above the ethmoidal bulla but does not enter the frontal sinus. (**b**) Sagittal CT delineates a supra bulla frontal cell extending through the frontal ostium into the frontal sinus with its posterior wall bordered by the anterior skull base (arrow). (**c**) As depicted in the sagittal plane, a supraorbital ethmoidal cell (arrow) shares the posterior wall of the frontal sinus (star). (**d**) The supraorbital ethmoidal cell (arrow) can give the appearance of a septated frontal sinus (star) in the coronal plane. (**e**) On axial CT, the same patient is seen to have bilateral supraorbital ethmoidal cells (arrows), which are located posterior and lateral relative to the frontal sinuses (stars)

ously known as suprabullar cell and frontal bullar cell, respectively. The supra bulla frontal cell extends into the posterior aspect of the frontal sinus such that the skull base forms its posterior wall. When an anterior ethmoid air cell in the vicinity of the anterior ethmoidal artery pneumatizes the orbital plate of the frontal bone extending along the orbital roof, it is described as a supraorbital ethmoid cell. This cell is posterior and lateral to the frontal sinus and drains into the lateral aspect of the frontal recess posterior and lateral to the true frontal sinus outflow tract. Because supraorbital ethmoidal cells frequently form part of the posterior wall of the frontal sinus, the impression of a septated frontal sinus may result on CT (Fig. 3.4). Clinically, disease in high frontoethmoidal cells as well as the supraorbital ethmoidal cell can be mistakenly thought to be in the frontal sinus. Correct localization of disease is imperative, as a frontal sinusotomy alone will not address disease in the supraorbital ethmoidal cell, which is more lateral and posterior to the true frontal sinus.

When evaluating the suprabullar region, it is also particularly important to identify the anterior ethmoidal artery to determine whether it is closely apposed to the anterior skull base or displaced inferiorly from the skull base by posterior pneumatization of the frontal sinus (Fig. 3.5). In some patients, the artery may pass through the superior ethmoidal space, pedicled on a mesentery of mucosa. The position of the anterior ethmoidal artery should be defined in every patient undergoing frontal sinus surgery. The anterior ethmoidal artery is a branch of the ophthalmic artery and passes into the nasal cavity along the anterior ethmoid skull base usually in the area superior to the ethmoidal bulla. Injury to the artery can lead to severe epistaxis as well as a rapidly expanding orbital hematoma. Endoscopically, the artery is identified in the area of the bulla lamella or the suprabullar area, with a suprabullar space present between the area of the frontal ostium and the artery. If multiple suprabullar or supraorbital cells are present, the artery is usually present between the first and second suprabullar or supraorbital ethmoidal cell, and this area should be very carefully dissected as hyperpneumatized frontal sinuses are more likely to have a pedicled ethmoidal artery.

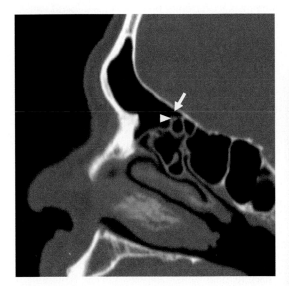

Fig. 3.5 Anterior ethmoidal artery. Sagittal sinus CT illustrates how posterior pneumatization of the frontal sinus (arrow) can inferiorly displace the anterior ethmoidal artery (arrowhead) from the skull base, which can be seen pedicled on a mesentery. The position of the artery is on the ethmoidal bone, typically in the area of the bulla lamella or suprabullar area

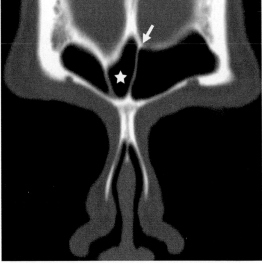

Fig. 3.6 Medial cells. As seen on coronal CT, the medial wall of a frontal septal cell (star) is the interfrontal septum (arrow)

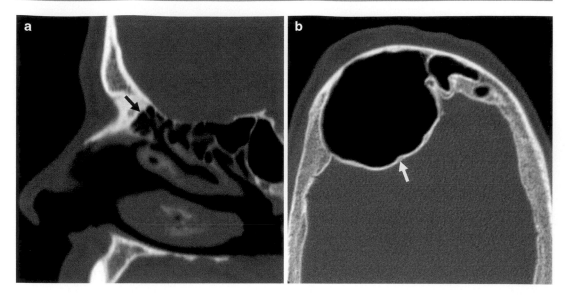

Fig. 3.7 Variants of frontal sinus pneumatization. (**a**) Sagittal noncontrast sinus CT depicts a case of marked frontal sinus hypoplasia (arrow). (**b**) Axial noncontrast sinus CT demonstrates pneumosinus dilatans with hyperpneumatization of the right frontal sinus causing abnormal convexity of the inner table (arrow)

Medial cells, which can cause the frontal sinus drainage pathway to deviate laterally and often posteriorly, can arise from the inferior frontal sinus or anterior ethmoidal complex (Fig. 3.6). Because of their association with the interfrontal sinus septum, these are recognized as frontal septal cells and can be associated with a pneumatized crista galli.

The degree of pneumatization of the frontal sinus (Fig. 3.7) and the adjacent ethmoidal cells is highly variable and also has significant consequences on surgical management. Developmental aplasia or hypoplasia of one or both frontal sinuses can occur. Small, hypoplastic frontal sinuses with severe inflammation or sclerosis are more likely to result in postoperative stenosis. The decision to operate on hypoplastic frontal sinuses with minimal disease should be carefully made based on the degree of symptomatology and the technical expertise of the surgeon. Additionally, if repeated endoscopic approaches have been unsuccessful, these sinuses may be more amenable to obliteration based on the small size and the presence of osteitic changes. Conversely, hyperpneumatized sinuses are usually associated with high frontoethmoidal cells that may require more skill, time, instrumentation, and navigation for complete dissection. In rare instances, frontal pneumosinus dilatans can be present leading to intracranial mass effect from remodeling of the inner table and placing the patient at risk for pneumocephalus.

The sinus CT scan is also used for intraoperative image guidance and navigation. While image-based navigation is not essential to use, the American Academy of Otolaryngology–Head and Neck Surgery includes surgery on the frontal sinuses as a criterion for considering intraoperative image guidance [6]. A critical benefit of the use of the image guidance systems is the ability to study the frontal recess and cell anatomy in a triplanar-linked view. The benefit of studying these views in understanding frontal recess anatomy cannot be overstated. If image guidance is not available, a variety of other commercially marketed radiology image viewers can also be utilized to study the three-dimensional anatomy of the frontal sinuses.

Characterization of Inflammatory Sinus Disease and any Associated Orbital or Intracranial Complications

The presence of frontal sinus mucosal thickening or fluid is taken as evidence of rhinosinusitis, though the acuity is indeterminate in the absence of prior studies for comparison. As defined by the American Academy of Otolaryngology–Head and Neck Surgery, the duration of sinonasal symptoms is utilized to characterize disease into acute or chronic [7]. The presence of fluid levels may indicate acute frontal sinusitis or an acute exacerbation of chronic frontal sinusitis. Fluid may layer on the posterior table or the frontal sinus floor, depending on whether imaging was performed in the sitting or supine positions. Isolated frontal sinus fluid may also be seen in patients with barotrauma. Sclerosis of the sinus walls supports the presence of chronic rhinosinusitis (past or present), but superimposed mucosal thickening can be acute, subacute, or chronic. Mucosal stripping from prior surgery can also result in sclerosis of the frontal recess. In the setting of rhinosinusitis, it is important to determine whether the frontal sinus drainage pathway is occluded and, if so, whether there is significant frontal sinus opacification suggesting clinically

meaningful outflow obstruction (Fig. 3.8). Even modest amounts of mucosal thickening can result in frontal recess obstruction, particularly when predisposed by narrowing from large adjacent air cells. It is important to define such anatomic variants and to also scrutinize the CT images for areas of rounded soft tissue opacification in the anterior ethmoidal region to suggest the presence of an obstructing polyp or mucocele, for example. In addition, it is critical to note whether obstruction is limited to the frontal sinus or whether anterior ethmoidal and maxillary sinus disease is present to indicate an ostiomeatal pattern of sinusitis (Fig. 3.9).

The frontal sinuses are intimately associated with both the orbits and anterior cranial fossa, thereby facilitating the development of orbital and intracranial complications of rhinosinusitis [8, 9]. The periorbita, which reflects into the eyelids anteriorly to become the orbital septum, provides a natural barrier to infection. However, the spread of infection can be direct or indirect, with the latter including bidirectional spread of infectious thrombophlebitis through the valveless venous network that drains the orbital and facial soft tissues. This can lead not only to orbital infection but also to cavernous sinus thrombosis and intracranial infection. As originally described by Chandler and colleagues, orbital complica-

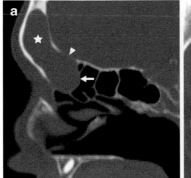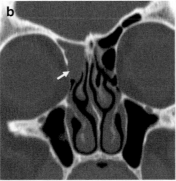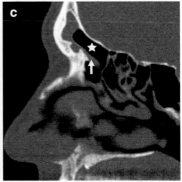

Fig. 3.8 Obstructive frontal sinusitis. (**a**) Sagittal noncontrast CT depicts an expansile anterior ethmoidal mucocele (arrow) with secondary obstruction of the frontal sinus (star). The anterior skull base (arrowhead) is thinned but not completely dehiscent. (**b**) On coronal noncontrast CT, a rounded structure in the right frontal recess causing frontal sinusitis was ultimately found to represent a polyp (arrow) at the time of surgery. (**c**) Sagittal noncontrast CT illustrates a large supraorbital ethmoidal air cell (star) significantly narrowing the frontal recess (arrow) and leading to obstructive frontal sinusitis

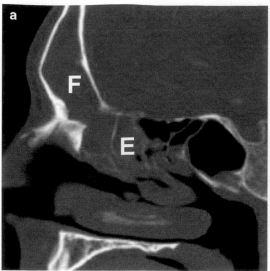
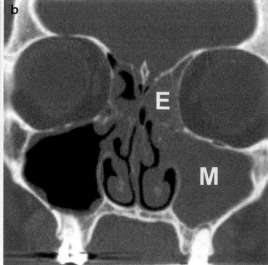

Fig. 3.9 Ostiomeatal pattern of sinusitis. (**a**) Sagittal and (**b**) coronal sinus CT illustrate an ostiomeatal pattern of obstructive sinusitis with complete opacification of the left frontal sinus (F), anterior ethmoidal air cells (E), and maxillary sinus (M)

tions of rhinosinusitis include preseptal cellulitis, orbital cellulitis, subperiosteal abscess, orbital abscess, and cavernous sinus thrombosis [10]. These infections are frequently associated with the ethmoid sinuses, though frontal rhinosinusitis can also seed orbital infection leading to a subperiosteal abscess in the superior orbit (Fig. 3.10). Intracranial complications of rhinosinusitis most commonly arise from the frontal sinuses. Because pneumatization of the frontal sinuses begins at about 6 years of age, such complications are uncommon in younger children in whom the frontal sinuses have yet to fully form. Frontal osteomyelitis with an associated subgaleal or subperiosteal abscess has been termed "Pott's puffy tumor" and is diagnosed with cross-sectional imaging as a rim-enhancing collection intimately associated with the outer table of the frontal bone (Fig. 3.11). Moreover, the osteomyelitis can be depicted on CT as areas of bone destruction, while MRI would demonstrate bone marrow edema and enhancement as a corollary. Infection can spread from the frontal sinuses along valveless emissary veins that cross the calvarium or through congenital or acquired

sites of bony dehiscence leading to meningitis, epidural abscess, subdural empyema, cerebritis, or brain abscess (Figs. 3.11, 3.12, and 3.13). CT is effective at screening for intracranial complications because of its widespread availability and rapid image acquisition, though MRI is most sensitive in the detection of small extra-axial collections and meningeal enhancement. In addition, when edema is seen in the brain on a noncontrast CT, MRI can distinguish cerebritis from abscess, as the latter will appear as a peripherally enhancing lesion with central restricted diffusion (Fig. 3.13). Likewise, the presence of restricted diffusion can also help confirm that subdural or epidural fluid collections are empyemas rather than hygromas (Fig. 3.12).

Both invasive and noninvasive forms of fungal sinusitis have characteristic imaging features [11]. Angioinvasive fungal sinusitis preferentially affects immunocompromised patients with underlying illnesses such as hematologic malignancies, diabetes, solid organ malignancies, and immunosuppression following solid organ or bone marrow transplantation. It can be identified on CT based on the presence of inflammatory

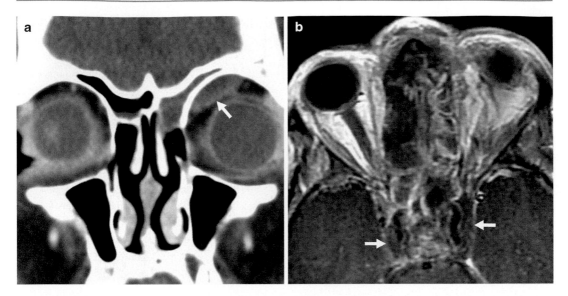

Fig. 3.10 Orbital complications of sinusitis. (**a**) Coronal contrast-enhanced CT demonstrates an opacified left frontal sinus with an adjacent rim-enhancing low-density collection (arrow) in the superior orbit, consistent with subperiosteal abscess that is contained by the periorbita. (**b**) In a separate case, contrast-enhanced T1-weighted MRI illustrates mild expansion of the cavernous sinuses with areas of non-enhancement, left greater than right, consistent with cavernous sinus thrombosis (arrows) in the setting of rhinosinusitis and left orbital cellulitis. The lateral wall of the cavernous sinus should normally be straight or concave, not bulging outward as in this case

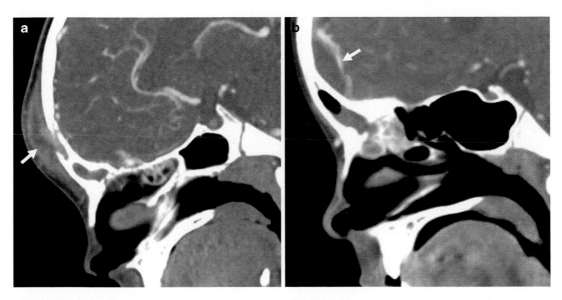

Fig. 3.11 Pott's puffy tumor and epidural abscess. (**a**) Sagittal contrast-enhanced CT demonstrates frontal sinus opacification with bone destruction involving the outer greater than inner tables. A rim-enhancing subgaleal collection with surrounding inflammatory fat stranding is consistent with Pott's puffy tumor (arrow). (**b**) In a different patient, sagittal contrast-enhanced CT illustrates a rim-enhancing lenticular-shaped collection along the inner table of an infected frontal sinus consistent with epidural abscess (arrow)

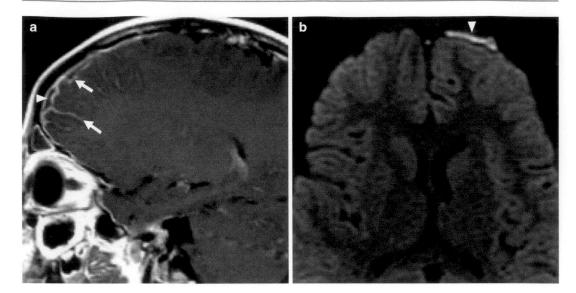

Fig. 3.12 Subdural empyema and meningitis. (**a**) Sagittal T1-weighted post-contrast MRI illustrates abnormal leptomeningeal enhancement (arrows) along the frontal lobe in the context of frontal sinusitis. A thin subdural rim-enhancing collection is also identified (arrowhead). (**b**) On axial diffusion-weighted MRI, the thin extra-axial collection has restricted diffusion (arrowhead), which is confirmatory that this represents a small subdural empyema

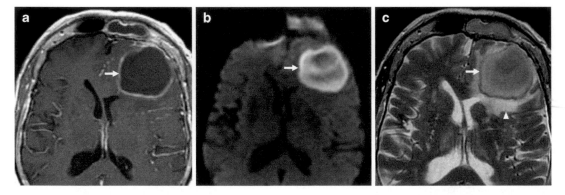

Fig. 3.13 Brain abscess. (**a**) A round rim-enhancing collection (arrow) is identified in the left frontal lobe in the setting of left frontal sinusitis on axial T1-weighted post-contrast MRI. (**b**) The presence of restricted diffusion (arrow) on an axial diffusion-weighted MRI sequence is consistent with pyogenic abscess. (**c**) On T2-weighted MRI, the abscess (arrow) is heterogeneous and not as hyperintense as cerebrospinal fluid, which is expected given its proteinaceous content. Surrounding T2 hyperintensity (arrowhead) in the left frontal white matter is secondary to vasogenic edema

changes in facial soft tissues or intracranial structures typically in the context of an at-risk patient with varying degrees of sinonasal opacification. In the early phase of disease, these findings often occur in the setting of intact bone because of spread along vascular channels. A CT-based seven variable model has been proposed based upon the presence of bone dehiscence, nasal septal ulceration, orbital invasion, and infiltration of periantral fat, pterygopalatine fossa, nasolacrimal duct, or lacrimal sac [12]. When one such variable was present, the positive predictive value for angioinvasive fungal sinusitis was 87%, while this increased to 100% with the presence of a second finding. Additionally, MRI often demonstrates T2 hypointensity in relation to the fungal elements, though this is not specific to fungal sinusitis and can also be seen with inspissated secretions. MRI can also depict non-enhancing tissue due to necrosis ("black turbinate" sign) [13] and can most effectively identify intracranial involvement in the form of direct brain or meningeal invasion, cavernous sinus thrombosis, or secondary infarcts when major intracranial arteries or veins are invaded (Fig. 3.14). Isolated frontal sinus involvement is uncommon, so these imaging features must be sought more broadly.

Noninvasive fungal sinus disease includes fungus ball and allergic fungal sinusitis [11]. Sinus fungal colonization in an immunocompetent patient can lead to fungus ball formation. Fungus balls typically appear as a non-aggressive rounded structure with heterogeneously increased density on CT (often partially calcified) and marked hypointensity on T2-weighted MRI (Fig. 3.15). They are usually isolated to a single sinus, with the maxillary and sphenoid sinus being the most common locations. The frontal

sinuses are uncommonly involved as a primary site for fungus ball formation but may also become secondarily obstructed and inflamed by a fungus ball involving the middle meatus. Allergic fungal sinusitis tends to be more generalized and often affects the frontal sinuses as a result. One or both frontal sinus may be involved with unilateral or bilateral disease on CT. Often found in association with nasal polyposis and allergic rhinitis, the most striking imaging feature is centrally increased density within the sinuses on CT. Although often heterogeneous and intermediate in signal on T1-weighted MRI, T2-weighted sequences exhibit central hypointensity that, at times, can be so dark that it mimics air (Fig. 3.16). It has been suggested that this is related to densely packed hyphae, high viscosity, and/or the ferromagnetic effect of iron and manganese. In these cases, it is critical to scrutinize all MRI sequences to avoid mistakenly attributing the marked T2 hypointensity to normal pneumatization.

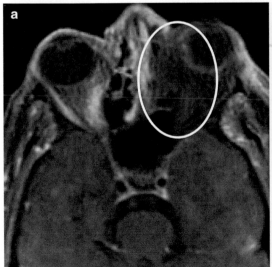
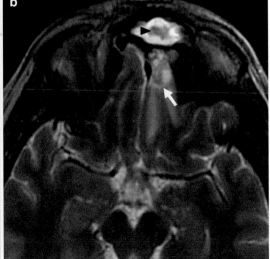

Fig. 3.14 Angioinvasive fungal sinusitis involving the frontal sinus. (**a**) Axial T1 post-contrast fat-suppressed MRI demonstrates a geographic area in the anterior left ethmoidal region and medial orbit in which normal expected contrast enhancement is lacking (oval). In the appropriate clinical setting, this is very suspicious for necrotic tissue due to angioinvasive fungal sinusitis. (**b**) More superiorly on axial T2-weighted MRI, the left frontal sinus is opacified with centrally hypointense material (arrowhead), a nonspecific finding that is consistent with fungal elements. Edema has developed within the inferior left frontal lobe consistent with intracranial invasion (arrow)

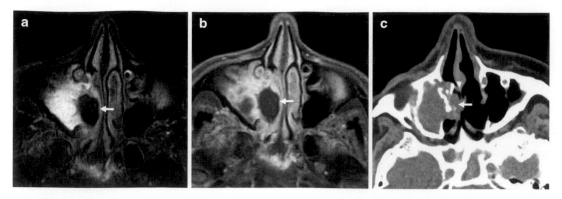

Fig. 3.15 Fungus ball. (**a**) Rounded structure in the right middle meatus is hypointense on T2-weighted MRI and (**b**) non-enhancing on axial T1 post-contrast fat-suppressed MRI, a finding which was found to represent a fungus ball (arrow) at the time of surgery. (**c**) As seen on axial noncontrast sinus CT, the fungus ball (arrow) demonstrates partial calcification. Although most commonly located in the maxillary and sphenoid sinuses, middle meatal involvement such as this can lead to frontal sinus obstruction

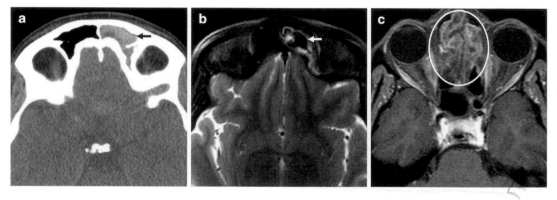

Fig. 3.16 Allergic fungal sinusitis. (**a**) Axial noncontrast CT demonstrates opacification of the left frontal sinus by high-density secretions (arrow). (**b**) Axial T2-weighted fat-suppressed MRI acquired on the same day as the CT illustrates how T2 hypointense (arrow) the secretions may be in the setting of allergic fungal sinusitis, an appearance which should not be mistaken for air. (**c**) Axial T1-weighted post-contrast sequence demonstrates exuberant enhancing anterior ethmoidal tissue (oval) consistent with sinonasal polyposis, a frequent association with allergic fungal sinusitis

Evaluation of the Postoperative Frontal Sinus

Postoperative CT is indicated following endoscopic sinus surgery if symptoms of rhinosinusitis persist or recur or if there is concern for surgical complications. Certainly, any bone defect abutting the anterior cranial fossa with adjacent soft tissue opacity within a sinus should be evaluated with MRI to exclude a posttraumatic or postoperative cephalocele, depending on the clinical history (Fig. 3.17). Similarly, the integrity of the lamina papyracea must be closely examined and any herniation of orbital fat into the frontal recess and ethmoidal cavity examined (Fig. 3.18). In patients who have undergone prior orbital decompression, iatrogenic frontal sinusitis can result from the decompressed orbit causing obstruction to the frontal sinus outflow.

A regimented approach for the postoperative evaluation of the frontal sinus should address the following questions:

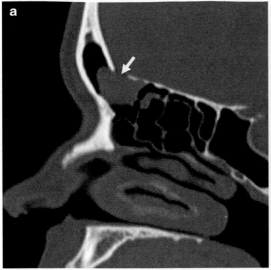
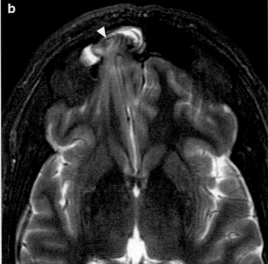

Fig. 3.17 Posttraumatic encephalocele. (**a**) A polypoid opacity is identified in the frontal sinus adjacent to a bone defect in the inner table (arrow) on sagittal noncontrast CT. (**b**) Axial T2-weighted MRI confirms that both brain and meninges have herniated through the osseous defect consistent with a meningoencephalocele (arrowhead). In this case, the patient had a remote history of craniofacial trauma

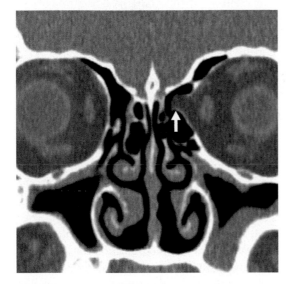

Fig. 3.18 Lamina papyracea defect. Preoperative evaluation for de novo and revision surgeries must include assessment of the lamina papyracea for any defects related to prior surgery or trauma. In this case, a remote medial orbital blow-out fracture has allowed a small amount of fat to protrude through a small defect in the lamina papyracea (arrow), a finding that may resemble a small polyp endoscopically

- What was the nature and extent of any previous procedure(s)? Specifically, is there evidence that the frontal sinuses were adequately addressed surgically?
- What structures were removed and was the resection complete or partial?
- Is the surgically modified frontal sinus drainage pathway patent? If not, is the occlusion secondary to the bone and/or soft tissue? Are there residual structures such as air cells or retained uncinate process along the frontal recess or within the frontal sinus causing meaningful narrowing?
- Are the frontal sinuses diseased and, if so, is opacification complete or partial? In the setting of opacification, are any expansile features present to raise concern for an underlying mucocele?
- Is there any loss of integrity of the skull base or orbital roof and medial wall?

In terms of recognizing the type of endoscopic surgery that has been previously performed, the initial step is to determine whether the frontal recess and sinus were directly approached or whether an attempt was simply made to improve frontal sinus drainage by indirectly addressing the anterior ostiomeatal complex with anterior ethmoidectomy, uncinectomy, and middle meatal maxillary antrostomy. If there is evidence of a previous endoscopic frontal sinus drainage procedure, the structures that were removed and the extent to which the surgery entered the frontal sinus are informative.

The Draf classification of frontal sinus surgery has been widely adopted and represents progressively more aggressive frontal resections [14, 15]. Draf type 1 focuses on eliminating any source of obstruction along the frontal recess inferior to the frontal sinus ostium. Although some differences in the procedure exist secondary to case-to-case anatomic variation, this would typically include complete removal of the uncinate process and, if needed, the anterior wall of the ethmoidal bulla and the medial lamella of the agger nasi cell. Draf type 2 procedures involve removing the same structures as Draf type 1 but extend more superiorly to widen the frontal sinus ostium. Draf type IIA usually entails removing all additional frontoethmoidal air cells along the superior limits of the frontal recess and any additional air cells that project into the frontal sinus, while Draf type IIB further removes the floor of the frontal sinus from the lamina papyracea to the nasal septum, including the anterior part of the middle turbinate. Draf type II procedures can be recognized in the sagittal plane by the widened opening from the frontal beak to the anterior skull base and in the coronal plane between the lamina papyracea and middle turbinate (or nasal septum if the middle turbinate was removed anteriorly). For the most severe cases of recalcitrant frontal sinus disease, the endoscopic modified Lothrop (Draf type III) procedure may have been performed. Recognition of this surgery is more straightforward, as the postoperative anatomy when viewed in the coronal plane has a very characteristic appearance that results from not only enlarging bilateral frontal sinus drainage but also establishing frontal sinus contiguity. Specifically, the superior aspect of the nasal septum and inferior portion of the interfrontal sinus septum are removed, along with bilateral Draf type IIB drainage.

The International Classification of the Extent of Endoscopic Frontal Sinus Surgery has more recently moved toward a stepwise approach in classifying the type and extent of previous frontal sinus surgery as follows [4]:

- *Grade 0*: Balloon sinus dilation (no tissue removal)
- *Grade 1*: Clearance of cell(s) in the frontal recess without any surgery within the frontal ostium
- *Grade 2*: Clearance of cell(s) directly obstructing the frontal sinus ostium
- *Grade 3*: Clearance of cell(s) pneumatizing through the frontal ostium into the frontal sinus without enlargement of the frontal ostium
- *Grade 4*: Clearance of cell(s) pneumatizing through the frontal ostium into the frontal sinus with enlargement of the frontal ostium
- *Grade 5*: Enlargement of the frontal ostium from the lamina papyracea to the nasal septum
- *Grade 6*: Removal of the entire floor of the frontal sinus with joining of the left and right ostia into a common ostium

As described at the point of publication, this classification was not unanimously agreed upon by all coauthors, in part because it can be argued that the frontal sinus lacks a true ostium and instead has more of a three-dimensional drainage channel. Nevertheless, this classification allows for an intuitive and methodical approach to the assessment of the postoperative frontal sinus, which can be viewed on a continuum from least to most aggressive. Because of its unique appearance on CT, grade 6 (modified Lothrop, Draf type III) is typically obvious, but less aggressive surgeries can be more challenging for the novice to identify. Because prior imaging is not always available in patients who are candidates for revision surgery, it may be difficult to know exactly what types of cells were previously cleared, thereby making it challenging at times to differentiate grades 2 and 3 (i.e., was a cell pneumatizing into the frontal sinus removed or was one ever developmentally present in the first place?).

In terms of radiologic description, the term "frontal sinusotomy" was initially most closely associated with Draf type II surgeries but has been used indiscriminately and should be avoided in the absence of an accompanying detailed description of findings, which can be viewed on a continuum (Fig. 3.19). It should, at minimum, be documented whether or not air cells have been resected

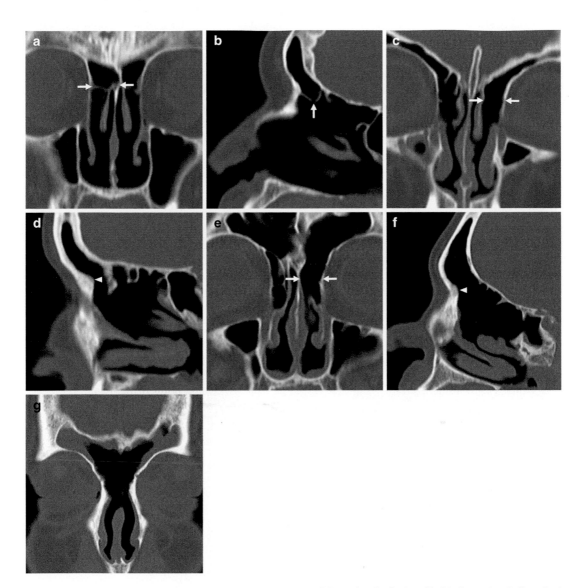

Fig. 3.19 Spectrum of endoscopic frontal sinus surgery. *Patient #1:* (**a**) Coronal and (**b**) sagittal CT images demonstrate evidence of previous endoscopic sinus surgery. Although ethmoidectomy has been performed and both the agger nasi cell and uncinate process have been resected, the most superior partitions along the frontal recess remain intact, and the frontal sinus has not been entered (arrows). *Patient #2.* (**c**) Coronal and (**d**) sagittal CT images illustrate complete anterior ethmoidectomy with widening of the floor of the frontal sinus from middle turbinate to lamina papyracea (arrows) though the frontal beak appears unaltered (arrowhead). *Patient #3.* (**e**) Coronal and (**f**) sagittal CT images show removal of all air cells along the frontal recess and within the frontal sinus. The frontal beak has been drilled down (arrowhead) to widen the frontal ostium in an anteroposterior direction, and the floor of the frontal sinus has been opened from nasal septum to lamina papyracea (arrows). *Patient #4.* (**g**) For refractory disease, coronal CT demonstrates maximum opening of the frontal sinuses with complete removal of all anterior ethmoidal cells, anterior parts of the middle turbinates, frontal sinus floors, and adjacent part of the frontal sinus septum and nasal septum

in the frontal recess, along the frontal ostium, and within the frontal sinus. As best seen in the sagittal plane, an assessment should be made as to whether the frontal beak has been drilled down to widen the frontal ostium. Lastly, the coronal plane nicely allows one to note whether a unilateral drill out has been performed because the widened opening from nasal septum to lamina papyracea is readily apparent. The types of endoscopic frontal sinus surgery and their nuances are described in much greater detail elsewhere in this textbook.

Once postoperative anatomy is understood, a determination needs to be made regarding the adequacy for treating frontal sinus disease. The potential need for revision endoscopic sinus surgery can be well depicted with CT. Common etiologies include mucosal disease, lateralized middle turbinate, scarring, neo-osteogenesis, and retained ethmoid, agger nasi, and frontal cells (Fig. 3.20), and patients frequently suffer from more than one of these [16–18]. The frontal sinuses are particularly prone to stenosis and recurrent mucosal disease following surgery, which can lead to functionally significant outflow obstruction given the limited dimensions of the frontal recess. Synechiae along the frontal recess, recurrent sinonasal polyposis, and mucosal thickening along an inadequately widened frontal recess all represent potential etiologies

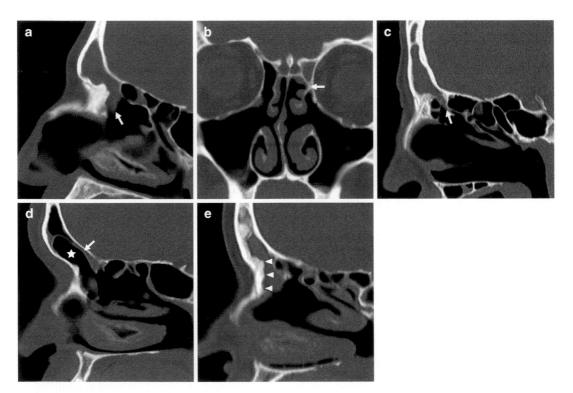

Fig. 3.20 Findings in revision frontal endoscopic sinus surgery. (**a**) Sagittal CT shows a lobulated opacity (arrow) in the surgically widened frontal recess causing frontal sinus obstruction. This was found to represent an inflammatory polyp at the time of revision surgery. (**b**) Coronal CT confirms that postoperative obstruction of the left frontal sinus is due to a lateralized middle turbinate (arrow). (**c**) A supra bulla cell is present posteriorly, and an agger nasi cell and a supra agger (type 1 frontal) cell are found anteriorly, as seen on sagittal CT. This combina-

tion of retained air cells results in narrowing of the frontal recess (arrow) with resultant frontal sinus opacification. (**d**) In spite of an anterior ethmoidectomy having been performed, a large supra agger frontal (type 3 frontal) cell is still present (star) and is seen to cause narrowing and elongation of the frontal ostium and recess (arrow) on sagittal CT. (**e**) Sagittal CT demonstrates postoperative neo-osteogenesis (arrowheads) along the frontal ostium and recess which, in conjunction with mucosal thickening and scarring, cause frontal sinus outflow obstruction

for obstructive sinusitis, though the CT appearance is nonspecific and does not reliably differentiate these. The same inflammatory milieu causing mucosal disease also predisposes to neo-osteogenesis, which is problematic as removal of neo-osteogenic bone often further propagates the process. Mucosal stripping at prior surgery may also result in neo-osteogenesis. Residual air cells along the frontal recesses or within the frontal sinuses proper may contribute to inadequate frontal sinus drainage, particularly when diseased or expanded due to mucocele formation. Ideally, a detailed preoperative assessment of frontal sinus and frontal recess anatomy in conjunction with computer-guided surgery would limit this as a cause for revision surgery. However, frontal sinus anatomy is complex, and frontoethmoidal cells may not have been fully addressed at prior surgery. Lateralization of the middle turbinate can also be seen to block frontal sinus drainage and is particularly well-recognized in the coronal plane. It is attributed to weakened middle turbinate support and/or overly aggressive resection causing synechiae formation between the lateral nasal wall and middle turbinate, thereby blocking the frontal recess.

Since the advent of endoscopic sinus surgery, the need for osteoplastic flaps with or without complete frontal sinus obliteration has declined considerably. However, patients with these procedures performed in the past may require continued care due to persistent symptoms or disease. In rare circumstances, posttraumatic deformity, tumor resection, mucocele repair, and severe cases of rhinosinusitis that are refractory or inaccessible to endoscopic approaches may still necessitate frontal sinus obliteration in the contemporary era [19–21]. Patients treated with an osteoplastic approach may show signs of anterior table bony fixation or resorption. Postoperative imaging in patients with prior obliteration is usually focused upon the identification of complications such as infection (recurrent rhinosinusitis, graft infection, cellulitis, osteomyelitis) and mucocele formation, with the latter being most common [22–24]. Long-term radiologic follow-up may be needed as

many patients with prior obliteration can present with mucoceles years to decades following the operation. Because the procedure involves stripping the mucosa and inserting some form of graft material, the lack of normal physiologic drainage poses a problem if the area is seeded by infection or residual mucosa continues to produce mucus. Multiple, loculated mucoceles may result in patients with prior obliteration. Such a pattern may also be seen in patients with complex craniofacial trauma status post repair. The appearance on imaging (Fig. 3.21) is largely dependent on the time that has elapsed since surgery and the type of graft material used (i.e., bone, fat, methyl methacrylate, hydroxyapatite cement). However, independent of graft material used, the obliterated frontal sinus cavities should be airless. On serial exams, CT should show no signs of bone irregularity, osteolysis, or progressive expansion. Frontal sinus obliteration performed with methyl methacrylate or hydroxyapatite cement has a very characteristic appearance because of its incredibly high density. When fat grafts are used, T2-weighted and T1-weighted post-contrast MRI must be obtained with fat suppression to null the signal attributable to the fat, since it is inherently bright on T1 and T2 fast spin-echo pulse sequences. Fat grafts exhibit a pattern of evolution on CT and MRI in that they transition from appearing similar to subcutaneous fat in terms of density and signal characteristics, respectively, to developing irregularly shaped areas of soft tissue related to scarring and fibrosis. Because this soft tissue within the graft can demonstrate T2 hyperintensity and enhancement, normal temporal evolution of the graft can be difficult to distinguish from inflammation, as these imaging features are similarly found in both symptomatic and asymptomatic patients [25]. However, any new inflammatory changes seen with MRI to extend into the surrounding calvarium, orbits, scalp, or cranial vault must be viewed with suspicion for infection. If any areas of bone expansion and remodeling are seen with CT, MRI can assess for an underlying mucocele (Fig. 3.22), as discussed in greater detail later in this chapter.

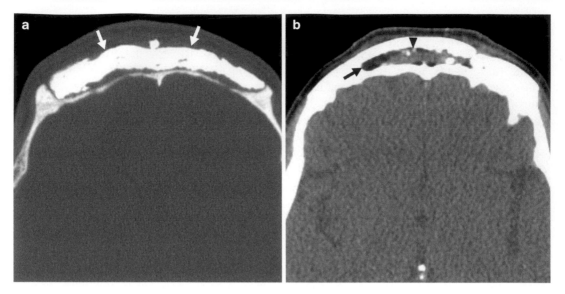

Fig. 3.21 Normal appearance of frontal sinus obliteration. (**a**) Axial noncontrast CT illustrates the incredibly high density of hydroxyapatite cement (arrows) when used for frontal sinus obliteration. (**b**) On axial noncontrast CT, the fat graft used for frontal sinus obliteration in a different patient does not maintain a homogeneous fat density. Areas of intermediate density similar to skeletal muscle (arrowhead) can develop secondary to scarring and fibrosis. Note the expected fat density in the right lateral aspect of this graft (arrow)

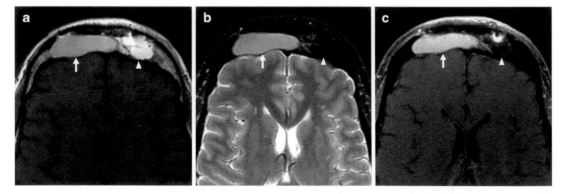

Fig. 3.22 Mucocele formation as a complication of frontal sinus obliteration. (**a**) Axial T1-weighted, (**b**) axial T2-weighted fat-suppressed, and (**c**) axial T1-weighted post-contrast fat-suppressed MRI sequences were acquired in a patient with worsening headaches several years following frontal sinus obliteration. Note the importance of the fat-suppression technique, as the mucocele (arrow) and residual fat graft (arrowhead) are both T1 hyperintense in (**a**), but the fat becomes dark in (**b**) and (**c**), both of which are fat-suppressed. In addition, it is important to compare the pre-contrast (**a**) and post-contrast (**c**) T1-weighted sequences to realize that the mucocele is intrinsically T1 hyperintense due to proteinaceous content and is not abnormally enhancing

Assessment of Expansile Mass-Like Lesions and Sinonasal Neoplasms

A detailed discussion of the imaging features of all sinonasal neoplasms is beyond the scope of this chapter, particularly given that primary neoplasms arising within the frontal sinuses are uncommon. Instead the goal is to present an imaging approach to mass-like lesions involving the frontal sinus and to understand the roles and limitations of CT and MRI.

CT is superior to MRI for the definition of the bone, and this is useful in several ways. Firstly, it is important to determine if there are any areas of osteolysis and, if so, to define the extent. When present, this should be characterized as to whether there is an indolent pattern of bone remodeling or an aggressive appearance of bone destruction. These should not be taken as synonymous with the presence of benign or malignant processes, respectively, as slow-growing neoplasms such as lymphoma and melanoma can smoothly remodel bone, while some benign lesions can have a more aggressive appearance [26]. Secondly, CT can more precisely define the integrity of the bone, which is useful for preoperative planning to differentiate rarefaction from complete dehiscence in areas such as the inner and outer tables of the frontal sinuses, the anterior skull base, and the orbital walls. Lastly, CT can effectively characterize the presence of internal calcification within a tumor, which can be helpful to differentiate cartilaginous and osteoid matrix, for example.

The assessment of an expansile or mass-like lesion involving the frontal sinus requires one to first make a determination as to whether a true neoplasm exists. Sinus opacification on CT can be secondary to inflammatory mucosal thickening and trapped secretions, while contrast-enhanced MRI is typically superior in delineating the presence and margins of an underlying sinonasal neoplasm [27, 28]. The prototypical expansile nonneoplastic lesion is a mucocele, of which over 90% occur in the frontal and ethmoid sinuses. CT demonstrates smooth bone expansion of the obstructed sinus that can lead to extension into the scalp, involvement of the anterior cranial fossa, and/or orbital deformity (Fig. 3.23). The appearance on MRI is variable because the degree to which the trapped secretions are hydrated dictates the MRI signal characteristics [29]. Mucoceles with proteinaceous inspissated secretions can be T1 hyperintense and T2 hypointense, while those with higher water content exhibit greater T1 and T2 prolongation. In cases of intrinsically T1 hyperintense mucoceles, it is imperative to review the pre- and post-contrast T1-weighted MRI sequences in conjunction with one another to avoid mistakenly diagnosing a mucocele as an enhancing tumor (Fig. 3.24).

When an area of osteolysis is identified and an underlying enhancing tumor is confirmed, imaging must then be used in an attempt to determine the extent of soft tissue involvement by a neoplastic process opposite the bone defect. For the frontal sinuses, the primary considerations most commonly involve the identification of dural and orbital involvement. For dural invasion, MRI is better suited due to its superior soft tissue contrast. Thin dural enhancement alone lacks

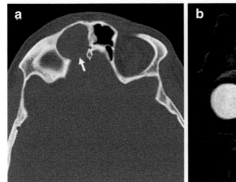 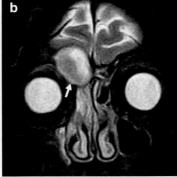 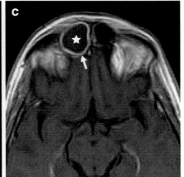

Fig. 3.23 Frontal sinus mucocele. (**a**) Axial noncontrast CT demonstrates expansion of the right frontal sinus with smooth bone remodeling and dehiscence of the inner table (arrow). (**b**) Coronal fat-suppressed T2-weighted sequence shows that the mucocele (arrow) is heterogeneous, some of which is brighter similar to cerebrospinal fluid, while other parts are darker similar to cerebral gray matter. Note the superomedial orbit deformity and remodeling of the floor of the anterior cranial fossa. (**c**) On axial post-contrast T1-weighted MRI, the central portion of the mucocele is hypointense and non-enhancing (star), while there is peripheral enhancement of the mucosa (arrow). Pyomucocele would need to be excluded on clinical grounds

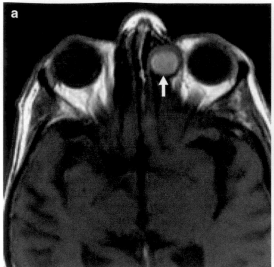 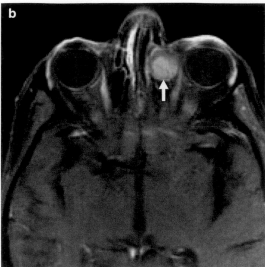

Fig. 3.24 Pitfall in mucocele imaging. (**a**) Axial T1-weighted MRI pre-contrast and (**b**) post-contrast depict an anterior left ethmoid mucocele (arrow). Because the inspissated proteinaceous secretions are very T1 hyperintense, they can be mistaken for enhancing tumor if care is not taken to closely compare the pre- and post-contrast images

sufficient specificity for confirmation of dural invasion, but, when associated with pial enhancement, focal dural nodularity, and/or dural thickness greater than 5 mm, the accuracy is significantly improved (Fig. 3.25) [30]. Intra-axial edema or enhancement within the inferior frontal lobes can be taken to mean frank brain invasion. CT and MRI play a complementary role in preoperatively predicting orbital invasion (Fig. 3.26), though MRI has been reported to underestimate orbital invasion more frequently than CT, potentially secondary to greater difficulty distinguishing the bone from the periorbita [31]. Abnormal signal or enhancement within extraocular muscles or muscle enlargement carries much greater specificity than sensitivity. Likewise, the suggestion of extraconal fat involvement on imaging is specific and has a high positive predictive value but lacks sensitivity. In contrast, bone dehiscence, adjacency to periorbita, and displacement of periorbita are more sensitive than specific. Because no imaging feature with CT or MRI accurately predicted orbital invasion with greater than 79% accuracy, there remains a role for intraoperative assessment in questionable cases [31].

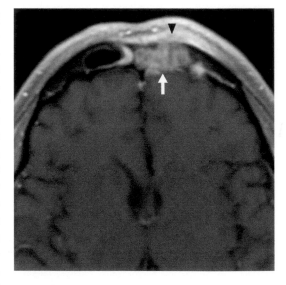

Fig. 3.25 Dural invasion. Axial T1-weighted post-contrast MRI with fat suppression demonstrates a small squamous cell carcinoma of the left frontal sinus. Focal dural thickening and nodularity (arrow) suggest dural invasion, which was confirmed surgically. Tumor also breaches the outer table to extend into the subgaleal scalp (arrowhead)

Because many sinonasal neoplasms have a nonspecific appearance and CT and MRI, imaging must focus primarily on planning a biopsy,

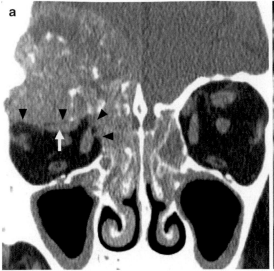
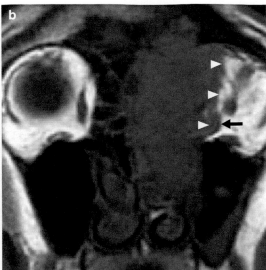

Fig. 3.26 Orbital invasion. (**a**) Coronal contrast-enhanced CT presents a large right frontal and ethmoidal squamous cell carcinoma causing extensive bone destruction. The mass significantly displaces the superior greater than medial periorbita with irregular infiltration of the adjacent extraconal fat (arrowheads). The superior rectus muscle (arrow) is displaced inferiorly but appears separated from tumor by a thin fat plane and does not appear enlarged. (**b**) Coronal T1-weighted MRI shows orbital invasion by an anterior ethmoidal squamous cell carcinoma that also involves the left frontal sinus. The periorbita is displaced, and there is irregular infiltration of the medial extraconal fat (arrowheads), partially blurring the margins of the inferiorly displaced medial rectus muscle (arrow). The bright T1 signal of the orbital fat provides a nice intrinsic source of contrast

determining resectability, and staging. However, in some instances, imaging features have been described that allow for more accurate diagnosis of tumors and tumor-like lesions of the frontal sinuses.

Inverted papilloma, an uncommon sinonasal tumor of ectodermal origin, most commonly arises from the lateral nasal wall but can infrequently develop within the frontal sinuses [32–35]. Although endoscopic resection can be achieved in many cases of frontal sinus inverted papilloma, it has been suggested that a more aggressive approach may be warranted in bilateral or secondary cases [34]. In addition to locally aggressive growth and its tendency for recurrence, there is an approximate 10–15% risk for the development of squamous cell carcinoma, of which approximately 60–70% are synchronous [36, 37]. A characteristic striated appearance, termed the "convoluted cerebriform pattern," has been described on T2-weighted and T1 post-

contrast MRI sequences (Fig. 3.27), while any areas of necrosis (non-enhancement) should raise concern for underlying carcinoma [38–40]. The CT appearance of inverted papilloma is nonspecific but plays a role not only for defining the location and severity of bone destruction but also for identifying the point of attachment. CT has been validated for determining the site of tumor origin through the identification of focal osteitis, which represents a bony strut at the point of tumor attachment [41–44]. Previously proposed staging systems for inverted papilloma all recognize involvement of the frontal sinuses and extension beyond the paranasal sinuses as higher stage disease, so these features should be specifically sought [45–47].

Osteomas are common benign bone-forming tumors of the paranasal sinuses, which are found in upward of 3% of sinus CT scans [48–51]. They can occur over a wide age range but are most commonly reported in the 4th to 6th decades of

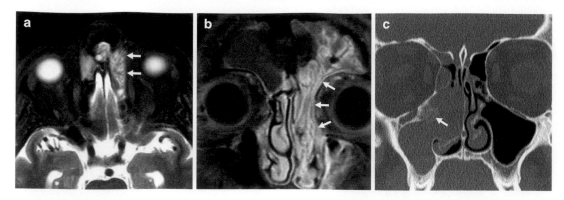

Fig. 3.27 Inverted papilloma. (**a**) Axial T2-weighted and (**b**) coronal T1-weighted post-contrast fat-suppressed MRI sequences demonstrate an anterior ethmoidal inverted papilloma (arrows) growing through the frontal recess into the left frontal sinus. Both images demonstrate a striated appearance (alternating bright and dark bands), which has been termed the convoluted cerebriform pattern. (**c**) In a different case, coronal noncontrast CT demonstrates focal osteitis along the orbital floor that corresponds to the site of inverted papilloma attachment (arrow)

life with a slight male predominance. Although osteomas can be found in any of the paranasal sinuses, most studies report the frontal sinuses to be most common, though an ethmoid predominance has also been described [48–51]. Osteomas are usually solitary and sporadic while multiplicity should raise the possibility of Gardner's syndrome [52]. Most osteomas range from a couple millimeters to several centimeters in size and tend to be slow growing [48]. Small osteomas are typically asymptomatic and incidentally detected, while larger frontal sinus lesions and those more intimately associated with the frontal sinus drainage pathway are more apt to cause sinus obstruction (mucoceles, infection, etc.), cosmetic deformity, headache, proptosis, or visual symptoms. The imaging appearance depends on composition as they can be made of dense cortical ("ivory") bone, cancellous ("mature") bone, or mixed (Fig. 3.28). Because ivory osteomas are comprised of dense lamellar bone with little fibrous stroma, they are very bright (dense) on CT and can be occult on MRI due to their dark signal. Osteomas can also histopathologically demonstrate osteoblastoma-like features, which have been associated with an increased likelihood of extension into an adjacent sinus/anatomic compartment and more frequent orbital involvement [51]. It should be noted that it can be difficult to accurately distinguish fibro-osseous

lesions with imaging [53]. Ossifying fibromas can have a very similar appearance to osteomas with variable amounts of cortical and cancellous bone, though ossifying fibromas are more common in the mandible [54].

Fibrous dysplasia, which is a skeletal disorder in which disorganized fibro-osseous tissue replaces medullary bone, can be monostotic or polyostotic. Sinonasal involvement in polyostotic craniofacial fibrous dysplasia and McCune-Albright syndrome is common [55]. Craniofacial fibrous dysplasia is characterized by thickening of the bone and expansion of the diploic space, which can encroach upon the frontal sinuses and orbits when the frontal bone is involved. Although it can be found as an incidental and asymptomatic finding, progressive bone expansion can lead to cosmetic deformity, impaired vision, and frontal sinus mucocele formation [56–58]. Familiarity with the imaging features of craniofacial fibrous dysplasia is important to prevent unnecessary biopsy [59–63]. When predominantly composed of bundles of spindle cells and trabeculae of immature woven bone, fibrous dysplasia has low signal on T1- and T2-weighted MRI and enhances (Fig. 3.29). The prototypical appearance on CT is "ground-glass opacity" in the context of a thinned and expanded, albeit intact, cortex. Moreover, the expanded bone tends to blend into adjacent normal bone. Consequently, an expansile lesion

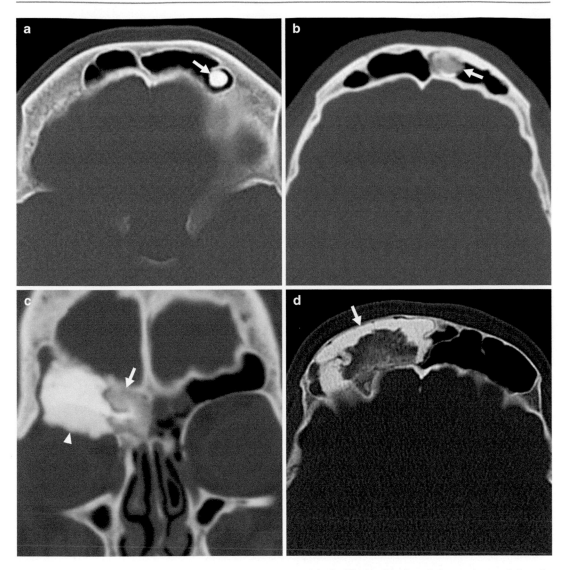

Fig. 3.28 Variable CT appearance of osteomas. (**a**) Tiny ivory osteoma (arrow) in the left frontal sinus demonstrates a characteristic homogeneous dense (i.e., bright) appearance. (**b**) Small mature osteoma (arrow) in the medial aspect of the left frontal sinus exhibits an intermediate density compatible with cancellous bone with minimal osteoblastic rimming. (**c**) A large mixed osteoma nearly completely fills the right frontal sinus and expands into the superior orbit. Note the more dense cortical bone laterally (arrowhead), compared with the less dense cancellous bone medially (arrow). (**d**) A pathologically confirmed ossifying fibroma (arrow) of the right frontal sinus underscores the challenge of diagnosing fibro-osseous lesions, as it looks very similar to a mixed osteoma on this axial sinus CT

found with MRI to be centered on a craniofacial bone should always be further evaluated with CT, as the characteristic ground-glass appearance could potentially obviate the need for tissue sampling. If there are no clinical indications for surgery, such pathognomonic cases can be followed with serial imaging during the period of somatic growth to monitor for progressive bone expansion. However, there are cases of fibrous dysplasia in which the imaging diagnosis is less certain because a heterogeneous and variable appearance occurs when there is less cellularity, fewer bony trabeculae, more cystic change and hemorrhage, and fewer collagen fibers [64]. This can lead to

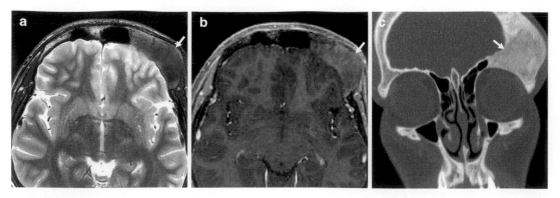

Fig. 3.29 Fibrous dysplasia. An area of frontal bone fibrous dysplasia (arrow) is identified lateral to the left frontal sinus. It demonstrates (**a**) hypointensity on axial T2-weighted MRI, (**b**) enhancement on axial T1-weighted post-contrast fat-suppressed MRI, and (**c**) a characteristic "ground-glass" appearance on coronal CT

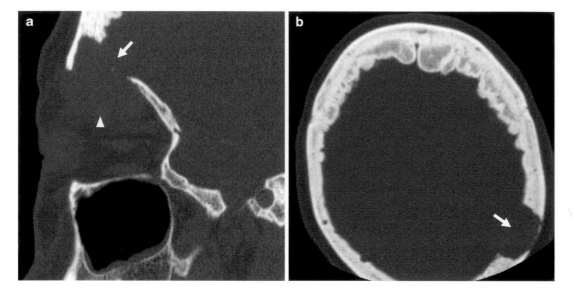

Fig. 3.30 Systemic cause of frontal sinus mass. (**a**) Sagittal noncontrast CT demonstrates a destructive frontal sinus mass eroding the inner table (arrow) and also invading into the superior orbit (arrowhead). (**b**) Axial noncontrast CT demonstrates a second lytic lesion in the left parietal calvarium (arrow). The patient was ultimately diagnosed with multiple myeloma

more T2 hyperintensity on MRI, heterogeneous enhancement, and areas of lower density on CT with less ground-glass opacity.

Lastly, although uncommon, the differential diagnosis of a destructive frontal sinus mass in an adult should always include the possibility of metastatic disease and multiple myeloma (Fig. 3.30) [65]. For example, an isolated metastatic lesion from renal cell carcinoma can occur concurrently or after treatment of the primary lesion or may be the first presentation of the disease. These lesions are hypervascular, and feasibility office biopsy of this lesion must be cautiously assessed. As such, it is worthwhile to review the medical record for any oncologic history, search for additional lesions on the available craniofacial imaging, and review any recent whole body imaging (positron emission tomography, bone scan, etc.) when available.

Summary

CT is the primary imaging modality that should be used for imaging the frontal sinus because of its widespread availability, high-resolution depiction of the bone, and multiplanar demonstration of anatomy. It can effectively screen for inflammatory sinus disease, provide a surgical roadmap for procedure planning, and help determine the candidacy of postoperative patients for revision surgery. MRI plays a complementary role with its superior soft tissue characterization and should be employed in cases of suspected intracranial complications of rhinosinusitis and for the characterization and local staging of neoplasms.

References

1. Kanowitz SJ, Shatzkes DR, Pramanik BK, Babb JS, Jacobs JB, Lebowitz RA. Utility of sagittal reformatted computerized tomographic images in the evaluation of the frontal sinus outflow tract. Am J Rhinol. 2005;19(2):159–65.
2. Kuhn FA. Chronic frontal sinusitis: the endoscopic frontal recess approach. Oper Tech Otolaryngol Head Neck Surg. 1996;7(3):222–9.
3. Wormald PJ. Surgery of the frontal recess and frontal sinus. Rhinology [Review]. 2005;43(2):82–5.
4. Wormald PJ, Hoseman W, Callejas C, Weber RK, Kennedy DW, Citardi MJ, et al. The international frontal sinus anatomy classification (IFAC) and classification of the extent of endoscopic frontal sinus surgery (EFSS). Int Forum Allergy Rhinol. 2016;6(7):677–96.
5. Bent JP, Cuiltysiller C, Kuhn FA. The frontal cell as a cause of frontal-sinus obstruction. Am J Rhinol. 1994;8(4):185–91.
6. Surgery AAoO-HaN. Position statement: intraoperative use of computer aided surgery. [11/18/2017]; Available from: http://www.entnet.org/?q=node/929.
7. Rosenfeld RM, Piccirillo JF, Chandrasekhar SS, Brook I, Ashok Kumar K, Kramper M, et al. Clinical practice guideline (update): adult sinusitis. Otolaryngol Head Neck Surg [Practice GuidelineResearch Support, Non-U.S. Gov't]. 2015;152(2 Suppl):S1–S39.
8. Hoxworth JM, Glastonbury CM. Orbital and intracranial complications of acute sinusitis. Neuroimaging Clin N Am [Review]. 2010;20(4):511–26.
9. Velayudhan V, Chaudhry ZA, Smoker WRK, Shinder R, Reede DL. Imaging of intracranial and orbital complications of sinusitis and atypical sinus infection: what the radiologist needs to know. Curr Probl Diagn Radiol [Review]. 2017;46(6):441–51.
10. Chandler JR, Langenbrunner DJ, Stevens ER. The pathogenesis of orbital complications in acute sinusitis. Laryngoscope. 1970;80(9):1414–28.
11. Ni Mhurchu E, Ospina J, Janjua AS, Shewchuk JR, Vertinsky AT. Fungal Rhinosinusitis: a radiological review with intraoperative correlation. Can Assoc Radiol J [Review]. 2017;68(2):178–86.
12. Middlebrooks EH, Frost CJ, De Jesus RO, Massini TC, Schmalfuss IM, Mancuso AA. Acute invasive fungal Rhinosinusitis: a comprehensive update of CT findings and design of an effective diagnostic imaging model. AJNR Am J Neuroradiol. 2015;36(8):1529–35.
13. Safder S, Carpenter JS, Roberts TD, Bailey N. The "black turbinate" sign: an early MR imaging finding of nasal mucormycosis. AJNR Am J Neuroradiol [Case Reports]. 2010;31(4):771–4.
14. Weber R, Draf W, Kratzsch B, Hosemann W, Schaefer SD. Modern concepts of frontal sinus surgery. Laryngoscope [Multicenter StudyValidation Studies]. 2001;111(1):137–46.
15. Weber RK, Hosemann W. Comprehensive review on endonasal endoscopic sinus surgery. GMS Curr Top Otorhinolaryngol Head Neck Surg [Review]. 2015;14:Doc08.
16. Huang BY, Lloyd KM, DelGaudio JM, Jablonowski E, Hudgins PA. Failed endoscopic sinus surgery: spectrum of CT findings in the frontal recess. Radiographics. 2009;29(1):177–95.
17. Otto KJ, DelGaudio JM. Operative findings in the frontal recess at time of revision surgery. Am J Otolaryngol. 2010;31(3):175–80.
18. Valdes CJ, Bogado M, Samaha M. Causes of failure in endoscopic frontal sinus surgery in chronic rhinosinusitis patients. Int Forum Allergy Rhinol. 2014;4(6):502–6.
19. Hahn S, Palmer JN, Purkey MT, Kennedy DW, Chiu AG. Indications for external frontal sinus procedures for inflammatory sinus disease. Am J Rhinol Allergy. 2009;23(3):342–7.
20. Konstantinidis I, Constantinidis J. Indications for open procedures in the endoscopic era. Curr Opin Otolaryngol Head Neck Surg [Review]. 2016;24(1):50–6.
21. Ochsner MC, DelGaudio JM. The place of the osteoplastic flap in the endoscopic era: indications and pitfalls. Laryngoscope [Evaluation Studies]. 2015;125(4):801–6.
22. Chandra RK, Kennedy DW, Palmer JN. Endoscopic management of failed frontal sinus obliteration. Am J Rhinol. 2004;18(5):279–84.
23. Kanowitz SJ, Batra PS. Citardi MJ. Comprehensive management of failed frontal sinus obliteration. Am J Rhinol [Comparative Study]. 2008;22(3):263–70.
24. Langton-Hewer CD, Wormald PJ. Endoscopic sinus surgery rescue of failed osteoplastic flap with fat obliteration. Curr Opin Otolaryngol Head Neck Surg [Review]. 2005;13(1):45–9.
25. Loevner LA, Yousem DM, Lanza DC, Kennedy DW, Goldberg AN. MR evaluation of frontal sinus osteo-

plastic flaps with autogenous fat grafts. AJNR Am J Neuroradiol. 1995;16(8):1721–6.

26. Som PM, Lawson W, Lidov MW. Simulated aggressive skull base erosion in response to benign sinonasal disease. Radiology. 1991;180(3):755–9.

27. Som PM, Shapiro MD, Biller HF, Sasaki C, Lawson W. Sinonasal tumors and inflammatory tissues: differentiation with MR imaging. Radiology. 1988;167(3):803–8.

28. Lanzieri CF, Shah M, Krauss D, Lavertu P. Use of gadolinium-enhanced MR imaging for differentiating mucoceles from neoplasms in the paranasal sinuses. Radiology. 1991;178(2):425–8.

29. Van Tassel P, Lee YY, Jing BS, De Pena CA. Mucoceles of the paranasal sinuses: MR imaging with CT correlation. AJR Am J Roentgenol. 1989;153(2):407–12.

30. Eisen MD, Yousem DM, Montone KT, Kotapka MJ, Bigelow DC, Bilker WB, et al. Use of preoperative MR to predict dural, perineural, and venous sinus invasion of skull base tumors. AJNR Am J Neuroradiol. 1996;17(10):1937–45.

31. Eisen MD, Yousem DM, Loevner LA, Thaler ER, Bilker WB, Goldberg AN. Preoperative imaging to predict orbital invasion by tumor. Head Neck [Comparative Study]. 2000;22(5):456–62.

32. Anari S, Carrie S. Sinonasal inverted papilloma: narrative review. J Laryngol Otol [Review]. 2010;124(7):705–15.

33. Sauter A, Matharu R, Hormann K, Naim R. Current advances in the basic research and clinical management of sinonasal inverted papilloma (review). Oncol Rep [Review]. 2007;17(3):495–504.

34. Walgama E, Ahn C, Batra PS. Surgical management of frontal sinus inverted papilloma: a systematic review. Laryngoscope [Review]. 2012;122(6):1205–9.

35. Schneyer MS, Milam BM, Payne SC. Sites of attachment of Schneiderian papilloma: a retrospective analysis. Int Forum Allergy Rhinol. 2011;1(4):324–8.

36. Barnes L. Diseases of the nasal cavity, paranasal sinuses, and nasopharynx. In: Barnes L, editor. Surgical pathology of the head and neck. 3rd ed. New York: Informa Healthcare USA, Inc.; 2009. p. 361–71.

37. Mirza S, Bradley PJ, Acharya A, Stacey M, Jones NS. Sinonasal inverted papillomas: recurrence, and synchronous and metachronous malignancy. J Laryngol Otol [Review]. 2007;121(9):857–64.

38. Ojiri H, Ujita M, Tada S, Fukuda K. Potentially distinctive features of sinonasal inverted papilloma on MR imaging. AJR Am J Roentgenol. 2000;175(2):465–8.

39. Maroldi R, Farina D, Palvarini L, Lombardi D, Tomenzoli D, Nicolai P. Magnetic resonance imaging findings of inverted papilloma: differential diagnosis with malignant sinonasal tumors. Am J Rhinol. 2004;18(5):305–10.

40. Jeon TY, Kim HJ, Chung SK, Dhong HJ, Kim HY, Yim YJ, et al. Sinonasal inverted papilloma: value of convoluted cerebriform pattern on MR imaging. AJNR Am J Neuroradiol [Validation Studies]. 2008;29(8):1556–60.

41. Yousuf K, Wright ED. Site of attachment of inverted papilloma predicted by CT findings of osteitis. Am J Rhinol. 2007;21(1):32–6.

42. Sham CL, King AD, van Hasselt A, Tong MC. The roles and limitations of computed tomography in the preoperative assessment of sinonasal inverted papillomas. Am J Rhinol [Comparative Study]. 2008;22(2):144–50.

43. Bhalla RK, Wright ED. Predicting the site of attachment of sinonasal inverted papilloma. Rhinology. 2009;47(4):345–8.

44. Kennedy DW. Radiological localization of Schneiderian papilloma. Int Forum Allergy Rhinol [Comment Editorial]. 2011;1(6):492.

45. Cannady SB, Batra PS, Sautter NB, Roh HJ, Citardi MJ. New staging system for sinonasal inverted papilloma in the endoscopic era. Laryngoscope [Review]. 2007;117(7):1283–7.

46. Han JK, Smith TL, Loehrl T, Toohill RJ, Smith MM. An evolution in the management of sinonasal inverting papilloma. Laryngoscope. 2001;111(8):1395–400.

47. Krouse JH. Development of a staging system for inverted papilloma. Laryngoscope. 2000;110(6):965–8.

48. Buyuklu F, Akdogan MV, Ozer C, Cakmak O. Growth characteristics and clinical manifestations of the paranasal sinus osteomas. Otolaryngol Head Neck Surg [Comparative Study Research Support, Non--U.S. Gov't]. 2011;145(2):319–23.

49. Earwaker J. Paranasal sinus osteomas: a review of 46 cases. Skeletal Radiol [Review]. 1993;22(6):417–23.

50. Erdogan N, Demir U, Songu M, Ozenler NK, Uluc E, Dirim B. A prospective study of paranasal sinus osteomas in 1,889 cases: changing patterns of localization. Laryngoscope [Comparative Study]. 2009;119(12):2355–9.

51. McHugh JB, Mukherji SK, Lucas DR. Sino-orbital osteoma: a clinicopathologic study of 45 surgically treated cases with emphasis on tumors with osteoblastoma-like features. Arch Pathol Lab Med. 2009;133(10):1587–93.

52. Alexander AA, Patel AA, Odland R. Paranasal sinus osteomas and Gardner's syndrome. Ann Otol Rhinol Laryngol [Case Reports]. 2007;116(9):658–62.

53. Som PM, Lidov M. The benign fibroosseous lesion: its association with paranasal sinus mucoceles and its MR appearance. J Comput Assist Tomogr. 1992;16(6):871–6.

54. MacDonald-Jankowski DS. Ossifying fibroma: a systematic review. Dentomaxillofac Radiol [Comparative Study Review]. 2009;38(8):495–513.

55. DeKlotz TR, Kim HJ, Kelly M, Collins MT. Sinonasal disease in polyostotic fibrous dysplasia and McCune-Albright syndrome. Laryngoscope [Research Support, N.I.H., Intramural]. 2013;123(4):823–8.

56. Atasoy C, Ustuner E, Erden I, Akyar S. Frontal sinus mucocele: a rare complication of craniofacial fibrous dysplasia. Clin Imaging [Case Reports]. 2001;25(6):388–91.

57. Derham C, Bucur S, Russell J, Liddington M, Chumas P. Frontal sinus mucocele in association with fibrous dysplasia: review and report of two cases. Childs Nerv Syst [Case Reports Review]. 2011;27(2):327–31.

58. Ricalde P, Horswell BB. Craniofacial fibrous dysplasia of the fronto-orbital region: a case series and literature review. J Oral Maxillofac Surg [Review]. 2001;59(2):157–67; discussion 67–8.
59. Atalar MH, Salk I, Savas R, Uysal IO, Egilmez H. CT and MR imaging in a large series of patients with craniofacial fibrous dysplasia. Pol J Radiol. 2015;80:232–40.
60. Camilleri AE. Craniofacial fibrous dysplasia. J Laryngol Otol [Case Reports]. 1991;105(8):662–6.
61. Casselman JW, De Jonge I, Neyt L, De Clercq C, D'Hont G. MRI in craniofacial fibrous dysplasia. Neuroradiology. 1993;35(3):234–7.
62. Hanifi B, Samil KS, Yasar C, Cengiz C, Ercan A, Ramazan D. Craniofacial fibrous dysplasia. Clin Imaging. 2013;37(6):1109–15.
63. Lisle DA, Monsour PA, Maskiell CD. Imaging of craniofacial fibrous dysplasia. J Med Imaging Radiat Oncol [Review]. 2008;52(4):325–32.
64. Jee WH, Choi KH, Choe BY, Park JM, Shinn KS. Fibrous dysplasia: MR imaging characteristics with radiopathologic correlation. AJR Am J Roentgenol. 1996;167(6):1523–7.
65. Abi-Fadel F, Smith PR, Ayaz A, Sundaram K. Paranasal sinus involvement in metastatic carcinoma. J Neurol Surg Rep. 2012;73(1):57–9.

Classification of Frontal Recess Cells and Extent of Surgery

4

Alkis James Psaltis and Peter-John Wormald

Introduction

Surgery to the frontal recess and sinus is considered amongst the most technically challenging aspects of endoscopic sinus surgery. Factors making surgery in this region difficult include the oblique orientation of the frontal recess, its narrow bony confines and the close proximity of the recess to the skull base and orbit. Poorly performed surgery in this region can result in suboptimal access to the frontal sinus proper, iatrogenic frontal sinusitis from cicatrization of the frontal recess and devastating complications, including cerebrospinal fluid (CSF) leak and orbital injury. A clear understanding of the anatomy of this region is therefore essential for safe and effective frontal sinus surgery. This chapter will review the anatomy of the frontal recess and introduce a newly published classification system for more intuitive frontal sinus anatomy classification and grading the extent of surgery. The purpose of this newly developed system is to assist sinus surgeons of all levels in their preparation and execution of frontal sinus surgery, and

facilitate clear communication between surgeons.

Current Classification Systems

Since Van Alyea's first description of "frontal cells" in 1941, numerous classification systems have been proposed to describe the cellular anatomy within this region [1–8]. To date, the two most commonly referenced systems include those proposed by Kuhn [1] and the system outlined in the recent European Position Paper on the Anatomical Terminology of the Internal Nose and Paranasal Sinuses [7]. The Modified Kuhn frontal classification system [9], probably the most commonly utilized system, classifies anterior ethmoidal cells according to their relationship to the agger nasi cell and any extension into the frontal sinus (see Table 4.1). The European system suggests classifying frontal cells as anterior or posterior and medial or lateral, with respect to the frontal recess/inner walls of the frontal sinus. Although useful as guides to the ethmoidal cellular position within the frontal region, current systems can be improved upon with respect to the precision and detail in describing cellular relationships in the frontal sinus drainage pathway.

To address deficiencies in contemporary classification systems, an international consortium of leading rhinologists have proposed an alternate, more precise classification system, the

A. J. Psaltis (✉) · P.-J. Wormald
Department of Otolaryngology Head and Neck Surgery, The University of Adelaide, Adelaide, SA, Australia

© Springer Nature Switzerland AG 2019
D. Lal, P. H. Hwang (eds.), *Frontal Sinus Surgery*, https://doi.org/10.1007/978-3-319-97022-6_4

Table 4.1 Modified Kuhn classification of frontal ethmoidal cells [9]

Type	Description
Agger nasi cell	*Cell that is either anterior to the origin of the middle turbinate or sits directly above the most anterior insertion of the middle turbinate into the lateral nasal wall*
Frontal ethmoidal cells	*An anterior ethmoidal cell that is in close proximity (touching) the frontal process of the maxilla*
Type I	Single frontal ethmoidal cell above agger nasi cell
Type II	Tier of frontal ethmoidal cells above agger nasi cell
Type III	Frontal ethmoidal cell that pneumatizes cephalad into the frontal sinus through the frontal ostium *but not extending beyond 50% of the vertical height of that frontal sinus on the CT scan (is usually found in the lateral region of the frontal ostium)*
Type IV	*A frontal ethmoidal cell that extends into the frontal sinus for more than 50% of the vertical height of the frontal sinus on the CT scan. Originally termed "an isolated cell in the frontal sinus"; however in our experience, isolated cells in the frontal sinus are extremely rare and seldom clinically important*
Supra bulla cells	These are Supra ultra ethmoidal cells *(cells above the bulla ethmoidalis)* that do not enter into the frontal sinus
Frontal bulla cells	This is a cell that originates in the supra bulla region but pneumatizes along the skull base into the frontal sinus, along the posterior wall of the frontal sinus
Intersinus septal cell (also termed "interfrontal sinus septal cell" in Kuhn classification)	This cell is associated with the frontal sinus septum and compromises the frontal drainage by occupying part of the frontal ostium. *It is always medially based and opens into the frontal recess*

The *modifications* from the original Kuhn classification are presented in *italics*

"International Frontal Sinus Anatomy Classification (IFAC)" [10]. The purpose of the IFAC is to provide a more precise nomenclature system based on the location of the cells relative to defined anatomical landmarks, and thus simplify and facilitate understanding of frontal recess cells and the frontal sinus drainage pathway. It is hoped that this classification will be easy to use, improve instruction of surgical steps, aid communication amongst surgeons and facilitate standardized reporting and comparison of surgical outcomes. The ultimate objective of IFAC is to improve surgical dissection and outcomes of frontal sinus surgery.

International Frontal Sinus Anatomy Classification (IFAC) System

The IFAC system uses consistent anatomical landmarks such as the agger nasi cell, the bulla ethmoidalis, the frontal sinus and the frontal ostium as points of reference for identifying and naming the more variable ethmoidal cells that pneumatize into the frontal sinus drainage pathway. Ethmoidal cells in the frontal region are further sub-grouped by location into anterior, posterior and medial cells based on their relationship to the frontal sinus drainage pathway, by using the above referenced landmarks. Anterior cells can displace the frontal drainage pathway medially, laterally, posteriorly or postero-medially, with the most commonly drainage pathway pushed medially. Posterior cells can displace the pathway anteriorly and depending upon on the presence and location of co-existent anterior cells drainage can result in either an anteromedial or anterolateral pathway. By virtue of their location, posterior cells are more likely to push the frontal sinus drainage pathway into an anteromedially. Cells associated with the frontal sinus septum always displace the drainage pathway laterally. Again, this may be further influenced by interplay with other co-existent cells. Table 4.2 summarizes the IFAC.

Table 4.2 International frontal sinus anatomy classification system

Cell position	Cell name	Definition
Anterior cells	Agger nasi cell (ANC)	Most anteriorly pneumatized ethmoidal cell that sits either anterior to the origin of the middle turbinate or directly above the most anterior insertion of the middle turbinate into the lateral nasal wall (Fig. 4.1)
	Supra agger cell (SAC)	Anterolateral ethmoidal cell or tier of cells, located above the agger nasi cell that do not pneumatize into the frontal sinus
	Supra agger frontal cell (SAFC)	Anterolateral ethmoidal cell, located above the agger nasi cell that pneumatizes into the frontal sinus
Posterior cells	Supra bulla cell (SBC)	A cell located above the bulla ethmoidalis that does not pneumatize into the frontal sinus
	Supra bulla frontal cell (SBFC)	A cell located above the bulla ethmoidalis that pneumatizes along the skull base into the frontal sinus
	Supraorbital ethmoidal cell (SOEC)	An anterior ethmoidal cell that pneumatizes around, anterior or posterior to the anterior ethmoidal artery over the roof of the orbit
Medial cells	Frontal sinus septal cell	A medially based cell that is attached to, or located in the interfrontal sinus septum

Anatomical Definitions used in IFAC

The Frontal Recess

The frontal recess is defined as the most antero-superior portion of the ethmoidal region that connects the anterior ethmoidal complex and the frontal sinus. Although the anatomy of the frontal recess may vary considerably due to variable pneumatization patterns of ethmoidal cells, its absolute boundaries remain consistent. The medial extent of the frontal recess is limited by the insertion of the vertical lamella of the middle turbinate into the lateral lamella of the cribriform plate. The lateral wall comprises of the maxillary process of the frontal bone, the lacrimal bone and the adjacent lamina papyracea. Anteriorly the frontal recess is bounded by the frontal process of the maxilla and frontal beak (bony thickening at the junction of the frontal bone and frontal process of the maxilla). Posteriorly the second part of the middle turbinate (basal lamella, oriented in the coronal plane) forms the boundary between the anterior and posterior ethmoidal cells. The bulla ethmoidalis and supra bulla cells significantly impact the anatomy of the frontal recess and on the drainage pathway of the frontal sinus. IFAC includes the bulla ethmoidalis and suprabullar cells as these are structures that significantly influence a bony partition from the anatomy of the frontal recess. If the anterior face of the bulla ethmoidalis reaches the skull base, it is termed the bulla lamella. If a bulla lamella is not present, the frontal recess will communicate directly with the suprabullar recess and sinus lateralis.

The Frontal Sinus Ostium

The frontal sinus ostium is the narrowest portion of the transition zone between the frontal sinus and the frontal recess located inferiorly. It is bounded by the thick frontal beak anteriorly, the skull base posteriorly, the insertion of the middle turbinate into the skull base medially and the lamina papyracea laterally. On computerized tomography (CT) imaging, it is best appreciated in the parasagittal plane as the "narrow neck" of the hour glass that is formed as the frontal sinus transitions into the frontal recess and ethmoid cavity.

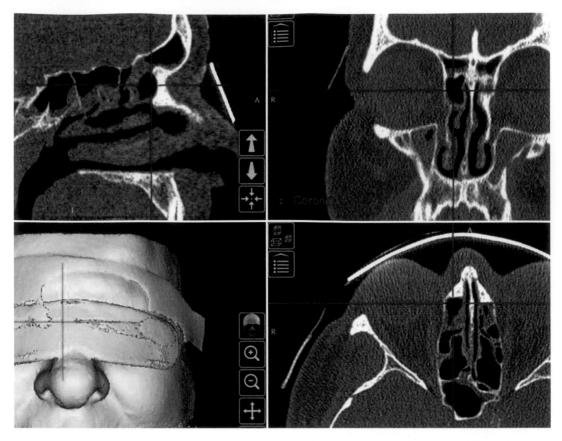

Fig. 4.1 Demonstrates an agger nasi cell (ANC), (red cross-hairs) in different planes. The lateral border of the ANC is formed by the orbit while the medial wall is usu- ally formed by the upward extension of the uncinate process. The frontal sinus typical drains posterior to the ANC. (Reproduced with permission from Wormald et al. [10])

Agger Nasi Cell

The agger nasi cell (ANC) is the term used for the most anteriorly positioned ethmoidal cell. This cell pneumatizes along the ascending intranasal portion of the frontal process of the maxilla, and is located at the axilla of the middle turbinate, i.e. at the junction of the anterior middle turbinate with the frontal process (see Fig. 4.1). Most commonly, the agger nasi cell is located just superior to the insertion of the middle turbinate into the lateral nasal wall, and forms an easily recognizable mound on the lateral nasal wall just anterior to the middle turbinate attachment. Its presence is almost universal, with radiological studies documenting its existence in 98% of subjects [1, 2]. The agger nasi cell thus is a consistent and useful landmark in preoperative planning and during surgical dissection.

Bulla Ethmoidalis

The *bulla ethmoidalis* (ethmoidal bulla) may not be a distinct cell as once thought. Rather it may be an airspace formed by pneumatization of the basal lamella of the middle turbinate. Its near-universal presence and consistent location makes the bulla ethmoidalis an invaluable landmark for endoscopic sinus surgery. The anterior face of the bulla ethmoidalis can pneumatize superiorly up to the skull base; if this is the case, the frontal sinus drainage pathway will always be anterior to this lamella. In some cases where the superior extent of the bulla ethmoidalis does not reach the skull base, a small airspace, referred to as the suprabullar recess, will be present. Cells that form above the bulla ethmoidalis and are in contact with the skull base are referred to as suprabullar cells. Ethmoidal cells that lie posterior the frontal sinus drainage pathway and pneumatize the roof of the orbit are named supraorbital ethmoidal cells. Since these cell types are located posterior to the frontal drainage pathway, they may both narrow the pathway and displace it anteriorly.

Anterior Cells

Anteriorly based cells may displace the frontal drainage pathway either medially, laterally, posteriorly or in some cases postero-medially or postero-laterally.

The *agger nasi cell* has a consistent location directly behind the frontal process of the maxilla, at or above the axilla of the middle turbinate (Fig. 4.1). Its relationship to the frontal process is best appreciated on parasagittal images, while coronal imaging demonstrates its close relationship to the middle turbinate. As stated before, the

agger nasi cell forms a reliable landmark that can be entered early and used as a reference when planning an approach to the frontal sinus. The frontal drainage pathway always lies posterior or medial to the ANC.

Supra agger cell (SAC) is a cell or a tier of cells located above the ANC and posterior to the frontal beak (Fig. 4.2). SACs are usually laterally based, as appreciated on the axial image. In this location, these cells will tend to displace the frontal drainage pathway medially or posteromedially. In the uncommon occurrence of a medially based SAC, the frontal drainage pathway will be displaced laterally. SACs do not pneumatize into the frontal sinus itself. Assessment of whether a cell transgresses into the frontal sinus is best achieved by viewing the coronal CT image. On a coronal CT scan, the frontal beak which marks the location of the frontal ostium is seen as a continuous shelf of the bone spanning the base of both frontal sinuses.

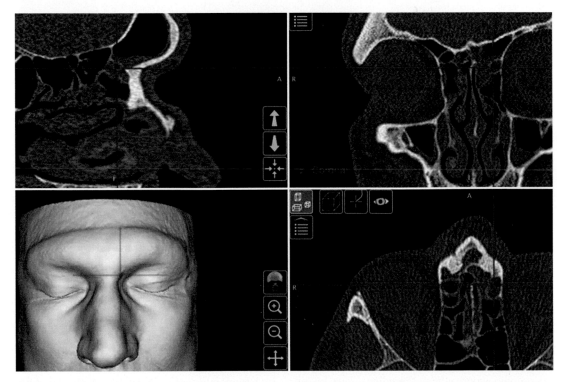

Fig. 4.2 A supra agger cell is demonstrated (red crosshairs) in different planes. SACs may exist as a single cell or a tier of cells that assume a position directly above an ANC. These cells do not pneumatize into the frontal sinus. This is best appreciated on the parasagittal CT scan. (Reproduced with permission from Wormald et al. [10])

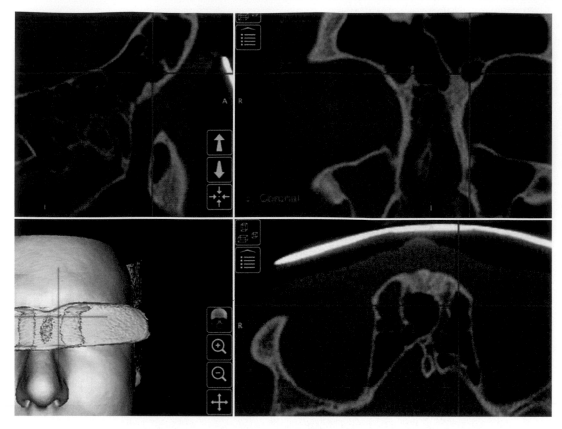

Fig. 4.3 Demonstrates a supra agger frontal cell (red cross-hairs) in different planes. As seen on both the coronal and sagittal images, these cells pneumatize beyond the frontal beak and into the frontal sinus. (Reproduced with permission from Wormald et al. [10])

Cells located below this shelf are SACs. Cells that pneumatize above this shelf of the bone and extend cranially to the frontal ostium area are termed supra agger frontal cells.

Supra agger frontal cells (SAFCs) are anterior or lateral ethmoidal cells that are located superior to ANCs and that pneumatize into the frontal sinus, above the frontal beak (Fig. 4.3). The extent of pneumatization of the SAFCs can be variable. Small SAFCs only extend into the floor of the frontal sinus, whereas large SAFCs may extend significantly into the frontal sinus. The size of the SAFC is important to assess as this will likely influence what technique is required for its removal. Small SAFCs can usually be addressed readily through endoscopic approaches. Complete removal of larger SAFCs may require more extended endoscopic approaches (i.e. unilateral or bilateral frontal drillout) or a combined external/endoscopic approach using trephination techniques.

Posterior Cells

Posteriorly based cells displace the frontal drainage pathway either medially, anteriorly or in some cases anteromedially.

The *bulla ethmoidalis* is a reliable and consistent landmark, present in almost all patients. Embryologically, this cell forms from the second lamella, and is thus located behind the uncinate process and ANC. The superior pneumatization of the bulla ethmoidalis can be variable as previously discussed, and in most patients, there are cells above the bulla ethmoidalis. Figure 4.4 demonstrates that the bulla ethmoidalis is located above the horizontal portion of the uncinate process.

A supra bulla cell (SBC) is a cell located directly above the bulla ethmoidalis. The posterior wall of this cell is the skull base. This cell can be appreciated both on the coronal and axial CT images (Fig. 4.5). SBCs stop short of pneumatizing into the frontal

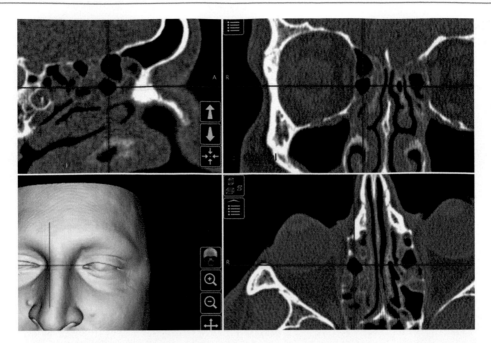

Fig. 4.4 The bulla ethmoidalis (red cross-hairs) is a consistent anatomical landmark seen behind the ANC. This cell is located above the horizontal portion of the uncinate process. Its superior pneumatization can be variable. (Reproduced with permission from Wormald et al. [10])

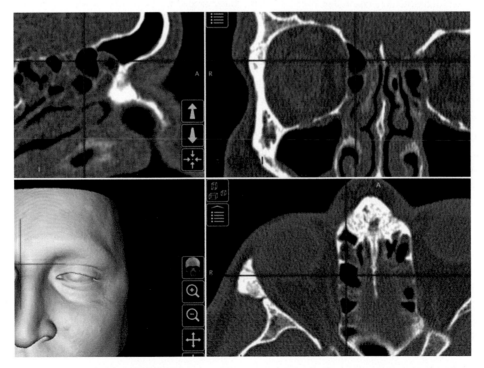

Fig. 4.5 This suprabullar cell (red cross-hairs) can be seen pneumatizing above the bulla ethmoidalis. Note that in this patient, the anterior wall of the suprabullar cell and the anterior wall of the bulla ethmoidalis are in almost direct continuity. The origin of the SBC from the skull base is an important distinguishing feature. (Reproduced with permission from Wormald et al. [10])

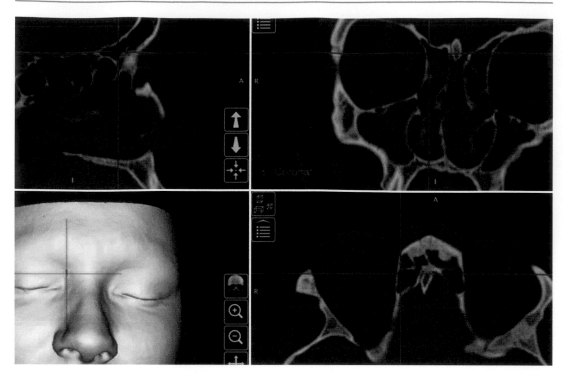

Fig. 4.6 Supra bulla frontal cells (red cross-hairs) can be considered as supra bulla cells that pneumatize into the frontal sinus. Like SBC they take origin from the skull base, but their anterior extension into the frontal sinus is what differentiates them from SBC. In this scan the SBFC can be seen displacing the frontal drainage pathway anteromedially. (Reproduced with permission from Wormald et al. [10])

sinus. If a SBC pneumatizes beyond the frontal ostium into the frontal sinus, it is termed a *supra bulla frontal cell* (Fig. 4.6). These cells typically narrow the frontal recess by displacing the frontal drainage pathway anteriorly or anteromedially.

A *supraorbital ethmoidal cell (SOEC)* is an ethmoidal cell that pneumatizes laterally into the orbital roof and may encroach upon the posterior aspect of the frontal sinus (Fig. 4.7). These cells can be confused with SBFC on axial imaging, as both have the skull base as the posterior wall. The anterior ethmoidal artery lies in close proximity to the first SOEC. Formal identification of the artery on preoperative review of CT scans is necessary to reduce the risk of intraoperative injury to the artery.

Frontal Septal Cell (FSC)

A *frontal septal cell*, referred to as an intersinus septal cell in previous classifications, arises from the frontal sinus septum that separates the right and left frontal sinuses (Fig. 4.8). If large, these cells can occupy a significant part of the drainage pathway and significantly narrow the pathway by pushing it laterally. The bony septation that forms the lateral wall of the cell and separates the frontal drainage pathway from the cell can be thick in patients, and prove difficult to remove with conventional hand-held instruments.

Classification of the Extent of Frontal Sinus Surgery

A wide spectrum of endonasal surgical procedures of the frontal sinus has been developed and defined. These are largely based on the sinusotomy classification outlined by Wolfgang Draf [3] (Table 4.3). Although the Draf classification is most commonly used nomenclature to describe endoscopic frontal sinus procedures, the descriptions of the Draf techniques vary in the literature.

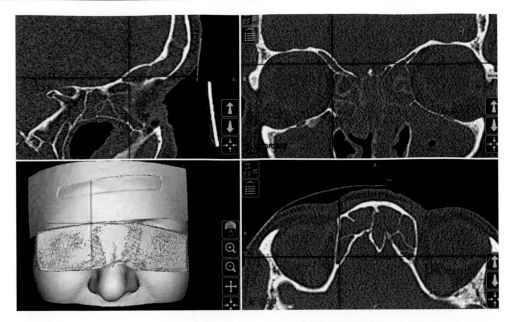

Fig. 4.7 Demonstrates a SOEC (red cross-hairs). On the axial scan, SOECs and SBFCs can be confused. The lateral pneumatization of the SOEC over the orbit as seen on the coronal and parasagittal scans is helpful in distinguishing SOEC from SBFC. These cells always displace the frontal drainage pathway medially or anteromedially. Note the pneumatization of the SOEC around the anterior ethmoidal artery. (Reproduced with permission from Wormald et al. [10])

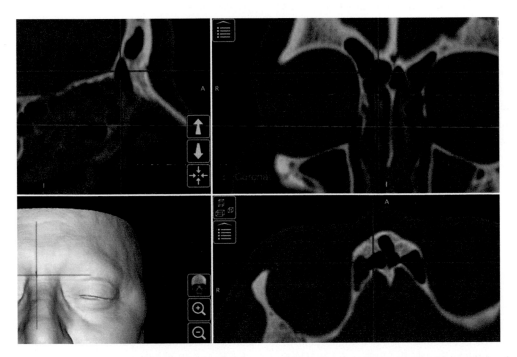

Fig. 4.8 A frontal sinus septal cell can be seen on the right side (red cross-hairs). This cell will always displace the frontal drainage pathway in a lateral or posterolateral direction. (Reproduced with permission from Wormald et al. [10])

Table 4.3 Endonasal frontal sinus drainage type I–III according to Draf [3]

Type	Extent of surgery
I	Anterior ethmoidectomy with drainage of the frontal recess without touching the frontal sinus outflow tract
IIa	Removal of ethmoidal cells protruding into the frontal sinus, creating an opening between the middle turbinate medially and the lamina papyracea laterally
IIb	Removal of the frontal sinus floor between the nasal septum medially and the lamina papyracea laterally
III	Type II drainage on both sides and removal of the upper part of the nasal septum and the lower part of the frontal sinus septum

Poor comprehension of descriptive details may lead to errors in performance of frontal sinus surgery, as well in the nomenclature used by the surgeon to document the technique performed for sinusotomy. These discrepancies also result in lack of standardized reporting and impact meaningful population-based assessment of surgical outcomes. A newer classification system defining the extent of frontal sinus surgery was recently proposed by an international consortium of tertiary rhinologists [10]. The purpose of this system was to facilitate accurate documentation of frontal sinus procedures. The frontal techniques are classified using a graduated approach based on the extent of surgery. It is hoped that such a system will enhance stepwise training of surgeons, improve discussions with patients regarding the difficulty of their surgery and standardize the reporting of frontal sinus surgery outcomes. The extent of endoscopic frontal sinus surgery (EFSS) classification system centers around the definition of the frontal ostium (as previously defined in the chapter). A grade 0 surgery has no removal of cells or tissue, and is limited to balloon catheter dilatation of the frontal drainage pathway (Grade 0; balloon ostioplasty). Grade 1–3 involve surgery to the cells below the frontal ostium (grade 1) (Fig. 4.9), within the frontal ostium (grade 2) (Fig. 4.10) and above the frontal ostium without removal of any frontal bone (grade 3) (Fig. 4.11). There is no removal of the bone around the frontal ostium in Grades 1-3, and only ethmoidal cells

are removed. Grades 4–6 involve removal of the frontal bone around the frontal ostium itself. Grade 4 (Fig. 4.12) is enlargement of the frontal ostium, most often by removal of the bony beak. Grade 5 (Fig. 4.13) is a unilateral frontal drill-out (akin to the Draf IIb procedure), and grade 6 (Fig. 4.14) is a bilateral frontal drillout (akin to the Draf III or modified Lothrop procedure). Table 4.4 lists each of the grades defined in the EFSS system.

Classification of the Complexity of Frontal Sinus Surgery

The international classification system of the radiological complexity (ICC) of frontal recess and frontal sinus surgery has also been recently proposed by an international consortium of tertiary rhinologists (Table 4.5). This system was developed for speed and for ease of use, as well as high intra- and inter-rater reliability. Through the use of well-defined radiological criteria, the proposers of the ICC believe that the complexity of frontal sinus surgery can be better documented, facilitating improvements in both training and commensurate reimbursement. Central to this system is the determination of the antero-posterior (AP) diameter of the frontal ostium on parasagittal CT imaging as well as the identification and documentation of ethmoidal cells pneumatizing the frontal outflow tract. In essence, frontal sinuses with wide anteroposterior dimension and limited superior extension of ethmoidal cells into the frontal sinus are likely to require less complex dissection than when the converse situation exists (narrow frontal dimensions and the presence of ethmoidal cells extending cranially into the frontal sinus) (Table 4.5).

Summary

Frontal recess anatomy has been historically difficult to understand, in part due to diverse nomenclature and classification systems used to describe the relevant anatomy. Use of consistent anatomical landmarks such as the agger nasi cell, the bulla

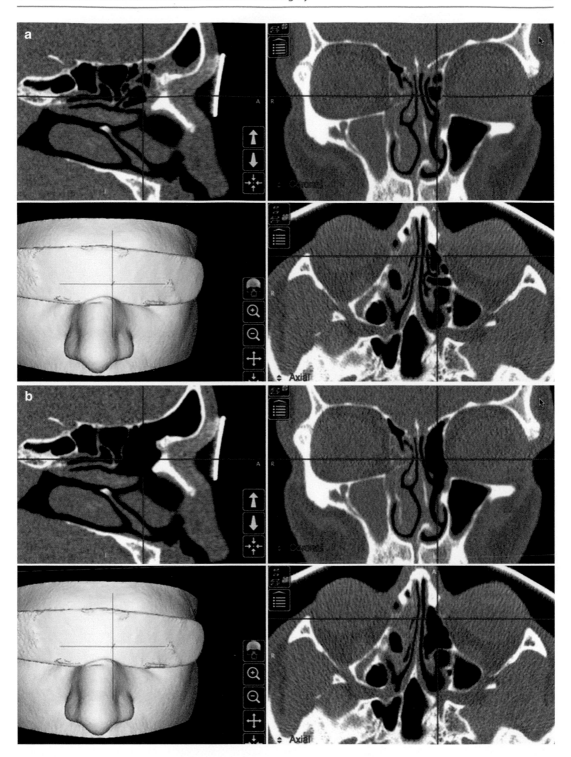

Fig. 4.9 (**a**, **b**) CT scan illustrating grade 1 extent of surgery. (**a**) The cells that need to be dissected do not encroach on the frontal ostium. (**b**) Surgery clears the frontal recess without instrumenting the frontal ostium. (Reproduced with permission from Wormald et al. [10])

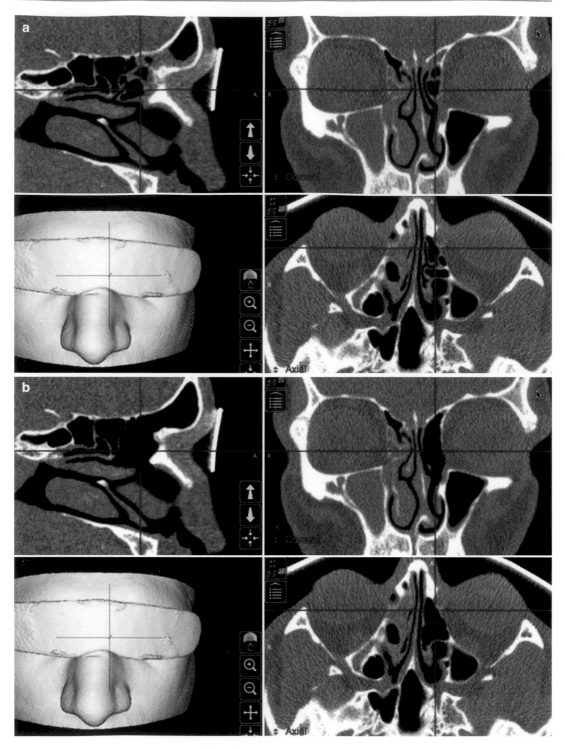

Fig. 4.10 (a, b) CT scan illustrating grade 2 extent of surgery. (a) The SAC encroaches on the frontal ostium without extending through the frontal ostium. (b) Removal of these cells opens the drainage pathway. (Reproduced with permission from Wormald et al. [10])

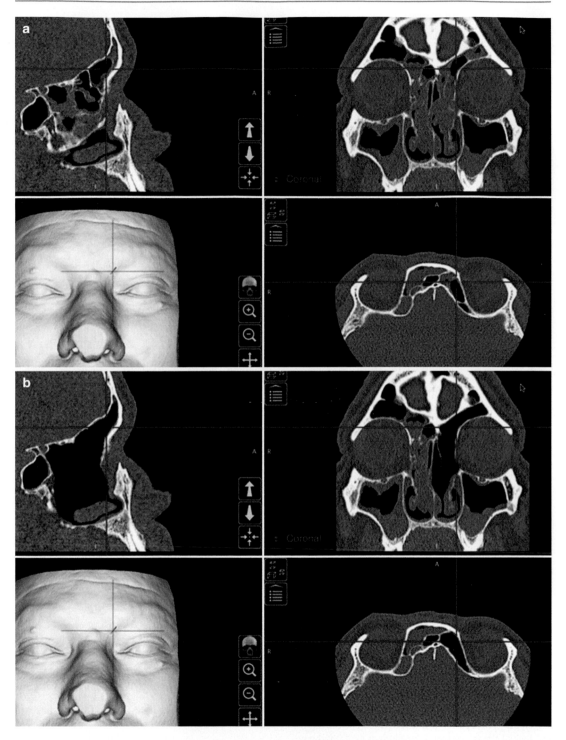

Fig. 4.11 (**a**, **b**) CT scan illustrating grade 3 extent of surgery. (**a**) The SAFC migrates through the frontal ostium into the frontal sinus. (**b**) Surgery involves removing the ethmoidal cell without any widening of the bony frontal ostium. (Reproduced with permission from Wormald et al. [10])

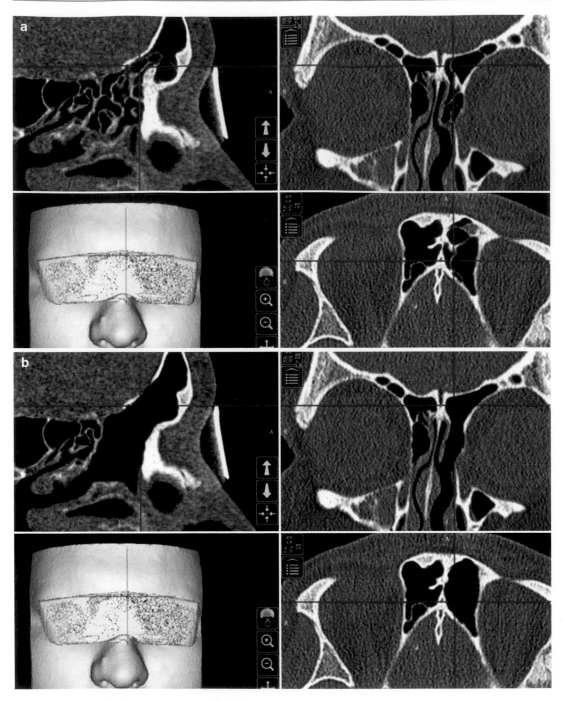

Fig. 4.12 (**a**, **b**) CT scan illustrating grade 4 extent of surgery. (**a**) There is a SAFC and a SBFC obstructing the drainage of the frontal sinus. In addition the frontal bony beak obstructs the drainage. (**b**) The frontal ostium has been enlarged by removal of the bone anterior to the frontal ostium. (Reproduced with permission from Wormald et al. [10])

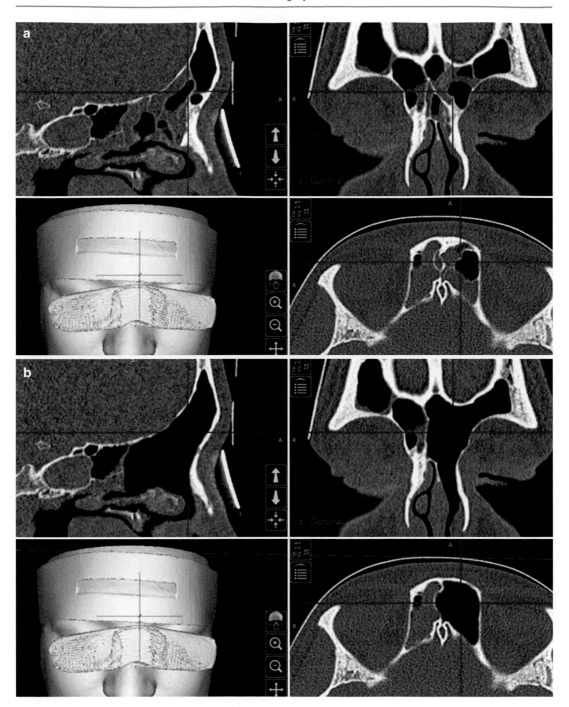

Fig. 4.13 (**a**, **b**) CT scans illustrating grade 5 extent of surgery. (**a**) There is an SAFC, an SBFC and an FSC all narrowing the drainage of the frontal sinus. (**b**) The frontal ostium has been widened by removal of the frontal beak and the floor of the frontal sinus between the lamina papyracea and the septum. (Reproduced with permission from Wormald et al. [10])

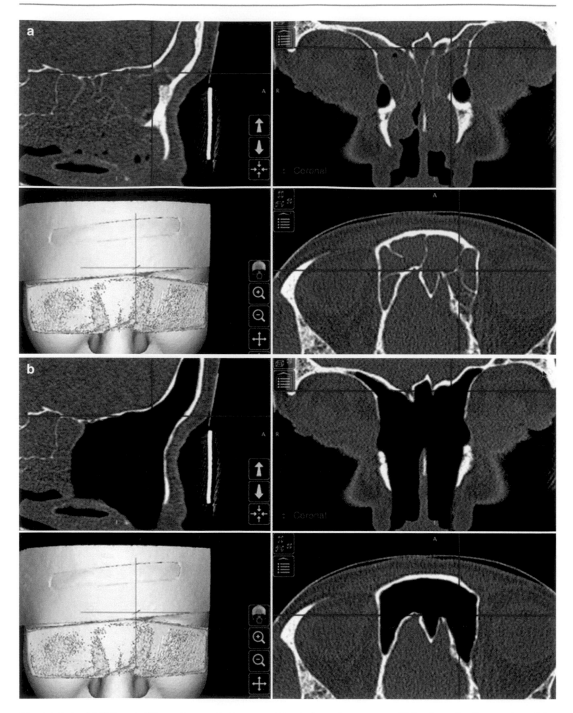

Fig. 4.14 (**a**, **b**) CT scans illustrating grade 6 extent of surgery. (**a**) Severe disease with previous surgery and narrow frontal ostium. (**b**) Surgery involved creation of an anterosuperior septectomy to remove the entire frontal beak, the entire floor of both frontal sinuses as well as the intersinus septum. This allows for the creation of the largest possible frontal neo-ostium incorporating both frontal sinuses (akin to the Draf III, frontal drillout or modified Lothrop procedure). (Reproduced with permission from Wormald et al. [10])

Table 4.4 International classification of extent of endoscopic frontal sinus surgery (EFSS) [10]

Grade	Technique	Typical cells involved
0	Balloon catheter assisted dilatation of the frontal outflow tract (no tissue removal)	
I	Clearance of frontal recess cells *not directly* obstructing the frontal sinus ostium	Small SACs or SBCs
II	Clearance of frontal recess cells *directly* obstructing the frontal sinus ostium	Small SACs or SBCs encroaching on or obstructing the frontal sinus drainage
III	Clearance of cells pneumatizing into the frontal sinus *without* bony enlargement of the frontal ostium	Small SAFC, SBFCs, FSCs
IV	Clearance of cells pneumatizing into the frontal sinus *with* bony enlargement of the frontal ostium	Large SAFC, SBFCs or FSCs with a narrow frontal ostium
V	Bony enlargement of the frontal ostium from the lamina papyracea to the nasal septum with the ipsilateral removal of the frontal sinus floor (Draf IIb or unilateral frontal drillout)	Large SAFCs, SBFCs, FCSs with a narrow frontal ostium
VI	Bony enlargement of the frontal ostium from one lamina papyracea to the other lamina papyracea, with removal of anterosuperior nasal septum and entire frontal sinus floor (Draf III or endoscopic modified Lothrop procedure or frontal drillout)	Large SAFCs, SBFCs, FCSs with a narrow frontal ostium

Table 4.5 International classification system of complexity of frontal sinus surgery

	Wide AP diameter ≥ 10 mm	Narrow AP diameter 9-6 mm	Very Narrow AP diameter ≤ 5 mm
Cells below ostium (Agger nasi, SAC, SBC)	Less complex (Grade 1)	Moderate complexity (Grade 2)	High complexity (Grade 3)
Cells encroaching into the ostium (SAFC, SBFC, SOEC, FSC)	Moderate complexity (grade 2)	High complexity (Grade 3)	Highest complexity (Grade 4)
Cells extending significantly into frontal sinus (SAFC, SBFC, SOEC, FSC)	High complexity (grade 3)	Highest complexity (Grade 4)	Highest complexity (Grade 4)

AP refers to the frontal ostium anterior-posterior (AP) diameter as measured from the frontal beak to the skull base at its narrowest distance on the parasagittal CT scan. Classification of the cells is based on the recent International Frontal Sinus Classification (IFAC) [10]

ethmoidalis and the frontal ostium, may help simplify concepts germane to comprehension of the frontal sinus drainage pathways. The authors of the IFAC and EFSS system hope that these new proposals will help surgeons better understand anatomical variations, surgical planning, instruction of trainees, reporting of surgical outcomes and communication with fellow surgeons.

References

1. Bent JPC-SC, Kuhn FA. The frontal cell as a cause of frontal sinus obstruction. Am J Rhinol. 1994;8:185–91.
2. Bolger WE, Butzin CA, Parsons DS. Paranasal sinus bony anatomic variations and mucosal abnormalities: CT analysis for endoscopic sinus surgery. Laryngoscope. 1991;101(1 Pt 1):56–64.
3. Draf W, Weber R, Keerl R, Constantinidis J. Current aspects of frontal sinus surgery. I: Endonasal frontal sinus drainage in inflammatory diseases of the paranasal sinuses. HNO. 1995;43(6):352–7.
4. Kuhn FA. Chronic frontal sinusitis: the endoscopic frontal recess approach. Oper Tech Otolaryngol Head Neck Surg. 1996;7(3):222–9.
5. Kuhn FA. An integrated approach to frontal sinus surgery. Otolaryngol Clin N Am. 2006;39(3):437–61. viii
6. Lee WT, Kuhn FA, Citardi MJ. 3D computed tomographic analysis of frontal recess anatomy in patients without frontal sinusitis. Otolaryngol Head Neck Surg. 2004;131(3):164–73.
7. Lund VJ, Stammberger H, Fokkens WJ, Beale T, Bernal-Sprekelsen M, Eloy P, et al. European position paper on the anatomical terminology of the internal nose and paranasal sinuses. Rhinol Suppl. 2014;(24):1–34.
8. Van Alyea OE. Frontal sinus drainage. Ann Otol Rhinol Laryngol. 1946;55(4):959. discussion
9. Wormald PJ, Chan SZ. Surgical techniques for the removal of frontal recess cells obstructing the frontal ostium. Am J Rhinol. 2003;17(4):221–6.
10. Wormald PJ, Hoseman W, Callejas C, Weber RK, Kennedy DW, Citardi MJ, et al. The international frontal sinus anatomy classification (IFAC) and classification of the extent of endoscopic frontal sinus surgery (EFSS). Int Forum Allergy Rhinol. 2016;6(7):677–96.

Instrumentation and Technology in Frontal Sinus Surgery

Pete S. Batra, Bobby A. Tajudeen, and Peter Papagiannopoulos

Rigid Endoscopy

The origins of nasal endoscopy can be traced to 1901, when Hirschmann attempted sinus endoscopy using a cystoscope [1]. Shortly thereafter, Reichert performed what is now regarded as the first endoscopic sinus procedure by manipulating the maxillary sinus using a 7 mm endoscope through an oroantral fistula. Maltz furthered the field by advocating for diagnostic evaluation of the sinonasal cavity with endoscopes, leading to the term, "sinoscopy" [1]. The development of the Hopkins rod system in the 1960s resulted in a major paradigm shift in the field. Walter Messerklinger was able to use rigid endoscopes to study the dynamics of mucociliary clearance, enhancing knowledge of paranasal anatomy and physiology. These concepts formulated the basis of functional endoscopic sinus surgery as popularized by Kennedy and Stammberger in the 1980s [2, 3].

The Hopkins rod-lens system provided a wide viewing angle, improved color perception and resolution, and facilitated greater light transmission, thus ushering the era of endoscopic sinus and skull base surgery [1]. Initially, endoscopy was performed directly through the endoscope eyepiece

given the suboptimal quality of the single-chip cameras. The development of three-chip cameras further enhanced the quality of the image, facilitating the use of video monitors for office and intra-operative endoscopy. The current high-definition video platforms provide enhanced clarity in visualization of endoscopic anatomy. Three-dimensional (3D) endoscopic platforms have now become available and have been successfully employed for endoscopic skull base surgery [4]. The overmagnification afforded by the currently available 3D systems has not been successful in maintaining proper spatial orientation for endoscopic frontal sinus surgery.

Standard rigid endoscopes are traditionally 4 mm in diameter with a standard length of 18 cm. Rigid endoscopes of 2.7 mm and 3.2 mm are also available for endoscopy in pediatric patients or adults with narrow nasal anatomy. While initially only zero degree scopes were available and used for endoscopic sinus surgery, currently a full array of angled endoscopes, including 30°, 45°, and 70°, are now widely available and used for sinus surgery. These greatly enhance the ability to visualize the frontal recess and frontal sinus proper [5]. Traditionally, the light post for angled endoscopes was placed opposite to the direction of visualization. The newer rigid endoscopes have the light post in the same direction as the angled endoscope ("reverse endoscopes"). This moves the light and camera cables away from the nares providing greater working room for frontal sinus surgery (Fig. 5.1).

P. S. Batra (✉) · B. A. Tajudeen
P. Papagiannopoulos
Department of Otorhinolaryngology – Head and Neck Surgery and Rush Sinus Program, Rush University Medical Center, Chicago, IL, USA

© Springer Nature Switzerland AG 2019
D. Lal, P. H. Hwang (eds.), *Frontal Sinus Surgery*, https://doi.org/10.1007/978-3-319-97022-6_5
73

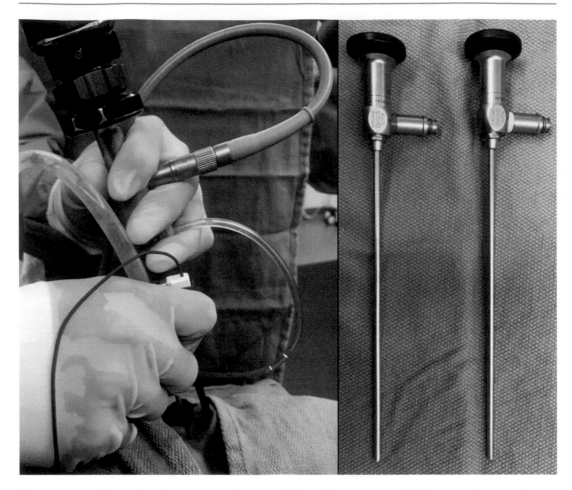

Fig. 5.1 Image (*left panel*) depicts execution of endoscopic frontal sinus surgery with 70° reverse telescope with camera and light cable facing upward; 30° and 70° reverse telescopes are also shown (*right panel*)

Frontal Instrumentation

Frontal dissection poses several challenges, including variable frontal recess anatomy, difficult visualization, narrow caliber space, proximity to vital structures such as the skull base and orbit, and the need for advanced and angled instrumentation. As such, sinus surgery failures occur mostly commonly in the frontal recess [6, 7]. Common findings at the time of revision frontal sinus surgery include edematous or hypertrophic mucosa, retained agger nasi cell, neo-osteogenesis within the frontal recess, lateral scarring of the middle turbinate, residual anterior ethmoid cells, and residual frontal cells. Many of the causes of failure result from poor surgical

technique and can be circumvented with delicate mucosal-sparing dissection technique utilizing the full array of frontal sinus instrumentation.

Hand Instrumentation

The use of through-cutting hand instrumentation is critical for sound surgical technique. Below is a list of commonly used hand instrumentation in frontal recess dissection:

- 45-degree mushroom punch – The 45° mushroom punch is particularly useful to enlarge an existing opening circumferentially (Fig. 5.2). In addition, it is the only frontal sinus hand

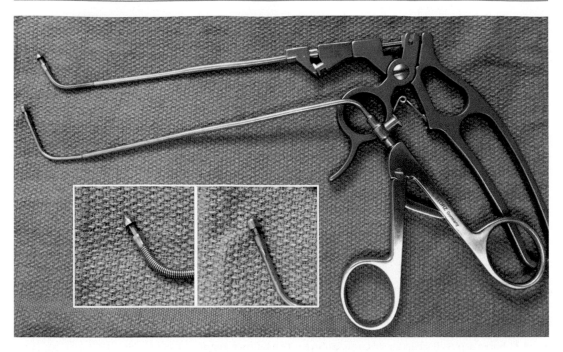

Fig. 5.2 Image illustrates 45° mushroom (*left panel insert*) and Hosemann (*right panel insert*) punches

instrument capable of removing horizontal partitions in an anterior to posterior direction in a through-cutting manner. This situation is commonly encountered in the posterior frontal recess. The Hosemann punch is similar to the 45° mushroom punch with much greater cutting strength (Fig. 5.2). This instrument is best used for the removal of osteitic bone of the frontal sinus floor.

- Bachert forceps – The Bachert forceps, also known as the "cobra," is the mainstay of frontal recess dissection. This instrument resembles a 45° Kerrison punch that punches back to the front (Fig. 5.3). The Bachert forceps is used to remove horizontal ledges, such as the cap of the agger nasi and frontal recess cells, in a back to front fashion.

- Through-cutting giraffe forceps – through-cutting giraffe forceps come in side-to-side and front-to-back varieties at both 45°and 90° angles (Fig. 5.4). These instruments are helpful in removing vertically oriented partitions such as the posterior wall (front-to-back) and medial wall (side-to-side) of the agger nasi, frontal, suprabullar, or frontal bullar cells.

- Non-through-cutting frontal giraffe forceps – These forceps also come in a side-to-side and front-to-back varieties at both 45° and 90° angles as well as different sizes (Fig. 5.5). They are useful to delicately remove loose remnants of bone. Additionally, they can be used to pull out thick eosinophilic mucin or foreign bodies following prior trauma.

- Frontal probes and curettes – A variety of supplementary frontal instruments including Kuhn probes/seekers and frontal curettes are also available (Fig. 5.6). Frontal seekers come in many versions and are generally ball-tipped, curved instruments that have extended length. They are very useful for high dissection of frontal recess cells. Additionally, fine probes can be useful in avoiding trauma to delicate mucosa in a small diameter frontal recess.

- Angled suction tips – A variety of angled narrow olive tip suctions are available in various sizes. The least traumatic option should be chosen depending on the width and the dissection. Additionally, malleable suctions that can be curved to the desired angled are also available.

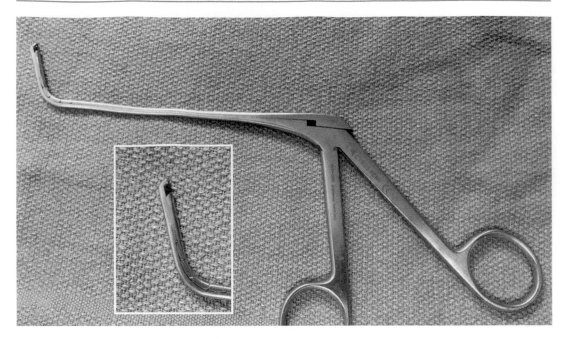

Fig. 5.3 Image depicts Bachert forceps, also known as chain Kerrison punch

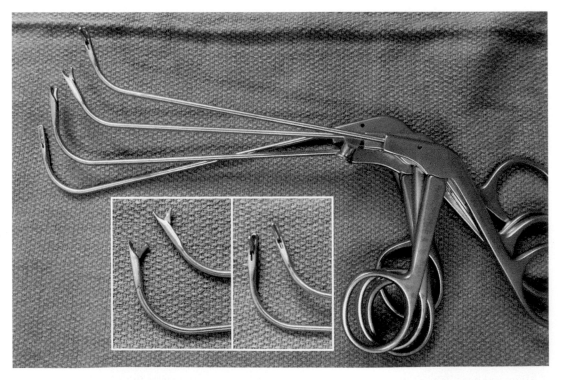

Fig. 5.4 Image shows side-to-side (*right panel insert*) and front-to-back (*left panel insert*) through-cutting giraffe forceps

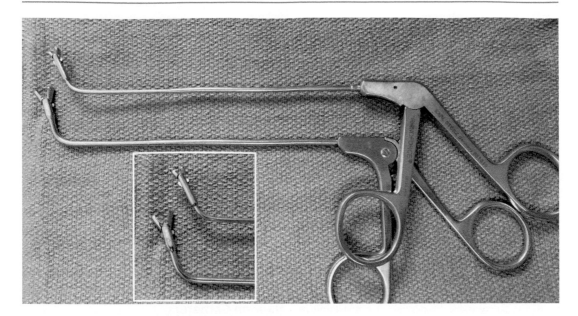

Fig. 5.5 Image illustrates non-through-cutting frontal giraffe forceps

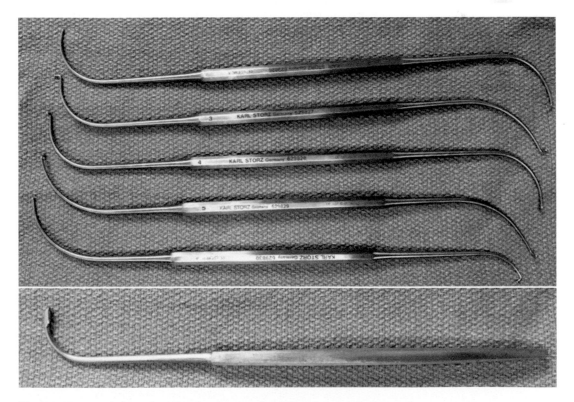

Fig. 5.6 Photograph shows frontal probes (*top panel*) and frontal curette (*lower panel*)

Powered Instrumentation

Powered instrumentation in frontal recess dissection includes microdebriders and drills. The microdebrider is a cylindrical instrument that has a hollow tube with an inner and outer portion. Both the inner and outer portions have a blade at their distal end. Continuous suction is applied to the instrument so cut tissue is captured and removed from the surgical field. Faster rotational speeds result in the removal of smaller fragments of tissue. Microdebriders are available in a variety of sizes and angulation. The 4 mm, 40° and 60° curved sinus blades are commonly utilized in frontal recess dissection (Fig. 5.7). A 2.9 mm 60° curved sinus microdebrider blade is also available for narrower frontal recesses. Sinus blades with rotatable blades are also available in 40°, 60°, and 90° angles; these can be used to address mucosal disease on the posterior and lateral aspects of the frontal sinus. The 40° angle microdebrider blade works best with 30° and 45° endoscopes, whereas the 60° and 90° microdebrider blades work well with 70° endoscopes. The microdebrider should be used judiciously in the frontal recess given the risk of denudation of mucosal surfaces and ensuing stenosis. It should

be utilized to clean up free mucosal edges after the use of through-cutting hand instrumentation.

Powered drills are also available in a variety of sizes and angles. The 70-degree diamond drill is the safest and most useful in frontal surgery (Fig. 5.8). Newer generations of powered drills allow for high-speed rotation at 30,000 rpm that significantly improves operative efficiency over lower-speed traditional drills. Drills are particularly useful when there is significant neo-osteogenesis or there is a prominent nasofrontal beak narrowing the frontal recess. Once the bone has been thinned with the drill, it is prudent to switch back to hand instrumentation to optimize both speed and safety.

Balloon Catheters

The role of balloon catheter dilation (BCD) of the frontal recess is primarily in the office setting or as an adjunct to traditional frontal recess dissection using standard instrumentation. The theoretical advantage of BCD is that it provides a unique opportunity to potentially achieve durable ostial and frontal outflow tract dilation with complete tissue preservation. The general technique

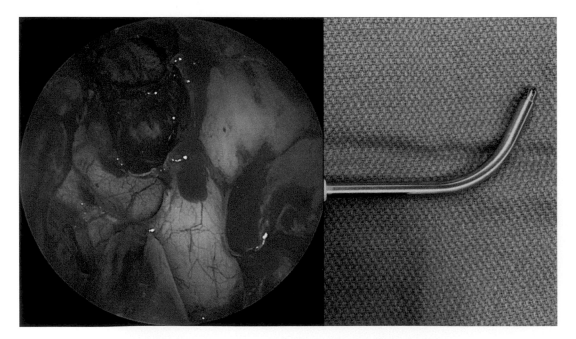

Fig. 5.7 Image demonstrates RAD-60 soft tissue shaver or microdebrider after left-sided frontal sinusotomy visualized with a 70° endoscope (left panel). The right panel demonstrates the curvature of the instrument

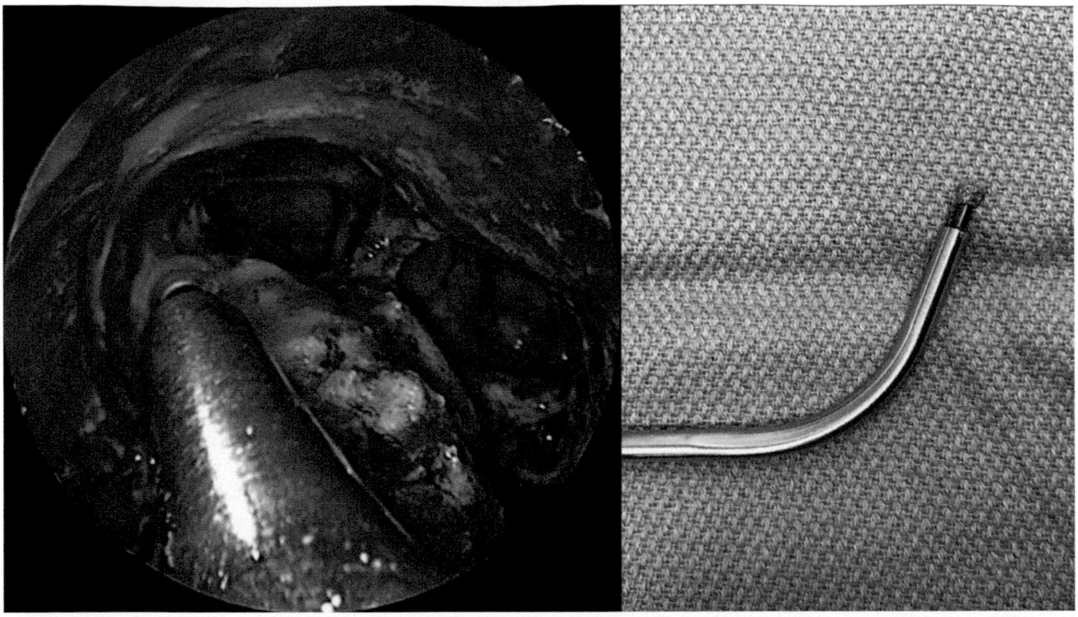

Fig. 5.8 Image depicts 70° diamond burr drill utilized for frontal drillout procedures for the removal of a frontal sinus osteoma. The right panel demonstrates the curvature of the drill

involves placement of a guidewire through the natural frontal sinus drainage pathway. Image guidance or light illumination can aid the identification process. Once proper placement of the device is confirmed, an appropriate diameter and length balloon are advanced and dilated to 10–12 atmosphere of pressure. Following dilation, irrigation can be performed, if required, through a variety of catheters. In the office setting, this completes the procedure. When used as an adjunct to frontal recess surgery, traditional instrumentation can then be used to remove obstructing frontal cells once a clear pathway to the frontal sinus has been established after BCD.

The largest study to date assessing the efficacy of in-office BCD included dilation of 268 frontal sinuses. Technical dilation of the frontal sinus was possible in 93.7% with 5 frontal sinuses (2%) requiring revision procedures [8]. Patients with greater disease burden (severe polyposis, scar tissue, etc.) were excluded from the study. In general, relative contraindications for BCD of the frontal sinus as a stand-alone procedure include cases with diffuse polyposis, extensive neo-osteogenesis of the frontal outflow tract, complex frontal pneumatization patterns, or questionable histology necessitating tissue removal for pathology.

Surgical Planning Software

Surgical planning for frontal recess/sinus surgery is essential for successful execution of the surgical steps. Triplanar review of the axial, coronal, and sagittal images facilitates understanding of the complex three-dimensional anatomy, including frontal recess pneumatization pattern and frontal sinus drainage pathway. Novel virtual 3D image viewing software (Scopis Building Blocks, Scopis GmbH, Berlin, Germany) may assist in better understanding of the anatomy and spatial orientation of the frontal recess/sinus [9]. Software tools allow the user to annotate relevant structures at their discretion. Further, specific cells in the frontal recess can be outlined by drawing boxes. This allows for the creation of building blocks concept on the CT scan in all three dimensions to better depict the frontal recess cells. The frontal sinus drainage pathway can also be drawn as a curvilinear line on the CT scan. Incorporation of virtual 3D planning surgical software has been demonstrated to augment understanding and spatial orientation of the frontal recess anatomy for trainees. This potential increase in trainee proficiency and comprehension theoretically may result in improved surgical skill and patient outcomes [9].

Surgical Navigation

Over the past two decades, intraoperative surgical navigation, also known as image-guided surgery (IGS), has been widely employed to improve surgical outcomes and reduce surgical morbidity. The registration process at the beginning of the surgical procedure aligns corresponding fiducial points in the preoperative CT imaging dataset and the intraoperative surgical field volume. Tracking with instruments or suctions in the surgical field affords the ability to correlate the CT anatomy with the endoscopic sinonasal anatomy allowing for better spatial orientation and execution of surgical steps [10]. Navigational accuracy, also known as target registration error (TRE), is defined by the relationship between the instrument tip and its measured position in the surgical field. Commercially available IGS systems provide a TRE within 1.5–

2.0 mm. Multiple retrospective studies have demonstrated that the IGS has been able to improve the completeness of endoscopic sinus surgery with a better safety profile.

The utility of IGS has been especially helpful in the context of endoscopic frontal sinus surgery given the narrow confines of the frontal recess and proximity to critical structures. This can be critical in the setting of extensive polyp disease or previous surgical manipulation resulting in loss of normal anatomic landmarks. Angled image guidance suctions can help identify residual frontal recess cells adjacent to the skull base and orbit. This may enhance surgeon confidence facilitating more comprehensive and safe frontal recess dissection and, in turn, improving long-term success rates of frontal sinus surgery (Fig. 5.9). Image guidance can also be an important adjunct in external frontal surgery, helping

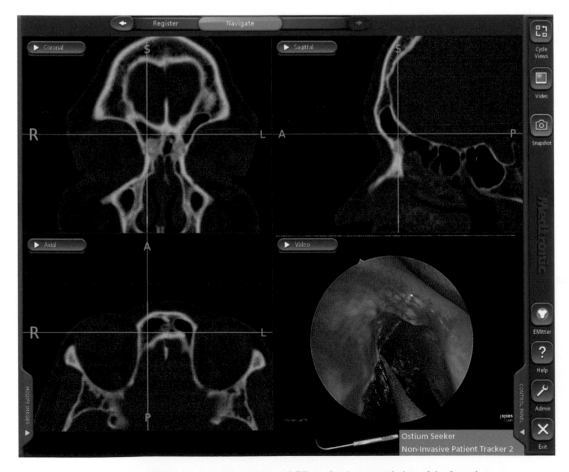

Fig. 5.9 Image illustrates triplanar image-guidance view of CT confirming cannulation of the frontal recess

identify the precise location for endoscopic frontal trephination or bony cuts for osteoplastic frontal sinusotomy.

Intraoperative CT Imaging

Despite the advantages of IGS, it relies on the preoperative CT dataset and cannot account for the anatomic alterations resulting from the intraoperative surgical manipulation. This can be especially challenging in longer cases when the system may be rendered least reliable during crucial portions of the procedure. Intraoperative CT imaging has the ability to circumvent limitations of surgical navigation by providing a near real-time update of the CT dataset. This has been loaded into IGS for further surgical planning and navigation to successful completion of surgery. Prospective clinical data suggests that intraoperative CT imaging may increase the completeness of surgery by identifying retained partitions [11]. Despite the initial promising results, intraoperative CT imaging systems are not widely available for frontal sinus surgery at the present time.

Summary

The advances in rigid endoscopy, frontal hand and powered instrumentation, and surgical navigation have ushered the modern era of endoscopic frontal sinus surgery. Indeed, the vast majority of primary and revision frontal sinus disease is now amenable to management by the endoscopic route. Careful understanding of the surgical instrumentation and IGS, including their advantages and limitations, is essential to successful execution of surgery. Intimate knowledge of frontal recess anatomy, requisite surgical experience, meticulous mucosal-sparing technique, and commitment to postoperative care remain critical to long-term success in frontal sinus surgery.

Financial Disclosures Batra: research grant (Medtronic), royalties (Springer), Optinose (Advisory Board), Sanofi Regeneron (Advisory Board)

Tajudeen: none

Papagiannopoulos: none

References

1. Govindaraj S, Adappa ND, Kennedy DW. Endoscopic sinus surgery: evolution and technical innovations. J Laryngol Otol. 2010;124:242–50.
2. Kennedy DW. Functional endoscopic sinus surgery. Technique. Arch Otolaryngol. 1985;111:643–9.
3. Stammberger H. Endoscopic endonasal surgery--concepts in treatment of recurring rhinosinusitis. Part II. Surgical technique. Otolaryngol Head Neck Surg. 1986;94:147–56.
4. Manes RP, Barnett S, Batra PS. Utility of novel 3-dimensional stereoscopic vision system for endoscopic sinonasal and skull-base surgery. Int Forum Allergy Rhinol. 2011;1:191–7.
5. Cohen NA, Kennedy DW. Endoscopic sinus surgery: where we are-and where we're going. Curr Opin Otolaryngol Head Neck Surg. 2005;13:32–8.
6. Otto KJ, DelGaudio JM. Operative findings in the frontal recess at time of revision surgery. Am J Otolaryngol. 2010;31:175–80.
7. Valdes CJ, Bogado M, Samaha M. Causes of failure in endoscopic frontal sinus surgery in chronic rhinosinusitis patients. Int Forum Allergy Rhinol. 2014;4:502–6.
8. Karanfilov B, Silvers S, Pasha R, Sikand A, Shikani A, Sillers M. Office-based balloon sinus dilation: a prospective, multicenter study of 203 patients. Int Forum Allergy Rhinol. 2013;3:404–11.
9. Agbetoba A, Luong A, Siow JK, Senior B, Callejas C, Szczygielski K, Citardi MJ. Educational utility of advanced three-dimensional virtual imaging in evaluating the anatomical configuration of the frontal recess. Int Forum Allergy Rhinol. 2016;7:143–8.
10. Citardi MJ, Batra PS. Intraoperative surgical navigation for endoscopic sinus surgery: rationale and indications. Curr Opin Otolaryngol Head Neck Surg. 2007;15:23–7.
11. Batra PS, Manes RP, Ryan MW, Marple BF. Prospective evaluation of intraoperative computed tomography imaging for endoscopic sinonasal and skull-base surgery. Int Forum Allergy Rhinol. 2011;1:481–7.

Endoscopic Techniques in Frontal Sinus Surgery

Devyani Lal and Peter H. Hwang

Introduction

Endoscopic frontal sinus is demanding [1, 2]. Surgery is technically challenging and carries a higher risk of complications, and postoperative stenosis may necessitate further revision surgery [3]. To perform surgery safely, effectively, and efficiently, the endoscopic frontal surgeon must commit to deepening their knowledge of the frontal anatomy. Additionally, ongoing review of the three-dimensional frontal recess anatomy on the patient's computerized tomography (CT) scans is critical for the surgeon to perform effective and safe frontal sinus surgery.

The development of contemporary endoscopic techniques was facilitated by the invention of endoscopes, powered instrumentation, surgical navigation, and ancillary technologies [1, 2, 4, 5]. The modern frontal sinus surgeon must utilize these tools to their advantage [1, 6, 7]. The surgeon should hone their skill in the use of angled endoscopes and instruments as well as meticulous tissue handling. Cadaveric dissection courses are crucial in gaining familiarity with the complex anatomy of the frontal recess as well as in dissection techniques.

In keeping with understanding of paranasal sinus physiology and mucociliary clearance, the objective of frontal sinus surgery for rhinosinusitis (RS) is to restore mucociliary function, ventilation and drainage [8]. The extent of surgery is influenced by disease pathophysiology as well as patient preference [9, 10]. Early endoscopic techniques were developed by Messerklinger, Wigand, and Draf [2, 4, 8]. These include the Draf I, Draf II, and Draf III (endoscopic modified Lothrop) procedures. These were later adopted, adapted and popularized by Kennedy and Stammberger [4]. The addition of powered instrumentation and image guidance was instrumental in the adoption of endoscopic techniques in frontal sinus surgery [6, 7]. Balloon-assisted dilatation is a relatively new endoscopic technique that has gained popularity [11]. Additionally, external frontal trephination techniques can be used as adjuncts to endoscopic frontal sinus surgery to address high or lateral frontal cells and disease ("above and below" technique) [12, 13].

Electronic Supplementary Material The online version of this chapter (https://doi.org/10.1007/978-3-319-97022-6_6) contains supplementary material, which is available to authorized users.

D. Lal (✉)
Department of Otolaryngology – Head and Neck Surgery, Mayo Clinic College of Medicine and Science, Mayo Clinic, Phoenix, AZ, USA

P. H. Hwang
Department of Otolaryngology – Head and Neck Surgery, Stanford University School of Medicine, Stanford, CA, USA

Frontal sinus surgery should be personalized and tailored to address the type and extent of pathology as well as the patient's anatomy. The contemporary frontal sinus surgeon must be familiar with the spectrum of surgical techniques and employ those that are most advantageous to the patient. Zealous postoperative care is also critical for successful outcomes. This chapter will detail the editors' techniques in performing endoscopic frontal sinus surgery.

Indications for Frontal Sinusotomy

The most common indication for frontal sinus surgery is chronic inflammatory disease that is unresponsive to medical therapy [14, 15]. Appropriate medical therapy (discussed in Chap. 29) should be employed prior to determining candidacy for sur-

gery; some patients will respond to such therapy and avoid surgery (Fig. 6.1). Other common indications for frontal sinus surgery include recurrent acute frontal sinusitis, recalcitrant or complicated acute frontal sinusitis, mucoceles, and tumors. A list of common indications is outlined in Table 6.1.

Office Assessment, Counseling, and Planning

During the initial office visit, a thorough review of clinical symptoms should be performed. Based on the disease state, appropriate medical therapy should be employed as indicated. If the patient will need surgery, a CT scan of the paranasal sinuses should be obtained and reviewed with the patient. Potential benefits from surgery, complications from unaddressed frontal disease

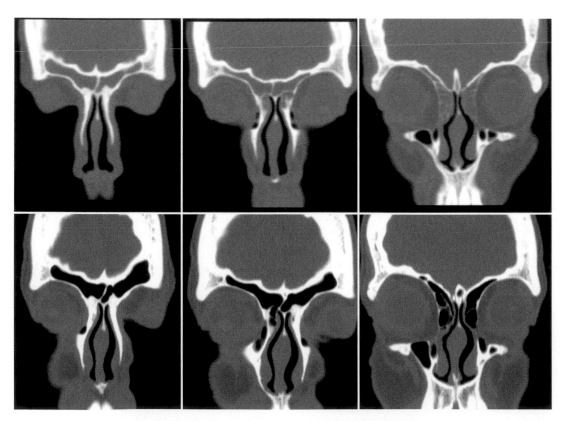

Fig. 6.1 Non-contrast sinus CT scan of a 34-year-old female meeting diagnostic criteria for chronic rhinosinusitis. The top panel shows coronal CT images sent in at the time of referral. The three bottom panels are correspond-ing posttreatment images taken after 6 weeks after completion of appropriate medical therapy. The posttreatment CT images show resolution of inflammatory changes in the paranasal sinuses

Table 6.1 Common indications of frontal sinus surgery

A. Chronic inflammatory disease
(a) Chronic rhinosinusitis (with or without nasal polyposis)
(b) Complications of chronic rhinosinusitis
(c) Noninvasive fungal ball
B. Acute inflammatory disease
(a) Acute frontal sinusitis unresponsive to medical therapy
(b) Recurrent acute frontal rhinosinusitis
(c) Acute frontal sinusitis with (impending) complications
(d) Acute invasive fungal rhinosinusitis
C. Mucocele
D. Frontal barosinusitis
E. Tumors of the frontoethmoidal region
(a) Benign tumors: osteoma, inverted papilloma, etc.
(b) Malignant tumors: primary and metastatic lesions
F. Cerebrospinal fluid leak and meningoencephalocele of the frontoethmoidal region
G. Frontal sinus trauma requiring surgical repair
H. Foreign body removal
I. Transfrontal approaches to pathology in other areas
(a) Anterior cranial base pathology
(b) Pathology of the medial and superior orbit
J. Pneumatocele of the frontal sinus

Table 6.2 Items for in-office review of CT while planning for frontal sinus surgery

A.	**Characterization of disease**
Pattern	Unilateral or bilateral Chronic or acute (mucosal thickening, fluid levels) Mucocele (expansile opacification with bony erosion into orbit skull base) Presence of polyps or mass Hyperdensity: fungus ball, allergic fungal disease, inspissated mucus Ostiomeatal complex disease
B.	**Frontal sinus anatomy**
Frontal sinus	Pneumatization: aplastic, hypoplastic, hyperpneumatized Frontal recess anatomy Frontal recess cells Width of the frontal recess (in sagittal and coronal planes)
Skull base	Integrity Height and slope of anterior ethmoidal roof Height, slope, and symmetry of cribriform plates (Keros classification) Position of anterior ethmoidal artery and if pedicled on a mesentery
Lamina papyracea	Integrity; healed fractures and any herniation into ethmoidal space
Uncinate	Position, rotation (any lateralization, scarring to lamina papyracea)
C.	**Intranasal anatomy**
Septum	Deviation, spurs, perforation
Middle turbinate	Pneumatization (concha bullosa), position (lateralization), paradoxical curvature, integrity (previous resection – total or partial)

(detailed in Chap. 23), and complications from frontal surgery (detailed in Chap. 24) should be discussed to facilitate decision-making. Correlation of symptoms with endoscopic and radiographic findings should be made. The pattern and extent of disease will help determine whether surgery is necessary and in managing expectations from surgery. This is especially important in uncomplicated disease when improvement in quality of life is the goal. Review of the CT scan prior to scheduling surgery is also critical in assessing the complexity of surgery and anticipating the need for additional time and equipment. Table 6.2 presents a checklist that can be used for reviewing the CT in the office. The presence of low-lying skull base, dehiscent skull base or lamina papyracea, and lateralized uncinate process may increase the risks associated with surgery. Narrow frontal recesses may impose higher risks of postoperative stenosis, as may osteoneogenesis. Anatomic variations such as extensively pneumatized frontoethmoidal cells may require additional operative time, instrumentation and navigation, as well as sup-plemental techniques such as frontal trephination or extended frontal sinusotomy. The presence of a dehiscent anterior ethmoidal artery may alert the physician to keeping the bipolar cautery or clips handy. A prominent deviated septum or large concha bullosa can impede endoscopic visualization of the frontal recess and may require management prior to frontal sinusotomy. Use of navigation systems should be considered in patients with complex frontal recess anatomy to facilitate comprehension of the anatomy, as well as to confirm landmarks during surgical dissection.

The patient is evaluated from the standpoint of general health status. Optimization of pulmonary and cardiac status may be necessary prior to scheduling surgery. Treatment of hypertension is also helpful in hemostasis intraoperatively and postoperatively. Cessation of anticoagulants or the use of "bridging" anticoagulant therapy should be coordinated in consultation with the prescribing physician. Patients with unstable asthma may benefit from perioperative corticosteroid therapy. The authors do not routinely use preoperative corticosteroids, but these may be of benefit in patients with florid nasal polyposis [16] or severely inflamed mucosa for optimizing the intraoperative field.

Surgical Anatomy: Brief Review

The anatomy and radiographic features of the frontal sinus are covered comprehensively in Chaps. 2, 3, and 4. A brief review pertinent to this chapter is presented in this section [17–20]. The frontal sinus drains into the nasal cavity through a space that lies between various ethmoidal structures (the frontal sinus drainage pathway; Fig. 6.2). The frontal sinus drainage pathway starts in the posteromedial aspect of the sinus (frontal infundibulum), which is a funnel-shaped structure (Fig. 6.2). The drainage pathway then narrows before widening again to open inferiorly into the nose, in an

hourglass configuration. The term frontal "ostium" has been conventionally used to refer to the narrowest part of the frontal sinus drainage pathway (Fig. 6.3). The term "frontal opening" has been recently proposed as a more accurate substitute for "frontal ostium," as the sinus does not have a true histomorphologic two-dimensional opening but a continuous three-dimensional space that opens into the frontal recess inferiorly (Fig. 6.3) [21]. The "frontal ostium' is the area in the frontal sinus drainage pathway that lies at the junction between the frontal infundibulum (when viewed from above) and the frontal recess (when viewed endoscopically from below). The frontal recess is the inferior part of the frontal sinus drainage pathway, inferior to the frontal sinus opening, comprising the most anterosuperior part of the ethmoidal complex [19]. The term "frontal recess" has sometimes been used to imply the entire frontal sinus drainage pathway, but this is inaccurate. The term "nasofrontal duct" is also incorrect, insofar as the histomorphology of the drainage pathway of the frontal sinus does not contain true ductal structures, and therefore the term "nasofrontal duct" has been abandoned. Instead, the drainage of the frontal sinus is a space that is convoluted and

a

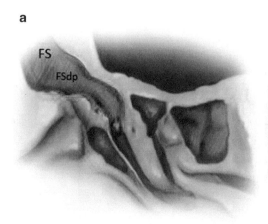

b

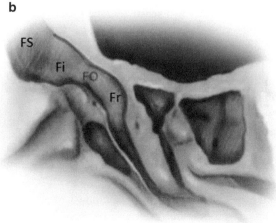

Fig. 6.2 (a) Frontal sinus drainage pathway (FSdp) is an hourglass-shaped three-dimensional space through which the frontal sinus (FS) drains into the nose. (b) The frontal sinus drainage pathway starts in the posteromedial aspect of the sinus (frontal infundibulum; Fi), which is a funnel-shaped structure. The term "frontal ostium" (FO) has been conventionally used to refer to the narrowest part of the frontal sinus drainage pathway. The frontal recess (Fr) is the inferior part of the frontal sinus drainage pathway, lying below the frontal ostium

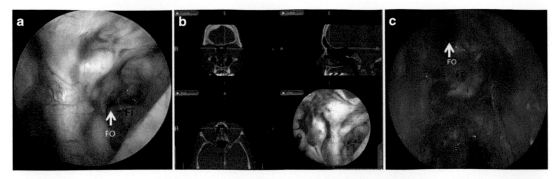

Fig. 6.3 (**a**) The left frontal infundibulum (Fi) as seen through a frontal trephination approach using a 30° endoscope looking inferiorly; note the full-shaped appearance of the frontal infundibulum as it progressively narrows into the "frontal ostium" (FO; white arrow). (**b**) Three-dimensional CT and endoscopic co-localization of the left frontal infundibulum as it approaches the frontal ostium area. (**c**) Left front recess (Fr) visualized through the nose with a 70° endoscope after removal of the agger nasi cell; the frontal recess narrows toward the frontal ostium (FO; white arrow)

shaped by configuration of ethmoidal air cells and structures. Drainage medial to the uncinate process, directly into the middle meatus, is the more commonly found configuration. When the uncinate attaches medially to the skull base or middle turbinate, the frontal recess first drains into the ethmoidal infundibulum, before eventually draining into the middle meatus.

The ethmoidal infundibulum is a three-dimensional space that lies lateral to the uncinate process, anterior and inferior to the ethmoidal bulla (bulla ethmoidalis), and medial to the orbit and maxillary sinus (Fig. 6.4). The superior configuration of the infundibulum is dependent on the superior attachment(s) of the uncinate process [17]. When the uncinate process attaches medially to the middle turbinate (Fig. 6.5a) or the skull base (Fig. 6.5b), the ethmoidal infundibulum is continuous superiorly with the frontal recess. When the uncinate process attaches laterally to the lamina papyracea (Fig. 6.5c), the ethmoidal infundibulum terminates superiorly in a blind pouch called "terminal recess." In this situation, the frontal recess opens medial to the uncinate process into the middle meatus (Fig. 6.5c). The uncinate process may have more than one superior attachment, and as many as six attachments have been described [22]. These superior attachments are important to recognize since they will determine how the frontal recess communicates into the nose.

The lateral and medial boundaries of the frontal recess thus vary with the superior attachment of the uncinate process. Depending on the uncinate attachment, the frontal recess is bound medially by the middle turbinate (Fig. 6.5c) or uncinate process (Fig. 6.5a, b). Laterally, it may be bound by the lamina papyracea (Fig. 6.5a, b) or the uncinate process (Fig. 6.5c). Anteriorly and posteriorly, the frontal recess is bound by the anterior ethmoidal complex. In the simplest configuration of ethmoidal pneumatization, the frontal recess is bound by the agger nasi anteriorly and the ethmoidal bulla posteriorly (Fig. 6.6). Widening of the frontal sinus drainage pathway can therefore be accomplished through removal of anterior ethmoidal cells, uncinate, and the vertical lamella of the middle turbinate. The absolute limits of frontal recess dissection are the lamina papyracea laterally and the skull base medially and posteriorly (Fig. 6.6). The anterior ethmoidal artery lies behind the frontal recess in the ethmoidal skull base, close to the attachment of the bulla lamella (if present), or in the posterior aspect of a suprabullar cell or supraorbital ethmoidal cell when these are present [23–25](Fig. 6.7). As ethmoidal partitions in the posterior part of the frontal recess are dissected, care must be taken to identify and preserve the anterior ethmoidal artery, especially when it is low lying. A pedicled ethmoidal artery is usually associated with the presence of hyperpneumatized ethmoidal cells [18, 25].

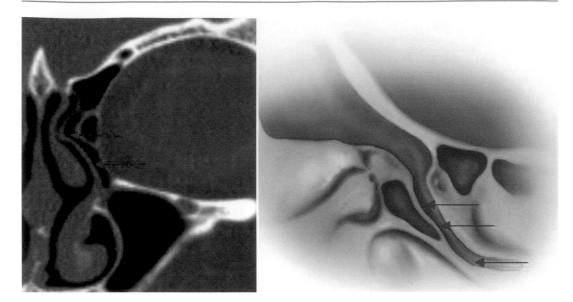

Fig. 6.4 The ethmoidal infundibulum (red arrows) is a three-dimensional space that lies lateral to the uncinate process, anterior and inferior to the ethmoidal bulla, and medial to the orbit and maxillary sinus. This is shown on the CT panel on the left and the schematic on the right side

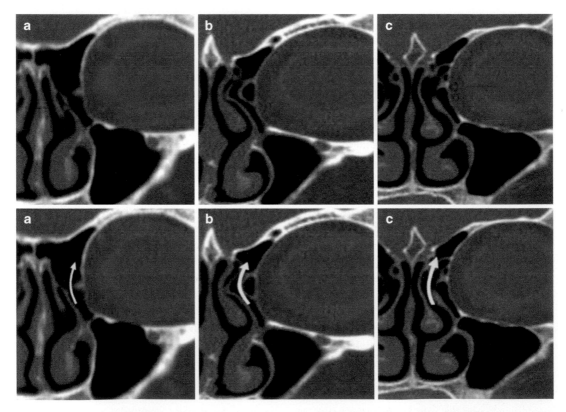

Fig. 6.5 The superior attachment of the uncinate process (red line) determines whether the frontal sinus drainage (yellow arrow) is into the middle meatus or the ethmoidal infundibulum. When the uncinate process attaches medially to the middle turbinate (**a**) or the skull base (**b**), the ethmoid infundibulum is continuous superiorly with the frontal recess. When the uncinate process attaches later- ally to the lamina papyracea, the frontal sinus drains medial to the uncinate process into the middle meatus (**c**). When the uncinate process attaches laterally to the lamina papyracea (C), the ethmoidal infundibulum terminates superiorly in a blind pouch called "terminal recess" (green arrow). In this last situation, the frontal recess drains medial to the uncinate process into the middle meatus (C)

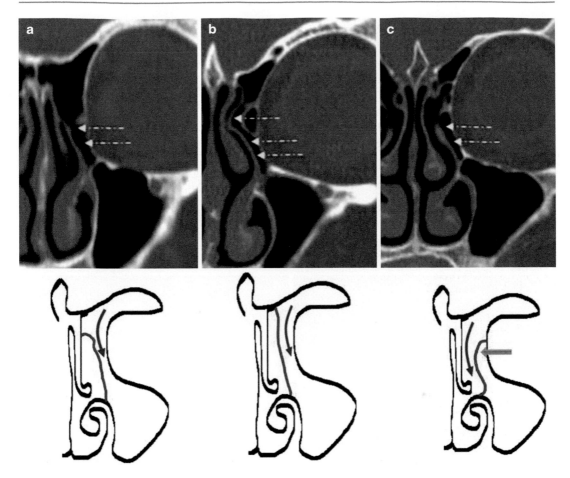

Fig. 6.5 (continued)

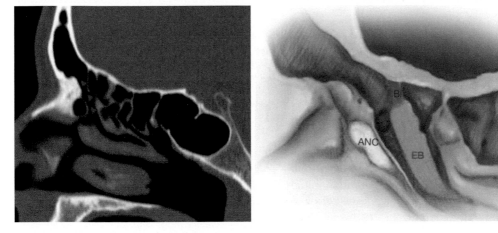

Fig. 6.6 Anteriorly and posteriorly, the frontal recess is bound by the anterior ethmoidal complex. In the simplest configuration, the frontal recess (red arrows) lies behind the agger nasi cell (ANC) and in front of the ethmoidal bulla (EB) and bulla lamella (Bl), when present

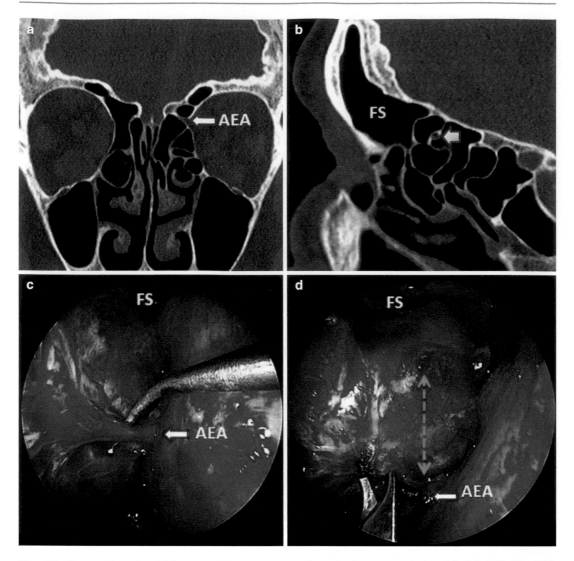

Fig. 6.7 The anterior ethmoidal artery (AEA) passes through the ethmoid skull base from the orbit to the ethmoidal roof, typically near the bulla lamella (white arrow). Occasionally, the artery may pass through the ethmoidal cells pedicled on a mesentery. Figures A and B show a pedicled left AEA on coronal and sagittal CT images, respectively. Images C and D show 30-degree and 70-degree endoscopic views, respectively, of the left AEA. The AEA is not present just behind the frontal ostium area but is typically located a distance (broken yellow arrow) posterior to the frontoethmoidal junction, in the suprabullar area. FS frontal sinus. The artery is being cauterized in this case as part of anterior skull base surgery, but typically should be left undisturbed if possible, in endoscopic sinus surgery

The presence of frontoethmoidal cells can complicate frontal anatomy and dissection. These cells belong to the anterior ethmoidal complex and lie both anterior and posterior to the frontal sinus drainage pathway. The detailed anatomy of these cells is discussed in Chaps. 2, 3, and 4; in this section, we will address the relevance of these cells in context to surgical dissection. Frontoethmoidal cells can often be mistaken for the frontal sinus during surgery and postoperative endoscopy. Additionally, when reviewing the sinus CT preoperatively, disease in frontoethmoidal cells may be mistaken to lie in the frontal sinus; failure to surgically dissect these diseased cells can lead to inadequate surgery.

Frontoethmoidal cells were first classified by Bent and Kuhn [26], and this classification was subsequently modified by Wormald [20]. A recent international consensus document was published in 2016 in an attempt to further simplify the classification of these cells (the International Frontal Sinus Anatomy Classification (IFAC)) [18]. The authors will be using the IFAC and modified Kuhn-Wormald [20] classifications in the chapter [18].

The cells that lie anterior to the frontal sinus drainage pathway are the agger nasi cell, the supra-agger cells (Kuhn Type 1, Kuhn Type 2 cells) and the supra-agger frontal cells (Kuhn Type 3 or Kuhn Type 4 cells) (Fig. 6.8). The agger nasi cell is the most anterior cell that can be seen in a coronal section, anterior to the middle turbinate insertion. While Kuhn described the Type 4 cell as an isolated cell within the frontal sinus, modern scanners with sagittal sections usually identify some confluence with the ethmoidal space [26]. Wormald therefore modified the Type 4 cell to identify a single supra-agger cell that extended more than halfway up the sagittal height of the frontal sinus [20].

The junction of the most anterior part of the middle turbinate with the agger nasi inferiorly is termed the "axilla." According to Nicolai (Chap. 2), all ethmoidal lamellae anterior to the ethmoidal bulla arise from derivatives of the first embryological lamella (uncinate process and agger nasi cell). Additionally, all lamellae anterior to the ethmoidal bulla and lateral to the vertical part of the middle turbinate are uncinate attachments; the agger nasi cell lies superior to the attachment of the vertical middle turbinate to the lateral nasal wall. When the axilla is removed, the anterior aspect of the agger nasi cells and the supra-agger cells can be opened. If the agger nasi bone is non-pneumatized or poorly pneumatized, an angled endoscope may be necessary to visualize the frontal recess above and behind the axilla of the middle turbinate. A well-pneumatized agger nasi bone is favorable, as removal of the agger nasi cell and associated anterior cells permits the use of a less angled endoscope to visualize the frontal recess. However, if cells extend well above the nasal beak area, then dissection becomes more challenging. Supra-agger cells

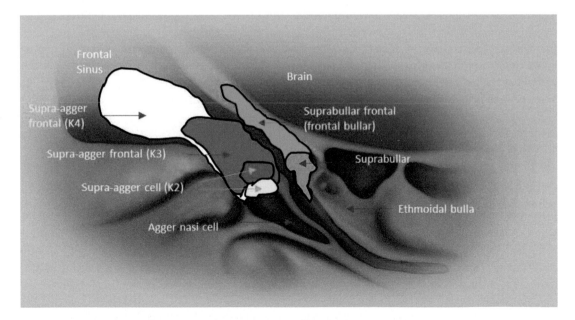

Fig. 6.8 Frontoethmoidal cells: The cells that lie anterior to the frontal sinus drainage pathway are the agger nasi cell, the supra-agger cells [Kuhn Type 1 ("K1") or Kuhn Type 2 ("K2") cells], and the supra-agger frontal cells [Kuhn Type 3 ("K3") or Kuhn Type 4 ("K4") cells]. Cells that are posterior to the frontal sinus drainage pathway are the ethmoidal bulla (bulla ethmoidalis), supra-bulla (suprabullar) cells, and supra-bulla frontal (frontal bullar) cells

that lie below the level of the nasal beak (Kuhn Type 1 and Kuhn Type 2) may be relatively simple to address in the hands of experienced surgeons. Supra-agger frontal cells extend into the frontal sinus above the nasal beak area (Kuhn Type 3 and Kuhn Type 4 cells) and may need more technical skills, time, and experience to dissect. The frontal septal cell (interfrontal sinus septal) lies between the right and left frontal sinuses; this cell may need to be dissected to address disease or to create an adequate frontal sinusotomy.

Cells that are posterior to the frontal sinus drainage pathway are the ethmoidal bulla, supra-bulla (suprabullar) cells and supra-bulla frontal (frontal bullar) cells (Fig. 6.8). Widening the frontal recess when these cells are present may require resecting the anterior wall of the posteriorly based cells using delicate angled cutting forceps or by curetting from a posterior-to-anterior direction from within the cells toward the frontal recess. In general, when dissecting frontoethmoidal cells, the goal of a surgical maneuver is to dissect away from the frontal recess so as to avoid mucosal injury and impaction of the outflow tract with bone fragments. However, in the presence of supra-bulla cells and supra-bulla frontal (frontal bullar) cells, dissection toward the frontal recess may become necessary to avoid injury to the skull base. Alternatively, the cells may be collapsed posteriorly toward the skull base, but this maneuver must be executed with extreme delicacy to avoid untoward complications.

When ethmoidal cells posterior to the frontal recess extend superolaterally to pneumatize the frontal plate above the orbit, they are called supraorbital ethmoid cells (Fig. 6.9). Supraorbital cells lie posterior and lateral to the true frontal sinuses. Multiple supraorbital cells can be present, and both anterior and posterior ethmoidal cells can pneumatize over the orbit. Each of these cells has a separate opening into the superior ethmoidal space, separated from each other by partitions which may need to be dissected. The most anterior supraorbital cell is separated from the frontal sinus by a partition, and its opening is posterior and lateral to the true frontal

sinus opening. In this situation, the anterior ethmoidal artery usually lies behind the first supra-orbital cell opening.

In summary, the frontoethmoidal cells influence the frontal sinus drainage path and can make surgical dissection more demanding. Predominance or pneumatization of medial cells pushes the frontal sinus drainage laterally, and conversely lateral frontoethmoidal cells push the sinus drainage pathway medially. The presence of frontoethmoidal cells posterior to the frontal recess will push the frontal sinus drainage pathway anteriorly, whereas prominent anterior cells conversely will push it posteriorly. The use of navigation systems may be helpful not only during intraoperative dissection but also importantly in preoperative planning. When surgical navigation is not available, other techniques can offer confirmation of successful entry into the frontal sinus. A mini-trephination through a small stab incision in the brow can serve as a portal for the frontal sinus to be flushed with saline irrigant; endoscopic confirmation of the egress of irrigant within the frontal recess can localize the frontal sinus drainage pathway. Transillumination is another option to distinguish frontoethmoidal cells from the frontal sinus. The true frontal sinus brilliantly transilluminates the forehead, whereas the frontoethmoidal cell transillumination is fainter and located closer to the medial canthal area (Fig. 6.10).

Intraoperative Preparation for Optimizing Surgical Field

The time before actual surgery is initiated is used for optimizing the surgical field. In the preoperative area, the patient is asked to spray a decongestant nasal spray (oxymetazoline hydrochloride 0.05%), two sprays in each nostril every 15 min for three times. Intraoperatively, a mean arterial pressure (MAP) of 55–70 mm Hg and a heart rate under 60 per min are aimed for, should the patient's general health and anesthetic techniques permit [27]. Figure 6.11 shows the setup in the operating room. The monitor is positioned across the surgeon, and a slave monitor is positioned

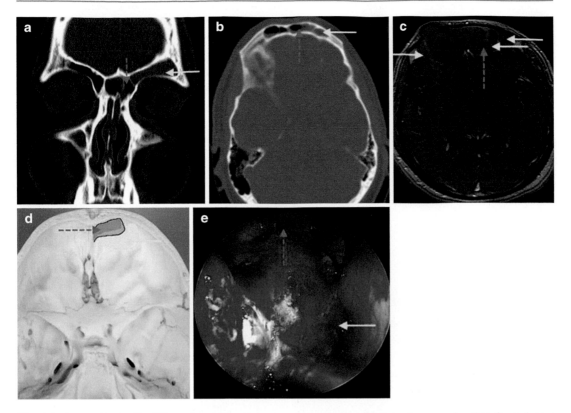

Fig. 6.9 Supraorbital cells: When ethmoidal cells posterior to the frontal recess pneumatize the orbital roof, they form supraorbital cell(s). (**a**) The presence pf a "partitioned" frontal sinus on a coronal CT scan should raise the possibility of a supraorbital cell (yellow arrow). (**b**) On axial CT scan, the supraorbital cell (yellow arrow) lies posterior and lateral to the true frontal sinus (blue dashed arrow). Images A and B belong to a patient who had two prior endoscopic frontal sinusotomy procedures and a frontal trephination procedure to address disease believed to lie in the frontal sinus; the presence of the supraorbital cell was not understood, leading to surgical failure. (**c**) Multiple supraorbital cells can be present, and both anterior and posterior ethmoidal cells can pneumatize over orbital roof. The MRI scan shows the presence of bilateral mucoceles that formed as a complication of prior frontal sinus obliteration. There are two supraorbital cell mucoceles (yellow arrows) on the left side and one on the right side. (**d**) Schematic showing the axial relationship of the frontal sinus (blue) and the supraorbital cell (yellow). Each supraorbital ethmoidal cell has its own opening into the nose. (**e**) A 70-degree endoscopy view of the left side; dissection of the frontal recess and supraorbital cell demonstrating that the frontal sinus (blue arrow) lies anterior and medial to the first supraorbital cell (yellow arrow). The suction tip is pointing at the location of the anterior ethmoidal artery, which usually lies behind the first supraorbital cell and not in the partition between the frontal sinus and the first supraorbital cell

across the surgical technician who is assisting. The patient is positioned supine with the head elevated 10–20° or in the "beach chair" position. This position reduces the MAP and central venous pressure and can reduce mucosal bleeding [28, 29]. The authors also use topical epinephrine pledgets (1:1000 concentration for healthy adult patients). To prevent accidental injection, this solution is always stained yellow with fluorescein dye (fluorescein eye strip), and all solutions on the field are labeled. Some surgeons use oxymetazoline hydrochloride 0.05% or 4% cocaine pledgets instead of epinephrine [30]. Prior to starting surgery, pledgets soaked with vasoconstrictor are placed in the nose with the help of a headlight or, preferably, under endoscopic visualization. Any bleeding due to mucosal trauma even at the time of placement of pledgets can significantly impact the surgical field, slow down surgery, and lead to poorer healing.

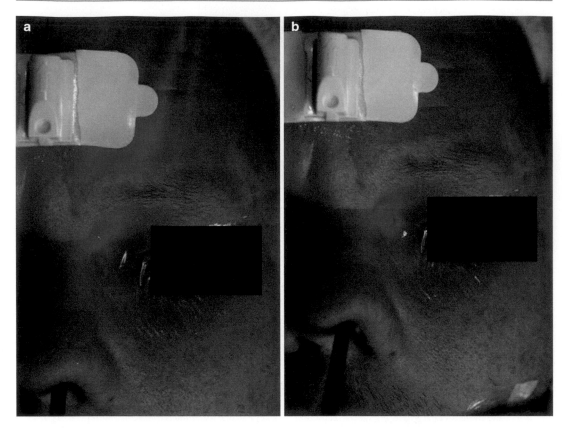

Fig. 6.10 Transillumination can be very helpful to confirm that the true frontal sinus has been dissected. Visualization of the frontal sinus with an angled endo- scopic brilliantly transilluminates the forehead (**a**), whereas the frontoethmoidal cell transillumination is fainter and confined to the medial canthal area (**b**)

The authors also have access to unipolar and bipolar cautery in the operating room. The range of hemodynamic metrics and dosages of medications that are presented here are for healthy adult patients; necessary modifications should be made for pediatric and high-risk populations [30].

Intraoperative Review of Sinus CT Scan

Frontal sinus surgery must not be performed if relevant CT images are not available in the operating room for review preoperatively as well as during surgery. Once pledgets have been placed intranasally, the authors spend the next 10–15 min reviewing the relevant anatomy on the sinus CT scan, as well as calibrating and verifying the navigation system (if being used); this period allows time for the decongestant to act on the nose and is also critical for developing a surgical plan. The superior uncinate attachment(s) and the frontal recess drainage pathway are studied, along with relationships of the relevant ethmoidal cells (Fig. 6.12). The three-dimensional anatomy of the frontal sinus drainage pathway is conceptualized by studying fine cut CT images in all three planes (coronal, sagittal, and axial). A mental three-dimensional rendering can be facilitated by use of the software for navigation systems. In revision surgery, causes of failure of prior surgery are also evaluated such as middle

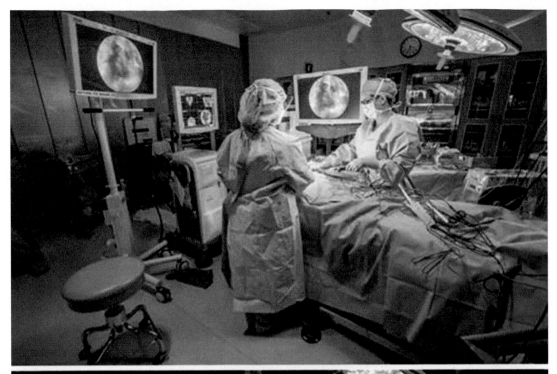

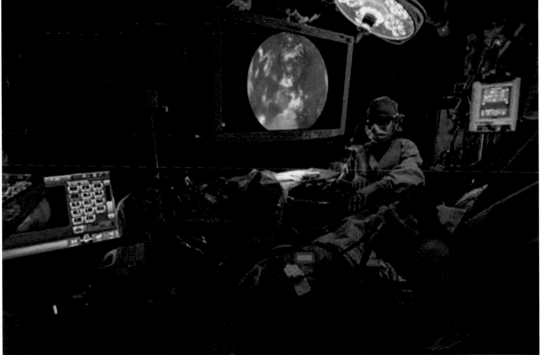

Fig. 6.11 Setup in the operating room showing positioning of two video monitors, as well as the navigation system. The surgeon should maximize ergonomics with the location of monitors and their own posture during surgery

Uncinate Process   Cap of Agger Nasi Cell

Anterior face of Ethmoidal Bulla   Frontal Ostium

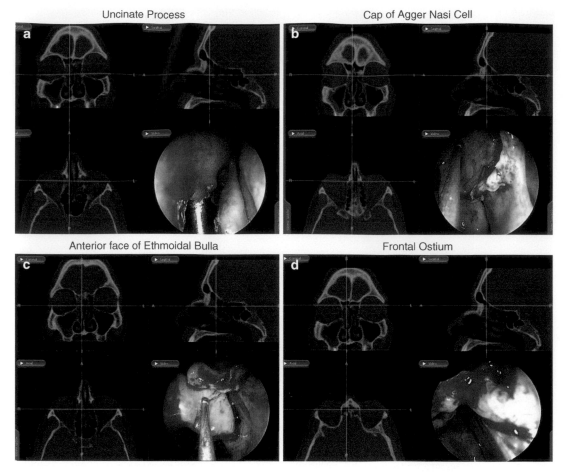

Fig. 6.12 The surgeon should learn to recognize the radiographic correlate of endoscopic anatomy on axial, coronal, and sagittal views; navigation system software can be very helpful for this process. In the following pictures, the probe points to the endoscopic landmark and the green crosshairs depict the radiographic correlate. (**a**) Right uncinate process. (**b**) Cap of the right agger nasi. (**c**) Anterior face of ethmoidal bulla. (**d**) Frontal ostium; the frontal recess lies inferior to the frontal ostium, between the agger nasi cell and the anterior face of the ethmoidal bulla

meatal scarring, lateralized middle turbinate, residual ethmoidal cells, recurrence of polyps, or osteoneogenesis. Table 6.3 lists the factors studied by the editors on the sinus CT scan. Next, the steps of dissection are planned. These include possible performance of a septoplasty to optimize visualization, instrumentation, and postoperative access, as well as the approach and sequence in which frontoethmoidal structures will be addressed.

Correlating CT Images with Endoscopic Anatomy

Once surgical dissection is initiated, the surgeon must correlate the understanding of the radiographic sinus anatomy with anatomical structures as they come into view. The use of the image guidance system can help confirm endoscopic visualized anatomical landmarks, especially in cases with distorted anatomy and revision surgery

Table 6.3 Detailed review of frontal recess anatomy on sinus CT scan at the time of surgery

Anterior boundary (Ethmoidal cells)	Agger nasi cell: presence, size Presence and number of frontoethmoidal cells Type I–IV/supra-agger or supra-agger frontal cells Size and pneumatization of nasal beak area
Posterior boundary (Ethmoidal cells)	Ethmoidal bulla (bulla ethmoidalis) Presence of suprabullar recess or bulla lamella Presence of supra bulla ethmoidal cells Supra-bulla (suprabullar) cell (Supra-bulla frontal (frontal bullar) cell Supraorbital ethmoidal cells (posterolateral to frontal recess)
Lateral	Lamina papyracea Integrity Healed fractures and any herniation into ethmoid space Shape Relative position to maxillary wall (medial or lateral)
Medial	Middle turbinate Pneumatization (concha bullosa) Position (lateralization) Paradoxical curvature Hypertrophy or atrophy Integrity (previous resection – total or partial) Cribriform plate Integrity Height, slope, and symmetry of the cribriform plates (Keros classification) Anterior ethmoidal artery: position and if on mesentery Frontal septal cell (interfrontal septal cell)
Superior	Integrity, height, and slope of anterior ethmoid roof Integrity and slope of the posterior frontal table
Uncinate	May be medial or lateral to true frontal recess based on superior uncinate attachment

(Fig. 6.13). Wormald introduced the concept of anatomical blocks to facilitate the reconstruction of the frontal recess in three dimensions [20]. Nicolai and colleagues [19] have recently outlined an excellent methodology of radiologically reviewing and addressing the frontal sinus drain-age pathway by the "agger-bullar classification ("ABC")" methodology. This is discussed in Chap. 2. The authors use a combination of both techniques, as illustrated in our videos. After reviewing CT imaging in all planes, the basal lamella of the middle turbinate is marked (blue) on the sagittal plane. Next, the frontal sinus drainage pathway (dotted line) is identified. Lastly, cells anterior and posterior to the frontal sinus drainage pathway are identified, named, and counted. The cells or spaces anterior or posterior to the frontal sinus drainage pathway are numbered, starting with the most inferior cell, and these must all be identified and dissected during frontal sinusotomy. Figures 6.14, 6.15, and 6.16 present three cases which illustrate the use of the "ABC" methodology. We then study the superior attachment of the uncinate process (Fig. 6.5). This information is then used to form a detailed understanding of the relevant anatomy to approach the frontal sinus dissection (Fig. 6.17), as illustrated in Video 6.1.

Extent of Frontal Sinus Surgery: Overview of the "Draf" Procedures

A commonly utilized classification on the extent of frontal sinus surgery is named after Prof. Wolfgang Draf, who developed micro-endoscopic procedures to establish frontal sinus drainage. Draf classified these procedures into three categories based on the extent of surgery on the frontal ostium and the frontal sinus floor. Draf I, Draf II, and Draf III techniques are further detailed in Table 6.4. The Draf III operation is also referred to as the endoscopic modified Lothrop procedure (EMLP), as it is the endoscopic adaptation of a procedure first described by Dr. Harold Lothrop in 1914 [31].

Prof. Draf described the Type I frontal sinusotomy to consist of removal of "obstructing disease inferior to the frontal ostium" [2]. The anterosuperior ethmoidal cells obstructing the frontonasal outflow tract in the frontal recess are removed without altering the frontal sinus ostium. This is the least aggressive of the frontal sinusotomy techniques in that it just exposes the fron-

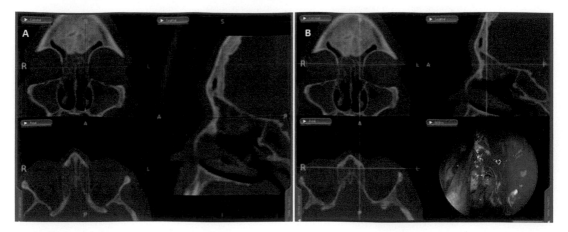

Fig. 6.13 Once the surgeon becomes familiar with the radiographic correlates, the sinus CT scan is studied in axial, coronal, and sagittal planes prior to surgery; this allows the surgeon to anticipate endoscopically viewed anatomy. (**a**) Scan studied in the planning phase showing the left uncinate process to attach to the skull base. (**b**) Intraoperatively, this radiographic analysis is endorsed by the endoscopic view

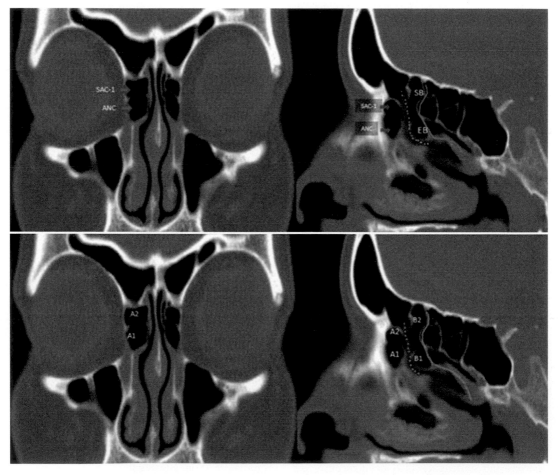

Fig. 6.14 Case 1: Radiographic review of right frontal sinus drainage pathway (yellow dotted line on sagittal views). The blue line marks the basal lamella of the middle turbinate (sagittal views). Top panel: Anteriorly, the patient has a large agger nasi cell (ANC) and a small supra-agger cell (SAC-1). Posteriorly, the frontal sinus drainage pathway is bound by a small ethmoidal bulla (EB) and a large supra-bulla cell. The bottom panel shows the "ABC" methodology; this patient has two anterior (A1, A2) and two posterior (B1, B2) cells or spaces that need to be dissected

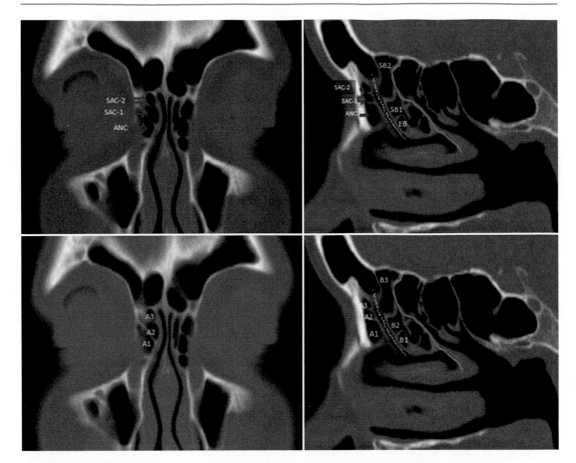

Fig. 6.15 Case 2: Radiographic review of right frontal sinus drainage pathway (dotted line on sagittal views). The blue line marks the basal lamella of the middle turbinate on sagittal views. Top panel: Anteriorly, the patient has a moderately sized agger nasi cell (ANC) and two small supra-agger cell (SAC-1, SAC-2). Posteriorly, the frontal sinus drainage pathway is bound by a small ethmoidal bulla (EB) and two supra-bulla cells (or space; SB1, SB2). The bottom panel shows the "ABC" methodology; this patient has three anterior (A1, A2, A3) and three posterior (B1, B2, B3) cells or spaces that need to be dissected

tal ostium without any actual manipulation (Fig. 6.18). The Draf II frontal sinusotomy comprises of formal enlargement of the frontal sinus ostium or outflow tract. This is further subclassified. The Draf Type IIA involves removal of those ethmoidal cells that intrude superior to the frontal ostium into the frontal sinus (frontal infundibulum) in addition to the Draf I procedure which involves removal of cells occupying the frontal recess (the part of the frontal sinus drainage pathway inferior to the frontal ostium) (Fig. 6.19). This maneuver results in enlarging the frontal drainage pathway, bounded laterally by the lamina papyracea and medially by the middle turbi-

nate. Dissection of frontoethmoidal cells in Draf I and Draf IIA procedures has also been described as the technique of "uncapping the egg" by Prof. Heinz Stammberger [1]. The Draf Type IIB drainage involves further medial resection of the frontal sinus floor to extend the medial boundary of the frontal sinusotomy to the nasal or interfrontal sinus septum, thereby creating a unilateral frontal sinusotomy with the widest width, extending from the lamina papyracea to the nasal or interfrontal sinus septum (Fig. 6.20). The Draf Type III frontal sinusotomy (endoscopic modified Lothrop procedure) creates a common drainage pathway of both the frontal

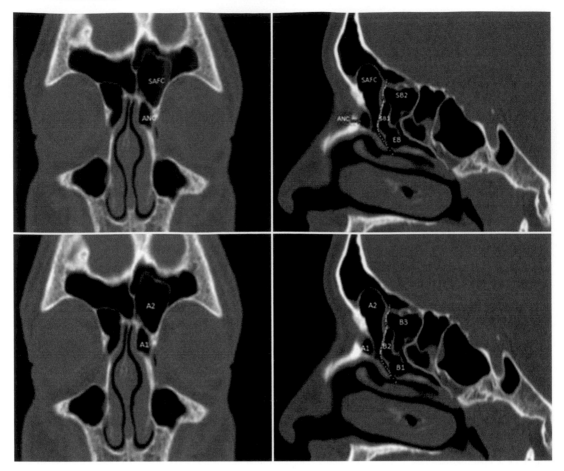

Fig. 6.16 Case 3: Radiographic review of left frontal sinus drainage pathway (yellow dotted line on sagittal views). The blue line marks the basal lamella of the middle turbinate on sagittal views. Top panel: Anteriorly, the patient has a small agger nasi cell (ANC) and a very large supra-agger frontal cell (SAC-1). The supra-agger frontal cell will require additional time and skill for dissection. Posteriorly, the frontal sinus drainage pathway is bound by a small ethmoidal bulla (EB) and two supra-bulla cells (or space; SB1, SB2). The bottom panel shows the "ABC" methodology; this patient has two anterior (A1, A2) and three posterior (B1, B2) cells or spaces that need to be dissected

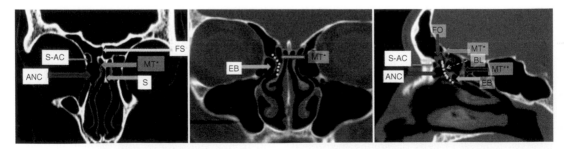

Fig. 6.17 CT review: The radiographic anatomy of the frontal sinus drainage pathway (broken yellow line) should be carefully reviewed and mentally labeled. Coronal and parasagittal CT images are presented here. The bright green arrow points to the bulla ethmoidalis (BE), dashed white arrow to the bulla lamella (Bl), and brown arrow to the agger nasi cell (ANC). The pink arrow points to the anterior vertical attachment of the middle turbinate (MT*), while the blue arrow points to the basal lamella (second part) of the middle turbinate (MT**). The frontal ostium (FO, red dumbbell) is pointed to by the red arrow. The orange arrow points to the supra-agger cell (S-AC). The ridged yellow arrow points to the interfrontal sinus septum (FS) and the light green arrow to the nasal septum (S)

Table 6.4 Endoscopic techniques in frontal sinus surgery

Procedure	Description
Draf I	Removal of ethmoidal partitions inferior to the frontal ostium (frontal recess) without formal instrumentation of the frontal ostium
Draf II	Complete removal of all anterior ethmoidal cells with formal instrumentation of the frontal ostium area
Draf IIA	Enlargement of the entire frontal drainage pathway to create a frontal ostioplasty extending laterally to the lamina papyracea and medially to the middle turbinate
Draf II B	The Draf Type IIA sinusotomy is further extended to a Draf IIB by further medial resection of the frontal sinus floor until the nasal or interfrontal septum. This extends the frontal ostioplasty from the lamina papyracea laterally to the nasal/ interfrontal septum medially. The procedure thereby creates a unilateral frontal ostioplasty with the widest width
Draf III (endoscopic modified Lothrop procedure)	Creation of a common drainage pathway for both frontal sinuses (and associated frontoethmoidal cells) into the nasal cavity. The technique involves removal of bilateral frontal sinus floor, all associated frontoethmoidal cells, interfrontal sinus septum, and adjacent superior nasal septum
"Above and below" technique	An endoscopic frontal ostioplasty supplemented by a frontal sinus external trephination
Balloon-assisted frontal sinusotomy	Use of a balloon as a standalone technique to dilate the frontal recess or to assist with conventional endoscopic frontal surgery

sinus (and associated frontoethmoidal cells) into the nasal cavity. This is achieved by removal of the frontal sinus floor on both sides between the lamina papyraceae along with resection of the interfrontal septum and cells and resection of the adjacent superior nasal septum. By marsupializing both frontal sinuses into one common cavity, the procedure creates maximal width possible, with the limits of the neo-ostium defined by the orbits laterally, the skull base posteriorly and the anterior frontal table anteriorly (Fig. 6.21).

Basic Steps in Endoscopic Frontal Recess Dissection

Surgical dissection of the frontal recess can be undertaken in several different ways. However, there are some universal principles that should be followed. Meticulous dissection with mucosal preservation in the frontal recess is critical to success. The surgeon must have access to specialized instrumentation specifically designed for frontal sinus surgery as discussed in Chap. 6. Figure 6.22a–d illustrates the basic frontal instrumentation in common use. Through-cutting instruments and powered microdebriders should be used to sharply cut mucosa without stripping it from the underlying orbit or skull base bone. Uncontrolled mucosal stripping and unnecessary exposure of bony surfaces predispose to reactive inflammation that can induce postoperative stenosis [3]. In general, one should aim for a minimum frontal sinusotomy diameter of 5 mm. We outline the basic steps in frontal recess dissection and the rationale for the technique commonly employed by the authors.

1. The patient is positioned and draped for endoscopic sinus surgery. The eyes are taped and draped into the field. Eyes are inspected and frequently palpated during surgery to ensure that there is no orbital hematoma. Palpation of the orbit can also help to delineate bony dehiscences of the lamina papyracea, as movement of displaced orbital contents may be visible in the ethmoidal and frontal dissection field.

2. Reverse-angled endoscopes can be useful for frontal sinus surgery (Fig. 6.23); the posts of the endoscope and the lens face in the same direction. This allows for freer range of movement for instrumentation and is also helpful when binarial four-hand instrumentation is needed.

3. Prior to any dissection, endoscopy and identification of visible structures and landmarks are conducted. In primary frontal sinus surgery, the uncinate process, the anterior maxillary line, the middle turbinate, the axilla of

Draf I

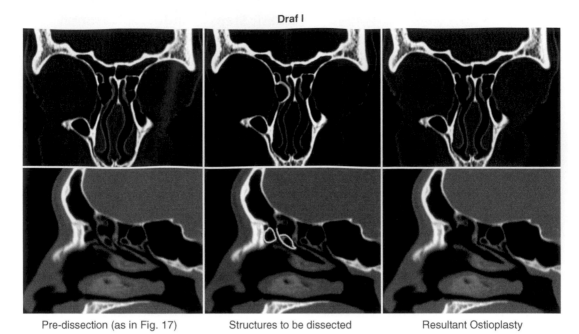

Pre-dissection (as in Fig. 17)   Structures to be dissected   Resultant Ostioplasty

Fig. 6.18 The Draf I procedure involves removal of "obstructing disease inferior to the frontal ostium." The anterosuperior ethmoidal cells obstructing the frontonasal outflow tract are removed to expose the frontal ostium without any actual manipulation. The schematic diagram shows the extent of resection of structures. Please refer to Fig. 6.17 for detailed labeling

Draf IIA

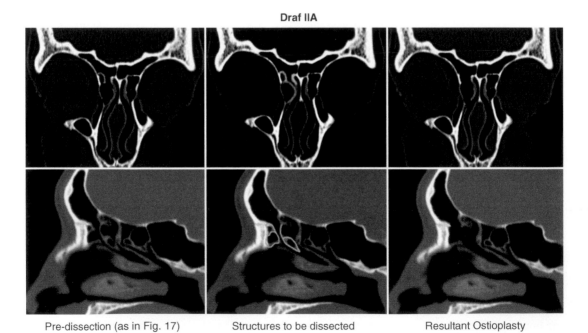

Pre-dissection (as in Fig. 17)   Structures to be dissected   Resultant Ostioplasty

Fig. 6.19 Draf II A procedure involves removal of those ethmoidal cells that intrude superior to the frontal ostium into the frontal sinus (i.e., the frontal infundibulum) in addition to the Draf I procedure which involves removal of cells occupying the frontal recess. The schematic diagram shows the extent of resection of structures as outlined in color. Please refer to Fig. 6.17 for detailed labeling

Draf IIB

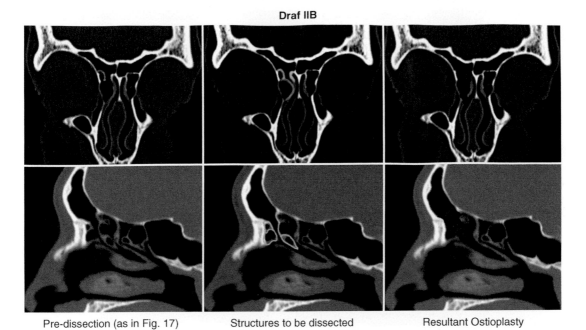

Pre-dissection (as in Fig. 17)   Structures to be dissected   Resultant Ostioplasty

Fig. 6.20 Draf IIB procedure further medial resection of the frontal sinus floor to extend the medial boundary of the frontal sinusotomy to the nasal septum, thereby creating a unilateral frontal sinusotomy with the widest width, extending from lamina papyracea to the nasal septum. The schematic diagram shows the extent of resection of structures. Please refer to Fig. 6.17 for detailed labeling

Draf IIIB

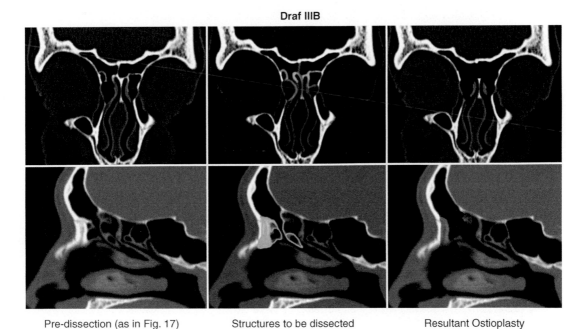

Pre-dissection (as in Fig. 17)   Structures to be dissected   Resultant Ostioplasty

Fig. 6.21 Draf III procedure involves removal of the frontal sinus floor on both sides between the lamina papyraceae along with resection of the interfrontal septum and cells and resection of the adjacent superior nasal septum. The schematic diagram shows the extent of resection of structures. Please refer to Fig. 6.17 for detailed labeling

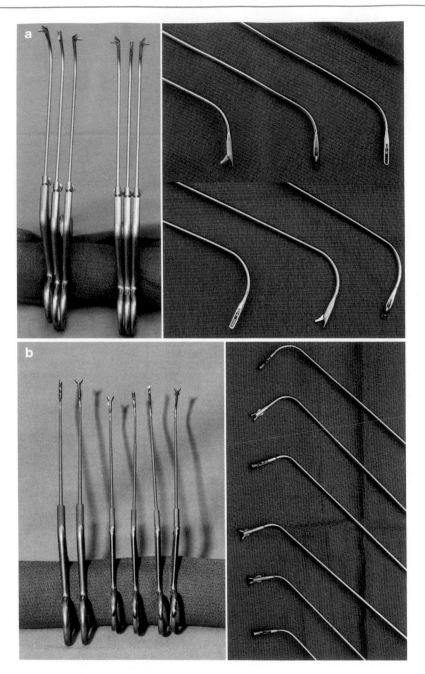

Fig. 6.22 Some basic frontal instrumentation. (**a**) Cutting giraffe instruments (45° and 90°) of different lengths. (**b**) Angled (45°, 60°, and 90°) giraffe instruments with cups (non-cutting) of different lengths. (**c**) Kerrison punches (a) and mushroom punches (b) of different sizes and lengths. (**d**) (a) Curettes of different angles (45°, 60°, and 90°); (**b**) frontal seekers in different lengths, angles (45°, 60°, and 90°), and directions. (c) Angled several angled suction tips of several sizes and a malleable suction that can be curved into the desired angle. (d) Microdebriders with different angled blades (40°, 60°) and sizes (2.9 mm, 4 mm)

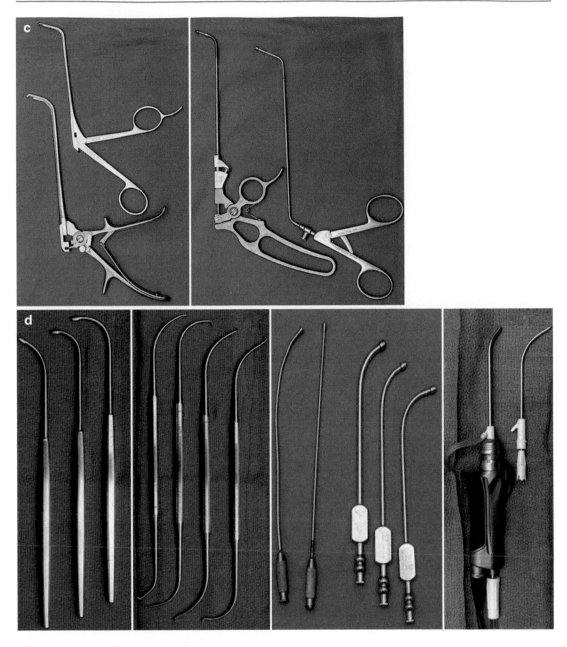

Fig. 6.22 (continued)

the middle turbinate, the ethmoidal bulla, the hiatus semilunaris, and the infundibulum are identified (Fig. 6.24). In revision frontal sinus procedures, the surgeon identifies remnants of the above structures (if any). In revision surgery where many of the structures have been lost, identifying the area of the anterior maxillary line/nasolacrimal duct, orbital floor, lamina papyracea, skull base, and residual ethmoidal structures becomes essential (Fig. 6.25). In revision surgery, causes of failure of prior surgery are also evaluated; these include middle meatal scarring, lateralized middle turbinate, residual

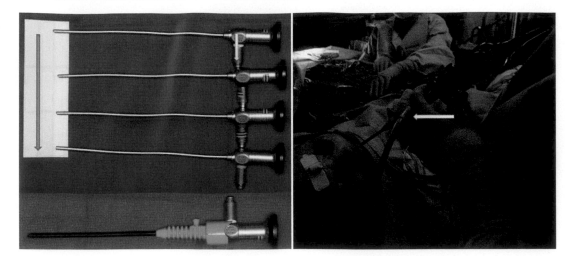

Fig. 6.23 Reverse-angled endoscopes facilitate frontal sinus surgery. The green arrows point to the direction of the post of the endoscope; in reverse-angled endoscopes, the post points to the direction of the lens used for visualization of the frontal sinuses (arrows). Reverse-angled Endo-Scrub sheaths are available for these endoscopes. The use of reverse-angled endoscopes helps keeps the light and camera cords away from the nostrils, facilitating instrumentation and binarial four-hand surgery

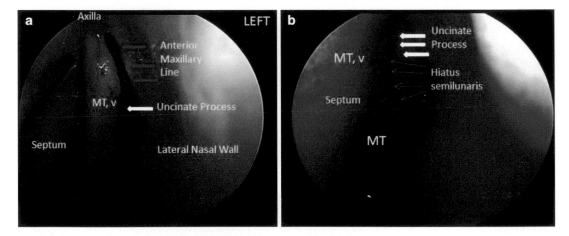

Fig. 6.24 Endoscopic landmarks for primary frontal sinus surgery primary for the left side are depicted. MT middle turbinate, MTv vertical part of the middle turbinate

ethmoidal cells, polyps, osteoneogenesis, tumor, etc. which are also identified.

4. The axilla of the middle turbinate is infiltrated with approximately 1 cc solution of lidocaine 1% epinephrine with 1:100,000 (Video 6.2). Squeeze-dried pledgets soaked in epinephrine 1:1000 are then placed in the middle meatus and the axilla of the middle meatus (Fig. 6.26). A 1 cm "relaxing" inci- sion in the basal lamella of middle turbinate medial to the ethmoidal bulla can help keep the middle turbinate medial and assist with visualization (video 6.3) [32].

5. If all paranasal sinuses are being addressed surgically, the authors undertake frontal recess dissection after maxillary antrostomy and spheno-ethmoidectomy have been completed. The most superior aspects of the

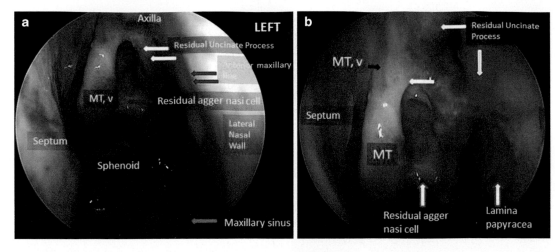

Fig. 6.25 Endoscopic landmarks for a patient requiring revision left frontal sinus surgery are depicted. MT middle turbinate, MTv vertical part of the middle turbinate. The vertical stub of the middle turbinate is its only remnant. The anterior and inferior parts of the agger nasi cell have also been previously removed

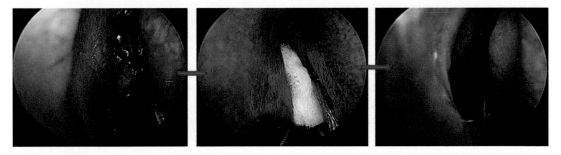

Fig. 6.26 Use of topical vasoconstrictor pledgets can significantly improve the surgical field. This is evident when comparing the pre-decongestion field (first image) with the post-decongestion state (third image) following placement of decongestant pledgets in the right middle meatus (center image)

uncinate process and ethmoidal bulla are preserved to assist with identification of the frontal recess pathway (Fig. 6.27). This sequence allows for identification of the lamina papyracea and ethmoidal skull base. By identifying the lamina papyracea early, inadvertent orbital penetration can be avoided.

6. If only frontal sinus dissection is to be undertaken, we proceed as follows: Using a zero-degree endoscope, a maxillary sinus seeker is introduced via the hiatus semilunaris into the ethmoidal infundibulum. The uncinate process is gently medialized to create distance from the orbit, and this maneuver also helps identify the anterior attachment of the uncinate process at the anterior maxillary line. The anterior maxillary line is the anterior limit of dissection to prevent injury to the nasolacrimal duct. Next, a retrograde uncinectomy is initiated via a pediatric backbiter at the junction of the upper two-thirds and the lower one-third of the vertical uncinate process, and the mid-third of the uncinate is then removed (Fig. 6.28). Starting the uncinectomy low and not blindly pushing into the infundibulum prevents inadvertent orbital penetration. Because the ethmoidal bulla and bulla lamella serve as the posterior limit of the frontal recess, it is not necessary to open the ethmoidal bulla prior to dissecting the frontal recess. This "intact bulla" technique offers a directed approach to

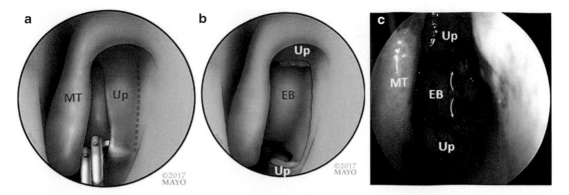

Fig. 6.28 (a) Schematic of the left middle meatus. The ethmoid infundibulum lies lateral to the uncinate process (Up). (a) The tine of the pediatric bite-biter lies lateral to the uncinate process (Up) in the ethmoidal infundibulum (EI). (b) The middle third of the left uncinate process has been removed to open the ethmoidal infundibulum (EI). (c) Endoscopic correlate of the schematic; the yellow arrows point to the superior and inferior aspects of the ethmoidal infundibulum lateral to the uncinate remnant. MT middle turbinate, EB ethmoidal bulla

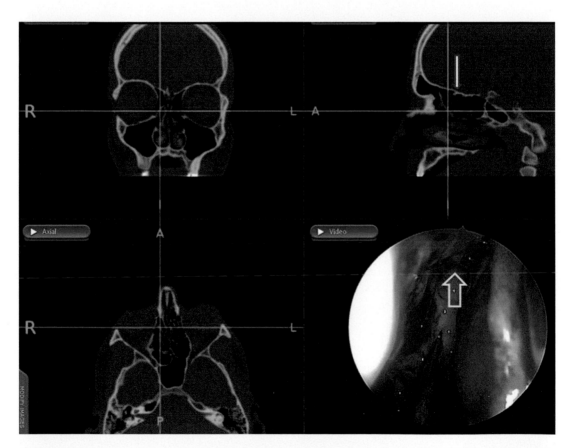

Fig. 6.29 Intact bulla technique: Because the ethmoidal bulla and bulla lamella serve as the posterior limit of the frontal recess, it is not necessary to open the ethmoidal bulla prior to dissecting the frontal recess. The navigation probe on the endoscopic image is laid on the anterior face of the ethmoidal bulla, and the yellow arrow points to the right frontal ostioplasty performed with the intact bulla technique. The green crosshairs on the radiographic triplanar views demonstrate that the intact bulla technique helps keep dissection anterior to the vulnerable lateral lamella of the cribriform plate, as well as the anterior ethmoidal artery (white arrow)

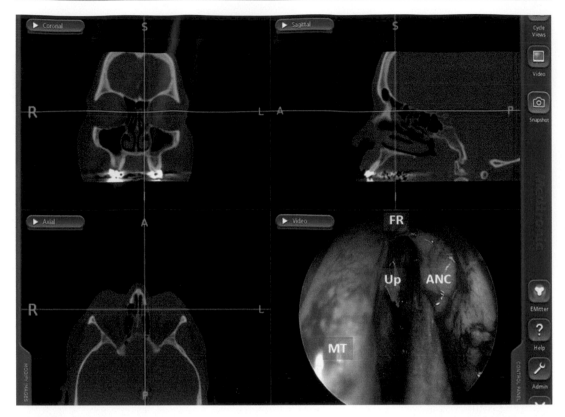

Fig. 6.30 The left uncinate process attaches superiorly to the skull base. Using the uncinate as guide for frontal recess dissection, the probe is passed lateral to the uncinate process and freely passes through the frontal ostium, as shown on the triplanar navigation imaging. Up uncinate process, MT middle turbinate, ANC agger nasi cell, FR frontal recess

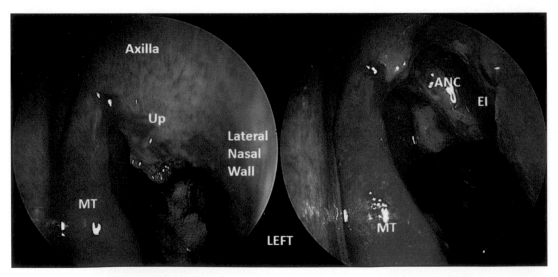

Fig. 6.31 Once spheno-ethmoidectomy has been concluded, the remnant uncinate and the area of the ethmoidal infundibulum are studied. The removal of the superior aspect of the uncinate process exposes the superior part of the ethmoidal infundibulum. Up uncinate process, MT middle turbinate, ANC agger nasi cell, EI ethmoidal infundibulum

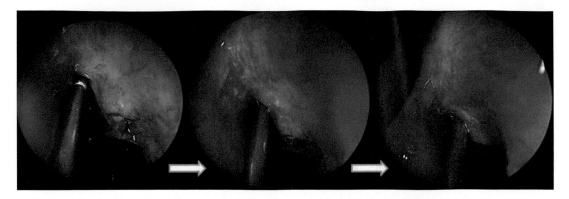

Fig. 6.32 When the uncinate attaches laterally to the lamina papyracea or ethmoidal bulla (first image), a probe advanced medial to the uncinate process will pass through the frontal recess between the superior attachment of the uncinate and the lateral lamella of the cribriform plate (second image). The probe must pass freely and without obstruction to confirm that it has entered the frontal ostium area (third image)

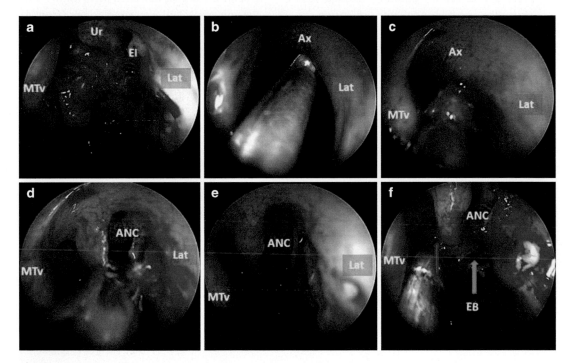

Fig. 6.33 Alternatively, using the zero-degree endoscopes, the superior part of the uncinate is removed to expose the superior aspect of the ethmoidal infundibulum (**a**). Next, the axilla of the middle turbinate is removed with a Kerrison rongeur (**b**, **c**), exposing the anterior wall of the agger nasi cell (**d**). Then the anterior wall and the inferior part of the agger nasi cell are removed (Fig. **e**). The frontal recess lies between the anterior face of the ethmoidal bulla and the posterior wall of the agger nasi cell (**f**). Ur, uncinate remnant; EI, ethmoidal infundibulum; Lat lateral nasal wall, ANC agger nasi cell, EB ethmoidal bulla, MT middle turbinate, MTv vertical part of the middle turbinate, Ax axilla. The left side is being dissected

bone can be drilled out to allow for a similar visualization [33]. It is not the authors' usual process to raise axillary flaps or drill the agger bone. However, when the agger nasi is well pneumatized, we do favor resecting the axilla with through-cutting forceps or rongeurs to improve visualization of the frontal recess and to facilitate dissection with less angled endoscopes and instruments. Removing the agger nasi cell early can also be used to perform an "intact bulla" frontal recess dissection, although clinical indications for this particular technique are for limited.

9. Next, the cap of the agger nasi cell is removed with a curved frontal curette by placing the curette carefully behind and above the agger nasi cell and collapsing the cell with an anteriorly and inferiorly directed trajectory ("uncapping the egg") (Fig. 6.34b,

c). The frontal sinus drainage pathway can be opened by completely removing the superior attachment of the uncinate process. Angled frontal giraffe instruments and the microdebrider are useful for this step (Fig. 6.34c, d). If supra-agger or supra-agger frontal cells are present, these must be identified (Fig. 6.34d). The frontal probe will not pass freely superiorly in the presence of these cells as it hits their cap and stops (Fig. 6.34e). The supra-agger cells and supra-agger frontal cells are removed sequentially, in a similar fashion to removal of agger nasi cell; these may require the use of 70-degree endoscope and more angled instruments (Fig. 6.35a–f; Video 6.5). The frontal ostium is identified after removal of the agger nasi cell, any supra-agger (frontal) cells, and superior uncinate attachments (Fig. 6.35f).

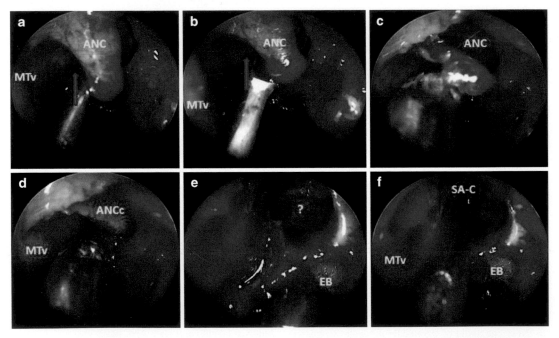

Fig. 6.34 A 30-degree endoscope and 45-degree frontal sinus seeker can be used to probe and identify the drainage pathway (**a**). Again, this must be done without any force, and the probe must never be pushed through a bony partition. (**b**) The agger nasi cell is pushed laterally, and then its cap is removed with the help of a curette (**b**) and microdebrider (**c, d**). (**e**) A large cell is encountered and may be confused with the frontal sinus. However,

figure **f** shows that the frontal probe stops after hitting the cap; this cell is therefore unlikely to be the true frontal sinus and is likely a supra-agger frontal cell (SA-C). EI ethmoidal infundibulum, Lat lateral nasal wall, ANC agger nasi cell, EB ethmoidal bulla, MT middle turbinate, MTv vertical part of the middle turbinate, Ax axilla, EB ethmoidal bulla. The left side is being dissected

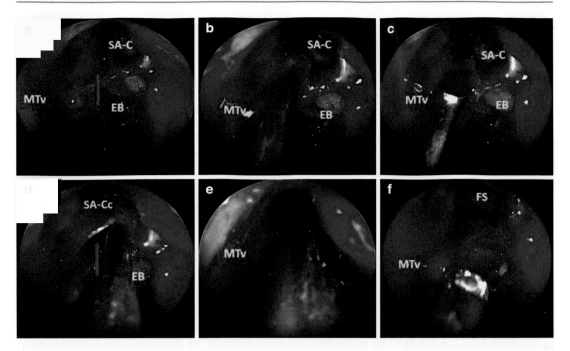

Fig. 6.35 The supra-agger cell is pushed laterally, (**a**) and then its cap is removed with the help of a curette (**b**) and microdebrider (**c, d**) similar to removal of the agger nasi cell. This brings into view the true frontal sinus. SA-C supra-agger frontal cell, EB ethmoidal bulla, MTv vertical part of the middle turbinate, EB ethmoidal bulla, FS frontal sinus. The left side is being dissected

10. The next step is removal of the ethmoidal partitions in the posterior aspect of the frontal recess (Fig. 6.36a–d, video 6.5) to conclude the dissection of the frontal sinus (Fig. 6.36e). These posteriorly based partitions may comprise portions of the bulla ethmoidalis, supra-bulla cell, or supra-bulla frontal cell. The ethmoidal skull base is easily identified in the posterior ethmoidal complex. The attachment of the basal lamella of the middle turbinate is then sharply dissected with through-cutting instruments. When dissecting the medial part of all superior ethmoidal cells, it is important to first identify the lateral lamella of the cribriform plate. The position of the anterior ethmoidal artery is carefully noted, and diligence is exercised when dissecting in this area. The artery is usually separated from the frontal ostium by a suprabullar recess or cell (Fig. 6.7). A curved frontal curette and frontal through-cutting instruments and 40-degree microde-

brider are used to carefully remove these ethmoidal partitions up to the area of the frontal ostium (Fig. 6.36).

11. Removal of all relevant ethmoidal partitions inferior to the frontal ostium concludes performance of a Draf Type I frontal sinusotomy (Video 6.1). If the area of the frontal ostium is formally widened by removal of the nasal beak and by widening the ostioplasty between the lamina papyracea laterally and the vertical attachment of the middle turbinate, then the ostioplasty is converted to a Draf IIA frontal sinusotomy. If ethmoidal partitions superior to the frontal recess are also removed, the Draf I is converted into the Draf IIA sinusotomy (Fig. 6.34, 6.35, and 6.36; Video 6.5).

12. If the ostioplasty is widened until the interfrontal septum or nasal septum by further removal to the frontal sinus floor medial to the vertical attachment of the middle turbinate, one then converts the Draf IIA procedure to Draf IIB procedure (Fig. 6.37a–c).

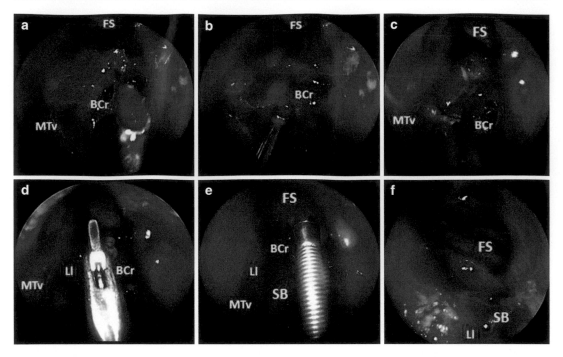

Fig. 6.36 The posterior frontal recess dissection is then performed by removing the remnant partitions of the bullar complex (**a–e**). Dissection must be performed with caution with visualization of the lateral lamella and the ethmoidal skull base. Through-cutting instruments, the angled microdebrider, and the mushroom punch are useful. The resultant ostioplasty (**f**) should have a smooth transition from the posterior frontal table to the anterior ethmoidal skull base. BCR bullar complex remnants, MTv vertical part of the middle turbinate, FS frontal sinus, SB skull base, Ll lateral lamella of the cribriform plate. The left side is being dissected

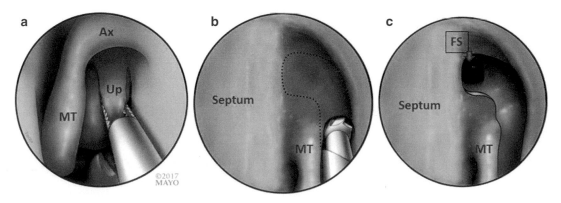

Fig. 6.37 Schematic showing a left Draf IIB procedure: if the Draf I or IIA ostioplasty (**a**) is widened to until the interfrontal septum or nasal septum. This is done by further removal of to the frontal sinus floor medial to the vertical attachment of the middle turbinate (**b, c**)

If there is extensive osteitis, severe inflammation, and extensive mucosal stripping found during a Draf IIA procedure, a Draf IIB procedure can be considered to maxi- mize the ostioplasty size and reduce the risk of stenosis. The Draf IIB procedure can be conducted with handheld instruments (Video 6.6). However, if thick bone is present in the nasal beak and floor area, use of a powered angle drill can help expedite the surgery (Video 6.7). Instruments that are useful for the Draf IIB procedure include the angled frontal mushroom punch and the angled frontal Kerrison rongeurs. Once a Draf IIA procedure has been completed, side-to-side angled frontal cutting instruments help precisely cut the vertical attachment of the middle turbinate that inserts on to the frontal sinus floor; the instrument should always be opened in a direction away from the skull base. Care must be undertaken not overshoot posteriorly past the frontal sinus floor as this can cause injury to the lateral lamella of the cribriform plate and result in a cerebrospinal fluid leak (Video 6.8). The angled mushroom punch, the angled Kerrison punch, or the powered drill can then be used to remove the frontal floor and nasal beak area. If bone of the nasal beak is demucosalized, the widest possible width in the anteroposterior (parasagittal) plane should be made, as bare bone is prone to osteitis and increased scarring. A mucosal graft or a stent (Silastic or drug-eluting) can also be considered.

13. Any pus or allergic mucin removed can be sent for bacteriologic and fungal cultures. Polyps can be removed using the 40- and 60-degree angled microdebriders. The head-rotatable microdebrider blades are useful for removing florid polyposis on the posterior frontal table. If there is minimal polypoid edema, this can be gently compressed to squeeze the fluid out, rather than removing the mucosa and risking inadvertent bone exposure. Polyps and tissue removed are sent for histopathological examination.

14. Gentle and copious irrigation of the frontal sinus is performed using a malleable suction to remove all bone chips, pus, and debris.

15. Hemostasis is achieved with the use of topical 1:1000 epinephrine and, where necessary, angled bipolar forceps.

16. At the conclusion of the procedure, if the middle turbinate shows a tendency toward lateralization, a medialization procedure can be performed. The medial aspect of the mid-

dle turbinate can be scarified to the septum after abrading the apposing areas of mucosa. The medialized position is held by placement of absorbable or nonabsorbable middle meatal spacers or sutures. The author uses a suture medialization technique (Video 6.9). Alternatives include trimming the anterior edge of the middle turbinate, especially when the turbinate has a paradoxical shape, or placing a middle meatal pack or stent to prevent middle turbinate lateralization.

Balloon-Assisted Frontal Sinusotomy

Balloon-assisted dilation is a technology that has become recently available for application in frontal sinus surgery. Balloon-assisted dilation of the frontal sinus drainage pathways can be performed to relieve ostial obstruction without removing tissue. Proponents cite advantages to include the mucosal-sparing approach, speedy healing, and decreased morbidity as well as its suitability for use in the office-based setting under local anesthesia. The frontal balloon can be used either as a tool for dissection during endoscopic frontal sinusotomy ("hybrid" technique; Video 6.10) or as a standalone tool. Chap. 10 details this technique.

Special Circumstances

1. Prudence must be exercised in dissection of ethmoidal partitions along the skull base, particularly when the anterior ethmoidal artery is exposed owing to extended pneumatization of the anterior ethmoid compartment. If the anterior ethmoid artery is injured and the lateral arterial stump retracts into the globe, it can result in a rapidly expanding orbital hematoma. If the artery is injured, it should be carefully cauterized both laterally and medially using bipolar cautery (Fig. 6.38). Use of a monopolar cautery can risk skull base injury and a cerebrospinal fluid leak.

2. When supra-agger cells are present, these can often be mistaken for the frontal sinus after

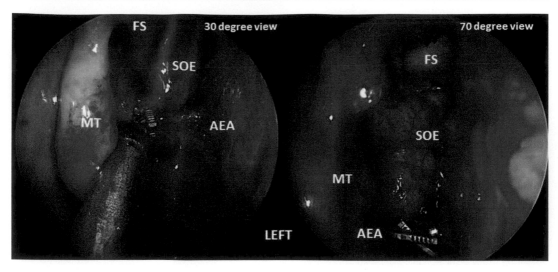

Fig. 6.38 Prudence must be exercised in dissection of partitions along the skull base, particularly when the anterior ethmoidal artery is exposed owing to extended pneumatization as in this patient with disease in the left supraorbital cell and frontal sinus. The anterior ethmoid artery was injured. Bleeding was quickly controlled with a bipolar cautery, and the arterial stump was clipped as well. FS frontal sinus, MT middle turbinate, SOE supraorbital ethmoidal cell, AEA anterior ethmoidal artery. The left side is being dissected

the agger nasi has been removed. By carefully reviewing the sagittal reconstructions of the frontal sinus on CT, one can anticipate the presence of these cells. The location of the supra-agger cells is always anterior and lateral to the true frontal sinus (Fig. 6.8). A 70-degree endoscope and 70–90-degree extended length frontal instruments may be necessary for high dissection (Video 6.5). Transillumination during dissection of these cells usually reveals a confined area of illumination around the medial canthal region. Once the true frontal sinus is opened, the full extent of the frontal sinus may be observed to be transilluminated (Fig. 6.10). Additionally, the visualization of a sagittal ridge in the roof of the sinus is also a good indication that the true frontal sinus has been opened up (Fig. 6.39); frontoethmoidal cells do not have these partitions. The use of computer-guided navigation can also help confirm the anatomical structures of the frontal recess and successful entry into the frontal sinus.

3. When supra-bulla frontal cells are present, the frontal ostium may not be visualized even after removal of the uncinate process and supra-agger cells. In this situation, the ethmoidal bulla has to be removed first, dissecting the skull base from a posterior to anterior direction. If a balloon-assisted surgery is being undertaken, the surgeon must be aware that the guidewire of the balloon may preferentially slide into a supra-bulla cell. If this cell is mistaken for the frontal sinus, not only will the true frontal sinus be missed, but anterior expansion from the balloon dilatation may collapse the cell supra-bulla frontal cell anteriorly, potentially exacerbating frontal sinus obstruction.

Draf III Approach (Endoscopic Modified Lothrop Operation)

The Draf Type III frontal sinusotomy (endoscopic modified Lothrop procedure) is used to create the widest possible common drainage pathway of bilateral frontal sinuses into the nasal cavity (Table 6.4). All associated frontoethmoidal cells are also incorporated into this common cavity (frontal septal cells, supra-agger frontal cells, supra-bulla frontal cells, etc.). This is achieved

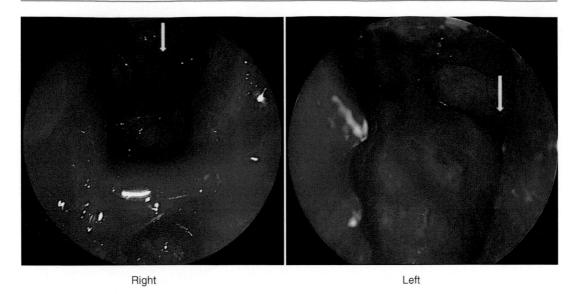

Right   Left

Fig. 6.39 Visualization of a sagittal ridge in the roof of the frontal sinus is also a good indication that the true frontal sinus has been opened up. The right and left frontal sinus are shown, with the arrow pointing to the ridges

by removal of the frontal sinus floor on both sides between the lamina papyracea, associated fronto-ethmoidal cells along with resection of the inter-frontal septum and adjacent superior nasal septum (Fig. 5.21). The goal is to marsupialize both frontal sinuses into one common cavity, creating the maximal width possible between the absolute limits: the orbits bilaterally, the skull base posteriorly, and the anterior frontal table. The endoscopic Draf III procedure can be performed by several different techniques such as the "inside-out," "outside-in," and "transseptal" approaches.

The "inside-out" technique is named so since the drilling begins within the frontal ostium and moves outward: toward the nasal beak anteriorly and toward the frontal process of the maxilla laterally. The "outside-in" technique starts with the drilling out of the nasofrontal beak area and the frontal floor and lastly incorporates the frontal ostia (Video 6.10) [34]. The outside-in Draf III technique is described in further detail in Chap. 8. The transseptal technique follows the nasal septal superiorly and uses an anterosuperior septectomy as the first step to initiate and identify the frontal sinuses [35–37].

The following steps detail the authors' approach to an "inside-out" approach (Figs. 6.40, 6.41, 6.42; Video 6.11).

1. Bilateral frontal sinusotomy is performed as detailed above.
2. An anterosuperior septectomy is performed in the area caudal to the floor of the frontal sinus. The size of the septectomy is approximately 1.5–2 cm in height and length. The septectomy should allow binarial view of the axilla and the vertical part of both middle turbinates. This septectomy should extend all the way dorsally to the attachment of the septum on the frontal sinus floor. Extending the inferior limit beyond the lower border of the middle turbinate is not necessary. The anterior limit of the septectomy should never extend beyond the nasal bone in order to prevent loss of dorsal nasal support. The posterior limits of the septectomy should not extend posterior to the resected stumps of the middle turbinate to avoid injury to the cribriform plate. Intraoperative computer-guided navigation is helpful in defining these limits. The septectomy is most easily demarcated

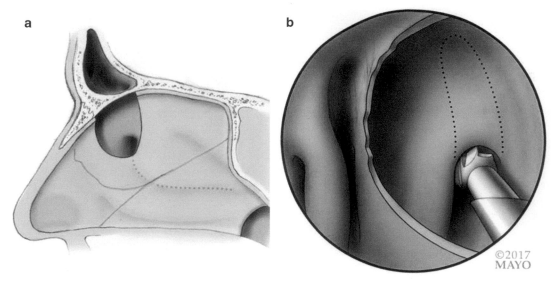

Fig. 6.40 Draf III procedure schematic. After bilateral frontal sinusotomy, an anterosuperior septectomy is performed in the area caudal to the floor of the frontal sinus. The size of the septectomy is approximately 1.5–2 cm in height and length. The anterior limit of the septectomy should never extend beyond the nasal bone in order to pre-vent loss of dorsal nasal support. The septectomy should allow binarial view of the axilla and the vertical part of both middle turbinates. This septectomy should extend all the way dorsally to the attachment of the septum on the frontal sinus floor. Extending the inferior limit beyond the lower border of the middle turbinate is unnecessary

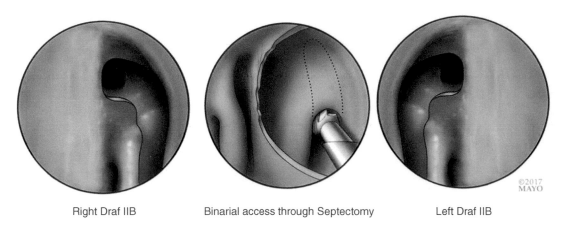

Right Draf IIB   Binarial access through Septectomy   Left Draf IIB

Fig. 6.41 The attachment of the anterior vertical part of the middle turbinate is trimmed to remove the attachment to the floor of the frontal sinus. A high-speed 30,000 rota-tions per minute (rpm) cutting 4 mm 40° angled burr is then inserted through the frontal ostium using a 30° or 45° endoscope. The nasal beak is then drilled out on each side

using an extended needle-tip monopolar cau-tery at a low coagulation setting. We also harvest the mucosa of the septectomy, if pos-sible, to use as a free mucosal graft. A unipo-lar cautery at low setting is used to coagulate the bleeding edges of the septectomy.

3. The attachment of the anterior vertical part of the middle turbinate is then trimmed to remove the attachment to the floor of the frontal sinus.
4. Next, the mucosa over the axilla of the mid-dle turbinate is removed with the microde-briders and the edges cauterized.

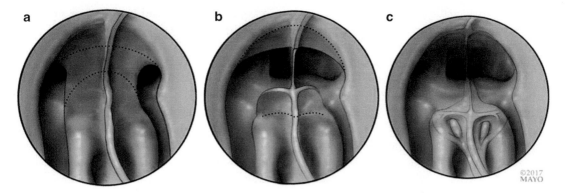

Fig. 6.42 The floor of the frontal sinus is then drilled medially toward the interfrontal septum (**a**). The junction of the bony septum with the floor and anterior table of the frontal sinus is then drilled out using high-speed coarse diamond burrs (15° and 40°) until a smooth transition between the anterior frontal table and the nasal bone is achieved (**b**). The frontal process of the maxilla is also drilled on each side, taking care not to breach the periosteum. The posterior projection along the posterior frontal table is carefully drilled down with the diamond burr, stopping anterior to the first olfactory filum (**c**). The interfrontal septum is removed to the frontal roof

5. A high-speed 30,000 rotations per minute (rpm) cutting 4 mm 40-degree angled burr is then inserted through the frontal ostium using a 30- or 45-degree endoscope. The nasal beak is then drilled out on each side.

6. The floor of the frontal sinus is then drilled medially, to the interfrontal septum.

7. The junction of the bony septum with the floor and anterior table of the frontal sinus is then drilled out using high-speed coarse diamond burrs (15° and 40°) until a smooth transition between the anterior frontal table and the nasal bone is achieved.

8. The frontal process of the maxilla is then drilled using a high-speed coarse diamond burr (15° and 40°). This should be thinned until the periosteum can be visualized, taking care not to breach it. The transmitted movement created by ballottement of the eye externally can be visualized endoscopically to ascertain that the bone has been thinned out to the periosteum.

9. All related frontoethmoidal cells (frontal septal cells, supra-agger, supra-agger frontal, supra-bulla frontal, and supra-bulla frontal cells) are incorporated into the frontal neo-ostium while taking care not to injure the anterior skull base and the anterior ethmoidal artery.

10. The posterior projection along the posterior frontal table is carefully drilled down with the diamond burr. Meticulous visualization while drilling is essential to not breach the skull base. The mucosa along this area can be gently dissected back to reveal the first olfactory filum, which is the posterior limit of the drilling. The navigation system can also be helpful in defining the posterior limit.

11. The interfrontal septum is then removed, extending dorsally all the way to the frontal roof. A more angled 60-degree drill and frontal 90-degree instruments can be helpful for this part of the dissection.

12. Multiple copious irrigations are carried out during drilling and at conclusion of surgery to flush out bone dust, debris, and pus.

13. The cavity is carefully inspected to ascertain hemostasis and confirm the integrity of the skull base. A Valsalva maneuver may be helpful at this time if there is concern regarding a possible cerebrospinal fluid leak.

14. Mucosal grafting is an optional maneuver performed at the conclusion of the procedure that may serve as a biological dressing and accelerate healing as well as inhibit osteoneogenesis and stenosis. The mucosal grafts from the septectomy are thinned out to make

them supple and laid over areas of exposed bone along the anterior frontal table. If septal grafts are not available, mucosal grafts can be harvested from the nasal floor.

15. A frontal stent can be fashioned with a thin Silastic sheeting to hold the mucosal graft in position. This stent must be positioned securely within the frontal sinus and across the septectomy to prevent dislodgement and can be secured to the nasal septum with a nonabsorbable suture. Alternatively, a commercially available corticosteroid-eluting stent (Propel) can also be used to hold the graft in position in patients where sustained release of local mometasone is desired. The stent is removed at approximately 2 weeks postoperatively. The use of frontal stents is discussed in depth in Chap. 22.

Frontal Sinusotomy Through the "Above and Below" Approach

This technique refers to the use of endoscopic surgery supplemented by a frontal trephination (Fig. 6.43). Frontal trephination is further detailed in Chap. 8. Frontal trephination is relatively easy and safe to perform in most patients. Relative contraindications for the frontal trephination procedure include hypoplastic frontal sinuses, exten-

sive osteoneogenesis and the presence of active vasculitis (Fig 6.43).

Applications of Different Frontal Sinusotomy Techniques

Once the decision to address the frontal sinus has been made, the surgeon and patient should determine which surgical approach to be utilized. This decision should be personalized for each patient. This section discusses the author's applications of different endoscopic frontal sinus techniques; a summary is also provided in Table 6.5. The authors practice a tiered approach, utilizing the least aggressive procedure that is likely to relieve symptoms and restore function.

Draf I Frontal Sinusotomy

This is the least aggressive of the frontal sinusotomy techniques in that it just exposes the frontal ostium without any actual manipulation (Fig. 6.18).

The Draf I frontal sinusotomy is indicated when the frontal sinus disease is the resultant from frontal recess outflow obstruction, and there is no significant disease or frontoethmoidal cells superior to the ostium that need to be addressed. The indication for the procedure is determined based on nasal endoscopy and CT scan, as well as

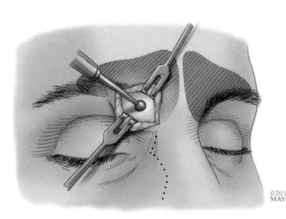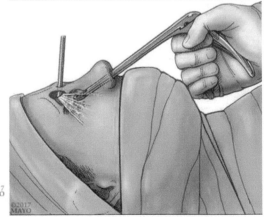

Fig. 6.43 The two panels show the use of frontal trephination for the "above and below" approach. Trephination is performed to augment instrumentation or visualization through the transnasal endoscopic approach

Table 6.5 Contemporary indications of endoscopic frontal sinus surgery

Procedure	Applications
Draf I	1. CRSsNP with minimal frontal recess disease 2. Acute frontal sinusitis 3. Recurrent acute frontal sinusitis
Draf II	1. Primary surgery for CRSsNP and CRSwNP 2. Revision surgery for CRSsNP and CRSwNP 3. Frontal mucoceles 4. Acute frontal sinusitis 5. Frontal barotrauma 6. Benign tumors 7. Recurrent acute frontal sinusitis
Draf IIA	1. Primary surgery for CRSsNP and CRSwNP 2. Revision surgery for CRSsNP and CRSwNP 3. Frontal mucoceles 4. Acute frontal sinusitis 5. Frontal barotrauma 6. Small frontoethmoidal osteoma 7. Recurrent acute frontal sinusitis 8. Pneumatocele of the frontal sinus
Draf II B	1. Revision surgery for CRSsNP and CRSwNP 2. Address a lateralized middle turbinate causing persistent frontal disease 3. Address middle turbinate remnants from prior resection that have scarred or lateralized, causing frontal sinusitis or mucocele 4. Neo-osteogenesis 5. Resection of frontoethmoidal osteoma 6. Resection of inverted papilloma 7. Endoscopic repair of frontal sinus trauma 8. Endoscopic repair of posterior frontal table CSF leak and meningoencephaloceles 9. Unilateral approach to the anterior cranial base 10. Unilateral approach to the medial and superior orbit
Draf III (endoscopic modified Lothrop procedure)	1. Revision surgery for CRSsNP associated with extensive scarring or neo-osteogenesis 2. Revision surgery for CRSwNP with recalcitrant disease subtype 3. Endoscopic repair of frontal sinus trauma 4. Endoscopic repair of posterior frontal table CSF leak and meningoencephalocele 5. Endoscopic resection of benign and malignant tumors involving the frontal sinus 6. As an approach to the anterior cranial base 7. As an approach to the medial and superior orbit

the disease subtype. For example, if frontal sinusitis is resultant from uncontrolled odontogenic sinusitis, this is likely to have originated first in the maxillary and then spreading contiguously to the frontal sinus via the ethmoid. Clearance of the maxillary and ethmoidal sinuses without formal frontal ostioplasty may be adequate to resolve the patient's disease. Abuzeid, Hwang, and colleagues prospectively studied 196 cases undergoing frontal sinusotomy and 30 cases treated with ethmoidectomy without formal instrumentation of the frontal recess (which they defined as a Draf 1 procedure). The study was able to demonstrate that for more limited disease, anterior ethmoidectomy alone could adequately treat milder frontal sinus disease. Formal frontal sinusotomy was more likely to be performed for more severe or recalcitrant forms of disease. A Draf I procedure may not be adequate if there is disease or obstructive cells superior to the frontal

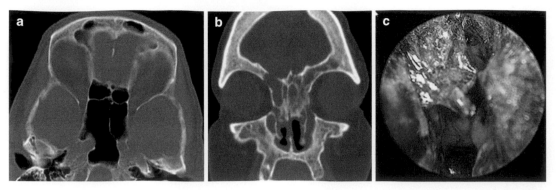

Fig. 6.44 Relative contraindications to frontal surgery include (**a**) small hypoplastic sinus with a narrow sagittal width, (**b**) extensive osteoneogenesis, and (**c**) active vasculitis as in this patients with granulomatosis with polyangiitis (formerly known as Wegener's granulomatosis)

ostium that need to be surgically addressed. Patients with nasal polyposis, eosinophilic mucin, supra-agger frontal cell, and supra-bulla frontal cells may require more extensive frontal sinus procedures.

The frontal sinus balloon dilatation technology can be used as a standalone procedure for patients with acute sinusitis, recurrent acute sinusitis, and stenosing frontal ostia. The balloon is also a tool that can be helpful in fracturing high frontoethmoidal cells and help with their dissection in conventional endoscopic frontal sinusotomy procedures. The procedure and indications are discussed in detail in Chap. 10.

Draf II A Frontal Sinusotomy

When the frontal sinusitis is resultant from frontal sinus pathology such as polyps, eosinophilic rhinosinusitis with mucin, or scarring from previous surgery or trauma, the Draf IIA frontal sinusotomy is our most common procedure of choice. When the frontal ostium is widened, the goal should be to create a minimum neo-ostium size of 5 mm or larger. When the anteroposterior (sagittal) width of the frontal recess is wide or the recess is populated by large, wide, ethmoidal cells, the Type IIA frontal sinusotomy results in a wide drainage pathway. Caution should be exer-

cised in performing a Draf IIA frontal sinusotomy in hypoplastic frontal sinuses, narrowed sagittal dimension, or excessive osteitis, as there may be higher risk of postoperative stenosis. In these situations, further widening of the frontal sinus drainage pathway may be necessary using the Draf IIB or Draf III procedures.

Draf II B Frontal Sinusotomy

The Draf Type IIB procedure creates a unilateral frontal sinusotomy with the widest width. The Draf IIB procedure is especially helpful when the residual stub of a previously resected middle turbinate lateralizes and closes off the frontal recess (Video 6.12). In this situation, the unstable middle turbinate needs to be resected to prevent restenosis. The Draf IIB procedure can also be helpful in cases of prominent frontal beak, which can be drilled off. Additionally, in cases of limited osteitis, the Draf IIB procedure may create a sufficiently wide ostioplasty that is unlikely to close down. It is our preference to perform a Draf IIB rather than a Draf III for neoplasms such as inverted papilloma when the pathology does not involve the interfrontal sinus septum (Video 6.13). This allows for preservation of an anatomic barrier against contralateral tumor spread should there be recurrence.

Draf III Frontal Sinusotomy (Endoscopic Modified Lothrop Procedure)

The Draf Type III frontal sinusotomy (endoscopic modified Lothrop procedure) creates the widest pathway for common drainage pathway for both frontal sinuses (and associated frontoethmoidal cells) into the nasal cavity. Indications for Draf III procedures may include (a) poorly controlled nasal polyposis; (b) extensive frontal recess osteitis; (c) repeated stenosis of less aggressive procedures; (d) management of frontal sinus cerebrospinal fluid leaks, encephaloceles, and trauma; (e) frontal mucoceles; (f) salvage of the previously obliterated frontal sinus; (g) access to the anterior skull base in cranial base surgery; and (h) establishment of gravitational drainage in "crippled frontal sinus with poor mucociliary function recovery after surgery. For most inflammatory sinus pathology (CRS) Draf III procedure should be employed if well-performed Draf II procedures and directed medical therapy have not succeeded in establishing adequate control of disease. In these situations, the sinonasal mucosa may have undergone irreversible damage leading to poor restoration of the normal pattern of mucociliary function. Causes of such failure can be severe inflammation, iatrogenic scar, and disease entities such as cystic fibrosis and primary ciliary dyskinesia.

The Draf III procedure can be performed "outside-in" or "inside-out." The "inside-out" approach is how we approached most of our Draf III procedures. However, this is difficult to perform in case of sagittally narrow frontal recesses and also takes longer in cases with dense osteitis of the frontal recess or where limited frontal recess landmarks exist. In these cases especially, we now perform the outside-in approach (Video 6.14).

Frontal Trephination

The frontal trephination can be customized to the disease and location being addressed. A "mini-trephination" or a formal, larger bony opening may be used. Historically, trephination was used for urgent management of acute frontal sinusitis or its related complications. In the contemporary era, the frontal trephination is applicable in a broader range of indications, as it also may provide an additional access portal for endoscopic visualization and instrumentation. Depending on the size of the trephination, endoscopes, instrumentation, or both simultaneously can be placed through the trephination. When trephination is performed to augment access through the transnasal endoscopic approach, the term "above and below approach" has been used for the technique. The frontal trephination is a valuable technique that has many contemporary indications where the procedure can be utilized with minimal morbidity. The mini-trephination can be used to evacuate pus in acute frontal sinusitis (severe or with complications), irrigate debris from the frontal sinus (Video 6.15), and endoscopically localize the frontal recess drainage pathway from below using colored dye flushed from above through the mini-trephination. The larger trephination can be used in combination with a transnasal endoscopic technique for removal of high frontoethmoidal cells or removal of disease (polyp, tumor, mucocele, etc.) in the lateral frontal sinus with or without endoscopic approach. The trephination is a valuable procedure for repair of frontal trauma and posterior table CSF leak and direct obliteration of a hypoplastic frontal sinus. It also provides access to the supraorbital area pathology.

Contraindications to Surgery

Patients must be medically stable to undergo surgery. A very narrow frontal recess (less than 5 mm from the nasal beak to the posterior frontal table) may make surgery challenging and is a contraindication for the inside-out Draf III (modified Lothrop approach). Supra-agger frontal cells may require accessory external techniques for removal through frontal trephination. Small hypoplastic frontal sinuses with severe inflammation and osteoneogenesis are prone to stenosis; repeated failures may be addressed by limited obliteration of these sinuses through a trephination approach (Fig. 6.44). Surgery in patients with active vasculitis should be avoided until the disease is well controlled or burnt out (Chap. 20).

Postoperative Care

Performing frontal sinusotomy commits the surgeon to following the patient closely. Patients are placed on oral antibiotics for 5–7 days after surgery, and this may be changed or extended based on intraoperative cultures. A tapering dose of oral corticosteroids is prescribed for most patients, and this may be extended for patients with severe tissue eosinophilia and nasal polyposis. In general, patients return for their first postoperative visit 1 week after surgery for endoscopic exam and possible debridement. Patients with narrow frontal openings are followed closely, sometime even weekly, and the surgeon should be prepared to promptly intervene to prevent irreversible stenosis. Once the size of the frontal sinusotomy shows stability, and the frontal recess mucosa appears to be healing satisfactorily, intervals for follow-up are extended. Postoperative care is detailed in Chap. 21. Chapter 12 details the management of the stenosing frontal sinus.

Summary

To perform surgery safely, effectively, and efficiently, the frontal surgeon must commit to mastering the frontal anatomy and instrumentation. Repeated review of the frontal sinus drainage pathway is conducive to comprehensively understanding the three-dimensional anatomy of the frontal sinus drainage pathway. Since the frontal recess anatomy is exceedingly variable, this review must be undertaken in a detailed fashion for every patient that will undergo surgery in the decision-making period, preoperatively and intraoperatively. Meticulous tissue handling and mucosal preservation along with complete and thorough dissection of ethmoidal structures in the frontal recess are critical to success. The decision to undertake surgery, the extent, and approach should be personalized.

References

1. Stammberger H. FESS: uncapping the egg. The endoscopic approach to frontal recess and sinuses. Tuttlingen, German: Storz GmbH; 2015.
2. Draf W, Weber R. Draf microendoscopic sinus procedures Am J Oto 1999.pdf. Am J Otolaryngol. 1993;14(6):394–8.
3. Stankiewicz JA, Donzelli JJ, Chow JM. Failures of functional endoscopic sinus surgery and their surgical correction. Oper Tech Otolaryngol Neck Surg. 1996;7(3):297–304.
4. Vining A, Eugenia W, David W. The transmigration of endoscopic sinus surgery from Europe to the United States.:10–3.
5. Stankiewicz JA, Lal D, Connor M, Welch K. Complications in endoscopic sinus surgery for chronic rhinosinusitis: a 25-year experience. Laryngoscope. 2011;121(12):2684–701.
6. Dalgorf DM, Sacks R, Wormald PJ, Naidoo Y, Panizza B, Uren B, et al. Image-guided surgery influences perioperative morbidity from endoscopic sinus surgery: a systematic review and meta-analysis. Otolaryngol Head Neck Surg (United States). 2013;149:17–29.
7. Wormald PJ. Salvage frontal sinus surgery: the endoscopic modified Lothrop procedure. Laryngoscope. 2003;113(February):276–83.
8. Stammberger H. Functional endoscopic sinus surgery. Philadelphia: B.C. Decker; 1991.
9. Snidvongs K, Pratt E, Chin D, Sacks R, Earls P, Harvey RJ. Corticosteroid nasal irrigations after endoscopic sinus surgery in the management of chronic rhinosinusitis. Int Forum Allergy Rhinol. 2012;2(5):415–21.
10. Snidvongs K, Kalish L, Sacks R, Sivasubramaniam R, Cope D, Harvey RJ. Sinus surgery and delivery method influence the effectiveness of topical corticosteroids for chronic rhinosinusitis: systematic review and meta-analysis. Am J Rhinol Allergy. 2013;27(3):221–33.
11. Sillers MJ, Melroy CT. In-office functional endoscopic sinus surgery for chronic rhinosinusitis utilizing balloon catheter dilation technology. Curr Opin Otolaryngol Head Neck Surg. 2013;21(1):17–22.
12. Patel ABAB, Cain RBRB, Lal D. Contemporary applications of frontal sinus trephination: a systematic review of the literature. Laryngoscope. 2015;125(9):2046–53.
13. Zacharek MA, Fong KJ, Hwang PH. Image-guided frontal trephination: a minimally invasive approach for hard-to-reach frontal sinus disease. Otolaryngol Head Neck Surg. 2006;135(4):518–22.
14. Orlandi RR, Kingdom TT, Hwang PH, Smith TL, Alt JA, Baroody FM, et al. International consensus statement on allergy and rhinology: rhinosinusitis. Int Forum Allergy Rhinol. 2016;6(November 2015):S22–209.
15. Fokkens W, Lund V, Mullol J. European position paper on rhinosinusitis and nasal polyps. Rhinology. 2007;(20):1–136.

16. Poetker DM, Jakubowski LA, Lal D, Hwang PH, Wright ED, Smith TL. Oral corticosteroids in the management of adult chronic rhinosinusitis with and without nasal polyps: an evidence-based review with recommendations. Int Forum Allergy Rhinol. 2013;3(2):104–20.

17. Lee WT, Kuhn FA, Citardi MJ. 3D computed tomographic analysis of frontal recess anatomy in patients without frontal sinusitis. Otolaryngol Head Neck Surg. 2004;131(3):164–73.

18. Wormald PJ, Hoseman W, Callejas C, Weber RK, Kennedy DW, Citardi MJ, et al. The international frontal sinus anatomy classification (IFAC) and classification of the extent of endoscopic frontal sinus surgery (EFSS). Int Forum Allergy Rhinol. 2016;0(0):1–20.

19. Pianta L, Ferrari M, Schreiber A, Mattavelli D, Lancini D, Bottazzoli M, et al. Agger-bullar classification (ABC) of the frontal sinus drainage pathway: validation in a preclinical setting. Int Forum Allergy Rhinol. 2016;6(9):981–9.

20. Wormald PJ. Surgery of the frontal recess and frontal sinus. Rhinology. 2005;43(2):82–5.

21. Lund VJ, et al. European position paper on the anatomical terminology of the internal nose and paranasal sinuses. Rhinol Suppl. 2014;24:1–34.

22. Landsberg R, Friedman M. A computer-assisted anatomical study of the nasofrontal region. Laryngoscope. 2001;111(12):2125–30.

23. Socher JA, Santos PG, Correa VC, De Barros E, Silva LC. Endoscopic surgery in the treatment of crista galli pneumatization evolving with localized frontal headaches. Int Arch Otorhinolaryngol. 2013;17(3):246–50.

24. Han JK, Becker SS, Bomeli SR, Gross CW. Endoscopic localization of the anterior and posterior ethmoid arteries. Ann Otol Rhinol Laryngol. 2008;117(12):931–5.

25. Jang DW, Lachanas VA, White LC, Kountakis SE. Supraorbital ethmoid cell: a consistent landmark for endoscopic identification of the anterior ethmoidal artery. Otolaryngol Head Neck Surg (United States). 2014;151(6):1073–7.

26. Bent JP, Guilty-Siller G, Kuhn FA. The frontal cell as a cause of frontal sinus obstruction. Am J Rhinol. 1994;8(4):185–91.

27. Nair S, Collins M, Hung P, Rees G, Close D, Wormald P-J. The effect of beta-blocker premedication on the surgical field during endoscopic sinus surgery. Laryngoscope. 2004;114(6):1042–6.

28. Tankisi A, Cold GE. Optimal reverse trendelenburg position in patients undergoing craniotomy for cerebral tumors. J Neurosurg. 2007;106(2):239–44.

29. Ko MT, Chuang KC, Su CY. Multiple analyses of factors related to intraoperative blood loss and the role of reverse Trendelenburg position in endoscopic sinus surgery. Laryngoscope. 2008;118(9):1687–91.

30. Higgins TS, Hwang PH, Kingdom TT, Orlandi RR, Stammberger H, Han JK. Systematic review of topical vasoconstrictors in endoscopic sinus surgery. Laryngoscope. 2011;121(2):422–32.

31. Lothrop HA. Frontal sinus suppuration: the establishment of permanent nasal drainage; the closure of external fistulae; Epidermization of Sinus. Ann Surg. 1914;59(A):937–57.

32. Getz AE, Hwang PH. Basal lamella relaxing incision improves endoscopic middle meatal access. Int Forum Allergy Rhinol. 2013;3(3):231–5.

33. Wormald PJ. The axillary flap approach to the frontal recess. Laryngoscope. 2002;112(3):494–9.

34. Chin D, Snidvongs K, Kalish L, Sacks R, Harvey RJ. The outside-in approach to the modified endoscopic lothrop procedure. Laryngoscope. 2012;122(8):1661–9.

35. Lanza DC, McLaughlin RB, Hwang PH. The five year experience with endoscopic trans-septal frontal sinusotomy. Otolaryngol Clin North Am. 2001;34:139–52.

36. McLaughlin RB, Hwang PH, Lanza DC. Endoscopic trans-septal frontal sinusotomy: the rationale and results of an alternative technique. Am J Rhinol. 1999;13(4):279–87.

37. Nishiike S, Yoda S, Shikina T, Murata J. Endoscopic Transseptal approach to frontal sinus disease. Indian J Otolaryngol Head Neck Surg. 2015;67(3):287–91.

Endoscopic Modified Lothrop Approach (Outside-In Technique)

E. Ritter Sansoni, Richard J. Harvey, and Raymond Sacks

Introduction

The modified endoscopic Lothrop procedure (MELP), Draf III, or common frontal sinusotomy is an adaptation of the procedure described by Harold Lothrop in 1914 [1]. Wolfgang Draf modified and popularized the approach in the 1990s, and it has since become an important procedure in the endoscopic sinus and skull base surgeon's armamentarium [2]. The technique is primarily used to treat a variety of frontal sinus pathologies; however, it is often combined with other approaches to manage lesions of the ventral skull base. The primary concept behind the MELP is that it converts the complex, varied, and limited frontal sinus outflow tracts into a simple, widely opened common frontal sinusotomy by removing the nasofrontal beak and frontal sinus floor. Creating a maximally opened common frontal sinusotomy allows for better access of topical therapies to the frontal sinus and improves surgical access to the frontal sinus and ventral skull base [3–5].

Indications

The most common indication for this procedure is for the management of medically recalcitrant inflammatory sinus disease with significant frontal sinus involvement (Table 7.1). As our understanding of the pathophysiology of chronic rhinosinusitis (CRS) has evolved, it is recognized that topical corticosteroids are an integral component of the treatment plan [6, 7]. However, the topical therapies must contact the affected sinuses to be effective. The primary benefit of the MELP in inflammatory sinus disease is that it allows for improved delivery of topical therapies to the frontal sinus when compared to more conservative frontal sinus approaches [3].

The common frontal sinusotomy is often employed as a secondary procedure for patients with recalcitrant or iatrogenic frontal sinus disease following prior endoscopic sinus surgery (ESS). However, in our opinion, it should be considered as a primary procedure in certain patient populations, such as those with eosinophilic CRS (Samter's triad, aspirin-exacerbated

E. Ritter Sansoni
Division of Rhinology and Skull Base Surgery, Department of Otolaryngology – Head and Neck Surgery, St Vincent's Hospital, Sydney, NSW, Australia

R. J. Harvey (✉)
Rhinology and Skull Base, Applied Medical Research Centre, UNSW, Sydney, NSW, Australia

Faculty of Medicine and Health Sciences, Macquarie University, Sydney, NSW, Australia

R. Sacks
Department of Otolaryngology, Macquarie University, Sydney, NSW, Australia

The University of Sydney, Sydney, NSW, Australia

© Springer Nature Switzerland AG 2019
D. Lal, P. H. Hwang (eds.), *Frontal Sinus Surgery*, https://doi.org/10.1007/978-3-319-97022-6_7

Table 7.1 Modified endoscopic Lothrop procedure indications

Inflammatory sinus disease (primary or salvage)	Eosinophilic rhinosinusitis (aspirin-exacerbated airway disease, Samter's triad, severe nasal polyposis) Ciliary dysfunction (primary or acquired) Failed frontal recess surgery Failed osteoplastic flap
Primary frontal sinus pathology[a]	Frontal sinus neoplasms Mucoceles Encephaloceles Cerebrospinal fluid leaks Anterior table fractures
Adjunct to ventral skull base procedures	Skull base resection of lesions adjacent or anterior to the anterior ethmoidal artery Skull base reconstruction with pericranial flap

[a]Excluding lesions of the lateral orbital roof unless combined with an orbital transposition

airway disease, extensive nasal polyposis) or ciliary dysfunction. This is especially true if there is concurrent lower airway inflammatory disease. These patients often have significant disease burden in the frontal recess and sinus which is associated with an increased risk of failing endoscopic frontal sinusotomy [8]. Other clinical scenarios where the MELP can be used include as a salvage procedure for failed osteoplastic flaps with frontal sinus obliteration or in cases of prior trauma with subsequent occlusion of the frontal outflow tract [9, 10].

Many frontal sinus lesions can be accessed through the Draf III cavity with the exception of those involving the lateral orbital roof [4]. However, the common frontal sinusotomy can be expanded with an orbital transposition to access more laterally based pathology [11]. It is therefore a good surgical approach to address selected cases of frontal sinus pathology including tumors, cerebrospinal fluid leaks, encephaloceles, and mucoceles.

Additionally, the MELP is an important adjunct to surgical approaches involving the ventral skull base. A Draf III should be performed during endoscopic skull base resections of lesions that approximate or are anterior to the anterior ethmoidal artery. There are two primary reasons for this: it improves surgical exposure, and it creates a simple, common neo-sinus that is easier to maintain in the postoperative period. A common frontal sinusotomy gives the surgeon a panoramic view of the entire cribriform plate and posterior table of the frontal sinus aiding in the resection and reconstruction [12]. Also, it permits the use of a zero-degree endoscope and straight instrumentation, which facilitate the triangulation of instruments [5]. The improved exposure during the resection also translates to easier tumor surveillance following treatment. Endoscopic endonasal approaches to the skull base create significant sinonasal dysfunction that is further compounded with adjuvant treatment. Performing a MELP decreases the risk of postoperative frontal sinus stenosis and mucocele formation and improves the delivery of nasal irrigations which optimize healing [3, 12, 13].

Contraindications

A medical contraindication for performing a MELP is in the setting of very active inflammatory disease of the upper or lower airway that requires very frequent or chronic use of systemic steroids. Topical medications are unlikely to be more efficacious, and these patients tend to heal poorly while the inflammatory condition is under suboptimal control. It is best to wait until the disease is at a stage where topical therapies will likely be the primary modality of disease control prior to creating a common frontal sinusotomy.

Few anatomic contraindications exist for the MELP. A frontal recess with an extremely narrow anterior-posterior dimension is often quoted as being a contraindication; however, the only instance where anatomy certainly precludes the common frontal sinusotomy is if the posterior table is <5 mm to the skin anterior the nasofrontal beak. This is only rarely seen in cases of craniofacial abnormalities or prior trauma, for example, uncorrected severely displaced naso-orbitoethmoidal fractures.

The Outside-In MELP

The outside-in technique is an evolution of the MELP that is more efficient than the traditionally described inside-out approach [14]. In the classic teaching, the removal of the nasofrontal beak and frontal sinus floor commences from within the frontal recess and sinus after the frontal recess has been dissected. However, this technique has several drawbacks because it requires frontal recess dissections, which often have significant disease burden or scarring, prior to creating the common frontal sinusotomy. This adds time to the procedure and necessitates the use of angled endoscopes, instruments, and drills. The outside-in approach avoids these issues since it does not navigate the complex anatomy of the frontal recess to identify the frontal sinus. Rather, known anatomical landmarks which serve as the boundaries for the common frontal sinusotomy cavity are identified early in the procedure, thus allowing the frontal sinus to be opened safely and efficiently with the use of a zero-degree endoscope and straight instruments [15].

The boundaries of the Draf III cavity are as follows:

- Posteriorly, the first olfactory neuron on each side demarcates the forward projection of the olfactory bulb.
- Laterally, the orbital plates of the frontal bone and periosteum of the skin covering the frontal process of the maxilla on both sides.
- Anteriorly, the plane of the anterior table of the frontal sinus.

Instrumentation

- A standard endoscopic sinus tray with a 2 mm, 40-degree Kerrison rongeur. No frontal sinus-specific instruments are required (Table 7.2).
- A zero-degree nasal endoscope. Wolfgang Draf described the technique using an operating microscope, proving that the procedure can be accomplished with a straight line of sight [2].

Table 7.2 Instrumentation

Standard endoscopic sinus tray
2 mm, 40° Kerrison rongeur
Zero-degree nasal endoscope
High-speed, self-irrigating drill with distal suction
4–5 mm coarse diamond burr
Needle tip monopolar electrocautery
Image guidance (optional)
0.5 mm thick Silastic sheet
NasoPore® dressing (Polyganics B.V., Netherlands)

- A 15-degree, high-speed, self-irrigating drill with a rough diamond burr. Drills that have an integrated distal suction and are capable of 30,000 rpm improve surgical efficiency. The rough diamond burr size should be 4 mm or greater.
- Image guidance is not necessary but helps to identify where to initiate the mucosal incisions. It is also useful when first learning the technique and for teaching purposes.
- Needle tip monopolar electrocautery with the tip bent at a 45° angle.
- 0.5 mm thick Silastic sheet to create the common frontal sinusotomy dressing.
- NasoPore® dressing (Polyganics B.V., Netherlands).

Procedure

Step 1: Patient Positioning and Setup

Patient positing and setup are critical to ensure the case proceeds as efficiently as possible. The importance of these initial steps cannot be overstated.

- Place the patient in the standard supine position with a shoulder roll to extend the neck. Neck extension changes the axis of the nasal cavity relative to the chest and allows for improved and more ergonomic access to the frontal sinus. This is true for all frontal sinus procedures.
- Secure the endotracheal tube to the right lower lip. This will ensure that the endotracheal tube and ventilator circuit are off the center of the patient's chest when the head is rotated toward the surgeon.

- Place cotton pledgets soaked in 1% ropivacaine and 1:2000 adrenaline into the nasal cavities as soon as possible. Make sure to place a pledget toward the nasofrontal beak on both sides.
- Set up the image guidance system. Image guidance is not required but is useful to judge where to initiate the mucosal incisions. It is also useful for teaching purposes and when first learning the outside-in technique since drilling through the thick bone of the nasofrontal beak may be unsettling.
- Place the bed at 15° reverse Trendelenburg to improve venous drainage.
- We prefer the anesthesiologist to use total intravenous anesthesia and maintain the patient bradycardic (55–65 bpm) with mean arterial pressures near 60 throughout the case.

Step 2: Define the Medial Orbital Wall

- An anterior ethmoidectomy, at minimum, must be completed to define the medial orbital wall prior to any drilling. However, depending on the indications for surgery, a complete sphenoethmoidectomy may be performed to identify the ventral skull base and anterior ethmoidal artery.

Step 3: Exposing the Nasofrontal Beak and Identifying the First Olfactory Neuron

- Using the navigation system, locate the point inferior to the nasofrontal beak and in the same coronal plane as the anterior table of the frontal sinus (Fig. 7.1). Alternatively, this point can be estimated by looking at the relationship to the middle meatus on sagittal imaging.
- Use the needle tip electrocautery, on a setting of 12 coagulation modes, to make a mucosal incision inferiorly along the frontal process of the maxilla and curve it slightly posteriorly toward the midportion of the middle meatus. Here, it will join the cut edge of mucosa from the uncinectomy (Fig. 7.2).

- Start at the same superior point and make a mucosal incision inferiorly along the septum; however, this incision should be several millimeters anterior to the later incision so that the incisions are staggered. Include any high septal deviation or prominent swell body in the area to be removed during the creation of the septal window.
- The inferior incision should go posteriorly until approximately the entrance of the middle meatus.
- Use the needle tip electrocautery to push through the septum at the anteroinferior junction of the septal incisions. This will make a mark in the contralateral septal mucosa which will simplify making symmetric mucosal flaps.
- Make the same mucosal incisions on the contralateral side and ensure that the incisions go all the way to the bone or cartilage.
- Use a Cottle elevator to raise the mucosal flaps. Start at the apex and then raise and reflect the lateral mucosa and then the septal mucosa posteriorly until the first olfactory neuron is identified.
- The first olfactory neuron is usually heralded by a small emissary vein that is just anterior to it. The vein is differentiated from the olfactory fascicle by its smaller caliber and lateral course. It is difficult to inadvertently avulse the first olfactory neuron since a sheath of dura accompanies it through the cribriform plate of the ethmoid (Fig. 7.3).

Step 4: Creating the Septal Window

- Use the microdebrider to remove the elevated mucosa and bipolar the mucosal edges.
- Place a Cottle elevator through the septum at the anteroinferior corner to create an opening in the septum. Then use a 2 mm Kerrison rongeur to cut through the cartilage and bone directly superior along the same line as the anterior septal incision.
- Use a straight heavy Mayo scissor of through-cutting instrument to make superior and inferior cuts in the exposed septum. Intermediate

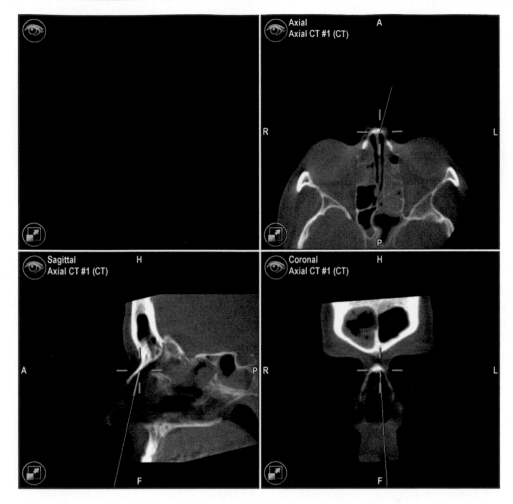

Fig. 7.1 Image guidance system demonstrating where to initiate the mucosal incisions

Fig. 7.2 Endoscopic view of the mucosal incisions. Note the relationship of the lateral incision (black arrow) with respect to the middle meatus and middle turbinate (MT). The septal incision (dashed line) is anterior to the lateral incision and includes the polypoid septal mucosa, which has been removed

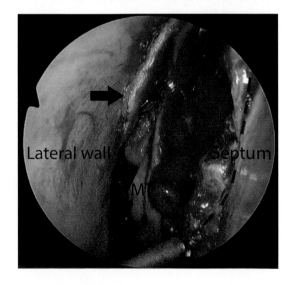

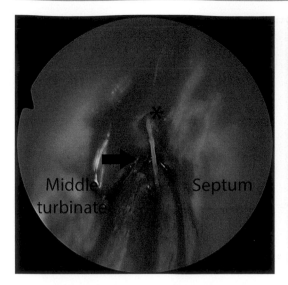

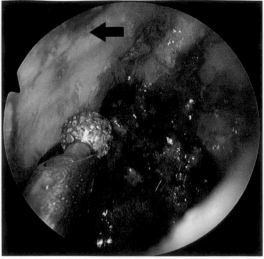

Fig. 7.3 Endoscopic view of the first olfactory neuron (black arrow) coming through the cribriform plate. A small emissary vein (asterisk) is typically seen just anterior to the neuron

Fig. 7.4 Endoscopic view of the exposed periosteum of the frontal process of the maxilla (black arrow). The locations of the first olfactory neurons (asterisks) are seen in this view

cuts can be made as needed. Remove the bone and cartilage from the septal window. It is best to remove all exposed cartilage and bone to decrease the amount of crusting in the postoperative period.

- Bipolar the cut mucosal edges to improve hemostasis.

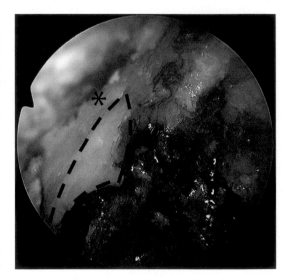

Fig. 7.5 Endoscopic view of the bone that is anterior to the frontal recess and superior to the axilla of the middle turbinate (MT). The bone inferior and medial to the exposed periosteum (asterisk) can be removed efficiently. The outlined area needs to be removed to obtain the maximum width of the ethmoid and Draf III cavities

Step 5: Drilling to Define the Lateral Limits of Dissection

- First, drill away the remaining crest of septum that remains attached superiorly below the nasofrontal beak and frontal sinus.
- Thin the bone of the lateral wall until the periosteum of the overlying skin is identified superiorly. The periosteum is whiter in color and bleeds more noticeably compared to the surrounding bone (Fig. 7.4).
- Exposing the periosteum superiorly ensures that any bone in a plane inferior and medial to it can be removed safely and efficiently. This includes the bone that is directly anterior to the frontal recess and superior to the axilla of the middle turbinate (Fig. 7.5).

- It is important to thin the bone inferomedially to the exposed periosteum to maximize the width of the dissection. Ideally, there should not be a prominent edge of bone as it transitions into the medial orbital wall. This will also make it easier to connect the frontal recess to the Lothrop cavity later in the case.

Step 6: Drilling Away the Nasofrontal Beak and Frontal Sinus Floor

- With the limits of dissection visible, the first olfactory neurons posteriorly and the exposed periosteum laterally drill away the nasofrontal beak in an inverted U-motion between the exposed periostea.
- This portion of the procedure may be disconcerting, but it is important to recognize that the frontal recess and sinus are between the burr and the skull base.
- Drill along a broad front to avoid tunneling into the frontal sinus. This includes removing the bone anterior to the frontal recess.
- The frontal sinus mucosa will become apparent as the bone is thinned (Fig. 7.6). Avoid the temptation to enter the sinus at this time because doing so will only create bleeding that will disturb the visual field. Instead, thin the surrounding bone.
- Enter the frontal sinus and use the equator of the burr to quickly remove the remaining

bone. Be cognizant of the depth of the drill to prevent unnecessary injury to the mucosa of the posterior table.

- Make the cavity as large as possible; doing so will minimize the risk of postoperative stenosis.

Step 7: Refining the Lothrop Cavity and Connecting the Frontal Recess

- Drill away the bone anterior to the frontal recess until it is thin enough to remove with hand instruments.
- Use a Kerrison rongeur to remove the bone in front of the frontal recess. Enter from the contralateral side to achieve the best angle. Also, remove any remaining frontal recess and anterior ethmoid partitions.
- Remove any frontal sinus partitions to create one simple sinus. Additionally, thin the bone at the transition of the lateral nasal wall to the orbital roof (Fig. 7.7). Doing so will "square-off" the cavity.
- With care, drill the bony septum almost to the level of the first olfactory neuron. This will

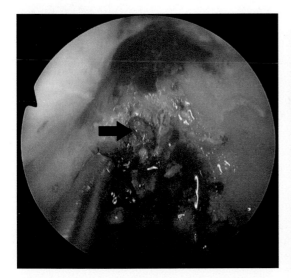

Fig. 7.6 Endoscopic view intact frontal sinus mucosa (black arrow). The surrounding bone should be thinned prior to entering the sinus. Note the inverted U-shape of the developing cavity

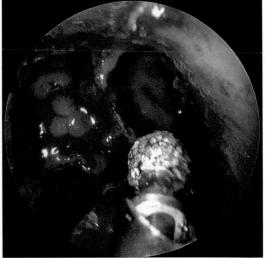

Fig. 7.7 Endoscopic view of the transition of the lateral wall of the nasal cavity to the orbital roof (dashed line). Thinning this bone will "square-off" the Draf III cavity

create a "T" where the septum joins the cribri-form plate of the ethmoid.

- Trim the heads of the middle turbinates back so they are posterior to the septal window. Doing so will stagger the mucosa so there is less chance of forming synechia at the entrance of the olfactory cleft. This will also maximize the width at the entrance of the ethmoid cavity allowing for improved access for topical therapies (Fig. 7.8).

Step 8: Closure and Dressings

- Mucosal grafts improve healing and diminish crusting [16]. Harvest mucosal grafts from the tail of the inferior turbinates and bipolar the donor sites. Thin the grafts by removing the submucosa; they should almost be transparent if done properly.
- Cut the 0.5 mm Silastic sheet in the shape of the template and place it into the sinonasal cavity with the limbs in the designated cavities (Fig. 7.9).
- Slide the mucosal grafts under the Silastic to cover the exposed bone of the lateral nasal

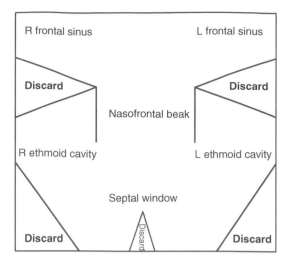

Fig. 7.9 Template to use for the Silastic dressing. The dressing may need to be altered slightly depending on the shape of the Draf III cavity

wall. This area is most prone to drying out and crusting since it is exposed to moving air during respiration.

- Place a third to one half of a NasoPore® into the septal window to provide support to the Silastic dressing. This will also help keep the grafts in place.

Postoperative Care

- Patients are discharged to home the same day as surgery unless there is another medical or social reason for hospital admission.
- Patients are prescribed a 10-day course of broad-spectrum or culture-directed antibiotics and a 21-day oral steroid taper.
- High-volume irrigations are started on postoperative day 1. A topical steroid is added to the irrigation immediately or after the oral steroid course is completed depending on the severity of disease.
- It is common to develop edema around the nasion and periorbital region. This is inflammation of the periosteum and responds well to nonsteroidal anti-inflammatory medications.

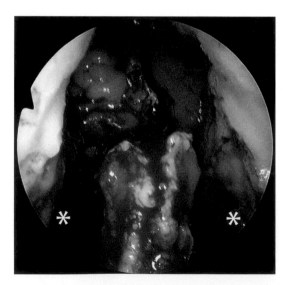

Fig. 7.8 Endoscopic view of the completed Draf III cavity. The anterior projection of the olfactory cleft is seen centrally. Note the smooth transition of the lateral limits of the Draf III cavity into the medial orbital walls (asterisks) of the ethmoid cavities

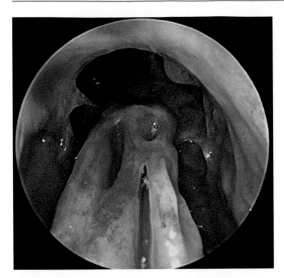

Fig. 7.10 Endoscopic view of a Draf III cavity 9 months following surgery in a patient with eosinophilic CRS. The patient uses a once-daily corticosteroid irrigation for disease control

- This first clinic visit is scheduled for 3 weeks following surgery. The Silastic dressing remains in place for at least 3 weeks.
- Remove any crusts and unfavorable synechiae during the initial visit. Remove any exposed bone flakes to improve the healing process and minimize crusting.
- The second clinic visit is 12 weeks following surgery. If there is unfavorable healing, surgical edema, or inflammatory disease, inject the tissue with 0.3–0.5 ml of triamcinolone 40 mg/ml. This will help settle inflammation and prevent cicatrix formation.
- A well-healed cavity is expected 3 months following surgery. Any local hypertrophic scar can be injected with triamcinolone 40 mg/ml with 1.25 inch, 25G needle on a 1 ml syringe (Fig. 7.10).

References

1. Lothrop HA XIV. Frontal sinus suppuration: the establishment of permanent nasal drainage; the closure of external fistulae; Epidermization of sinus. Ann Surg. 1914;59:937–57.
2. Draf W. Endonasal micro-endoscopic frontal sinus surgery: the Fulda concept. Oper Tech Otolaryngol Head Neck Surg. 1991;2:234–40.
3. Barham HP, Ramakrishnan VR, Knisely A, et al. Frontal sinus surgery and sinus distribution of nasal irrigation. Int Forum Allergy Rhinol. 2016;6:238–42.
4. Timperley DG, Banks C, Robinson D, Roth J, Sacks R, Harvey RJ. Lateral frontal sinus access in endoscopic skull-base surgery. Int Forum Allergy Rhinol. 2011;1:290–5.
5. Liu JK, Christiano LD, Patel SK, Tubbs RS, Eloy JA. Surgical nuances for removal of olfactory groove meningiomas using the endoscopic endonasal transcribriform approach. Neurosurg Focus. 2011;30:E3.
6. Rudmik L, Hoy M, Schlosser RJ, et al. Topical therapies in the management of chronic rhinosinusitis: an evidence-based review with recommendations. Int Forum Allergy Rhinol. 2013;3:281–98.
7. Snidvongs K, Pratt E, Chin D, Sacks R, Earls P, Harvey RJ. Corticosteroid nasal irrigations after endoscopic sinus surgery in the management of chronic rhinosinusitis. Int Forum Allergy Rhinol. 2012;2:415–21.
8. Chandra RK, Palmer JN, Tangsujarittham T, Kennedy DW. Factors associated with failure of frontal sinusotomy in the early follow-up period. Otolaryngol Head Neck Surg. 2004;131:514–8.
9. Wormald PJ, Ananda A, Nair S. Modified endoscopic lothrop as a salvage for the failed osteoplastic flap with obliteration. Laryngoscope. 2003;113:1988–92.
10. Smith TL, Han JK, Loehrl TA, Rhee JS. Endoscopic management of the frontal recess in frontal sinus fractures: a shift in the paradigm? Laryngoscope. 2002;112:784–90.
11. Karligkiotis A, Pistochini A, Turri-Zanoni M, et al. Endoscopic endonasal orbital transposition to expand the frontal sinus approaches. Am J Rhinol Allergy. 2015;29:449–56.
12. Batra PS, Kanowitz SJ, Luong A. Anatomical and technical correlates in endoscopic anterior skull base surgery: a cadaveric analysis. Otolaryngol Head Neck Surg. 2010;142:827–31.
13. Jo HW, Dalgorf DM, Snidvongs K, Sacks R, Harvey RJ. Postoperative irrigation therapy after sinonasal tumor surgery. Am J Rhinol Allergy. 2014;28:169–71.
14. Chin D, Snidvongs K, Kalish L, Sacks R, Harvey RJ. The outside-in approach to the modified endoscopic Lothrop procedure. Laryngoscope. 2012;122:1661–9.
15. Knisely A, Barham HP, Harvey RJ, Sacks R. Outside-in frontal drill-out: how I do it. Am J Rhinol Allergy. 2015;29:397–400.
16. Illing EA, Cho do Y, Riley KO, Woodworth BA. Draf III mucosal graft technique: long-term results. Int Forum Allergy Rhinol. 2016;6:514–7.

Frontal Trephination: Indications, Anatomy, Techniques, and Outcomes

Garret W. Choby and Jayakar V. Nayak

Introduction

Given the challenging anatomy of the frontal recess and critical neighboring structures, surgery to the frontal sinus is undertaken in a measured and calculated manner. Historically, frontal sinus surgery was exclusively approached externally. Techniques have ranged from obliterative surgery to external fronto-ethmoidectomy to trephination [1–3]. However, the majority of these procedures were associated with a high failure rate and/or revision rate, as well as complications, including injury to the orbit and cerebrospinal fluid (CSF) leak [2, 3].

With the advent of the endoscopic era as pioneered by Messerklinger and Stammberger, endoscopic techniques to address frontal sinus disease were developed [4, 5]. This progress was fundamentally assisted by the development of angled scopes, endoscopic instrumentation, and endonasal powered tools, along with the high-resolution computed tomography (CT) imaging and improved understanding of frontal recess anatomic variants. Endoscopic approaches soon became the workhorse techniques for approaching a wide range of frontal sinus pathologies.

Despite the utility of endoscopic techniques, external approaches still retain a vital role in frontal sinus surgery to treat such entities as frontal sinus trauma, CSF leaks, complicated rhinosinusitis, mucoceles with orbital involvement, and tumors with superior or lateral sites of origin. Frontal sinus trephination serves as a readily employed option in this armamentarium to address both inflammatory and noninflammatory conditions of the frontal sinus, as well as an adjunct to endoscopic techniques. Trephination allows direct external access to the frontal sinus via a well-masked curvilinear incision in the shadow line of the brow. Entry into the sinus can range from a simple 1–2 mm entry site to permit irrigation from above, to a 2–3 cm bone plate removal for tumor or intracranial access. This chapter describes the indications, techniques, and outcomes of this procedure.

G. W. Choby
Division of Rhinology and Endoscopic Skull Base Surgery, Department of Otolaryngology – Head and Neck Surgery, Stanford University School of Medicine, Stanford, CA, USA

Division of Rhinology and Endoscopic Skull Base Surgery, Department of Otorhinolaryngology – Head and Neck Surgery, Mayo Clinic, Rochester, MN, USA

J. V. Nayak (✉)
Division of Rhinology and Endoscopic Skull Base Surgery, Department of Otolaryngology – Head and Neck Surgery, Stanford University School of Medicine, Stanford, CA, USA

© Springer Nature Switzerland AG 2019
D. Lal, P. H. Hwang (eds.), *Frontal Sinus Surgery*, https://doi.org/10.1007/978-3-319-97022-6_8

Indications

The original indication for trephination was treatment of acute complications of advanced frontal sinus infection, such as the classically misnamed Pott's puffy "tumor." For inflammatory disease, the trephination is commonly used as an adjunctive open technique to endoscopic frontal sinus approaches ("above and below" technique) to help identify the true frontal outflow tract or allow access to pathology that is outside the reach of endoscopic instruments. To identify the frontal outflow tract endoscopically via a combined "above and below" approach, saline or fluorescein can be dripped through the trephination site and be visualized endoscopically in the nose, as the trephine access point is far superior to the frontal outflow tract (Fig. 8.1a). In highly recalcitrant disease, some practitioners favor temporary placement of a small cannula through the external trephine site to allow for instillation of irrigants, antimicrobials, or other medications (Fig. 8.1b). Indications for frontal sinus trephination are outlined in Table 8.1 [6–9].

Table 8.1 Indications for frontal sinus trephination

Inflammatory disease	Anatomic/noninflammatory disease
Acute frontal sinusitis	CSF leak
Pott's puffy "tumor"	Neoplasm (benign or malignant)
Chronic frontal sinusitis	Bony anomaly (fibrous dysplasia, osteoma)
Frontal sinus mucocele	Intracranial tumor
Allergic fungal rhinosinusitis	Posterior table trauma
Inability to identify frontal outflow tract endoscopically	Frontal recess stenosis

Techniques

- General considerations:
  - Frontal sinus trephination can be carried out under local anesthesia or general anesthesia. Most surgeons, however, prefer general anesthesia for patient comfort and to prevent inadvertent patient movement during the procedure.

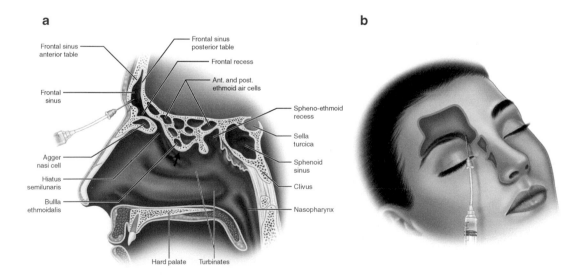

Fig. 8.1 Frontal sinus relationships when considering trephination. (**a**) Sagittal illustration of frontal sinus outflow tract, narrowed anteriorly by the agger nasi cell and posteriorly by the ethmoid air cell complex. A trephination drill and/or an indwelling indwelling catheter can pass through the frontal sinus the frontal sinus anterior table and terminate within the frontal sinus. Illustration of indwelling irrigation stent for delivery of irrigant or medication through frontal trephination. (**b**) Catheter entering through external trephination in the medial aspect of the brow

- General anesthesia is also indicated due to the frequent need for combining open trephination with endoscopic techniques.
  - Important anatomic landmarks should be identified including the superior orbital rim and supraorbital notch.
    - The supraorbital notch is palpable in the superior orbital rim, in line with the pupils. This landmark corresponds to the supraorbital foramen, through which passes the supraorbital bundle of nerve and vessels. The trephine entry will always be medial to this site.
- Approximating the incision and trephination site:
  - Considerations in selecting incision site:
    - The ideal location of the trephination is in the inferomedial portion of the pneumatized frontal sinus, at the apex of the "frontal bossing" anterior projection of the frontal sinus (Fig. 8.1a).
    - This entry site will preclude any possibility of direct entrance into the outflow tract (which is always far more inferior and medial).
    - The proposed site of entry should be at a portion of the frontal sinus that has adequate anterior-posterior depth from the posterior table and skull base to avoid inadvertent intracranial injury.
  - Traditional approach:
    - Occipitofrontal and "6-foot Water's view" radiographs can be obtained and projected to match the actual size of a given patient's skull prior to surgery (Fig. 8.2). The outline of the frontal sinus can be traced over the patient's forehead to approximate the pneumatized sinus. Alternatively, if a plain film X-ray can be printed, the impression/outline of the frontal sinus anatomic borders can be cut out of this film, placed onto the patient's skin, and traced as a general "template" for the frontal anatomy. This technique is rarely used in the modern era but can be utilized in selected situations.
  - Surface anatomic landmark approach:
    - A straight horizontal line can be drawn from the apex of the supraorbital notch to the contralateral supraorbital notch. A perpendicular line is then drawn vertically to bisect this horizontal line. The proposed site of incision should be approximately 1 cm lateral to the midline along this horizontal line (Fig. 8.3a). This technique is also rarely used in the modern era.

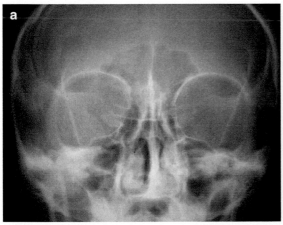
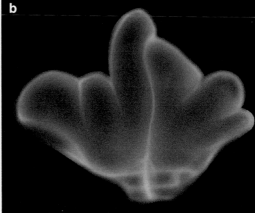

Fig. 8.2 Fronto-occipital radiograph/6-foot Water's view of the frontal sinus. (**a**) Plain film X-ray printed to demarcate frontal sinus borders. Note the small dimensions of the frontal sinus compared to the surrounding frontal bone. (**b**) If the plain film is cut using scissors, a general "template" for the frontal sinus is created, which can be used to mark out the location of the frontal sinus prior to external frontal procedures

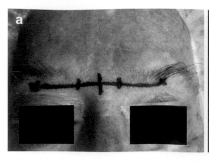 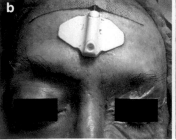 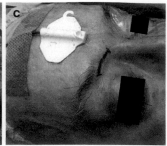

Fig. 8.3 Planning the incision for frontal trephination, (a) anatomic approach between supraorbital notches; (b, c) 1.5 cm curvilinear incision over the right medial brow, within the natural shadow line of the orbital socket, over the right frontal sinus as confirmed with a computer-assisted navigation probe. This is seen from the frontal (b) and 45-degree angled (c) views

- Computer-assisted navigation approach:
  - High-resolution CT and MRI scanning with computer-assisted navigation have significantly improved the accuracy and ability to verify the perimeter of the frontal sinus preoperatively [10].
  - After confirming accurate registration, the navigation probe can be used to mark out the entire border of the frontal sinus over the patient's skin to confirm localization (if required).
  - Alternatively, a 1.0–1.5 cm curvilinear incision is marked out within the medial eyebrow, and the navigation probe confirms the location of the proposed entry into the frontal sinus anterior table, as well as distance from the posterior table.
  - Once safely created, the trephine can also be carried out laterally or medially as dictated by the location of the pathology to be addressed. Again, computer-assisted navigation and careful study of the preoperative CT scan will guide this site selection.
- Frontal trephination procedure:
  - Local anesthetic should be infiltrated into the soft tissue of the medial brow on the affected side:
    - Avoid direct injection of the supraorbital artery or vein.
    - Injection should be carried out after completion of computer-assisted navigation surface registration so that the contour of the skin surface will not be altered by infiltration, thus affecting the accuracy of registration.

- A 1.0–1.5 cm curvilinear incision is carried out just below the medial eyebrow or within the medial eyebrow itself, within the "shadow line" of the orbital socket (Fig. 8.3b, c).
  - To avoid damaging the hair follicles, ensure that the blade is beveled parallel to the direction of hair follicles. Avoid using monopolar cautery near hair-bearing areas.
  - Avoid violation of the supraorbital neurovascular bundle during incision. The site of proposed incision should be medial to these structures as noted previously.
  - An alternative skin incision site may be useful in patients with prominent glabellar rhytids. In these patients, an incision can be carried out in the depth of a variably oriented glabellar rhytid, which may have some aesthetic postoperative benefit [11].
- Once incision site hemostasis is attained, the dissection should be taken down through the deep soft tissue and muscle to the periosteum. The latter should be elevated over the proposed trephination site with a Freer or Cottle elevator (Fig. 8.4a).
- The proposed trephination site is again confirmed with the computer-assisted navigation probe.
- A high-speed drill with a cutting or diamond drill bit is used to create a 3–4 mm trephination into the anterior table of the frontal sinus (Fig. 8.4b).
  - As the bone thins during drilling, it is important to slowly alleviate pressure to avoid plunging "through and through,"

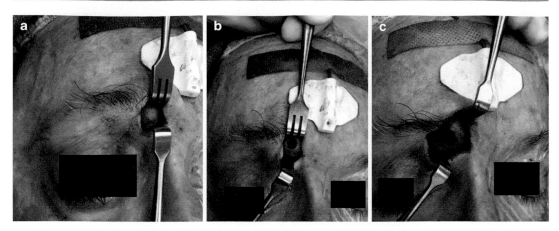

Fig. 8.4 Frontal trephination procedure. (**a**) Dissection through soft tissue to expose the periosteum; (**b**) circular trephine created through the anterior table with diamond drill bit. Sinus cavity visualized. (**c**) Trephine expanded with Kerrison rongeur for wider access in this patient with a frontal neoplasm

i.e., into the posterior table of the frontal sinus.

- Depending on the indication, the site of trephination can be further widened with the drill or a Kerrison rongeur to allow passage of the endoscope or other instruments into the frontal sinus (Fig. 8.4c).
- If the trephination is intended to be stented open for long-term infiltration of topical medications, a pediatric nasogastric feeding tube or biliary T-tube can be trimmed to size and sutured into place (Fig. 8.1).
  - There are also a variety of commercial products available that provide instrumentation to assist with the trephination and a transient, implantable irrigation cannula.

Outcomes

A number of limited studies have examined short- and long-term outcomes of frontal sinus trephination. Crozier et al. used trephination to assist endoscopic attempts to repair frontal sinus CSF leaks having extensive superior or lateral extension. In this study, they demonstrated excellent results with no recurrences found during their mean follow-up period of 37 months [6, 12]. In several small series, resection of inverted papilloma of the frontal sinus via a trephination approach had excellent results with no recurrence noted during the follow-up period in 80–100% of patients [6–8, 13]. Osteoma removal has also been shown to be successful with this approach in a series of ten patients [14]. Batra et al. demonstrated excellent frontal sinus outflow patency in 19/22 (86%) patients during a follow-up period of 16.2 months who underwent combined endoscopic and trephination approaches for complex frontal sinus indications [6, 9]. Gallagher and Gross reported frontal outflow tract patency in 15/16 patients undergoing frontal trephination for complex frontal sinusitis during a mean follow-up interval of 3.8 months [6, 15].

With regard to complications of trephination, facial/periorbital cellulitis has been cited as the most common complication, occurring in 2–4% of reported patients. CSF leak was reported in 0.5%–20% of patients depending on the series. Other rarely seen complications include proptosis, excessive bleeding, and orbital complications such as retrobulbar hematoma or corneal abrasion [6, 8, 9, 14, 15]. In rare instances, the curvilinear incision has been reported to heal as a taut web. Although we have not seen this in our practice, and the patient shown in Figs. 8.3 and 8.4 healed well, a zigzag incision line can be alternatively used for the medial brow incision.

In the modern era, the feasibility and safety of this procedure have been well-established. Lee et al. studied the average size and depth of adult frontal sinuses and reported that 85% of patients studied have sufficient depth of their frontal sinuses to accommodate standard frontal sinus trephination instruments (~7 mm). However, up to 15% of patients may have hypoplastic frontal sinuses with at least one point that is <7 mm in anterior-posterior depth between the anterior and posterior tables. On average, males have been shown to have deeper frontal sinuses than females ($p < 0.001$) [16]. Plitcher et al. described similar findings in a review of sinus CT imaging and also noted that the deepest (safest) point of most adult frontal sinuses is close to the midline, which is the most anterior projection of frontal bone bossing [17]. In all cases, the preoperative CT scan must be carefully studied to assess the size and depth of the frontal sinus to avoid complications such as inadvertent posterior table penetration or orbital transgression.

Summary

The frontal sinus has historically been the most difficult sinus to access and successfully treat long term due to its anatomic complexities, narrow outflow tract, and critical nearby structures. Although endoscopic approaches have become the mainstay in virtually all sinus practices, external techniques including frontal trephination retain a crucial role for the comprehensive sinus surgeon in specific situations. Frontal sinus trephination is a safe adjunctive procedure to treat lesions with superior or lateral origin or extension that are otherwise unreachable from a purely endoscopic perspective.

References

1. Ochsner MC, DelGaudio JM. The place of the osteoplastic flap in the endoscopic era: indications and pitfalls. Laryngoscope. 2015;125(4):801–6. https://doi.org/10.1002/lary.25014.
2. Silverman JB, Gray ST, Busaba NY. Role of osteoplastic frontal sinus obliteration in the era of endoscopic sinus surgery. Int J Otolaryngol. 2012;2012:501896. https://doi.org/10.1155/2012/501896.
3. Isa AY, Mennie J, McGarry GW. The frontal osteoplastic flap: does it still have a place in rhinological surgery? J Laryngol Otol. 2011;125(2):162–8. https://doi.org/10.1017/S0022215110002288.
4. Stammberger H. Endoscopic endonasal surgery-concepts in treatment of recurring rhinosinusitis. Part II. Surgical technique. Otolaryngol Head Neck Surg. 1986;94(2):147–56.
5. Kennedy DW. Functional endoscopic sinus surgery. Technique. Arch Otolaryngol Chic Ill 1960. 1985;111(10):643–9.
6. Patel AB, Cain RB, Lal D. Contemporary applications of frontal sinus trephination: a systematic review of the literature. Laryngoscope. 2015;125(9):2046–53. https://doi.org/10.1002/lary.25206.
7. Zacharek MA, Fong KJ, Hwang PH. Image-guided frontal trephination: a minimally invasive approach for hard-to-reach frontal sinus disease. Otolaryngol Head Neck Surg. 2006;135(4):518–22. https://doi.org/10.1016/j.otohns.2006.05.033.
8. Fishero BA, Chen PG, Payne SC. Modified glabellar rhytid incision for frontal sinus trephination. Laryngoscope. 2014;124(12):2676–9. https://doi.org/10.1002/lary.24765.
9. Crozier DL, Hwang PH, Goyal P. The endoscopic-assisted trephination approach for repair of frontal sinus cerebrospinal fluid leaks. Laryngoscope. 2013;123(2):321–5. https://doi.org/10.1002/lary.23499.
10. Cohen AN, Wang MB. Minitrephination as an adjunctive measure in the endoscopic management of complex frontal sinus disease. Am J Rhinol. 2007;21(5):629–36. https://doi.org/10.2500/ajr.2007.21.3083.
11. Walgama E, Ahn C, Batra PS. Surgical management of frontal sinus inverted papilloma: a systematic review. Laryngoscope. 2012;122(6):1205–9. https://doi.org/10.1002/lary.23275.
12. Sautter NB, Citardi MJ, Batra PS. Minimally invasive resection of frontal recess/sinus inverted papilloma. Am J Otolaryngol. 2007;28(4):221–4. https://doi.org/10.1016/j.amjoto.2006.09.003.
13. Seiberling K, Jardeleza C, Wormald P-J. Minitrephination of the frontal sinus: indications and uses in today's era of sinus surgery. Am J Rhinol Allergy. 2009;23(2):229–31. https://doi.org/10.2500/ajra.2009.23.3298.
14. Batra PS, Citardi MJ, Lanza DC. Combined endoscopic trephination and endoscopic frontal sinusotomy for management of complex frontal sinus pathology. Am J Rhinol. 2005;19(5):435–41.
15. Gallagher RM, Gross CW. The role of minitrephination in the management of frontal sinusitis. Am J Rhinol. 1999;13(4):289–93.
16. Lee AS, Schaitkin BM, Gillman GS. Evaluating the safety of frontal sinus trephination. Laryngoscope. 2010;120(3):639–42. https://doi.org/10.1002/lary.20803.
17. Piltcher OB, Antunes M, Monteiro F, Schweiger C, Schatkin B. Is there a reason for performing frontal sinus trephination at 1 cm from midline? A tomographic study. Braz J Otorhinolaryngol. 2006;72(4):505–7.

External Techniques in Frontal Sinus Surgery

9

Devyani Lal, Rami James N. Aoun,
John M. DelGaudio, and Naresh P. Patel

Introduction

External techniques for frontal sinus surgery are often thought of as "historical" approaches that have been supplanted by endoscopic approaches. While the vast majority of frontal sinus pathology may be addressed by endoscopic techniques, select pathology may still warrant external frontal surgery [1, 2]. Given the relative rarity of such indications, it is important to maintain familiarity and skill with these techniques. Even as the indications of such approaches continually evolve, external techniques remain a valuable tool in the armamentarium of the contemporary sinus surgeon. However, our philosophical approach to open frontal sinus surgery has dramatically evolved in intent and execution. The primary aim with these techniques may be to restore sinus function, minimize tissue destruction, and preserve mucosa. Where possible, this approach eschews sacrifice of sinus mucosa and obliteration of the sinuses. Instead of obliterating the frontal sinus, the preferred goal of these external techniques is also to restore sinus function (functional "external" sinus surgery). In rare and select cases, external approaches may still need to be utilized for destruction and obliteration of the affected frontal sinus.

External approaches to the frontal sinus were initially developed to manage life-threatening complications of acute or chronic sinusitis. Historically, surgery for inflammatory frontal sinus disease was dangerous and controversial [3, 4]. The history, development, and evolution of frontal sinus surgery and external techniques are elegantly described in Chap. 1. This chapter will provide a focused review of indications and technical nuances.

External or open procedures that are most commonly utilized for frontal sinus surgery are frontal sinus trephination, external frontoethmoidectomy, external frontal sinusotomy with or without the osteoplastic flap, and frontal sinus cranialization. With the exception of the cranialization procedure, the other techniques can be conducted with either a function-preserving or an ablative approach. Where possible, it is our approach to use functional

D. Lal (✉)
Department of Otolaryngology – Head and Neck Surgery, Mayo Clinic College of Medicine and Science, Mayo Clinic, Phoenix, AZ, USA

R. J. N. Aoun · N. P. Patel
Department of Neurological Surgery, Mayo Clinic, Phoenix, AZ, USA

J. M. DelGaudio
Department of Otolaryngology – Head and Neck Surgery, Emory University School of Medicine, Atlanta, GA, USA

© Springer Nature Switzerland AG 2019
D. Lal, P. H. Hwang (eds.), *Frontal Sinus Surgery*, https://doi.org/10.1007/978-3-319-97022-6_9

external techniques by themselves or as an adjunct to a functional endoscopic approach. The frontal trephination technique can be a useful adjunct to endoscopic techniques or used as a stand-alone external procedure. This technique is discussed in detail in Chap. 8.

When performed meticulously, external approaches to the frontal sinus have an excellent cosmetic outcome and safety profile. The attendant morbidity rates and revision surgery rates can also be low.

Over the last three decades, innovative endoscopic surgical techniques have been developed which can address many frontal sinus pathologies that were historically only approachable by external means [5, 6]. A recent study reported that the utilization of open frontal technique has decreased by a third between 2000 and 2011, while endoscopic frontal sinus procedures increased around threefold over the same time period [7]. External approaches to the frontal sinus constitute approximately 5% of the total number of surgeries and have been in steady decline over the past two decades [7]. These techniques however remain an important tool in the arsenal of otolaryngologists when dealing with complex, traumatic, neoplastic, and chronic frontal sinus disease refractory or not amenable to endoscopic approaches [2, 6–9].

Indications

In general, external frontal techniques for inflammatory sinus disease are reserved for those that have failed multiple prior endoscopic procedures or where the disease is far lateral and inaccessible through endoscopic approaches (Table 9.1) [1]. As technology, instrumentation, and surgical

Table 9.1 Contemporary indications of external frontal sinus techniques

Combined approach with endoscopic procedures
Laterally located or endoscopically inaccessible frontal sinus disease
Frontal sinus diseases refractory to endoscopic surgery
Traumatic injuries to the frontal sinus
Sinonasal malignancy

skills evolve, the indications for external approaches do as well [5, 6, 8–11]. For instance, recent studies report excellent outcomes and low failure rates for endoscopic approaches to lateral frontal sinus pathologies and posterior frontal table fractures [10, 11]. The indications of specific external techniques will be discussed with the specific procedures.

Preoperative Work-Up and Planning

Detailed evaluation and meticulous preoperative planning are necessary to undertake external frontal sinus surgery. All patients should undergo nasal endoscopy and a thin-cut multiplanar paranasal sinus computerized tomography (CT) evaluation prior to surgery. Once the indications for surgery have been established, a thorough review of the anatomy as well as the location of the disease is conducted. The extent of frontal pneumatization should be carefully studied on the sinus CT scan in all three planes (coronal, axial, and sagittal). Special attention is directed to the sagittal width (depth) to assess safety and feasibility of any external approach that will involve sawing or drilling through the anterior frontal table. Sequela from prior surgical management should be carefully studied. The location of the anterior ethmoidal artery is determined, and note is made if it is pedicled within the ethmoidal space. The slope, symmetry, depth, and integrity of the anterior skull base should be carefully studied.

The presence of soft tissue infection, mucocele, mucopyocele, and cranial nerve abnormality is examined and documented. Note is made of any aberrant anatomy as well as bony erosion of the orbit, skull base, and anterior and posterior frontal table. Magnetic resonance imaging (MRI) is critically valuable in cases where tumor is suspected to rule out orbital, dural, and perineural invasion [12]. However, even in patients with inflammatory sinus disease, an MRI can be very helpful in distinguishing a potential mucocele from tumor and differentiating between mucoceles and fat in patients who have undergone prior obliteration procedures [5].

Anatomic Considerations in External Frontal Sinus Surgery

A comprehensive understanding of frontal sinus anatomy is essential before attempting any open operation. The frontal sinus has complex anatomy and is intimately related to the orbit and the cranial cavity; these can be inadvertently injured. The paired frontal sinuses are located in the anteromedial inferior portion of the frontal bone. The frontal sinus is bordered by a relatively thick anterior table and a thinner posterior table, which separates the sinus from the frontal lobe of the brain. Medially, the intersinus septum separates the two frontal sinuses. The frontal sinuses are typically unequal in size. In approximately 10% of the population, one or both frontal sinus may be aplastic or hypoplastic. Disease in hypoplastic sinuses may be more challenging to address surgically as there is limited room for instrumenation (Fig. 9.1). The floor of the frontal sinus forms the medial orbital roof. The anterosuperior ethmoidal cells can be variably pneumatized, which can influence the drainage pathway of the frontal sinus. Occasionally the interfrontal septum is also pneumatized [13, 14]. The frontal sinuses open into the nasal cavity through a funnel-shaped recess (frontal recess) from the inferomedial aspect of the sinus; this area is conventionally termed the "frontal ostium" [13]. If the intent of surgery is function-restoring, then the frontal sinus mucosa, especially in the frontal recess, should be handled with great care. Details of frontal sinus anatomy are discussed in the relevant chapters.

Complications and Caveats

Meticulous surgical technique can minimize complications and postoperative sequelae. Multiple studies have demonstrated that in well-selected patients, external frontal sinus approaches have excellent outcomes, safety, and low revision rates [2, 5, 9]. Excellent cosmesis can be achieved by careful attention to indications, contraindications, and surgical detail [15] (Fig. 9.2). Two cardinal strategies can help avoid complications. Mucosal preservation and careful dissection of the frontal recess and frontal ostium in non-obliterative surgeries are critical (Fig. 9.3). In obliterative surgery, all mucosal lining should be completely removed and the frontal ostium and recess completely plugged (Fig. 9.4).

Common complications for external techniques include problems with cosmesis. Poorly positioned incisions and poor suture techniques can also lead to alopecia and broad scars (Fig. 9.5). Frontal bossing or depression can result from poorly positioned or poorly healed bone flap (Fig. 9.6). Exposure of hardware (Fig. 9.7) and chronic frontal osteomyelitis with fistulae (Fig. 9.8) can result from infection of the obliterated sinus. Scarring of the frontal recess due to

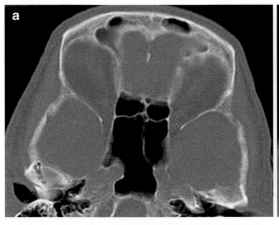 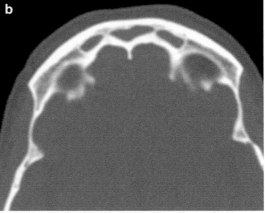

Fig. 9.1 Disease in hypoplastic frontal sinuses (**a**) or in sinuses with very narrow anteroposterior width (**b**) can be technically challenging to address both endoscopically and externally

Fig. 9.2 A bicoronal incision that is well placed, executed, and closed can heal with acceptable cosmesis, as shown in this patient with male pattern baldness

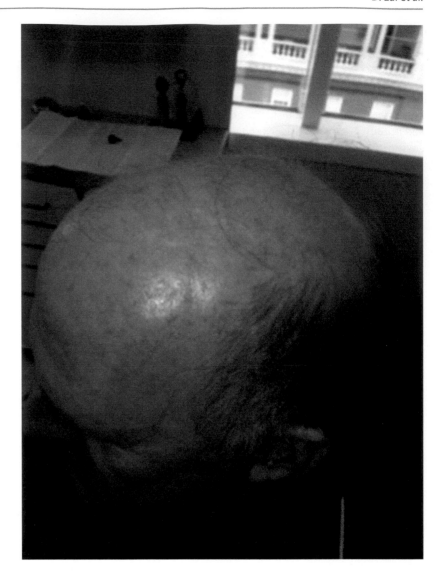

adhesions or neo-osteogenesis can cause disease recalcitrance, recurrent infection, or secondary mucoceles (Fig. 9.9). Fat donor site morbidity such as scar and infection can occur. Cerebrospinal fluid (CSF) leak, brain injury, and orbital injury can result. Neurological injuries can result from injuries to the supratrochlear, supraorbital, and frontal branch of facial nerve [16–18]. Long-term complications include chronic neuralgic pain, forehead numbness, and recurrent mucoceles (Fig. 9.9) [4]. Other surgical complications include infections and abscess formation, myocardial infarctions, cardiovascular accidents, venous thromboembolic disease, and pulmonary disease.

Intraoperative Preparation

The patient is laid supine. It may be helpful to have the head positioned on a horseshoe headrest. Surgical pinning is not necessary, unless mandated by image guidance needs. Turning the surgical table 90° or 180° away from the anesthesia machine allows the surgeon free access to the frontal area (Fig. 9.10). The surgical field is prepared and draped in a sterile fashion. The eye is taped shut with transparent adhesive tape and draped into the field (Fig. 9.11a). A corneal shield or tarsorrhaphy may be beneficial to minimize covering of the eye (Fig. 9.11b). The nose is

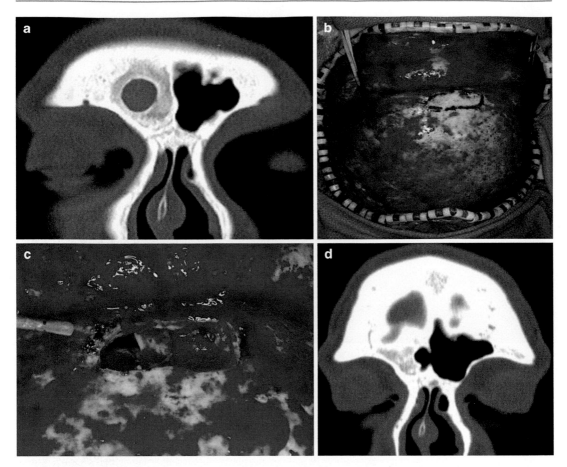

Fig. 9.3 Functional external sinus surgery: Mucosal preservation and careful dissection of the frontal recess and frontal ostium in non-obliterative surgeries are critical. (**a**) CT sinus showing right frontal mucocele. (**b**) Given the hypoplastic nature of the right frontal sinus, a functional external approach via a bicoronal incision and osteoplastic flap approach was chosen over an endoscopic approach. (**c**) After the anterior frontal table was removed, the right frontal disease was addressed, and the interfrontal sinus septum was removed. Mucosa in both frontal sinuses was preserved, and the right frontal sinus was then marsupialized into the left frontal sinus to drain into the nose. (**d**) Postoperative sinus CT imaging shows bilateral functional frontal sinuses. In this situation, the functional external approach was advantageous over the endoscopic approach; the endoscopic approach would have required prolonged drilling, more extensive surgery for ethmoidectomy, longer healing time and more demanding postoperative debridement. This case is discussed in further detail in the chapter and Figs. 9.35, 9.36 and 9.37

decongested with topical pledgets as described in the endoscopic technique chapter (Chap. 6). Intraoperative image guidance is utilized in our practice to map out the extent of the frontal sinuses and plan the surgical approach (Fig. 9.12). The patient tracker and image guidance system is set up in a such way so as to not interfere with the operative field (Fig. 9.13a). The use of a fixed reference frame for image guidance which is screwed away from the field can be helpful (Fig. 9.13b). If image guidance is not available, the use of a 6-feet Caldwell (occipitofrontal) view or transillumination has been described (Fig. 9.14) [1].

Surgical Technique

The next section describes the indications and technique for specific procedures.

Frontal Sinusotomy with Osteoplastic Flap

Historically, the osteoplastic approach has been used concomitantly with frontal obliteration [4]. However, the osteoplastic approach can be utilized without frontal obliteration as a

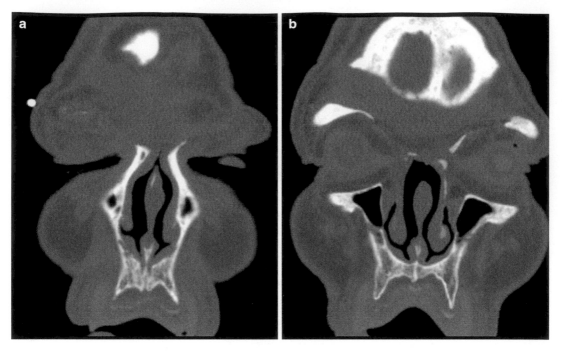

Fig. 9.4 CT scan images showing bilateral frontal sinus obliteration with muscle. In obliterative surgery, all mucosal lining should be completely removed and the frontal ostium and recess completely plugged to prevent postoperative mucocele formation

Fig. 9.5 The bicoronal scar in this patient is wide and has led to local alopecia. Additionally, the anterior placement of the scar has now made it visible secondary to age-related male pattern baldness in this patient

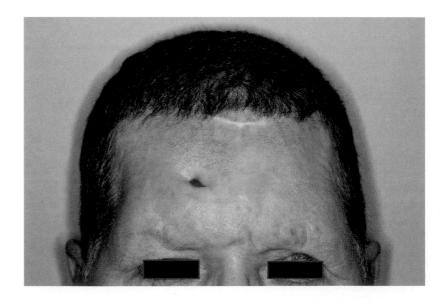

Fig. 9.6 Depression of the forehead is noted after radiation therapy in this patient who underwent an osteoplastic flap procedure along with left orbital exenteration

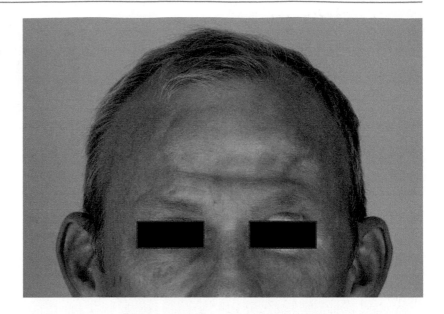

Fig. 9.7 Exposed hardware from a poorly healed osteoplastic flap

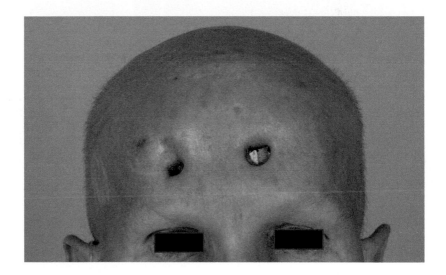

function-restoring technique with preservation of the mucosa and following principles employed in functional endoscopic sinus surgery. In general, this technique can be used to address a variety of frontal pathologies that are not amenable to an endoscopic approach [9, 15, 19]. Indications for which this procedure can be considered are listed in Table 9.2. When the frontal sinus function is determined to be unsalvageable, the decision to obliterate is made. In the contemporary era, this is a rare procedure applied to frontal sinuses with dense scar tissue, extensive osteoneogenesis, or recurrent failure from functional endoscopic or external approaches. Many frontal mucoceles and tumors can be managed without obliteration [9]. The advantage of not obliterating the sinus,

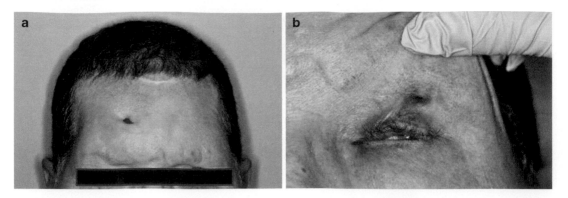

Fig. 9.8 Chronic frontal osteomyelitis with multiple fistulae in this patient who had previously undergone frontal sinus obliteration procedure with hydroxyapatite

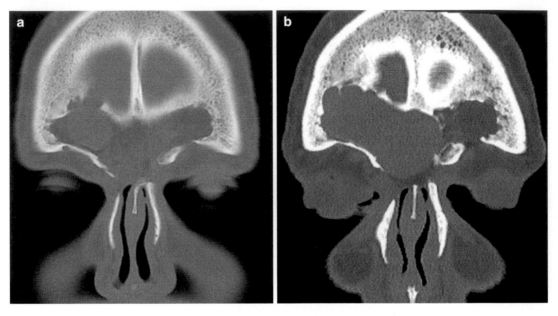

Fig. 9.9 Mucocele formation suspected after frontal sinus obliteration procedure with fat graft in year 2000. (**a**) Right frontal mucocele in year 2002. (**b**) Same patient with expansion of the prior mucocele noted at evaluation in year 2016

such as in cases of inverted papilloma, is the capability of endoscopic visualization of recurrence [20]. When the decision to obliterate the frontal sinus is made, the diseased mucosa is removed, and the frontal inlet/ostium is obliterated.

Caution should be exercised in employing the osteoplastic flap technique if the viable bone in the frontal sinus is reduced by 50% and in the presence of fulminant acute frontal sinusitis or Pott's puffy tumor. These situations may jeopar-

dize bone flap survival (Fig. 9.6). Other paranasal sinuses should be addressed prior to undertaking the osteoplastic technique. The patient should be counseled about risks specific to this procedure. The most common intraoperative complications for frontal sinusotomy procedures are orbital fat exposure, inadvertent fracture of anterior table, malpositioning of the anterior wall, and dural tears [18]. The most common postoperative complications reported are numbness extending along the forehead to

Fig. 9.10 The patient is laid supine. It may be helpful but is not necessary to have the head positioned on a horseshoe headrest. Surgical pinning is not necessary. Turning the surgical table 90° or 180° away from the anesthesia machine allows the surgeon free access to the frontal area

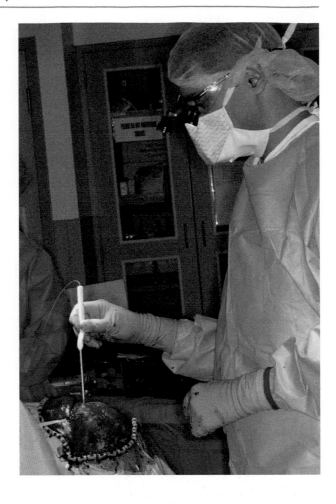

the top of the head (due to temporary or permanent injury to the supraorbital and supratrochlear nerves), mucocele formation, persistent neuralgia, frontal bossing or depression, and epistaxis. Other complications include fat necrosis, donor site wound complications, alopecia at the incision line, a visible scar in balding patients, bone flap necrosis, cosmetic deformity, orbital injury, CSF leak, and intracranial infections and injury. The choice of the obliteration material should be made carefully, with autologous abdominal fat being most commonly used in the contemporary era. Frontal sinus obliteration with hydroxyapatite and other foreign material may be associated with increased rates of infection, flap necrosis, and graft extrusion (Fig. 9.8) [5].

Steps:

1. The patient is placed supine on the operating room table. All pressure points should be padded.
2. The operating table is turned 180° (or 90°) away from the anesthesia machine (Fig. 9.15).
3. The head is placed on a gel doughnut or a horseshoe headrest (Fig. 9.10).
4. The patient's hair should be conservatively clipped on either side of the proposed incision. Alternatively, rubber bands may be used to sweep away longer hair (Fig. 9.16). The planned incision line drawn is with a sterile marking pen in a

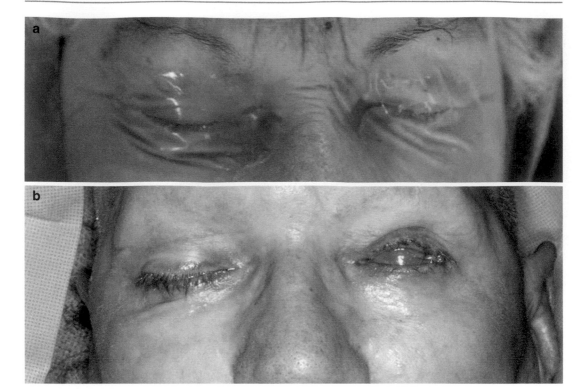

Fig. 9.11 The eye is taped shut with transparent adhesive tape and draped into the field (**a**). Alternatively, a corneal shield can be used if performing trephination or external frontoethmoidectomy (**b**)

standard bicoronal fashion, extending from the tragus of the ipsilateral ear up over the crown of the head, parallel to and behind the hairline, coronally toward the tragus of the contralateral ear (Fig. 9.17). Other incisions that can be utilized are the pretrichial, mid-forehead, and brow incisions. Gullwing incisions, which are bilateral brow incisions connected through a glabellar incision, result in a transection of the supraorbital nerves and an obvious scar (Fig. 9.18). This is rarely performed any longer.

5. An image guidance system can be used at this time to perform a registration and check external landmarks for accuracy (Fig. 9.13a). The use of a fixed reference frame for image guidance away from the field is helpful (Fig. 9.13b). This can be screwed through a small incision in an area away from the sur-

gical and incision site. This placement holds steady during the procedure.

6. The patient should then be prepped and draped in standard surgical sterile fashion.

7. The incision line is injected with 1% lidocaine and epinephrine 1:100,000 at least 10 minutes before the procedure begins.

8. A #10 blade is used to incise down through the skin into subcutaneous soft tissue along the previously marked incision line. The knife is beveled so as to not transect through hair follicles (Fig. 9.19a).

9. A needle-tip Bovie cautery is then used to deepen the incision down to the temporalis fascial layer bilaterally as well as down toward the calvarium in the middle (Fig. 9.19b).

10. Raney clips may be used to secure hemostasis, but these are not essential (Fig. 9.20). By working in small segments, the skin and the

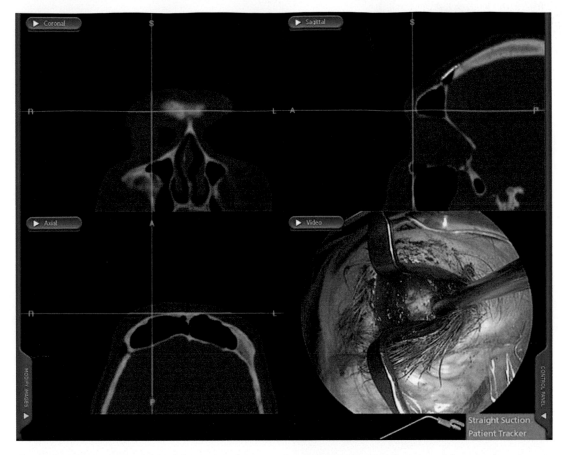

Fig. 9.12 Image guidance with triplanar views is extremely valuable in planning the external frontal approach, as in this case of frontal trephination via a lateral brow approach

deeper layers can be incised and vascular control obtained before proceeding to the adjacent segment (Fig. 9.19a, b).

11. The bicoronal scalp flap is then elevated forward by creating a plane between the temporalis fascia and the scalp on the lateral sides and subperiosteally in the midline. It is extended low down to the area of the glabella, preserving the supraorbital and supratrochlear neurovascular bundle (Fig. 9.21).

12. Alternatively, the bicoronal flap may be elevated superficial to the pericranium (Figs. 9.21b and 9.22). The pericranium can be incised beyond the borders of the bone flap and left attached to the inferior part of the bone flap (Fig. 9.23). Closure of the pericranium will help to seat the bone flap, obviating the need for plates and screws (Fig. 9.24).

13. The flap is retracted anteriorly using 2-0 Vicryl suture attached to rubber bands attached to Allis clamps or dural retractor hooks (Fig. 9.25). Care should be taken not to create holes in the pericranial flap, should it be needed for use later for obliteration, skull base defect repair, or cranialization.

14. Using three-dimensional intraoperative navigation, the bilateral frontal sinuses can be mapped out on the patient's frontal bone (Figs. 9.10 and 9.12). Alternatively, delineation can be done utilizing an onlay template created preoperatively utilizing 3D models extracted from CT scans [25]. If these are not available, a template can be planned using the X-ray film of a 6-feet Caldwell (occipito-frontal) view which has been sterilized (Fig. 9.14). The X-ray film is cut along the

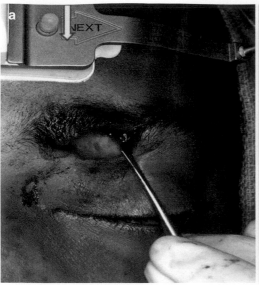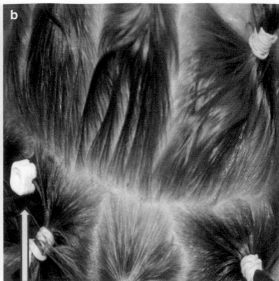

Fig. 9.13 The image guidance reference frame should be placed away from the planned incision site (yellow arrows). (**a**) Conventional forehead frame for a frontal trephination via the brow. (**b**) A fixed reference frame for image guidance can be screwed through a small incision in an area away from the surgical and incision site into the skull bone (Dynamic Reference Frame, Medtronic, Minneapolis, MN)

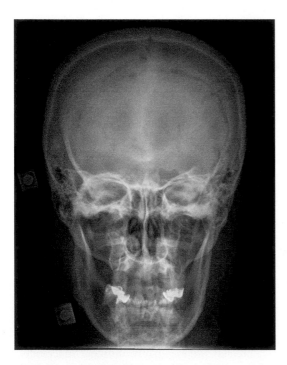

Fig. 9.14 If image guidance is not available, a 6-feet Caldwell Luc (occipitofrontal) view X-ray can be used for planning the osteotomy. The X-ray film is sterilized, and then the outline of the frontal sinus is cut out and placed over the anterior frontal table to help map the osteoplastic flap. This approach is no longer used in our practice

borders of the frontal sinus and placed on the forehead to plan the limits of the osteotomy. Transillumination methodology has also been described to map the frontal sinus extent but is not accurate. Image guidance has been demonstrated to be superior to both of these modalities [26].

15. A sterile marking pen may be used at this point to mark the landmarks and limits of the planned osteotomy (Figs. 9.26 and 9.27).

16. Next, a high-speed drill with 1.8–2.0 mm bit is used to create a trephination into either side of the frontal sinus (Fig. 9.26). A bone flap is then created in an oval fashion by following the contours of the drawn lines (Fig. 9.27). Beveling the edges of the bone flap inferiorly directs the saw away from the intracranial contents and also creates a contour that allows the anterior table flap to rest back in place without falling into the sinus when replaced (Fig. 9.23). Entry into one of the frontal sinuses is then straightforward. A small osteotome and mallet are used to complete the osteotomy such that the bone flap could be removed in a single piece. If the bone flap is fractured due to prior trauma or

Table 9.2 Indications for frontal sinusotomy with osteoplastic flap (with or without obliteration)

Frontal mucoceles with the following characteristics: far lateral extension and osteoneogenesis, mucoceles with multiple loculations in the setting of prior frontal sinus obliteration, extensive frontal recess neo-osteogenesis
Posterior frontal table cerebrospinal fluid (CSF) leaks and/or encephalocele, where endoscopic visualization or reach of instrumentation is suboptimal
Frontal fractures: complex or comminuted anterior and posterior table fractures
Larger frontoethmoidal osteoma and bony tumors
Inverted papilloma: far lateral and supraorbital attachments, multifocal sites of involvement, attachment to anterior frontal table where endoscopic visualization or reach of instrumentation is suboptimal
Malignancy of the frontal sinus: primary or metastatic
Osteomyelitis unresponsive to medical therapy
Pneumatocele resulting in cosmetic deformity

disease, or during elevation, all pieces should be carefully preserved. Alternatively, the bone flap can be left pedicled on the pericranium inferiorly (Fig. 9.23). This allows replacement of the bone flap and closure using only sutures to re-approximate the pericranial incision (Fig. 9.24). [15]

17. The intersinus septum is then removed by using the high-speed drill as well as Kerrison rongeurs (Fig. 9.28).

18. Care should always be taken to allow the patient's normal mucosa to remain wherever possible if the frontal sinus will not be obliterated or cranialized. After the frontal sinus is cleared of disease, attention should be directed toward ensuring patent drainage of the two frontal sinuses (Fig. 9.28) followed by reconstruction. Usually this is done via an external Lothrop procedure and by widening the frontal recess (Fig. 9.29).

19. If obliteration of the frontal sinus is to be performed, then all frontal mucosa should be meticulously stripped from the bone. A diamond burr may be used to remove microscopic fragments of mucosa till a smooth contour of the bone is defined (Fig. 9.30). Magnification with a microscope or an endoscope is very helpful in assuring that all mucosa has been removed.

20. For obliteration, autologous fat graft is procured from the abdomen or thigh and then inserted into the frontal pneumatized space to obliterate it. Fibrin glue may be used to hold the fat in place. An alternative is hydroxyapatite cement to obliterate the space, but this is now discouraged due to long-term problems with infection and extrusion. A third option is a free muscle flap. The frontal ostia are tightly packed to inhibit nasal mucosa ingrowth into the frontal sinus.

21. The preserved osteoplastic flap is then brought back into the field to seal the space. The bone flap is secured in position using multipoint fixation consisting of mini plates and mini screws. If the bone flap is fractured, all pieces should be carefully repositioned and then plated or wired together (Fig. 9.31). A small amount of Gelfoam should be placed in the gaps around the bone flap in order to help prevent the bone flap from depressing and prevent significant influx of air. In cases where the bone flap cannot be replaced, a mesh plate can be used as a scaffold to bridge any gap or hole in the calvarium (Fig. 9.32), or hydroxyapatite cement can be used to recreate the anterior table contour.

22. Next, the scalp flap and calvarium are irrigated using antibiotic solution and thoroughly dried. A medium-sized vacuum drain is placed in the subgaleal space and tunneled out percutaneously and secured to the skin using a 3-0 nylon suture.

23. The Raney clips are then removed, and a 2-0 Vicryl suture is used in an interrupted fashion to close the galea aponeurotica. Skin staples are used to close the skin. This is

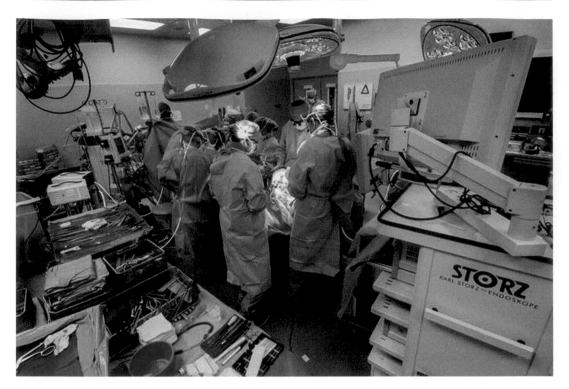

Fig. 9.15 The patient is placed supine on the operating room table. The operating table is turned 180° (or 90°) away from the anesthesia machine (towards the left side of the picture) such that the surgeons can stand free of the anesthesia apparatus near the head of the patient (towards right right of the picture)

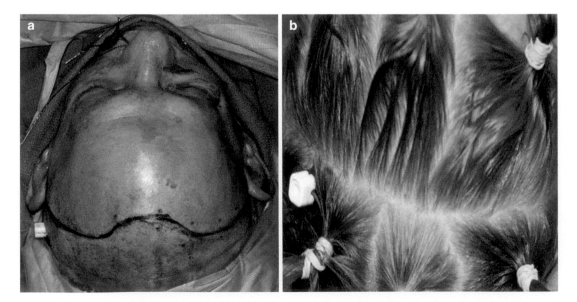

Fig. 9.16 The patient's hair should be conservatively clipped on either side of the proposed incision, unless they prefer to shave the whole head (**a**). Alternatively, rubber bands may be used to sweep away longer hair (**b**)

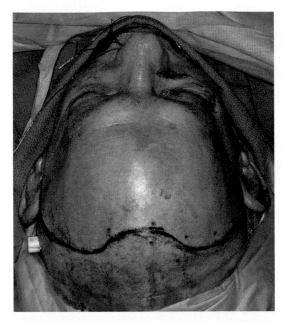

Fig. 9.17 The planned incision line is drawn with a sterile marking pen in a standard bicoronal fashion, extending from the tragus of the ipsilateral ear up over the crown of the head parallel to and behind the hairline coronally toward the tragus of the contralateral ear. The bicoronal incision is marked as an inverted "V" shape. This configuration helps maintain more vascularity at the middle part of the scalp flap. If a pericranial flap is needed, the scalp incision can be planned more posteriorly

Fig. 9.18 Figure showing a bilateral brow incision connected through a glabellar incision. This is rarely performed any longer as it results in a transection of the supraorbital nerves and an obvious scar

followed by the application of bacitracin ointment and a sterile dressing. A wrap is then performed, and care is taken not to depress the midline area between the orbits.

Caveats with Frontal Sinus Obliteration Procedure

Relative contraindications for frontal sinus obliteration include posterior table erosion, orbital roof erosion (Fig. 9.33), hyperpneumatized supraorbital ethmoidal cells, and inverting papilloma or tumor involving the frontal sinus. In these cases, complete removal of the mucosa is difficult and may result in CSF leak or orbital injury and residual or recurrent tumor become buried and not recognizable.

Patients should be counseled on immediate and long-term complications. Immediate complications include pain, forehead and scalp numbness due to injury to the supraorbital and supratrochlear vessels, as well as poorly healed skin scar, alopecia, and forehead depression or bossing. CSF leak and brain injury may also occur. In the long term, patients are at risk of developing mucoceles; these

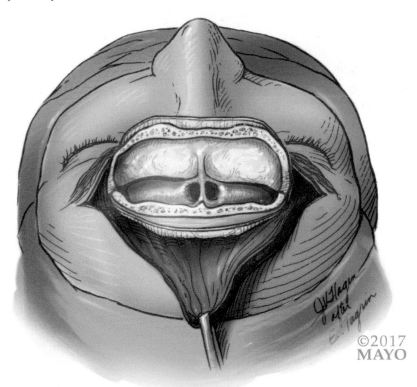

©2017
MAYO

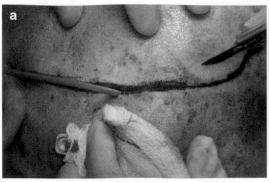

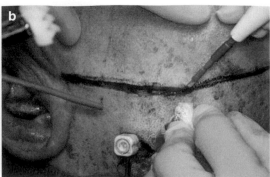

Fig. 9.19 (**a**) A #10 blade is used to incise down through the skin into subcutaneous soft tissue along the previously marked incision line. The knife is beveled so as to not transect through hair follicles. (**b**) Next, a needle-tip Bovie cautery is used to deepen the incision

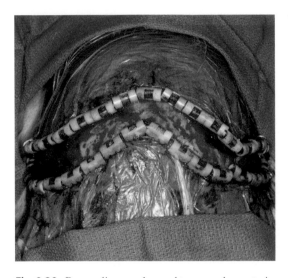

Fig. 9.20 Raney clips may be used to secure hemostasis, but are not essential

arise from residual microscopic mucosa and may appear after several years from the original procedure. Additionally, mucosa from the nose may also grow into the sinus from the frontal recess, which must be carefully occluded. Patients are also at risk of long-term pain, hyperesthesia, and paresthesia. Long-term follow-up of patients who have undergone obliteration is mandated since mucoceles can occur decades after this procedure due to regrowth of mucosa from the frontal recess or within the frontal sinus itself (Fig. 9.9). Multiple loculated mucoceles may form, and distinguishing these from fat may be difficult even with MRI scans (Fig. 9.34) [18, 21].

Osteoplastic Flap Without Obliteration: Case Illustration

A 49-year-old male with myelofibrosis and upcoming bone marrow transplant was referred for a lesion in the right frontal sinus. Differential diagnoses included frontal mucocele, infection, or a neoplastic mass. CT and MRI imaging were performed (Fig. 9.35a–d). CT images of the right frontal sinus showed it to be hypoplastic, with dense, thick bone that would need to be drilled via an endoscopic transnasal approach to the sinus. However, the left frontal sinus appeared to be well pneumatized with a wide frontal sinus drainage pathway opening into the nose (Fig. 9.35d). We anticipated that this patient with poor immunological status and medical status needed a relatively quick procedure. Therefore, we elected to approach the frontal sinus lesion via an osteoplastic flap approach. Access to the frontal sinus was performed according to the technique above. After the osteoplastic flap was removed (Fig. 9.36a), we confirmed that the true right frontal sinus was hypoplastic. The bony lesion was filled with mucoid material that was negative for malignancy on frozen section histopathology. Mucus and dysplastic bone were sent for culture and histopathology. The mucosa of the right frontal sinus itself appeared to be healthy. The left frontal sinus was noted to be well pneumatized, with

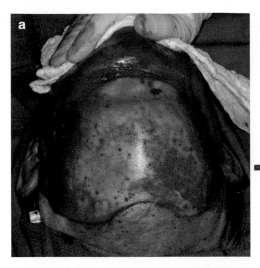

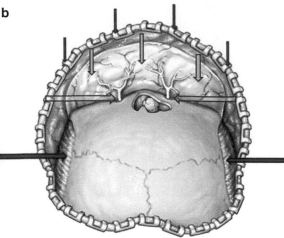

Fig. 9.21 The incision is deepened down to the temporalis fascial layer bilaterally as well as the calvarial bone in between (**a**). Alternatively, the scalp incision is only incised to the layer of the pericranium. The posterior edge of the scalp incision is then back-elevated such that a longer pericranial flap can be harvested. The bicoronal scalp flap is then elevated forward by creating a plane between the temporalis fascia laterally and the scalp subperiosteally in the midline. It is extended low down to the area of the glabella, preserving the supraorbital and supratrochlear neurovascular bundles. (**b**) A schematic of the extent of the elevation of flap. Laterally, the flap is elevated to the junction with the temporalis fascia (red arrows), and anteriorly to the glabella, carefully identifying and preserving the supraorbital and supratrochlear neurovascular bundles (yellow arrows). In the schematic, the pericranium has been elevated as a separate layer (green arrows) from the skin and subcutaneous layer (blue arrows)

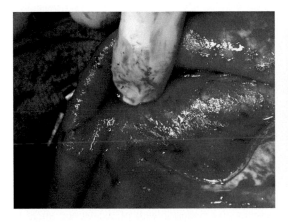

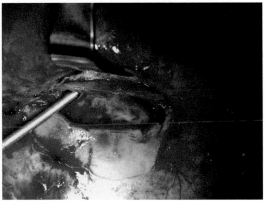

Fig. 9.22 As shown in Figure 9.21b, the bicoronal flap may be elevated superficial to the pericranium, and the pericranium can be incised beyond the borders of the bone flap (step 12; Fig. 9.21)

Fig. 9.23 The pericranium can be left attached to the inferior part of the bone flap

healthy mucosa and with a wide drainage pathway (Fig. 9.36b). We therefore elected not to obliterate the right frontal recess but instead marsupialize the right frontal sinus into the left frontal sinus (Fig. 9.36b). Meticulous attention was paid to avoid any frontal mucosa trauma.

Using upturned Kerrison rongeurs and drills, the interfrontal sinus septum was taken down, as well as the walls of the interfrontal sinus cell. At the conclusion of surgery, a nice drainage pathway from the right frontal sinus across the interfrontal sinus septa into the left frontal sinus and

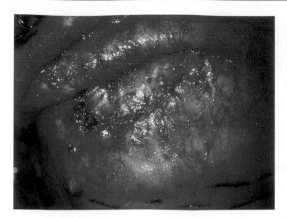

Fig. 9.24 In this alternate scenario (Figs. 9.22 and 9.23), the closure of the pericranium will help seat the bone flap. If the flap is very well seated, this may minimize the need for plates and screws

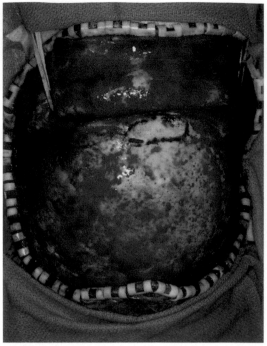

Fig. 9.25 The bicoronal soft tissue flap is retracted anteriorly using 2-0 Vicryl suture attached to rubber bands attached to Allis clamps or dural hooks. Care should be taken not to create holes in the pericranial flap should it be needed for use later for obliteration, skull base defect repair, or cranialization

therefore into the nose was created. The cavity was then irrigated thoroughly to remove bone dust and chips while avoiding any trauma to the sinus mucosa. The osteoplastic flap was then replaced by plating with three two-hole plates. The bicoronal flap was then closed in layers. Three-month follow-up imaging showed the osteoplastic flap to be well healed and the newly created pathway between the right and left sinuses to be adequate for bilateral frontal sinus function (Fig. 9.37). The procedure, thus, was a modification of the historical external Lothrop procedure.

Frontal Sinus Cranialization

Frontal sinus cranialization involves removal of the posterior frontal table (Fig. 9.38). In the contemporary era, it is not indicated for chronic frontal disease and may be used in frontal sinus trauma with comminuted posterior table fractures.

Cranialization of the frontal sinus consists of meticulous removal of the sinus mucosa and the posterior wall of the frontal sinus, causing the frontal lobe to occupy the frontal sinus, abutting the anterior table and floor of the frontal sinus [22]. Donald and Bernstein first described the cranializa-

tion of the frontal sinus in 1978 for managing posterior frontal table trauma [23]. Cranialization is approached in a similar fashion to the osteoplastic flap technique. Once the frontal mucosa has been meticulously removed, additional steps are undertaken. In addition to removing the intersinus septum, the posterior wall of the frontal sinus is also removed. The frontal lobe of the brain reconfigures and expands into the frontal sinus. At that point the frontal sinus becomes an epidural space for the brain. The frontal ostium area is obliterated with fat, muscle, or a flap (Fig. 9.3). Some authors have advocated using the pericranial flap technique for cranialization of the frontal sinus [22]. They propose that adding an extra layer between the intracranial space and the frontal sinus bone provides additional protection. If needed, the pericranial flap can be dissected off from the scalp

Fig. 9.26 Marking pen tracing directly on calvarium is utilized to plan the bone flap osteotomy. Next, a high-speed drill with 1.8–2.0 mm bit is used to create a trephination into either side of the frontal sinus

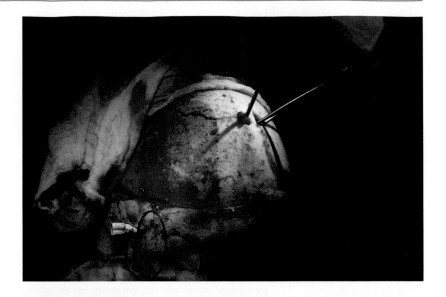

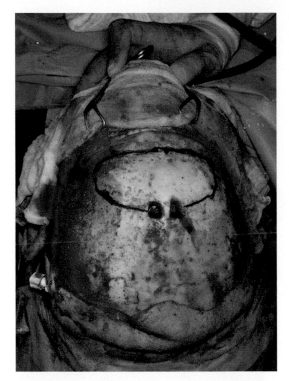

Fig. 9.27 A bone flap is then created in an oval fashion by following the contours of the drawn lines. Beveling the edges of the bone flap inferiorly directs the saw away from the intracranial contents and also creates a contour that allows the anterior table flap to rest back in place without falling into the sinus when replaced

flap after deepening the incision on the scalp to the calvarium. Alternatively, the scalp incision is deepened but not through the pericranium. The scalp and the pericranial flaps are raised as separate flaps (see Fig. 9.21).

In the modern era, cranialization is not usually utilized for inflammatory sinus disease [11]. Indications for contemporary use include frontal sinus malignancy involving the posterior table and comminuted fractures of the posterior frontal table, along with the need for cranialization in some neurosurgical approaches [22].

Cranialization: Case Illustration

A 66-year-old patient with history of renal cell carcinoma presented with a frontal forehead bulge and headache (Fig. 9.39). CT and MRI imaging revealed a contrast-enhancing mass suggestive of metastatic renal cell carcinoma that had eroded through the anterior and posterior tables of frontal sinus (Fig. 9.40). The mass infiltrated into the soft tissue of the forehead anteriorly and the dura posteriorly. Palliative gross total resection of the frontal sinus tumor

Fig. 9.28 A common cavity is created by removing the intersinus septum with the high-speed drill as well or Kerrison rongeurs. Care should always be taken to preserve mucosa if the frontal sinus will not be obliterated or cranialized (blue arrow showing the functional drainage path into the nose)

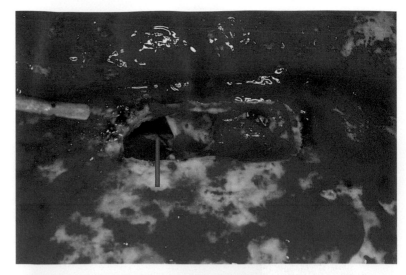

Fig. 9.29 After the frontal sinus is cleared of disease, attention should be directed toward ensuring patent drainage of the two frontal sinuses (arrows). Usually this is done via an external Lothrop procedure and by widening the frontal recess

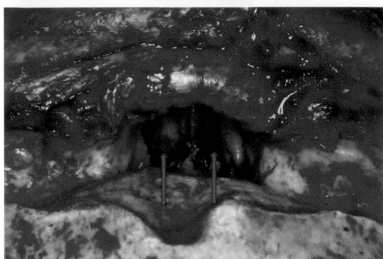

Fig. 9.30 If obliteration of the frontal sinus is to be performed, then all mucosa should be meticulously stripped off from the bone under magnification. A diamond burr may be used to remove microscopic fragments of mucosa till a smooth contour of the bone is defined

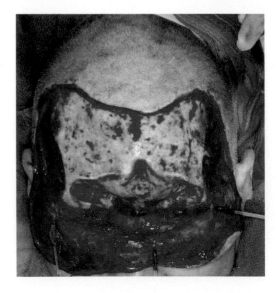

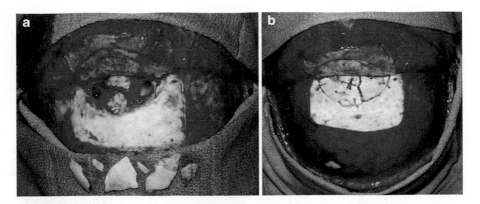

Fig. 9.31 If the bone flap is fractured, all pieces should be carefully repositioned and then plated or wired together

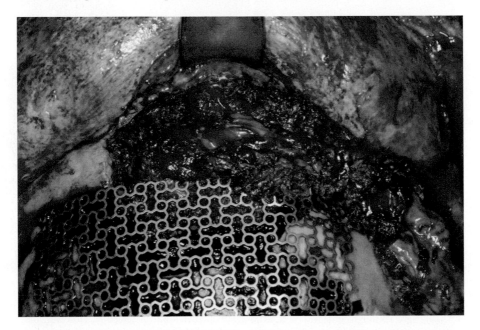

Fig. 9.32 In cases where the bone flap cannot be replaced, a mesh plate can be used as a scaffold to bridge any gap or hole in the calvarium

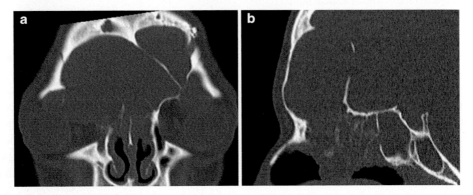

Fig. 9.33 CT scan of a patient with multiple mucoceles in a previously obliterated cavity. The coronal and sagittal views show extensive erosion of the orbital roof and the posterior frontal tables. This situation is a relative contra-indication for frontal sinus obliteration as complete removal of the mucosa is difficult and may result in cerebrospinal fluid leak or orbital injury

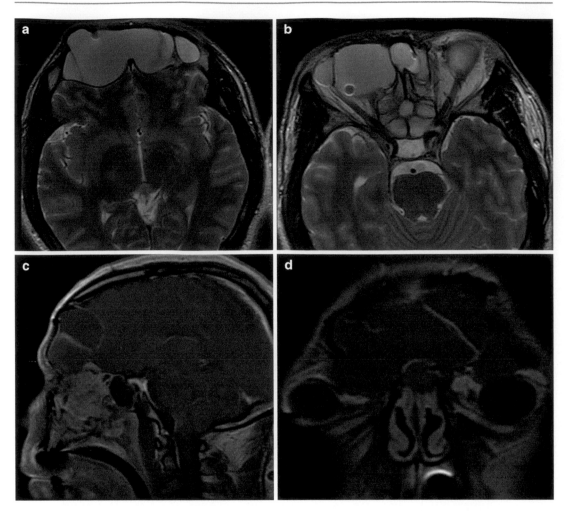

Fig. 9.34 MRI scan images showing multiple loculated mucoceles in a patient who underwent frontal sinus obliteration over 5 years ago. T2-weighted images (**a**, **b**, axial views) show the mucocele to be bright and rich in fluid as opposed to fat which is dark on this sequence. Images **c**, **d** show T-1 weighted images with contrast in sagittal (**c**) and coronal (**d**) planes; the lining of the mucocele is bright, while the fluid itself is dark. Fat is noted to be bright in the left medial orbit on image **d**. However, distinguishing mucocele from fat may be difficult even with MRI scans when the mucocele content becomes inspissated with the passage of time

was planned via an external approach using a bicoronal skin incision. As the skin flap was reflected inferiorly over the anterior table of the frontal sinus, there was gross macroscopic tumor that had already invaded through the anterior table wall extending to the underlying skin (Fig. 9.41). The tumor was freed from the skin anteriorly. The temporalis fascia was preserved and the pericranium was retracted with the scalp. A Leyla bar was set up so that the flap would be reflected superiorly-anteriorly with no pressure on the eyes. The orbital rims were subsequently exposed. The tumor was quite vascular. Two burr holes were placed on both sides of the sinus about 2 cm superior to the tumor (Fig. 9.41), and a number 3 Penfield was used to separate the

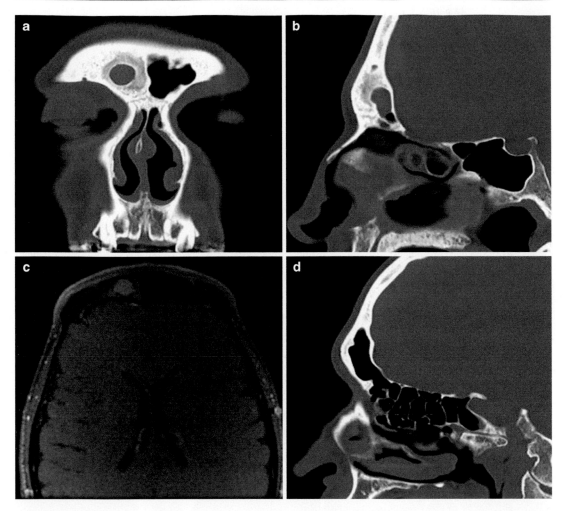

Fig. 9.35 (**a**) Coronal section CT scan of patient demonstrating complete opacification of a hypoplastic right frontal sinus. (**b**) Axial section MRI T-1 weighted sequence with contrast shows a discrete cyst or mass in right frontal sinus. (**c**) Sagittal section CT scan demonstrating opacified and hypoplastic right frontal sinus. CT images of the right frontal sinus show dense, thick bone that will need to be drilled via an endoscopic transnasal approach to the sinus. (**d**) Sagittal section CT scan demonstrating a well pneumatized and healthy left frontal sinus with a wide frontal sinus drainage pathway

dura from bone. A craniotome was used to fashion the craniotomy. Above this, the bone had been eroded significantly by the tumor. The bone flap was placed in antibiotic solution. However, after inspecting the inside of the bone, it was noted that it had been eroded by the tumor. Gross total resection of the tumor was achieved. After the tumor was removed off the frontal lobe dura, a small dural tear near the crista galli was patched with a pericranial graft. There was no obvious tumor invasion into the orbital contents. Bipolar cautery was used to gently coagulate the periorbita without entering the orbits bilaterally. The frontal sinus mucosa was removed entirely using the diamond burr to drill down to the bone. The epidural space was subsequently lined with fibrillar collagen, and then a mesh was used to replace the frontal bone (Fig. 9.42a). The osteoplastic bone flap could not be used since it was involved by tumor. The mesh nicely

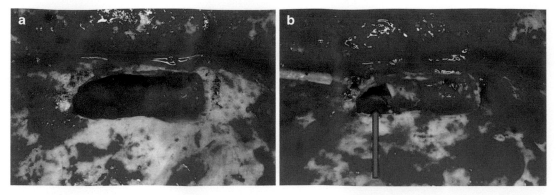

Fig. 9.36 An osteoplastic flap with a bicoronal approach was used for the patient in Fig. 9.35. Mucoid material was found and evacuated from the right frontal sinus, and the underlying mucosa was found healthy. The left frontal sinus was completely healthy with a wide frontal sinus drainage pathway; its ostium and recess can also be visualized (arrow). We therefore elected not to drill the right frontal recess but instead marsupialize the right frontal sinus into the left frontal sinus

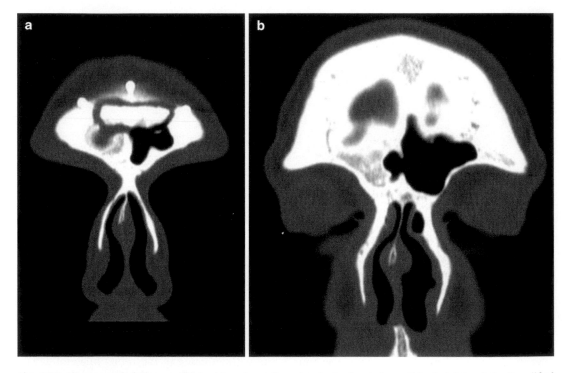

Fig. 9.37 Three-month follow-up CT imaging shows the osteoplastic flap to be well healed (**a**) and the "modified external Lothrop" common cavity to be adequately ventilated by the left frontal sinus drainage pathway (**b**)

contoured the frontal area. A gap was kept so that a vascularized free flap could be placed into it and under the dura. There was no evidence of bleeding into the epidural space prior to the flap being placed. The free flap was subsequently harvested from the left leg vastus lateralis muscle (Fig. 9.42b, c). It was fitted into the defect, completely obliterating the frontal sinus space and contouring the mesh plate (Fig. 9.42d). The vascular pedicle was anastomosed to the tempo-

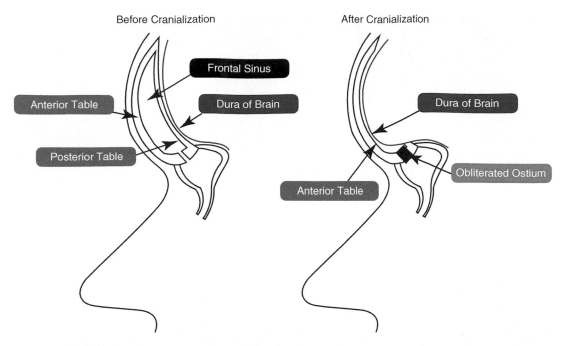

Fig. 9.38 Schematic representation of frontal sinusotomy with cranialization. The anterior border of the frontal lobe dura approximates the posterior wall of the anterior table after cranialization

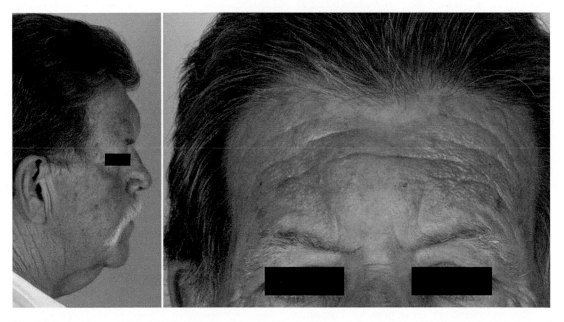

Fig. 9.39 A 66-year-old male with history of renal cell carcinoma presented with a frontal forehead bulge and headache

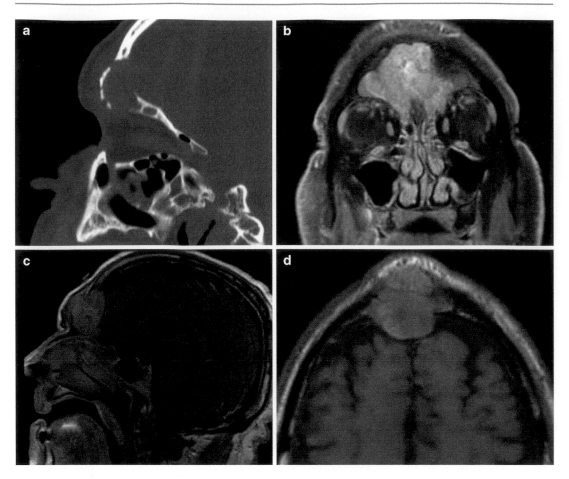

Fig. 9.40 (**a**) Sinus CT scan demonstrating an expansile mass of frontal sinus eroding the anterior, posterior, and inferior (orbital) walls on sagittal view. (**b, c, d**) T-1 weighted MRI sequence with gadolinium contrast shows a large con- trast-enhancing mass in the bilateral frontal sinus with extension into adjacent structures in the coronal (**b**), axial (**c**), and sagittal (**d**) sections; the contrast-enhancing mass infiltrates the soft tissue anteriorly and the dura posteriorly

ral artery and vein. Once the flap had been placed, there did not appear to be any significant pressure on the dura. Two drains were placed in the scalp wound well away from the vascular pedicle and were sutured into place. The head wound was then closed with 3-0 Vicryl suture in the deep dermal plane and running 4–0 and 5–0 Prolene to approximate the skin. The patient had no intraoperative or postoperative complica- tions. Pathology confirmed the mass to be renal cell carcinoma metastasis. Follow-up images showed excellent cosmetic results, even after completion of postoperative radiation therapy (Fig. 9.43).

External Frontoethmoidectomy

External frontoethmoidectomy is a procedure that has rare indications in the contemporary era (Table 9.3). Instead, most transorbital incisions that are now utilized are for access to the anterior skull base and the ethmoidal arteries [24, 25]. The procedure is briefly presented here for a compre- hensive coverage of external techniques for frontal sinus surgery.

In contrast to the anterior approach for external frontal sinusotomy, the external frontoethmoidec- tomy approach utilizes a lateral transorbital approach instead (Fig. 9.44). Access to the frontal sinus occurs through the medial superior aspect of

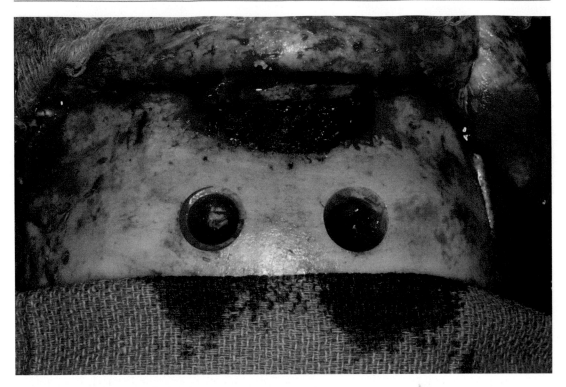

Fig. 9.41 Burr holes are placed on each side of the sinuses. The tumor can be visualized clearly already invading through the anterior table wall and extending into the skin

the orbit, through the lacrimal bone, and through anterior ethmoidal cells into the floor of the frontal sinus (Fig. 9.44b). Figure 9.45 demonstrates the difference in approach between a direct frontal trephination technique and the external frontoethmoidectomy approach. Access from the external frontoethmoidectomy approach is through relatively thin bones when compared to the anterior table of the frontal sinus. Important anatomic landmarks for this procedure include the medial canthus ligament, the lacrimal sac and its fossa, the trochlea, and finally the ethmoidal, supraorbital, and supratrochlear vessels. These are at risk of injury during external frontoethmoidectomy.

A transorbital approach to the frontal sinus was first described by Jansen in 1902 [1]. Although Lynch's name is most closely associated with the external frontoethmoidectomy procedure, Knapp described it first in 1908, ahead of Lynch's description in 1921 [1]. The original surgery begins with an external skin incision. The more modern iteration of the Lynch procedure is the Neel-Lake mod-

ification described in 1976 [26]. This procedure commences with intranasal ethmoidectomy, before any external approach is implemented. The external approach is then conducted via a modified Killian incision (Fig. 9.44a). This incision starts inferior to the medial portion of the eyebrow and in a curvilinear fashion courses medial to the medial canthus and ends 1 cm caudal to medial canthus at the caudal margin of the nasal bone. Incorporation of a "W" notch or stair-step in the incision can reduce the likelihood of unfavorable scar contracture ("bowstring" deformity). The incision is then deepened to the periosteum. The periosteum is elevated from the lower portion of the incision, the nasal process of the maxilla, medial wall and roof of orbit, nasal bone, and supraorbital ridge. Care must be taken to preserve the supratrochlear nerve and the supraorbital artery and nerve bundles. The medial canthal ligament is mobilized from the lacrimal fossa with both its limbs. It is tagged with a suture and retracted. The trochlea and the lacrimal sac are displaced from

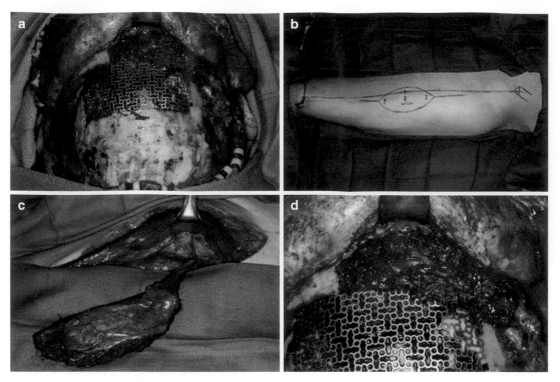

Fig. 9.42 (**a**) The mesh plate is used to replace the osteo-plastic flap that has been invaded by the tumor. (**b**) The vastus lateralis muscle flap is marked on the patient's thigh after measuring the defect harvesting. (**c**) The appro-

priately sized muscle flap is harvested. (**d**) The muscle flap is micro-anastomosed to the superficial temporal vessels in the neck as free tissue transfer and slid under the mesh. The muscle flap obliterates the frontal sinus

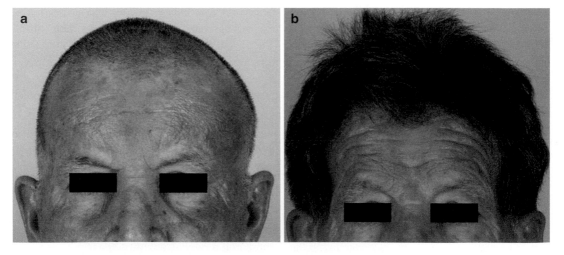

Fig. 9.43 (**a**) Image of patient at 1 month follow-up. Frontal defect is not visualized anymore. (**b**) Patient at 6 months follow-up shows excellent cosmesis even after completion of postoperative radiation therapy

Table 9.3 Indications for considering external frontoethmoidectomy

Previous endoscopic frontal sinus failure (obliterative or non-obliterative)
Patients with extensive neo-osteogenesis with a localized pyomucocele or mucocele
Traumatic injuries
Access to the ethmoidal arteries
Access to the anterior skull base
Local osteomyelitis

the underlying bone and also retracted with the rest of the globe laterally. This provides a good bony exposure to the medial orbit and brings the frontoethmoidal suture into view. The anterior and posterior ethmoidal arteries are identified. The anterior ethmoidal artery is cauterized with a bipolar, while the posterior is left intact unless posterior ethmoidectomy will also be conducted. The frontoethmoidal suture and ethmoidal vessels are

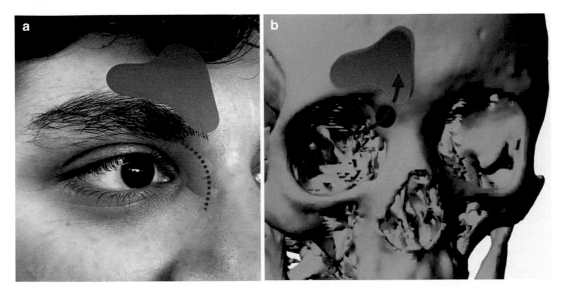

Fig. 9.44 (**a**) Schematic demonstrating the relationship between the modified Killian incision (red dotted line, Figure A) with the anterior ethmoidal (light green) and the frontal (gray) sinuses. (**b**) Schematic diagram demonstrating the frontoethmoidectomy approach through the medial orbit and through the ethmoidal cells into the floor of the frontal sinus (red arrow)

Figs. 9.45 This figure illustrates the difference between a direct frontal trephination through the brow (shown here) versus through a Lynch or Killian approach (broken line) that would be used to enter the frontal sinus through the medial orbit and anterior ethmoidal cavity

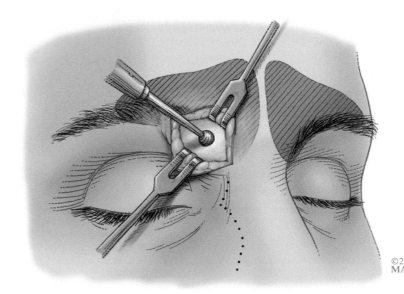

©2017
MAYO

the superior limits of the dissection. These landmarks correspond to the floor of the anterior cranial fossa. The osteotomy is extended from the lacrimal groove of the lacrimal bone to the lamina papyracea of the ethmoid bone. Subsequently intranasal anterior ethmoidectomy is performed, and the agger nasi and frontoethmoidal cells are removed. The frontal recess may be widened if occluded, by extending the opening from the frontal sinus posteriorly to the vertical attachment of the middle turbinate. The frontal sinus mucosa is generally preserved, as is the middle turbinate. The floor of the frontal sinus can be accessed at this point, and a portion of it is removed using a Kerrison rongeur. An endoscope may be used to visualize the frontal sinus. A rim of the frontal sinus floor medially and laterally is usually spared. A piece of Silastic sheeting is cut and rolled on itself. The free end of it is inserted into the frontal sinus and the other end through the recess along the nasal septum to which it is secured by a nylon suture. The periosteum is sutured back with nonresorbable sutures in order to secure the trochlea and medial canthal ligament in place. The subcutaneous tissue and skin are subsequently sutured with resorbable sutures. Interrupted simple sutures are utilized to supplement closure. The Silastic sheet is removed 6 weeks postoperatively. In contrast to the conventional Lynch procedure, the modified Lynch procedure preserves the frontal process of the maxilla, a portion of the frontal sinus floor, and spares the normal frontal mucosa as well as the middle turbinate. This prevents the orbital content from collapsing medially or herniating superiorly into the frontal sinus. Preserving the mucosa and middle turbinate decreases scar formation and osteoneogenesis in addition to preserving function.

The most common complications of external frontoethmoidectomy include proptosis, diplopia, restricted ocular movements, and latero-inferior displacement of the orbital contents. Other complications include lacrimal sac injuries and infections, vision loss from optic nerve injury, supraorbital or supratrochlear nerve injury causing sensory dysfunction, pseudohypertelorism from failure of medial canthal ligament reattachment, retrobulbar hematomas secondary to improper control of the ethmoidal vessels, and dural leaks secondary to anterior cranial fossa entry [26].

Other Techniques

The historical external Lothrop approach is now rarely utilized, except in modified forms (Fig. 9.36). Techniques such as the Riedel's technique which exteriorized the frontal sinus are now rarely indicated or performed as well. These have been supplanted by endoscopic techniques. The Riedel's technique involves removal of the anterior table of the frontal sinus if it is destroyed and unsalvageable due to fractures, tumors, or infection. The skin of the forehead is then allowed to collapse into the posterior frontal table, thus "exteriorizing" the sinus. This procedure was lifesaving for infections such as Pott's puffy tumor in the historical ear. Removal of the anterior table however leads to a significant cosmetic deformity due to collapse and retraction of the forehead skin into the posterior table (Fig. 9.46). In the contemporary era, most infectious frontal pathology is addressed by other procedures. If the anterior table has to be removed, the table is reconstructed by modern procedures such as microvascular free flaps [27]. We present an

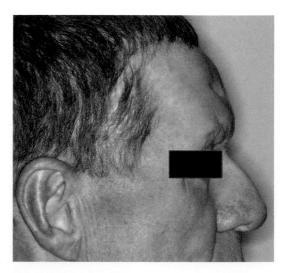

Fig. 9.46 Removal of the anterior frontal table however leads to a significant cosmetic deformity due to collapse and retraction of the forehead skin into the posterior table

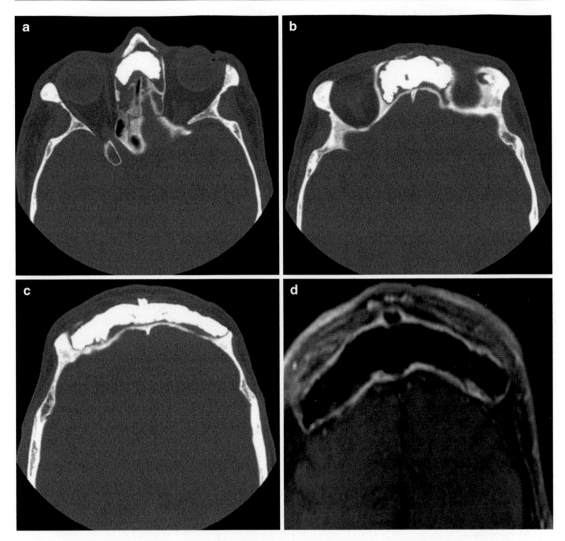

Fig. 9.47 Imaging from a patient who had undergone prior frontal sinus obliteration with hydroxyapatite a decade ago. Axial CT images (**a–c**) show the frontal sinus cavity to be occupied by hyperdense material. The anterior frontal table is completely eroded. The axial T1 with contrast MRI image (bottom right, **d**) shows regrowth of sinus mucosa in the lining of the frontal sinus, as demonstrated by the contrast enhancement along the periphery of the sinus. The overlying skin and soft tissue appear inflamed

illustrative case of a patient who had undergone prior frontal sinus obliteration with hydroxyapatite a decade ago (Fig. 9.47). He then developed frontal osteomyelitis with draining fistula and destruction of the anterior frontal table (Fig. 9.48).We addressed this frontal sinus pathology with an external approach (Fig. 9.49). After a bicoronal incision was made, the anterior table was found to be completely eroded. The

hydroxyapatite was removed. The residual frontal sinus mucosa was removed, and then the underlying bone was polished using 4 mm coarse diamond burr. If the overlying skin was then allowed to heal over this defect, this would have resulted in the classic Riedel's exteriorization technique, as well as a marked cosmetic deformity (Fig. 9.49d). Instead, the anterior table was reconstructed using an anterolateral thigh free

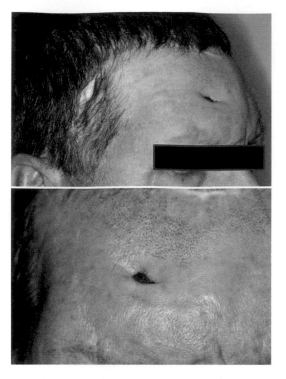

Fig. 9.48 The hydroxyapatite is infected and extruding through the forehead fistula

flap which was used to obliterate the frontal sinus, as well as to ensure satisfactory cosmesis (Fig. 9.50).

Frontal Sinus Trephination

This technique is still very valuable in the contemporary era and often underutilized [8]. The procedure is described in detail in Chap. 8. The frontal trephination technique can be used in isolation to address isolated frontal disease or can be used in conjunction with an endoscopic technique (the "above and below" approach; Fig. 9.51). The trephination can be performed through the brow (Fig. 9.52a) or the forehead (Fig. 9.52b). A conventional incision with a drill to remove the anterior frontal table can be used (Fig. 9.52a). Alternatively, a commercially available handheld mini-trephine is also available that can be used to cannulate a blunt tipped metal catheter into the anterior frontal table, which can be used to flush the frontal sinus intraoperatively or postoperatively (Fig. 9.52b).

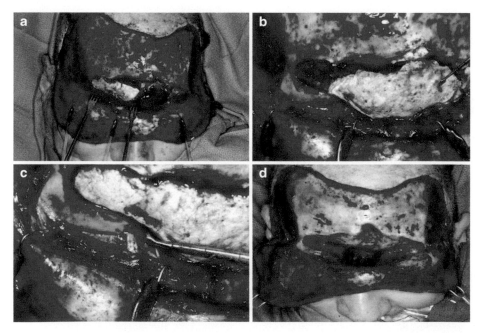

Fig. 9.49 (**a**) A bicoronal scalp incision was used. (**a–c**) The remnant anterior table and hydroxyapatite were removed. (**d**) Left as such, the resultant cavity would be a classic Riedel's exteriorization technique. However, to optimize cosmesis, a free flap was undertaken to reconstruct the forehead soft tissue. This involved obliteration of the frontal sinus cavity with free muscle transfer. The frontal sinus mucosa was therefore meticulously removed, polishing the underlying bone with a 4 mm coarse diamond burr

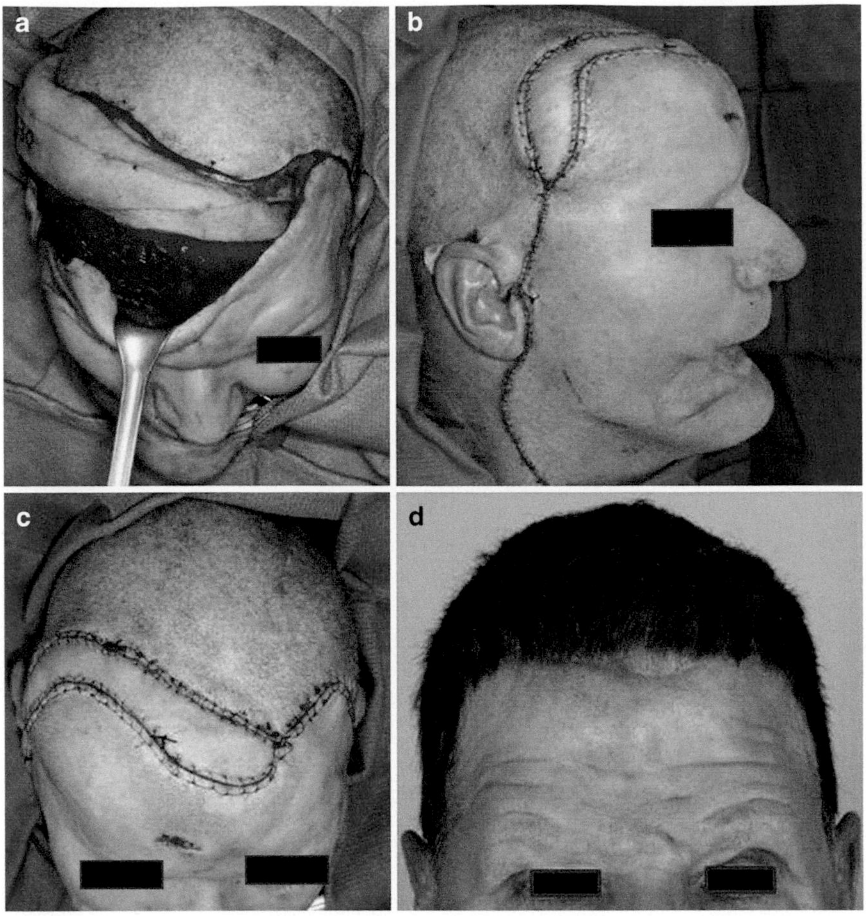

Fig. 9.50 (**a**) The frontal sinus defect was reconstructed using a microvascular free flap harvested from the anterolateral thigh; a skin paddle is left to monitor the flap vitality. (**b**) The flap is inset. (**c**) The overlying skin fistula is excised and sewed. (**d**) The flap is well healed and inset after 2 years, with excellent cosmesis

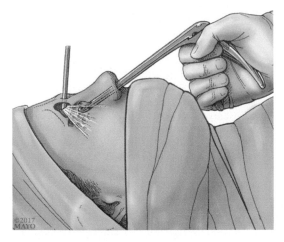

Fig. 9.51 Schematic explaining the "above and below" approach. Both the trephination and endonasal approaches are used simultaneously in this approach. Endoscopy and passage of instrumentation can be conducted through either the trephination or the endonasal approach

Summary

External techniques in frontal sinus surgery remain an integral part of the rhinologic armamentarium in the contemporary era of endoscopic sinus surgery. The vast majority of inflammatory frontal sinus pathology is managed superiorly using endoscopic techniques. External frontal sinus techniques can be associated with higher burden of immediate and long-term postoperative complications and sequela. However, even in cases where endoscopic techniques can be successfully performed but require lengthier operative time or morbidity, open procedures may provide a faster, definitive option. Since endoscopic techniques have supplanted the vast majority of external techniques, it is becoming increasingly difficult to maintain skills in external techniques. Educational programs must recognize

a   b

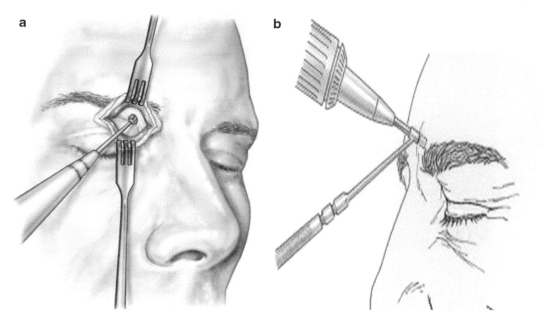

Fig. 9.52 The placement of the trephination can be personalized and is chosen based on the anatomy and pathology to be addressed. Trephination can be performed through a brow incision (**a**) or the anterior forehead (**b**) using a small incision and drill (**a**) or with a commercially available mini-trephination system (**b**)

that decreasing performance of external approaches for frontal surgeries may compromise their trainees' exposure to such modalities of treatment. External frontal techniques may be invaluable for recalcitrant inflammatory sinus disease that are not adequately addressed by prior endoscopic procedures or where the disease is far lateral and inaccessible through endoscopic approaches. Patients with malignancies, benign tumors, fractures, and CSF leaks may also require external frontal approaches.

References

1. Lawson W, Ho Y. Open Frontal Sinus Surgery. Otolaryngol Clin N Am. 2016;49(4):1067–89. https://doi.org/10.1016/j.otc.2016.03.027.
2. Hahn S, Palmer JN, Purkey MT, Kennedy DW, Chiu AG. Indications for external frontal sinus procedures for inflammatory sinus disease. Am J Rhinol Allergy. 2009;23(3):342–7. https://doi.org/10.2500/ajra.2009.23.3327.
3. Jacobs JB. 100 years of frontal sinus surgery. Laryngoscope. 1997;107(11 Pt 2):1–36.
4. Ramadan HH. History of frontal sinus surgery. Arch Otolaryngol Head Neck Surg. 2000;126(1):98–9. https://doi.org/10.1007/3-540-27607-6_1.
5. Courson AM, Stankiewicz JA, Lal D. Contemporary management of frontal sinus mucoceles: a meta-analysis. Laryngoscope. 2014;124(2):378–86. https://doi.org/10.1002/lary.24309.
6. Cervantes SS, Lal D. Crista galli mucocele: endoscopic marsupialization via frontoethmoid approach. Int Forum Allergy Rhinol. 2014;4(7):598–602. https://doi.org/10.1002/alr.21321.
7. Svider PF, Sekhsaria V, Cohen DS, Eloy JA, Setzen M, Folbe AJ. Geographic and temporal trends in frontal sinus surgery. Int Forum Allergy Rhinol. 2015;5(1):46–54. https://doi.org/10.1002/alr.21425.
8. Patel AB, Cain RB, Lal D. Contemporary applications of frontal sinus trephination: a systematic review of the literature. Laryngoscope. 2015;125(9):2046–53. https://doi.org/10.1002/lary.25206.
9. Ochsner MC, DelGaudio JM. The place of the osteoplastic flap in the endoscopic era: indications and pitfalls. Laryngoscope. 2015;125(4):801–6. https://doi.org/10.1002/lary.25014.
10. Conger BT Jr, Illing E, Bush BWB. Management of lateral frontal sinus pathology in the endoscopic era. Otolaryngol neck Surg. 2014;151(1):159–63.
11. Chaaban MR, Conger B, Riley KO, Woodworth BA. Transnasal endoscopic repair of posterior table fractures. Otolaryngol Head Neck Surg. 2012;147(6):1142–7. https://doi.org/10.1177/0194599812462547.
12. Neel GS, Nagel TH, Hoxworth JM, Lal D. Management of orbital involvement in sinonasal and ventral skull base malignancies. Otolaryngol Clin N

Am. 2017;50(2):347–64. https://doi.org/10.1016/j.otc.2016.12.010.

13. Lee WT, Kuhn FA, Citardi MJ. 3D computed tomographic analysis of frontal recess anatomy in patients without frontal sinusitis. Otolaryngol Head Neck Surg. 2004;131(3):164–73. https://doi.org/10.1016/j.otohns.2004.04.012.

14. van Alyea OE. Frontal cells: an anatomic study of these cells with consideration of their clinical significance. Arch Otolaryngol. 1941;34:11–23.

15. Healy DY, Leopold DA, Gray ST, Holbrook EH. The perforation technique: a modification to the frontal sinus osteoplastic flap. Laryngoscope. 2014;124(6):1314–7. https://doi.org/10.1002/lary.24460.

16. Orlandi RR, Kingdom TT, Hwang PH, et al. International consensus statement on allergy and rhinology: rhinosinusitis. Int Forum Allergy Rhinol. 2016;6(November 2015):S22–S209. https://doi.org/10.1002/alr.21695.

17. Bartley J, Eagleton N, Rosser P, Al-Ali S. Superior oblique muscle palsy after frontal sinus minitrephine. Am J Otolaryngol Head Neck Med Surg. 2012;33(1):181–3. https://doi.org/10.1016/j.amjoto.2011.04.008.

18. Weber R, Draf W, Keerl R, et al. Osteoplastic frontal sinus surgery with fat obliteration: technique and long-term results using magnetic resonance imaging in 82 operations. Laryngoscope. 2000;110(June):1037–44. https://doi.org/10.1097/00005537-200006000-00028.

19. Rivera T, Rodríguez M, Pulido N, García-Alcántara F, Sanz L. Current indications for the osteoplastic flap. Acta Otorrinolaringol (English Ed). 2016;67(1):33–9. https://doi.org/10.1016/j.otoeng.2015.01.004.

20. Lawson W, Patel ZM. The evolution of management for inverted papilloma: an analysis of 200 cases. Otolaryngol - Head Neck Surg. 2009;140(3):330–5. https://doi.org/10.1016/j.otohns.2008.11.010.

21. Loevner LA, Yousem DM, Lanza DC, Kennedy DW, Goldberg AN. MR Evaluation of Frontal Sinus Osteoplastic Flaps. Am J Neuroradiol. 1995;16(9):1721–6.

22. Donath A, Sindwani R. Frontal sinus cranialization using the pericranial flap: an added layer of protection. Laryngoscope. 2006;116(9):1585–8. https://doi.org/10.1097/01.mlg.0000232514.31101.39.

23. Donald PJ, Bernstein L. Compound frontal sinus injuries with intracranial penetration. Laryngoscope. 1978;88:225–32.

24. Ramakrishna R, Kim LJ, Bly RA, Moe K, Ferreira M. Transorbital neuroendoscopic surgery for the treatment of skull base lesions. J Clin Neurosci. 2016;24:99–104. https://doi.org/10.1016/j.jocn.2015.07.021.

25. Berens AM, Davis GE, Moe KS. Transorbital endoscopic identification of supernumerary ethmoid arteries. Allergy Rhinol (Providence). 2016;7(3):144–6. https://doi.org/10.2500/ar.2016.7.0167.

26. Neel HB, McDonald TJ, Facer GW. Modified lynch procedure for chronic frontal sinus diseases: rationale, technique, and long-term results. Laryngoscope. 1987;97(11):1274–9.

27. Raghavan U. The place of Riedel's procedure in contemporary sinus surgery. J Laryngol Otol. 2004;118(9):700–5.

Balloon-Assisted Frontal Sinus Surgery

10

Anali Dadgostar, Fahad Al-Asousi, and Amin R. Javer

Introduction

Chronic rhinosinusitis (CRS) is a significant health issue, affecting approximately 16% of the adult population, ranking it as one of the most prevalent ailments in the Western world [1, 2]. In the United States, CRS has been estimated to generate annual health-related costs of more than $5 billion [2]. Obstruction of the sinus ostia is considered one of the mechanisms that contribute to development and maintenance of CRS by impairing ventilation and drainage of the sinus cavities. In patients with CRS, the frontal sinus is frequently affected and has a major contribution to the impact of the disease on quality of life, making it a high priority target for medical and surgical intervention. Treatment of CRS involves medical treatment, surgical treatment, or a combination of both. Surgical therapy is typically offered after a course of appropriate medical therapy. The most frequently used surgical approach is functional endoscopic sinus surgery (FESS) with the goal of establishing patency of the sinus drainage pathways and enhancing mucosal clearance [3]. Although shown to be very effective, FESS typically requires general anesthesia and carries the risk of scarring and

adhesions within the ostiomeatal anatomy [6]. The word "functional" emphasizes the preservation of normal mucosal clearance via the natural anatomic drainage pathways [4, 5]. Nowhere is this principle more important than in the frontal recess. Here, preservation of mucosa is paramount to prevent restenosis (recurrence of narrowing) and consequent complex and potentially hazardous revision procedures.

The concept of dilating an ostium via a high-pressure balloon was originally developed and promoted in the fields of cardiology, vascular surgery, and urology. The introduction of high-pressure balloon dilation catheter technology in 2005 to create sinus ostia enlargement led to development of the "balloon sinuplasty" procedure. Balloon catheter-assisted dilatation has emerged over the years as another viable option in the treatment of low-grade sinus disease. A body of data now supports the concept that transnasal dilation to open and remodel sinus ostia is an effective treatment of CRS [7–10]. The majority of the initial balloon catheter-assisted dilatation procedures were completed using general anesthesia and fluoroscopy to navigate the balloon catheter to the treatment site and often performed as a hybrid procedure in conjunction with FESS. Technological innovation, improvements in balloon catheter-assisted dilatation techniques, and a long history of experience with this procedure now facilitate use of balloon catheters under local anesthesia with endoscopic guidance rather

A. Dadgostar · F. Al-Asousi · A. R. Javer (✉)
St. Paul's Sinus Centre, St. Paul's Hospital,
Department of Otolaryngology – Head and Neck
Surgery, Vancouver, BC, Canada

© Springer Nature Switzerland AG 2019
D. Lal, P. H. Hwang (eds.), *Frontal Sinus Surgery*, https://doi.org/10.1007/978-3-319-97022-6_10

than fluoroscopy [11, 12]. Balloon ostial dilatation (BOD) refers to solely dilating natural drainage pathways of the maxillary, frontal, and sphenoid sinuses, without removing any tissue. Because of its mucosal-sparing nature, BOD typically results in less bleeding and more rapid healing, requires fewer postoperative debridements, and may allow for earlier return to work. Office-based dilatation eliminates the risks associated with general anesthesia, is more convenient for patients, and offers the potential for considerable cost savings [13].

Frontal Sinus Considerations and Indications

Before consideration for surgery, patients should have failed appropriate medical therapy, have persistent symptoms of at least 12 weeks, and demonstrate evidence of chronic rhinosinusitis on computed tomography (CT). Currently, there is no evidence to support using BOD or any other instrumentation to operate on frontal sinuses without inflammatory disease. Patient selection is paramount – the patient must demonstrate the ability to tolerate endoscopic assessment and instrumentation of the sinonasal cavity in the office setting [13]. It is prudent to review the CT images preoperatively to identify any potential anatomic variations such as middle turbinate concha bullosa, paradoxical curvature of the middle turbinate, and nasal septal deviation that would make sinus access difficult and uncomfortable for the patient even with appropriate anesthesia.

Frontal sinus disease management remains one of the most difficult undertakings in endoscopic sinus surgery. Anatomic studies have demonstrated that the underlying problem in chronic frontal sinusitis is not the sinus but rather its drainage pathway through the frontal recess. The frontal recess is an inverted funnel-like area that connects the frontal ostium superiorly to the anterior ethmoidal space inferiorly. It is usually pneumatized by a variety of frontal recess cells, which may cause anatomical frontal recess obstruction and be the primary cause of chronic

frontal sinusitis [14–17]. The complex anatomy and its anterosuperior location render endoscopic frontal recess dissection and visualization difficult, therefore predisposing it to surgical failure. The frontal sinus is the most challenging of the major paranasal sinuses to obtain good surgical results. This is mainly due to its unique and varied anatomy, acute angle of access, and proximity to critical structures (olfactory fossa, skull base, and orbit). Surgical failures on the frontal sinus are often secondary to significant mucosal trauma during frontal sinusotomy, leading to scar formation. The critical goal of operating on the frontal recess is not only to relieve obstruction of the outflow tract and treat the existing disease from an anatomical perspective but, also and more importantly, prevent recurrence of disease. This goal is inherently easier to achieve in primary surgical intervention. Unfortunately, iatrogenic causes have a large role in recurrent frontal sinusitis, with neo-osteogenesis and recurrent polyposis also being significant factors [18]. Frontal sinus surgery should encompass an understanding of the underlying abnormality (inflammatory vs neoplastic), the unique anatomy of the frontal recess, the need for adequate exposure for postoperative monitoring and care in the clinic, and the long-term impact of the particular procedure utilized.

It is important to understand the underlying disease process of each patient before proceeding with BOD. As stated, the aim of this technology is to restore the natural sinus drainage pathways in a minimally invasive way. The potential advantage is reduced incidence of the scarring often associated with surgical manipulation and mucosal stripping. Within the frontal sinus outflow tract, BOD allows for greenstick fracturing and lateral displacement of the medial and superior wall of obstructing frontal cells, medial displacement of an obstructing intersinus septal cell wall, and/or dilating soft tissue stenosis in previously operated patients. Therefore, rather than excising inflamed tissue and adjacent bone, in theory, the balloon compresses the mucosa and causes microfractures of the underlying obstructive bony wall, thereby creating ostial patency. Ostial patency alone however may not be enough to assure an ideal outcome. For example, BOD should not be performed if there is suspicion or pathologic confirmation of neoplastic disease. In patients with CRSwNP or eosinophilic and CRS, BOD alone may also not be sufficient. In such cases, tissue removal and surgical widening of the outflow tract by removal of frontal recess cells are necessary to address disease and facilitate local drug delivery. Narrow recesses and dense neo-osteogenesis of the frontal sinus outflow tract may impede easy access to the frontal sinus ostium. In these situations, BOD may be used in conjunction with traditional FESS techniques ("hybrid technique") to conduct frontal sinus surgery.

Technology

Several commercial devices are currently available for balloon dilation of the frontal sinus. Although the basic principles of BOD are the same regardless of the device used, there may be specific technical differences that the user must be become familiar with. Currently, there are four manufacturers of BOD devices approved by the US Food and Drug Administration (FDA), namely, Acclarent (Irvine, California, USA), Entellus (Plymouth, Minnesota, USA), Medtronic (Minneapolis, Minnesota, USA), and Smith & Nephew (Cordova, Tennessee, USA). Some utilize the Seldinger technique (whereby a catheter is advanced and positioned over a guidewire) for balloon placement. The delivery catheter, which is specifically angulated at 70 degrees for the frontal sinus, is endoscopically positioned at the entrance of the ostium. The guidewire is passed through the catheter into the sinus and the balloon advanced over it, positioned to straddle the ostium. It is then transiently inflated to a high pressure (up to 12 atmospheres), thereby pushing the bony partitions obstructing the recess out of the way. Some manufacturers provide devices specifically designed for some of the unique features of frontal sinus outflow tract anatomy, mimicking a frontal sinus seeker. They also provide further ability to change the trajectory of the tip of the wire, which improves proper ostial cannu-

lation, subsequent balloon advancement, and dilation of the frontal sinus outflow tract. For hybrid technique with FESS, the ethmoid cells have been dissected and the anterior ethmoid artery is localized, using standard instrumentation. Next, the balloon is inserted under direct endoscopic visualization into the frontal recess. Image guidance can be used concurrently to confirm correct positioning in the frontal sinus. The balloon is then inflated.

Procedure

Diligent patient counseling and preparation is key for achieving success with balloon dilatation. High-resolution tri-orthogonal CT scan imaging should be reviewed prior to commencing the procedure to examine and conceptualize the drainage pathway of the frontal sinus. The procedure is usually performed with the patient in a sitting position. The patient is prepared by application of topical 4% lidocaine combined with topical oxymetazoline cotton pledgets medial and lateral to the middle turbinate to allow for gentle medial displacement of the middle turbinate once anesthesia is achieved. A 0-degree or 30-degree endoscope is typically used at the beginning to allow for a broad field of visualization. Visualization of the sinus guide placement for the guidewire may be facilitated by angled endoscopes, which are also used to examine the frontal ostium after the dilatation has been performed. Access to the frontal sinus is best achieved if the tip of the 70-degree sinus guide is placed between the uncinate process and the face of the ethmoid bulla in the parasagittal plane. The distal tip should be visible near the upper third of the ethmoid bulla and not passed into the frontal recess to allow the guidewire to explore a broader area in search of the pathway into the frontal sinus (Fig.10.1). At this point, the guidewire is advanced into the frontal sinus. If the guidewire does not easily pass into the frontal sinus, it is retracted back into the sinus guide, the sinus guide is repositioned, and attempted cannulation is repeated. The latest technologies use image guidance of the distal tip of the wire to confirm its position within the frontal ostium (Fig. 10.2). Once proper placement of the device is confirmed, an appropriately sized balloon (diameter and length are considerations) is advanced and dilated to 10–12 atmospheres of pressure. Once the frontal sinus is successfully accessed, balloon advancement and dilatation are performed and may be repeated more proximally or distally within the frontal sinus outflow tract depending on the frontal anatomy and length of balloon chosen. On completion of the procedure,

the patient is observed for 20–30 min to watch for acute complications and discharged with follow-up instructions as with traditional FESS.

Discussion

Current 1-year follow-up studies of balloon sinus dilatation reveal significant reduction in sinonasal symptoms and healthcare use after balloon dilation, very low rate of revision surgery, and efficacy similar to FESS in the treatment of CRS in patients with chronic sinus disease [19, 20]. Chandra et al. [21] reported on long-term outcomes of the REMODEL (randomized evaluation of maxillary antrostomy versus ostial dilation efficacy through long-term follow-up) study and performed a meta-analysis of the long-term outcomes of stand-alone balloon sinus dilatation. They found comparable outcomes from 6 to 24 months between the FESS and balloon dilatation groups including SNOT-20 scores, number of acute infections, and antibiotic prescriptions. The meta-analysis concluded that balloon dilatation produced faster recovery, less postoperative pain, and fewer debridements than FESS. A recent report including 37 patients with CRS demonstrated feasibility of in-office BOD

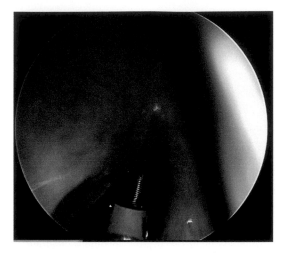

Fig. 10.1 Positioning of the sinus guide and advancement of the guidewire

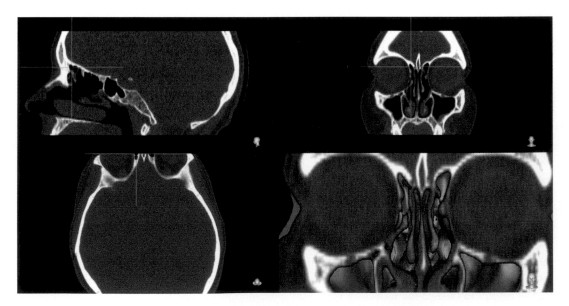

Fig. 10.2 Image guidance confirmation of the distal tip of the wire within the frontal sinus

for all sinuses, technical success, procedure tolerability, and clinical and statistical improvement in patient symptoms [22].

BOD technology provides the advantage of use in the office setting. Office setting utilization has the obvious advantages of the elimination of the risks and recovery of general anesthesia and avoidance of the associated costs with the hospital outpatient department or ambulatory surgical facility. In-office BOD has been shown to be safe and well tolerated with outcomes similar to those achieved in traditional venues [22–24]. A recent survey of members of the American Rhinologic Society suggests that surgeons are more accepting of balloon catheter technology now compared with 5 years ago, and many of them believe that their use of such technology will increase in the future [25].

Two studies have retrospectively examined patients undergoing office-based revision frontal sinus balloon dilation. Eloy et al. [26] reported retrospectively on five patients who had office-based dilation of a stenosing frontal neo-ostium using transnasal balloon dilation instrumentation. All five patients were reported to be asymptomatic at a mean follow-up of 5 months with patent drainage pathway. Unfortunately, the study lacked a validated quality of life instrument upon which to base patient symptom outcomes. In a retrospective study performed by Luong et al. [27], six patients undergoing office-based dilation for postoperative frontal sinus ostium stenosis using either a lacrimal dilation catheter or a sinus dilation catheter were assessed. Using topical anesthesia and endoscopic visualization, they found that durable patency was achieved in all six frontal sinuses dilated, with only one patient requiring a second dilation due to ostium contraction >50% during the follow-up range of 4–9 months. The patient-reported outcomes are limited by lack of a baseline questionnaire and use of a non-validated survey.

Chan et al. [28] studied five patients with chronic frontal sinusitis who had failed medical management and also presented with ipsilateral anterior ethmoid sinusitis. After balloon dilation of the frontal stenosis without ethmoidectomy, all patients showed complete radiographic clearing of both the dilated frontal sinus and the anterior ethmoid. Catalano et al. [29] examined the use of balloon dilatation of the frontal recess for the treatment of CRS in 20 patients with advanced frontal sinus disease that had failed medical therapy. They found that pretreatment and posttreatment Lund-Mackay scores showed significant improvement in patients with certain subsets of chronic rhinosinusitis, particularly those patients with chronic rhinosinusitis without nasal polyposis.

Several studies have examined frontal sinus patency rates post-FESS. Chan and colleagues [30] examined 294 frontal sinuses operated using traditional FESS techniques. Long-term patency was achieved in 88%. In another study examining 100 frontal sinuses operated using FESS techniques, Askar and colleagues [31] reported long-term patency in 90%. The largest study to date including in-office BOD of the frontal sinuses reported that 251 of 268 frontal sinuses were successfully dilated (93.7%) with 5 frontal sinuses requiring revision procedures (2%) [23]. BOD can also be used in conjunction with traditional FESS techniques as a hybrid procedure. Javer et al. performed a single-blinded, randomized, controlled, prospective study of 30 patients undergoing FESS for CRS. Patients underwent a hybrid approach with balloon dilatation on one side and traditional frontal sinusotomy for the opposite side. The results demonstrated reduced blood loss and operative time in the hybrid balloon technique with patency comparable to traditional frontal sinusotomy at 1 year postoperatively [32].

Balloon catheter dilatation is not commonly utilized in the pediatric population. In a recent survey of the American Rhinologic Society (ARS) membership, 90% performed adenoidectomy as a first step. BOD was not frequently used with only 17% performing it in the pediatric population. Overall, 66% never or rarely used it and only 3% always or almost always used it [33].

Although it may appear that BOD achieves higher patency rates, it is important to realize that patients undergoing BOD typically have a lower burden of disease than those undergoing traditional FESS procedures. This emphasizes the importance of carefully selecting the appropriate procedure for each unique clinical situation.

Complications

Balloons can be associated with the same complications that are associated with traditional ESS. In 2016, Prince and Bhattacharyya reviewed adverse events reported with the use of balloons in sinuses on the openFDA database [34]. Of the 114 reported adverse events, there were 72 cases of patient injury. These included 4 deaths, 17 cases of skull base injury, and 15 CSF leaks (frontal and sphenoid). Orbital injury was the most common complication with 13 patients requiring lateral canthotomy and 3 requiring medial orbital decompression. Device malfunction was reported in 36 cases (device fracture). In addition, since tissue is not removed, histopathology is also not available as a consequence of using this technique.

Summary

Balloon catheter-assisted dilatation is a new and important tool available for addressing frontal sinus disease. Prior to undertaking BOD, it is important to understand the significance of carefully selecting the appropriate procedure for the unique clinical situation with assessment of the underlying disease process, patient anatomy, and technique. Balloon-assisted frontal sinus dilatation serves as a stand-alone or complementary procedure for the treatment of medically refractory chronic rhinosinusitis.

Acknowledgments We would like to recognize the efforts our research coordinator, Christopher Okpaleke, for his assistance with this manuscript.

References

1. Adams PF, et al. Current estimates from the National Health Interview Survey, 1996. Vital Health Stat 10. 1999;200:1–20.

2. Blackwell DL, et al. Summary health statistics for US adults: National Health Survey, 1997. Vital Health Stat 10. 2002;205:1–109.

3. Fokkens W, Lund V, Mullol J. European position paper on rhinosinusitis and nasal polyps 2007. Rhinol Suppl. 2007;20:1–136.

4. Kennedy DW, Zinreich SJ, Rosenbaum AE, Johns ME. Functional endoscopic sinus surgery. Theory and diagnostic evaluation. Arch Otolaryngol. 1985;111(9):576–82.

5. Stammberger H. Endoscopic endonasal surgery - concepts in treatment of recurring rhinosinusitis. Part II. Surgical technique. Otolaryngol Head Neck Surg. 1986;94(2):147–56.

6. Lee JM, Grewal A. Middle meatal spacers for the prevention of synechiae following endoscopic sinus surgery: a systematic review and meta-analysis of randomized controlled trial. Int Forum Allergy Rhinol. 2012;2(6):477–86.

7. Kuhn FA, Church CA, Goldberg AN, et al. Balloon catheter sinusotomy: one-year follow-up outcomes and role in functional endoscopic sinus surgery. Otolaryngol Head Neck Surg. 2008;139(3S3):S27–37.

8. Vaughan WC. Review of balloon sinuplasty. Curr Opin Otolaryngol Head Neck Surg. 2008;16:2–9.

9. Bolger WE, Brown CL, Church CA, et al. Safety and outcomes of balloon catheter sinusotomy: a multicenter 24-week analysis in 115 patients. Otolaryngol Head Neck Surg. 2007;137:10–20.

10. Brodner D, Nachlas N, Mock P, Truitt T, Armstrong M, Pasha R, Jung C, Atkins J. Safety and outcomes following hybrid balloon and balloon-only procedure using a multifunction, multisinus balloon dilation tool. Int Forum Allergy Rhinol. 2013;3(8):652–8. Epub 2013 Feb 19.

11. Stankiewicz J, Tami T, Truitt T, et al. Transantral, endoscopically guided balloon dilation of the ostiomeatal complex for chronic rhinosinusitis under local anesthesia. Am J Rhinol Allergy. 2009;23:321–7.

12. Karanfilov B, Silvers S, Pasha R, et al. Office-based balloon sinus dilation: a prospective, multicenter study of 203 patients. Int Forum Allergy Rhinol. 2013;3(5):404–11.

13. Prickett K, Wise S, DelGaudio J. Cost analysis of office-based and operating room procedures in rhinology. Int Forum Allergy Rhinol. 2012;2:207–11.

14. Kuhn FA, Bolger WE, Tisdal RG. The agger nasi cell in frontal recess obstruction: an anatomic, radiologic and clinical correlation. Oper Tech Otolaryngol Head Neck Surg. 1991;2:226–231.5.

15. Bent JP, Cuilty-Siller C, Kuhn FA. The frontal cell in frontal sinus obstruction. Am J Rhinol. 1994;8:185–191.6.

16. Owen RG, Kuhn FA. The supraorbital ethmoid cell. Otolaryngol Head Neck Surg. 1997;116:254–261.7.

17. Merritt R, Bent JP, Kuhn FA. The intersinus septal cell. Am J Rhinol. 1996;10:299–302.

18. Philpott CM, Mckiernan DC, Javer AR. Selecting the best approach to the frontal sinus. Indian J Otolaryngol Head Neck Surg. 2011;63(1):79–84.

19. Bikhazi N, Light J, Truitt T, Schwartz M, Cutler J, REMODEL Study Investigators. Standalone balloon dilation versus sinus surgery for chronic rhinosinusitis: a prospective, multicenter, randomized, controlled trial with 1-year follow-up. Am J Rhinol Allergy. 2014;28(4):323–9.
20. Gould J, Alexander I, Tomkin E, Brodner D. In-office, multisinus balloon dilation: 1-year outcomes from a prospective, multicenter, open label trial. Am J Rhinol Allergy. 2014;28(2):156–63.
21. Chandra RK, Kern RC, Cutler JL, Welch KC, Russell PT. REMODEL larger cohort with long-term outcomes and meta-analysis of standalone balloon dilatation studies. Laryngoscope. 2016;126(1):44–50.
22. Albritton F, Casiano R, Sillers M. Feasability of in-office endoscopic sinus surgery with balloon sinus dilation. Am J Rhinol Allergy. 2012;26(3):243–8.
23. Karanfilov B, Silvers S, Pasha R, et al. Office-based balloon sinus dilation: a prospective multi-center study of 203 patients. Int Forum Allergy Rhinol. 2013;3:404–11.
24. Cutler J, Truitt T, Atkins J, et al. First clinic experience: patient selection and out- comes for ostial dilation for chronic rhinosinusitis. Int Forum Allergy Rhinol. 2011;1(6):460–5.
25. Halderman AA, Stokken J, Momin SR, Smith TL, Sindwani R. Attitudes on and usage of balloon catheter technology in rhinology: a survey of the American Rhinologic Society. Am J Rhinol Allergy. 2015;29(5):389–93.
26. Eloy JA, Friedel ME, Eloy JD, Govindaraj S, Folbe AJ. In-office balloon dilation of the failed frontal sinusotomy. Otolaryngol Head Neck Surg. 2012;146:320–2.
27. Luong A, Batra PS, Fakhri S, Citardi MJ. Balloon catheter dilatation for frontal ostium stenosis in the office setting. Am J Rhinol. 2008;22:621–4.
28. Chan Y, Melroy CT, Kuhn FA. Is anterior ethmoid disease really responsible for chronic frontal sinusitis? Presented at the annual meeting of the American Rhinologic Society Annual Meeting, Chicago; 2008.
29. Catalano PJ, Payne SC. Balloon dilation of the frontal recess in patients with chronic frontal sinusitis and advanced sinus disease: an initial report. Ann Otol Rhinol Laryngol. 2009;118(2):107–12.
30. Chan Y, Melroy C, Kuhn C, et al. Long-term frontal sinus patency after endoscopic frontal sinusotomy. Laryngoscope. 2009;119(6):1229–32.
31. Askar M, Gamea A, Tomoum M, et al. Endoscopic management of chronic frontal rhinosinusitis: prospective quality of life analysis. Ann Otol Rhinol Laryngol. 2015;124(8):638–48.
32. Hathorn IF, Pace-Asciak P, Habib AR, Sunkaraneni V, Javer AR. Randomized controlled trial: hybrid technique using balloon dilation of the frontal sinus drainage pathway. Int Forum Allergy Rhinol. 2015;5(2):167–73.
33. Beswick DM, Ramadan H, Baroody F, Hwang PH. Practice patterns in pediatric chronic rhinosinusitis: a survey of the American Rhinologic society. Am J Rhinol Allergy. 2016;30:418–23.
34. Prince A, Bhattacharyya N. An analysis of adverse event reporting in balloon sinus procedures. Otolaryngol Head Neck Surg. 2016;154(4):748–53.

Management of the Stenosing Frontal Recess

Rickul Varshney and Jivianne T. Lee

Introduction

Functional endoscopic sinus surgery (FESS) has been employed as an effective intervention for treatment of medically refractory chronic rhinosinusitis (CRS), with reported success rates of 76–98% [1–3]. However, achieving long-term, positive outcomes can be challenging and is contingent upon optimization of the wound healing environment during the postoperative period [4]. Local complications such as scarring, middle turbinate lateralization, and stenosis of surgically enlarged ostia can lead to recurrent sinonasal obstruction and eventual surgical failure. Residual inflammation can also impede mucosal recovery and incite polypoid disease, further compromising surgical results. Consequently, revision FESS rates ranging from 10% to 37% have been reported [5, 6].

The frontal sinus is particularly vulnerable to surgical failure given its narrow outflow and difficult accessibility to topical therapies. Patency rates after frontal sinusotomy (Draf IIA) can range anywhere from 67.6% to 92% [7] and may diminish over time [8], highlighting the need for diligent surveillance following surgery. The most common causes of frontal sinus surgery failure are [8–10]:

- Medialization of the middle turbinate
- Incomplete anterior ethmoidectomy
- Mistaking the terminal recess as the frontal sinus
- Incomplete removal of the agger nasi or frontal cells
- Recurrence of polyps
- Scarring, stenosis, or neo-osteogenesis of the frontal ostium

This chapter aims to address management of the stenosing frontal recess. A broad spectrum of therapeutic options have been developed to manage this condition including postoperative debridement, balloon sinus dilation (BSD), frontal stents, bioabsorbable implants, and in-office revision frontal sinusotomy; all of which will be discussed in this chapter.

Electronic Supplementary Material The online version of this chapter (https://doi.org/10.1007/978-3-319-97022-6_11) contains supplementary material, which is available to authorized users.

R. Varshney, MD
Department of Otolaryngology, McGill University, Montreal, QC, Canada

J. T. Lee, MD (✉)
Department of Head and Neck Surgery, University of California Los Angeles David Geffen School of Medicine, Los Angeles, CA, USA

Postoperative Debridement

There is strong evidence to indicate that postsurgical endoscopic debridement of the sinonasal cavity prognosticates disease recidivism and potential need for revision FESS (Table 11.1). Consequently, meticulous postoperative care following FESS has been recognized to be just as critical as the surgery itself in ensuring long-term positive outcomes and frontal ostial patency. Rudmik et al. performed an evidence-based review and recommended debridements as part of routine postoperative care following FESS, although the optimal frequency of these interventions was not defined [15]. The latter was echoed in a systematic review by Green et al. [16].

- Diligent postoperative surveillance with removal of crusts and early lysis of adhesions may help prevent frontal recess stenosis and potentially reduce the need for revision frontal sinus surgery.
- The timing of such debridements will be contingent upon the patient's degree of stenosis and tendency to rescar.
- Such procedures frequently require use of endoscopic frontal sinus instruments typically used in the operating room to re-enlarge the frontal ostium.
- Curved suctions, seekers, and angled through-cutting/grasping/punch forceps are extremely useful when performing frontal sinus debridements in the office setting to remove scar bands obstructing the frontal recess and reopen stenotic frontal ostia (Fig. 11.1).

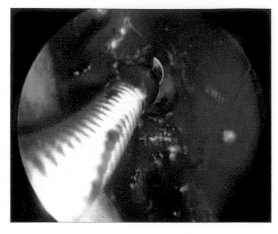

Fig. 11.1 Endoscopic image of in-office frontal sinus debridement with a 70-degree rigid scope. Hosemann punch forceps are being used to enlarge a stenotic frontal ostium

Table 11.1 Studies assessing the impact of post-FESS debridements on surgical outcomes

Authors	Year	Intervention	Outcomes
Gaskins [11]	1994	970 endoscopic ethmoidectomies (6–70-month follow-up)	10.5% adhesion incidence. Scar formation at 2-week to 48-month post-FESS (mean 8.69 months). 4.1% required revision surgery
Bugten et al. [12]	2006	60 FESS patients randomized to either postoperative saline irrigation alone ($n = 31$) or saline irrigation and debridements ($n = 29$). Debridement group had slightly more patients with frontal recess surgery	Significantly fewer crusts in debridement group at 12-day post-FESS. Less adhesions at 12 weeks in debridement group
Bugten et al. [13]	2008	Follow-up from above study with follow-up at 56 weeks	Debridement group demonstrated significantly more improvement in nasal congestion and sneezing
Lee et al. [14]	2008	Post-FESS patients allocated to 3 groups (10 in each group): group 1 (debridement twice a week), group 2 (once a week) or group 3 (once every 2 weeks)	At 4-week follow-up, VAS scores for symptoms of patient discomfort were significantly different (group 3 had worst scores). At 6-month follow-up, sinonasal outcome test-20 scores and objective endoscopic findings had no statistical difference. 1-week intervals for debridements likely optimal

FESS functional endoscopic sinus surgery, *VAS* visual analog scale

Balloon Sinus Dilation

Introduced in 2005, balloon sinus dilation (BSD) has been used to treat stenosing frontal ostia both intraoperatively and postoperatively in the clinic setting (Table 11.2) [17]. In-office BSD of frontal ostia has been shown to be both safe and tolerable [17]. Such in-office procedures offer the additional advantages of patient convenience, cost savings, and avoidance of general anesthesia [18, 19]. Currently, there are four manufacturers of BSD devices approved by the US Food and Drug Administration (FDA), namely, Acclarent (Irvine, California, USA), Entellus (Plymouth, Minnesota, USA), Medtronic (Minneapolis, Minnesota, USA), and Smith and Nephew (Cordova, Tennessee, USA).

- BSD of postoperative frontal ostia would most ideally be performed in the slowly stenosing frontal recess, with persistent visualization of a patent frontal ostium to allow easy cannulation (Fig. 11.2) [20].
- A wide variety of tools are currently available to help navigate balloons and ensure proper placement into stenosed frontal ostia including malleable instrumentation, transillumination, lighted seekers, guidewires, etc.
- In-office navigation can also be used to confirm proper balloon placement, which will be discussed later in this chapter.
- Once the balloon is verified to be in the correct location, sequential dilations may be performed in the same setting to incrementally increase the size of the frontal ostium.
- However, due to the potential for frontal ostia to restenose following BSD, close follow-up is still necessary to ensure patency is maintained and redilation is not required.

Table 11.2 Studies in which BSD was used to treat stenotic frontal ostia

Authors	Year	Intervention	Outcomes
Eloy et al. [20]	2012	5 patients that failed conventional frontal sinusotomies (DRAF IIa and IIb) were treated with in-office BSD due to persistent frontal headaches	Mean duration between the two procedures was 6.9 months All patients successfully treated and patent frontal drainage pathway seen at a mean follow-up of 5 months
Luong et al. [21]	2008	6 patients with postoperative frontal recess stenosis were managed with in-office BSD using either a lacrimal balloon or a sinus balloon catheter	One ostium contracted and required redilation All frontal sinuses were patent on endoscopic examination and functional based on the absence of symptoms at follow-up from 4 to 9 months
Wycherly et al. [22]	2010	BSD to address frontal sinus ostia stenosis under general anesthesia (24 ostia in 13 patients)	Patency rate of 86% at 13-month follow-up 16% required revision surgery

BSD Balloon sinus dilation

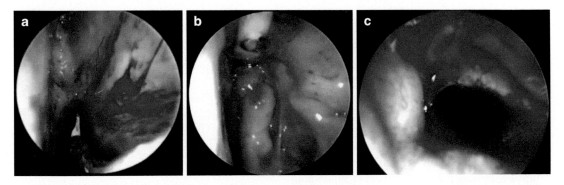

Fig. 11.2 Endoscopic images depicting (**a**) placement of a malleable seeker into a stenotic frontal ostium, (**b**) balloon dilation of the frontal ostium, and (**c**) frontal ostium post-dilation

Stenting or placement of a drug-eluting implant may also be useful in helping to preserve ostial patency following balloon dilation.

- Multiple studies have demonstrated the effectiveness of BSD in the treatment of frontal ostial stenosis (Table 11.2). Thus, BSD has emerged as an integral part of our treatment armamentarium for frontal stenosis, particularly in the office setting.

Frontal Sinus Stents

The role of frontal sinus stents in the prevention and management of frontal recess stenosis following sinus surgery remains controversial. The benefits of stenting include (1) separation of mucosal healing edges to reduce synechiae and stenosis, (2) occupying dead space so that it does not fill with blood and crusts, and (3) serving as a potential matrix for reepithelialization [23]. The disadvantages include (1) risk of biofilm formation, (2) chronic infection, (3) persistent foreign body, and (4) potential discomfort from stent removal [24].

Indications

- Frontal sinus stents have been recommended in cases where scarring and restenosis is anticipated.
- Hosemann et al. demonstrated that a neo-ostium of less than 5 mm and patients with aspirin sensitivity or nasal polyposis were at higher risk for stenosis [25].
- It has also been shown that mucosal healing after sinus surgery can take up to 3 months [4]. Therefore, stents may ideally need to be kept in place until the healing process and reepithelialization along the frontal drainage pathway have occurred.
- However, the optimal type and duration of stent placement are still unclear. Studies have reported successfully leaving stents in place anywhere from 5 days to 17 years [26] without complications.

- Stents may also be placed following balloon ostial dilation to maintain frontal patency.

Types

There are a myriad of frontal sinus stents that have been developed (Table 11.3):

- Two of the most commonly used are the Freeman and Rains stents, both of which have demonstrated positive clinical outcomes (Table 11.4). The Freeman (InHealth Technologies, Carpinteria, California, USA) is a 20 mm bi-phalanged hollow silicone tube [27], while the Rains stent (Smith & Nephew ENT, Memphis, Tennessee, USA) is a soft, silicone rubber tube [28].
- More recently, silastic sheets have been recommended for use as frontal sinus stents. Their pliability allows the stent to conform to the shape of the frontal ostium and prevents undue pressure on the mucosa [32]. Bednarski et al. utilized silastic sheets varying from 0.01 to 0.04 inches thickness in this manner. Thinner sheets were rolled in a tubed fashion and placed into the frontal ostium following unilateral frontal sinusotomy in instances where greater than 40% of the mucosa was denuded [32] (Fig. 11.3). Thicker sheets were used for Draf III procedures and cut into a U-shaped configuration for placement in the common frontal sinus outflow tracts.
- Drug-eluting stents have also been introduced:
  - An ethylvinyacetate rolled up sheet that elutes dexamethasone was placed in three frontal ostia (Draf II or Draf III), kept in

Table 11.3 Types of frontal sinus stents

| Gold |
| Tantalum foil |
| Polyethylene terephthalate |
| Rains stent |
| Freeman stent |
| Polymeric silicone (silastic) sheets |
| Double J stent |
| T-tube stent |

Table 11.4 Studies examining the efficacy of various frontal sinus stents

Authors	Year	Stent	Patients	Duration of placement	Outcomes
Freeman et al. [27]	2000	Freeman stent (silicone)	46 patients undergoing ESS	Mean f/u 29 months	All stents remained patent 6 patients required frontal obliteration
Rains [28]	2001	Rains stent (silicone)	67 patients undergoing ESS	Mean removal at 35 days (5 patients with long-term placement)	94% patency rate (failures in AFS cases) at follow-up 8–48 months
Mansour [29]	2013	Double J stent	5 patients undergoing ESS	6 months	4 of 5 patients (6 of 7 sinuses) with patent frontal outflow Tract after 10 to 36 months' follow-up
Rotenberg et al. [30]	2016	T-tube stent	30 patients undergoing ESS	4 weeks	1 patient had restenosis at mean follow-up 7.3 months
Orlandi et al. [31]	2008	Rains stent	9 patients undergoing ESS	Stent at least 6 months	Mean follow-up 33.8 months 7 still had stent (2 removed because of infection or discomfort), remaining patients have patent stents and asymptomatic

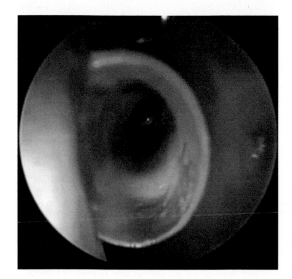

Fig. 11.3 Endoscopic image illustrating a silastic stent in the frontal sinus

place for 3–4 weeks, and removed in the office with good postoperative results [33].
- A doxycycline-releasing stent was used in a pilot study on ten patients undergoing frontal sinus surgery with an ostial diameter of 5–7 mm [34]. On one side a doxycycline-releasing stent was placed and on the other a non-drug-eluting stent. After 6 months, the side with the drug-eluting stent was found to have lower matrix metalloproteinase-9 concentrations, improved endoscopic appearance, and superior ostial patency than controls.
- Thereafter, other drug-eluting absorbable materials have been employed following frontal recess dissection such as the polylactide implant, which will be discussed in the subsequent section.

Drug-Eluting Implants

Steroid-Eluting Spring Implant

The polylactide sinus implant is a steroid-eluting, bioabsorbable stent (Intersect ENT, Menlo Park, California, USA) that is comprised of 370 μg mometasone furoate embedded in a polymer matrix [35]. It is available in two sizes, one with a diameter of 5.2 mm (Propel) and a smaller version with a diameter of 4 mm (Propel mini) (Fig. 11.4).

Many studies have shown that intraoperative placement of these implants is feasible and safe [36–38] with significant benefits in postoperative healing. Han et al. performed a meta-analysis of two randomized controlled trials which demon-

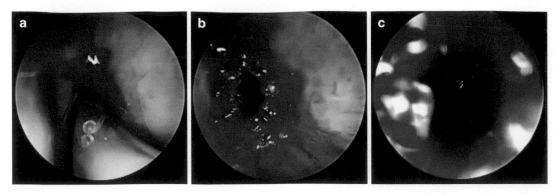

Fig. 11.4 Endoscopic photographs showing deployment of the steroid-eluting spring implant into the frontal sinus (**a**), with its inferior edge circumferentially abutting the frontal ostium (**b**) and the remainder interfacing with the mucosa of the frontal sinus (**c**)

strated a reduced need for postoperative interventions, adhesions, and oral steroids with use of the implant [36, 38, 39].

Although originally designed for the ethmoid cavity, the implant was recently FDA approved for use in the frontal sinus and has been successfully employed to address frontal ostial stenosis both in the office and operating room settings. Janisiewicz et al. treated two patients with prior FESS and recurrent frontal ostial stenosis with in-office placement of the implant following frontal balloon dilation (Fig. 11.4) [40]. Smith et al. performed a prospective, randomized controlled trial of 80 patients undergoing frontal surgery who received an implant on one side and no implant on the other [41]. At 30- and 90-day follow-up, the treatment side had a reduced need for postoperative interventions as well as decreased use of oral steroids. The implanted side also demonstrated significant improvements in inflammation and patency rates at 30-day follow-up compared to controls.

Steroid-Eluting Eight-Pronged Implant

Recently, a novel version of the steroid-eluting implant (SINUVA, Intersect ENT, Menlo Park, California, USA) has been developed specifically for treatment of recurrent nasal polyposis in the office setting. Unlike the implants currently available, this model is arch-shaped with eight prongs, has a stiffer composition, and elutes a

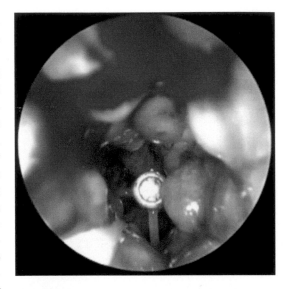

Fig. 11.5 Endoscopic photograph depicting placement of the eight-pronged steroid-eluting implant for in-office treatment of recurrent nasal polyposis

higher dosage of mometasone furoate (1350 μg versus 370 μg) over a longer period of time (3 months vs. 30 days) [42].

- Forwith et al. performed a RCT of 100 patients in which significant reduction in ethmoid obstruction, polyp grade, and need for revision surgery was observed with the implant versus controls after 3–6 months of follow-up [43].
- Such an implant may be useful in the future in cases where the frontal recess is obstructed by recurrent nasal polyps within the ethmoid bed (Fig. 11.5).

In-Office Revision Frontal Surgery

In-office management of sinonasal pathologies has expanded significantly in recent years. Reports of sinus mucoceles [44, 45], mucus recirculation [46], and inverted papilloma recurrences [47] being treated with in-office procedures have all been published. With adequate analgesia, revision frontal sinusotomy can also be performed in the clinic setting to address frontal recess obstruction. Angled thru-cut, grasping, and punch forceps are used to resect remaining ledges and adhesions to reopen the frontal sinus outflow tract (Video 11.1). Consequently, it is helpful to have the full complement of endoscopic frontal sinus instruments available when performing in-office revision FESS, similar to the operating room. In-office navigation and microdebriders are also useful, particularly when addressing frontal recess stenosis in the context of prior surgery or performing revision polypectomy.

In-Office Navigation

Although traditionally developed for the operating room, surgical navigation systems specifically designed for use in the office setting have been recently introduced. Such technology is especially useful when performing revision frontal procedures in the clinic to facilitate verification of key landmarks in patients with altered anatomy.

- The Fiagon system is an electromagnetic image guidance platform (Fiagon GmbH, Berlin, Germany) with an extremely compact footprint. This allows the unit to fit into the shelf of a standard endoscopy tower (Fig. 11.6a). Such space-saving attributes have made this system ideal for use in the clinic setting. In addition, the navigation device has the unique ability to track both rigid and flexible instruments including guidewires, balloon catheters, malleable pointers, and bendable suctions.

- A compact version of the Fusion System (Medtronic, Minneapolis, Minnesota, USA), another electromagnetic image guidance platform, has also been developed. Although it does not have the capability of navigating flexible instrumentation, it is able to track the electromagnetic balloon dilation device (NuVent, Medtronic, Minneapolis, Minnesota, USA) [42], which is comprised of a rigid sinus seeker with built-in calibration to enable surgical navigation (Fig. 11.6b).

- With the advent of in-office navigation, sinus surgeons now have additional tools in their

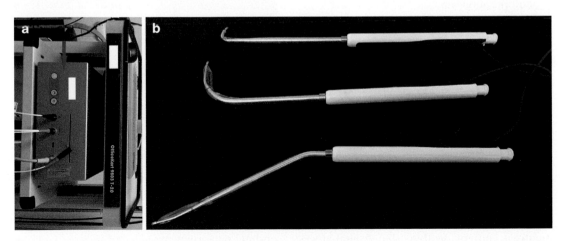

Fig. 11.6 In-office electromagnetic surgical navigation system. (**a**) Its compact size allows the unit (arrow) to fit easily into the shelves of a standard clinic endoscopy tower. (**b**) Rigid sinus seekers with trackable balloons and built-in calibration for surgical navigation. (**c**) In-office balloon dilation of the frontal sinus outflow tract under image guidance

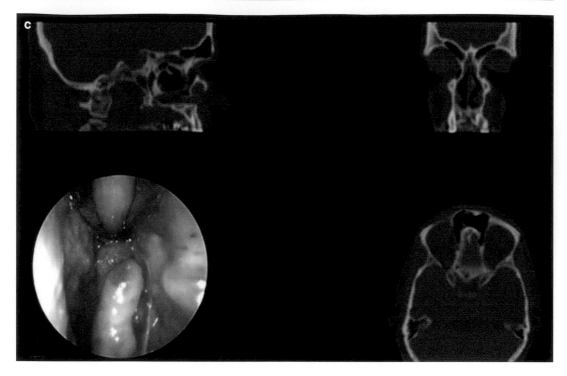

Fig. 11.6 (continued)

armamentarium to ensure adequate placement of balloon catheters and other malleable instrumentation through a stenotic frontal recess (Fig. 11.6c). This is particularly important when accessing the frontal sinus in patients with complex anatomy or a history of multiple surgeries.

In-Office Microdebriders

New microdebriders specifically developed for use in the office setting have also been introduced. The vacuum-powered microdebrider (PolypVac, Laurimed, Redwood City, California, USA) is a disposable, handheld device that can be used to address frontal recess obstruction secondary to polyp recurrence. It has a 3.5 mm malleable tip with a 360° rotatable shaft, which allows angled debridement of recurrent polyps within the frontal recess (Fig. 11.7). The power of the device is dependent on the suction strength, especially in cases of fibrotic polyps. A minimum airflow gauge

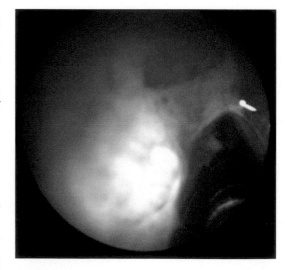

Fig. 11.7 Endoscopic image depicting use of a malleable in-office microdebrider to remove polyps obstructing the frontal recess

reading of 48 l/min has been recommended for optimal performance [42].

Gan et al. used this vacuum-powered microdebrider on 68 patients with nasal polyposis who were either awaiting surgery or had postoperative recurrence of polyps [48]. Eighty-seven percent of patients underwent successful polypectomy. Although the majority of polyps were within the nasal cavity and ethmoid sinuses, 4% were within the frontal sinuses. Ninety-seven percent of patients reported a comfort level of "fair" to "excellent," with a mean surgical time of only 3 minutes per side. No complications were reported.

More recently, two other microdebriders (Nexus, Medtronic, Jacksonville, Florida, USA; Karl Storz, Tuttlingen, Germany) have been recently developed for use in the clinic setting. Both have the same functionality as their counterparts currently in the OR but with a smaller footprint (Nexus) in the case of the former and reusable blades (Karl Storz, Tuttlingen, Germany) in the case of the latter. Such devices can be used for the treatment of recurrent polyps in the ethmoid bed or within the frontal recess with possible concurrent navigation (Video 11.2).

It should be noted that the various strategies and technologic innovations presented in this chapter to address frontal recess/ostial stenosis are not mutually exclusive. In many cases, these various devices and procedures are used in tandem to treat the multifactorial etiology of the disease. A combination of in-office microdebriders, cold steel instruments, stents, drug-eluting implants, navigation, etc. can be used together in the same setting (Videos 11.1 and 11.2).

Revision Frontal Surgery

Ultimately, if in-office procedures are not sufficient to address stenotic frontal ostia, revision FESS is required in the operating room. The reported revision rates for FESS range from 10% to 37% [5, 6]. There is usually a natural progression in the approach to frontal sinusotomy with Draf II failures treated with an endoscopic modified Lothrop/Draf III procedure and frontal sinus obliteration used as a last resort. These frontal sinus procedures are discussed in other chapters of this textbook.

Summary

There are a myriad of approaches in the management of frontal recess stenosis. It is important to follow patients judiciously during the postoperative period and ensure adequate endoscopic visualization of the frontal outflow tract in order to recognize stenosis early. Once discovered, depending on etiology, a wide variety of tools and devices can be used either individually or in combination to treat synechiae, inflammation, scarring, or recurrent polyps that may obstruct frontal sinus outflow following sinus surgery. Endoscopic debridements, BSD, frontal sinus stents, drug-eluting implants, in-office revision ESS, etc. could all conceivably be used in the same patient depending on the clinical course of the disease. Although a challenge, maintenance of frontal ostium patency can be achievable by a good understanding of the available modalities in the armamentarium of the rhinologist as described in this chapter.

References

1. Senior BA, Kennedy DW, Tanabodee J, Kroger H, Hassab M, Lanza D. Long-term results of functional endoscopic sinus surgery. Laryngoscope. 1998;108(2):151–7.
2. Ragab SM, Lund VJ, Scadding G. Evaluation of the medical and surgical treatment of chronic rhinosinusitis: a prospective, randomised, controlled trial. Laryngoscope. 2004;114(5):923–30.
3. Bhattacharyya N. Symptom outcomes after endoscopic sinus surgery for chronic rhinosinusitis. Arch Otolaryngol Head Neck Surg. 2004;130(3):329–33.
4. Hosemann W, Wigand ME, Gode U, Langer F, Dunker I. Normal wound healing of the paranasal sinuses: clinical and experimental investigations. Eur Arch Otorhinolaryngol. 1991;248(7):390–4.
5. Wynn R, Har-El G. Recurrence rates after endoscopic sinus surgery for massive sinus polyposis. Laryngoscope. 2004;114(5):811–3.
6. Mendelsohn D, Jeremic G, Wright ED, Rotenberg BW. Revision rates after endoscopic sinus surgery: a recurrence analysis. Ann Otol Rhinol Laryngol. 2011;120(3):162–6.
7. DeConde ASST. Outcomes after frontal sinus surgery: an evidence-based review. Otolaryngol Clin N Am. 2016;49(4):1019–33.
8. Friedman M, Bliznikas D, Vidyasagar R, Joseph NJ, Landsberg R. Long-term results after endoscopic

sinus surgery involving frontal recess dissection. Laryngoscope. 2006;116(4):573–9.

9. Chan Y, Melroy CT, Kuhn CA, Kuhn FL, Daniel WT, Kuhn FA. Long-term frontal sinus patency after endoscopic frontal sinusotomy. Laryngoscope. 2009;119(6):1229–32.

10. Friedman M, Landsberg R, Schults RA, Tanyeri H, Caldarelli DD. Frontal sinus surgery: endoscopic technique and preliminary results. Am J Rhinol. 2000;14(6):393–403.

11. Gaskins R. Scarring in endoscopic ethmoidectomy. Am J Rhinol. 1994;8(6):271–4.

12. Bugten V, Nordgard S, Steinsvag S. The effects of debridement after endoscopic sinus surgery. Laryngoscope. 2006;116(11):2037–43.

13. Bugten V, Nordgard S, Steinsvag S. Long-term effects of postoperative measures after sinus surgery. Eur Arch Otorhinolaryngol. 2008;265(5):531–7.

14. Lee JY, Byun JY. Relationship between the frequency of postoperative debridement and patient discomfort, healing period, surgical outcomes, and compliance after endoscopic sinus surgery. Laryngoscope. 2008;118(10):1868–72.

15. Rudmik L, Soler ZM, Orlandi RR, Stewart MG, Bhattacharyya N, Kennedy DW, Smith TL. Early postoperative care following endoscopic sinus surgery: an evidence-based review with recommendations. Int Forum Allergy Rhinol. 2011;1(6):417–30.

16. Green R, Banigo A, Hathorn I. Postoperative nasal debridement following functional endoscopic sinus surgery, a systematic review of the literature. Clin Otolaryngol. 2015;40(1):2–8.

17. Sillers MJ, Lay KF. Balloon catheter dilation of the frontal sinus ostium. Otolaryngol Clin N Am. 2016;49(4):965–74.

18. Rees CJ, Halum SL, Wijewickrama RC, Koufman JA, Postma GN. Patient tolerance of in-office pulsed dye laser treatments to the upper aerodigestive tract. Otolaryngol Head Neck Surg. 2006;134(6):1023–7.

19. Prickett KK, Wise SK, DelGaudio JM. Cost analysis of office-based and operating room procedures in rhinology. Int Forum Allergy Rhinol. 2012;2(3):207–11.

20. Eloy JA, Friedel ME, Eloy JD, Govindaraj S, Folbe AJ. In-office balloon dilation of the failed frontal sinusotomy. Otolaryngol Head Neck Surg. 2012;146(2):320–2.

21. Luong A, Batra PS, Fakhri S, Citardi MJ. Balloon catheter dilatation for frontal sinus ostium stenosis in the office setting. Am J Rhinol. 2008;22(6):621–4.

22. Wycherly BJ, Manes RP, Mikula SK. Initial clinical experience with balloon dilation in revision frontal sinus surgery. Ann Otol Rhinol Laryngol. 2010;119(7):468–71.

23. Chen PG, Wormald PJ, Payne SC, Gross WE, Gross CW. A golden experience: fifty years of experience managing the frontal sinus. Laryngoscope. 2016;126(4):802–7.

24. Perloff JR, Palmer JN. Evidence of bacterial biofilms on frontal recess stents in patients with chronic rhinosinusitis. Am J Rhinol. 2004;18(6):377–80.

25. Hosemann W, Kuhnel T, Held P, Wagner W, Felderhoff A. Endonasal frontal sinusotomy in surgical management of chronic sinusitis: a critical evaluation. Am J Rhinol. 1997;11(1):1–9.

26. Hunter B, Silva S, Youngs R, Saeed A, Varadarajan V. Long-term stenting for chronic frontal sinus disease: case series and literature review. J Laryngol Otol. 2010;124(11):1216–22.

27. Freeman SB, Blom ED. Frontal sinus stents. Laryngoscope. 2000;110(7):1179–82.

28. Rains BM. Frontal sinus stenting. Otolaryngol Clin N Am. 2001;34(1):101–10.

29. Mansour HA. Double j stent of frontal sinus outflow tract in revision frontal sinus surgery. J Laryngol Otol. 2013;127(1):43–7.

30. Rotenberg BW, Ioanidis KE, Sowerby LJ. Development of a novel t-tube frontal sinus irrigation catheter. Am J Rhinol Allergy. 2016;30(5):356–9.

31. Orlandi RR, Knight J. Prolonged stenting of the frontal sinus. Laryngoscope. 2009;119(1):190–2.

32. Bednarski KA, Kuhn FA. Stents and drug-eluting stents. Otolaryngol Clin N Am. 2009;42(5):857–66. x.

33. Hosemann W, Schindler E, Wiegrebe E, Gopferich A. Innovative frontal sinus stent acting as a local drug-releasing system. Eur Arch Otorhinolaryngol. 2003;260(3):131–4.

34. Huvenne WZN, Tijsma E, Hissong B, Huurdeman J, Holtappels G, Claeys S, Van Cauwenberge P, Nelis H, Coenye T, Bachert C. Pilot study using doxycycline-releasing stents to ameliorate postoperative healing quality after sinus surgery. Wound Repair Regen. 2008;16(6):757–67.

35. Wei CC, Kennedy DW. Mometasone implant for chronic rhinosinusitis. Med Devices (Auckl). 2012;5:75–80.

36. Murr AH, Smith TL, Hwang PH, Bhattacharyya N, Lanier BJ, Stambaugh JW, Mugglin AS. Safety and efficacy of a novel bioabsorbable, steroid-eluting sinus stent. Int Forum Allergy Rhinol. 2011;1(1):23–32.

37. Forwith KD, Chandra RK, Yun PT, Miller SK, Jampel HD. Advance: a multisite trial of bioabsorbable steroid-eluting sinus implants. Laryngoscope. 2011;121(11):2473–80.

38. Marple BF, Smith TL, Han JK, Gould AR, Jampel HD, Stambaugh JW, Mugglin AS. Advance II: a prospective, randomized study assessing safety and efficacy of bioabsorbable steroid-releasing sinus implants. Otolaryngol Head Neck Surg. 2012;146(6):1004–11.

39. Han JK, Marple BF, Smith TL, Murr AH, Lanier BJ, Stambaugh JW, Mugglin AS. Effect of steroid-releasing sinus implants on postoperative medical and surgical interventions: an efficacy meta-analysis. Int Forum Allergy Rhinol. 2012;2(4):271–9.

40. Janisiewicz A, Lee JT. In-office use of a steroid-eluting implant for maintenance of frontal ostial patency after revision sinus surgery. Allergy Rhinol. 2015;6(1):68–75.

41. Smith TL, Singh A, Luong A, Ow RA, Shotts SD, Sautter NB, Han JK, Stambaugh J, Raman A. Randomized controlled trial of a bioabsorbable

steroid-releasing implant in the frontal sinus opening. Laryngoscope. 2016;126:2659.

42. Varshney R, Lee JT. New innovations in office-based rhinology. Curr Opin Otolaryngol Head Neck Surg. 2016;24(1):3–9.

43. Forwith KD, Han JK, Stolovitzky JP, Yen DM, Chandra RK, Karanfilov B, Matheny KE, Stambaugh JW, Gawlicka AK. Resolve: bioabsorbable steroid-eluting sinus implants for in-office treatment of recurrent sinonasal polyposis after sinus surgery: 6-month outcomes from a randomized, controlled, blinded study. Int Forum Allergy Rhinol. 2016;6(6):573–81.

44. Barrow EM, DelGaudio JM. In-office drainage of sinus mucoceles: an alternative to operating-room drainage. Laryngoscope. 2015;125(5):1043–7.

45. Eloy JA, Shukla PA, Choudhry OJ, Eloy JD, Langer PD. In-office balloon dilation and drainage of frontal sinus mucocele. Allergy Rhinol. 2013;4(1):e36–40.

46. DelGaudio JM, Ochsner MC. Office surgery for paranasal sinus recirculation. Int Forum Allergy Rhinol. 2015;5(4):326–8.

47. Sham CL, Woo JK, van Hasselt CA, Tong MC. Treatment results of sinonasal inverted papilloma: an 18-year study. Am J Rhinol Allergy. 2009;23(2):203–11.

48. Gan EC, Habib AR, Hathorn I, Javer AR. The efficacy and safety of an office-based polypectomy with a vacuum-powered microdebrider. Int Forum Allergy Rhinol. 2013;3(11):890–5.

Identifying and Addressing Causes of Failure in Frontal Sinus Surgery

12

Theodore A. Schuman and Brent A. Senior

General Considerations

Incidence of Failure in Frontal Sinus Surgery

When frontal sinus surgery is performed, creation of a stable, patent frontal outflow tract is critical to optimizing patient outcomes. The importance of frontal recess patency is threefold: provide symptom improvement, allow direct access of topical therapeutic agents including corticosteroid and saline irrigations to sinus mucosa, and prevent long-term complications including mucocele formation.

Advances in endoscopic instrumentation (microdebrider, high-definition cameras, angled instrumentation, high speed drills), image-guided technology, and adjuvant therapies (topical steroid irrigations, drug-eluting stents) and a more nuanced understanding of the anatomy and function of the frontal sinus have led to an improved

ability to effectively manage frontal disease while minimizing morbidity.

DeConde and Smith (2016) reviewed 25 years of frontal sinus surgery outcomes studies and reported a trend in improving success of frontal sinus surgery in each subsequent decade. Historically, primary open approaches to the frontal sinus led to short-term patency but unacceptably high long-term restenosis rates of approximately 30%. By comparison, endoscopic frontal sinus patency rates following Draf IIA surgery range from 67.6% to 92% in the last 10 years, with most studies demonstrating a success rate in the mid-80% range [1].

Askar et al. (2015) prospectively evaluated 60 patients undergoing 100 Draf IIA sinusotomy procedures for chronic frontal sinusitis; 80% were revision. Overall rate of frontal sinus ostial patency was 90% at 6 months or greater, with no significant difference in surgical success in primary vs. revision, polyp vs. non-polyp, and asthmatic vs. non-asthmatic patients. Physical, emotional, and functional domains of the Rhinosinusitis Disability Index (RSDI) improved in all groups [2].

Despite progress in surgical management of frontal sinus disease, all surgical approaches, endoscopic and open, can fail, leading to persistent symptoms, impaired quality of life, and need for revision surgery.

T. A. Schuman
Rhinology and Skull Base Surgery, Department of Otolaryngology – Head and Neck Surgery, University of North Carolina at Chapel Hill,
Chapel Hill, NC, USA

B. A. Senior (✉)
Division of Rhinology, Allergy, and Endoscopic Skull Base Surgery, Department of Otolaryngology – Head and Neck Surgery, University of North Carolina at Chapel Hill, Chapel Hill, NC, USA

© Springer Nature Switzerland AG 2019
D. Lal, P. H. Hwang (eds.), *Frontal Sinus Surgery*, https://doi.org/10.1007/978-3-319-97022-6_12

Surgical Failure Can Occur Due to Multiple Reasons

Technical Issues

1. Circumferential removal of frontal recess mucosa leading to cicatricial scarring and new bone formation
2. Failure to remove all cells impinging on the frontal drainage pathway
3. Overly aggressive drilling resulting in exposed bone and excessive crusting, leading to subsequent scar and new bone formation
4. Recurrence/progression of disease, including nasal polyposis and osteitis [1]
5. Inadequate postoperative irrigation or debridement

Anatomic Considerations

The unique anatomy of the frontal sinus outflow tract predisposes this region to surgical failure.

The acute nasofrontal angle makes effective visualization and instrumentation difficult. In the coronal plane, the frontal drainage pathway lies between two critical structures – the orbit and the midline skull base. In the sagittal plane, the anterior-posterior diameter of the frontal outflow tract is variable and influenced by a number of factors:

1. Patient age
2. Frontal sinus development
3. Comorbidities, for example, hypoplastic sinuses in a patient with cystic fibrosis
4. Prominence of anterior frontal beak
5. Size of agger nasi cell and ethmoidal bulla (bulla ethmoidalis)
6. Presence and size of additional cells impinging upon the frontal recess:
   (a) Frontoethmoidal cells
   (b) Suprabullar (suprabullar cells)
   (c) Frontal septal (interfrontal septal) cells

Careful preoperative review of CT scans is critical to ensure removal of all cells while preserving sinonasal mucosa and nearby neurovascular structures. Image guidance technology may be useful for optimizing extent of dissection, especially in cases of revision surgery, extensive polyposis, or alteration of expected anatomic landmarks.

Patient Factors

Patient factors for failure include non-compliance with treatment, inadequate postoperative irrigation, and debridement. Some biological subtypes are also associated with uncontrolled mucosal inflammation. Chronic mucosal inflammation has been increasingly recognized as a central component in the pathophysiology of chronic rhinosinusitis. Surprisingly, the data linking uncontrolled inflammation to the failure of frontal surgery is sparse. In a large, single-center study of 109 patients undergoing primary Draf IIA surgery, Naidoo et al. (2012) found no evidence for increased ostial restenosis in patients with nasal polyposis, eosinophilic mucin, asthma, allergy, or elevated Lund-Mackay score [3]. Similarly, Chandra, Palmer, Tangsujarittham, and Kennedy (2004) found no relationship between frontal sinus surgery failure and asthma, nasal polyposis, aspirin sensitivity, and allergic fungal sinusitis. In this study, however, a significantly higher rate of failure was demonstrated in patients with advanced radiologic disease on preoperative CT [4].

Specific Causes of Frontal Sinus Surgery Failure

Valdes, Bogado, and Samaha (2014) reviewed 109 revision frontal sinusotomies in 66 patients and found persistent mucosal edema, neo-osteogenesis, and technically incomplete surgery to be common causes of surgical failure (see Table 12.1). Most patients had more than one etiology of persistent frontal disease after prior surgical intervention [5]. Otto and DelGaudio (2010) reviewed 289 revision frontal sinusotomies in 149 cases and reported similar findings, with many patients having more than one cause for

Table 12.1 Computed tomography (CT) findings of patients who underwent revision frontal sinus surgery

CT findings	Percent of patients who underwent revision frontal sinus surgery
Residual agger nasi	73.4%
Residual ethmoid cells except agger nasi	32.2%
Bulla ethmoidalis	21.1%
Suprabullar cells	9.2%
Frontobullar cells	2.7%
Residual frontal cells	24.8%
Edematous mucosa	92.7%
Neo-osteogenesis in the frontal recess	45.9%
Lateral scarring of middle turbinate	47.7%

Adapted from Valdes et al. [5]

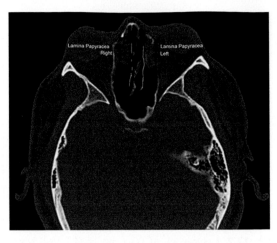

Fig. 12.1 Graphical plot of residual right and left ethmoid cells found on the lamina papyracea in 55 patients undergoing revision sinus surgery. (Figure and legend used with permission from Gore et al. [7])

frontal failure. Mucosal edema (67%) and osteo-neogenesis (7%) indicated ongoing inflammation. Technical factors leading to frontal surgery failure were identified in 75% of patients, including lateralized middle turbinate (30%), scarring of the frontal recess (12%), and retained cells including agger nasi (13%), frontoethmoidal (8%), and other ethmoidal cells (53%) [6]. Gore, Ebert, Zanation, and Senior (2012) reviewed the CT scans of 55 patients undergoing revision FESS and found retained anterior ethmoidal cells (65% of sides), agger nasi cell (52%), and uncinate processes (46%) to be common findings. Residual ethmoidal cells were more common along the skull base and lamina papyracea and on the patient's right side. Figure 12.1 demonstrates the distribution of residual anterior ethmoidal cells in this series [7]. Specific factors are discussed below.

reported a significant relationship between the size of the Draf IIA sinusotomy and odds of persistent frontal ostial patency after primary sinus surgery. Ostial size >4.8 mm was strongly correlated with surgical success, whereas stenosis of the neo-ostium was noted to be more likely with A-P diameter <3.7 mm. Restenosis was clinically significant, with most surgical failure patients demonstrating persistent symptoms, polyps, and infection [3]. Hosemann et al. (1997) reported that a drop in ostial size below 5 mm was associated with an increase in stenosis rate from 16% to 30%. A 2 mm frontal ostium was associated with a 50% incidence of surgical failure [8]. The surgeon cannot control the patient's underlying anatomy, but meticulous surgical technique and resection of all cell partitions is crucial in optimizing frontal sinus surgery outcomes.

Small Ostial Size

The size of the postsurgical frontal ostium is determined by the patient's anatomy and the completeness of surgery. Careful review of preoperative computed tomography (CT) scans allows for identification of frontal sinuses prone to restenosis due to small anterior-posterior (A-P) diameter (see Fig. 12.2). Naidoo et al. (2012)

Middle Turbinate Lateralization

Lateralization of the intact middle turbinate may lead to lasting obstruction of the frontal sinus outflow tract (see Fig. 12.3). Partial resection of the middle turbinate can result in scarring of the turbinate remnant to the nasal sidewall, across the frontal recess. Frontal sinus obstruction, stasis of secretions, and increased

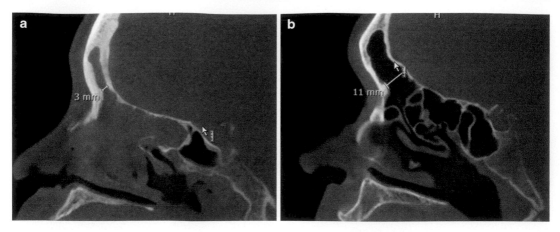

Fig. 12.2 Comparison of large and small frontal sinus ostia. (**a**) Sagittal reconstructions of preoperative thin-cut sinus CT demonstrate a narrow diameter between the anterior and posterior tables of the frontal recess. The resulting neo-ostia would be expected to be small, placing this patient at increased risk for restenosis following frontal sinus surgery. (**b**) In contrast, this patient has a wide A-P diameter of the frontal recess, with a correspondingly decreased risk of surgical failure

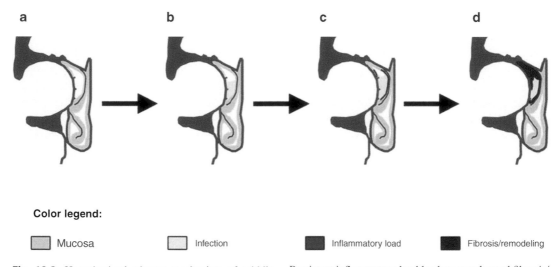

Color legend:

☐ Mucosa   ☐ Infection   ◼ Inflammatory load   ◼ Fibrosis/remodeling

Fig. 12.3 Hypothesized adverse mechanism of middle turbinate lateralization (MTL). (**a**) Postoperative middle turbinate lateralization occurs as a side effect of sinus surgery. (**b**) MTL harbors repeated infections that do not clear easily as well as reduces penetration of topical medication, leading to a persistent inflammatory load (**c**). (**d**) Persistent inflammatory load leads to accelerated fibrosis/remodeling in the region, which eventually involves the frontal recess and frontal sinus ostium, ending in frontal scarring and stenosis. (Figure and legend used with permission from Bassiouni et al. [9])

inflammation may result, necessitating revision frontal sinus surgery.

Bassiouni et al. (2015) examined 151 patients after complete endoscopic sinus surgery (ESS) and found no correlation between middle turbinate lateralization (MTL) and symptoms. Survival analysis, however, revealed MTL to be more common in patients requiring revision surgery [9].

Numerous techniques have been described to avoid MTL including suture conchopexy, controlled synechiae, metal clips, middle meatal spacers, and absorbable implants. Long-term outcomes of these interventions are unclear [9].

Middle turbinate resection is a viable option in properly selected patients with extensive inflammatory disease. Soler et al. reported improved olfaction and endoscopic appearance in patients undergoing bilateral middle turbinate resection when compared to a cohort with MT preservation [10]. If the middle turbinate is resected, care must be taken to avoid lateral scarring of the residual axillary tissue.

Incomplete Removal of the Uncinate Process

Incomplete uncinectomy indicates failure to appropriately open the ostiomeatal complex, a key concept in successful ESS. Residual uncinate process tissue high in the middle meatus may result in scarring and/or mechanical obstruction of the frontal recess. Frequently, incomplete uncinectomy also results in failure to open the true maxillary ostium, which may lead to circular flow of maxillary secretions and persistent maxillary sinusitis, which may in turn contribute to concordant frontal sinus disease.

Retained Cells

Agger Nasi Cell
Valdes, Bogado, and Samaha (2014) reported that of the surgeon-dependent factors leading to failure of frontal sinus surgery, retention of the agger nasi cell was most common, occurring in 73.4% of patients [5]. The agger nasi intrudes into the frontal recess from an anterior position. The roof of the agger nasi may lie high in the frontal recess and be missed, especially without the use of angled endoscopes and careful preoperative review of CT scans. Failure to completely remove the agger nasi cell can result in persistent symptomatic opacification of the frontal sinus after prior ESS (see Fig. 12.4).

Ethmoidal Bulla (Bulla Ethmoidalis)
Residual ethmoidal bulla was noted in 21.1% of patients undergoing revision frontal sinus surgery [5]. The ethmoidal bulla impinges upon the posterior aspect of the frontal recess and if incompletely resected may scar to other remnant structures.

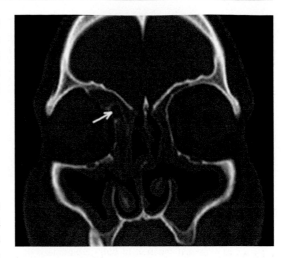

Fig. 12.4 Residual right agger nasi cell with accompanying Type I frontal cell. Also seen is an uncorrected septal deviation. (Figure and legend used with permission from Gore et al. [7])

Suprabulla (Suprabullar) Cells
Anterior ethmoidal cells superior to the ethmoidal bulla (bulla ethmoidalis) may extend up the posterior table and intrude into the posterior aspect of the frontal recess. Failure to adequately resect these cells was noted in 9.2% of frontal sinus surgery revisions [5]. Figure 12.5 demonstrates a patient undergoing revision Draf IIA frontal sinusotomy with resection of a residual suprabulla (suprabullar) cell.

Frontoethmoidal Cells
Bent, Guilty-Siller, and Kuhn (1994) described four classes of frontoethmoidal cells based upon their number and location [11]. These cells sit superiorly to the agger nasi and may extend well into the frontal sinus proper. As an alternative to the Bent and Kuhn system, Wormald et al. (2016) published the International Frontal Sinus Anatomy Classification (IFAC), in which expert consensus was used to create a new classification of anterior ethmoid cells impinging upon the frontal recess [12]. In the IFAC system, cells are classified by location (anterior, posterior, or medial) and presence of extension into the frontal sinus (see Fig. 12.6). Failure to recognize the presence and incomplete removal of frontoethmoidal cells may result in surgical failure and recurrence of symptoms. A 24.8% incidence of

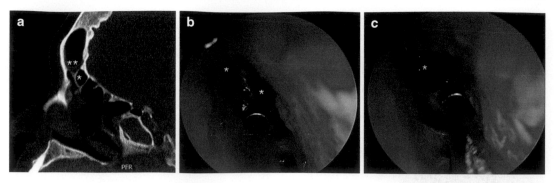

Fig. 12.5 Revision Draf IIA frontal sinusotomy with resection of residual suprabulla frontal cell. (**a**) Preoperative sagittal reconstruction of thin-cut sinus CT demonstrates residual anterior ethmoid cell originating superior to expected location of bulla ethmoidalis and extending along posterior table of left frontal sinus, consistent with a suprabulla frontal cell *(single white asterisk)*. Mucoperiosteal thickening in the distal frontal sinus suggests ongoing inflammation *(double white asterisk)*, and this patient had persistent symptoms despite medical management and prior functional endoscopic sinus surgery. (**b**) Intraoperative view of left frontal recess using 45-degree endoscope at time of revision surgery. The roof of the suprabulla frontal cell is noted posterolaterally *(single white asterisk)*, obstructing the majority of the frontal outflow tract. A small, edematous frontal ostium was located anteromedially, which in this image has already been dilated with a curette *(single yellow asterisk)*. (**c**) View using 45-degree endoscope after definitive removal of residual suprabulla frontal cell. Note dramatic increase in frontal ostial size in reference to 4 mm olive-tipped frontal sinus suction *(single yellow asterisk)*. (Images courtesy of Brent A. Senior, MD)

Cell type	Cell name	Definition	Abbreviation
Anterior cells (push the drainage pathway of the frontal sinus medial, posterior or posteromedially)	Agger nasi cell	Cell that sits either anterior to the origin of the middle turbinate or sits directly above the most anterior insertion of the middle turbinate into the lateral nasal wall.	ANC
	Supra agger cell	Anterior-lateral ethmoidal cell, located above the agger nasi cell (not pneumatizing into the frontal sinus).	SAC
	Supra agger frontal cell	Anterior-lateral ethmoidal cell, that extends into the frontal sinus. A small SAFC will only extend into the floor of the frontal sinus, whereas a large SAFC may extend significantly into the frontal sinus and may even reach the roof of the frontal sinus.	SAFC
Posterior cells (push the drainage pathway anteriorly)	Supra bulla cell	Cell above the bulla ethmoidalis that does not enter the frontal sinus.	SBC
	Supra bulla frontal cell	Cell that originates in the supra-bulla region and pneumatizes along the skull base into the posterior region of the frontal sinus. The skull base forms the posterior wall of the cell.	SBFC
	Supraorbital ethmoid cell	An anterior ethmoid cell that pneumatizes around, anterior to, or posterior to the anterior ethmoidal artery over the roof of the orbit. It often forms part of the posterior wall of an extensively pneumatized frontal sinus and may only be separated from the frontal sinus by a bony septation.	SOEC
Medial cells (push the drainage pathway laterally)	Frontal septal cell	Medially based cell of the anterior ethmoid or the inferior frontal sinus, attached to or located in the interfrontal sinus septum, associated with the medial aspect of the frontal sinus outflow tract, pushing the drainage pathway laterally and frequently posteriorly.	FSC

Fig. 12.6 International Frontal Sinus Anatomy Classification (IFAC) Air cells impinging upon the frontal recess are characterized by location anterior, posterior, or medial to the frontal outflow tract. In addition, cells are identified based upon presence or lack of extension into the frontal sinus proper. (Figure used with permission from Wormald et al. [12])

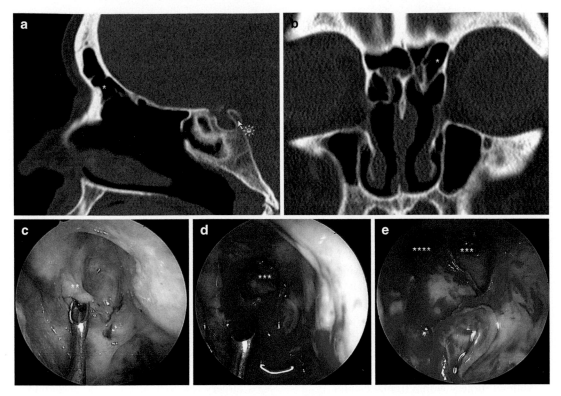

Fig. 12.7 Revision Draf IIA frontal sinusotomy with resection of Bent-Kuhn Type III/supra-agger frontal cell. (**a**) Preoperative sagittal reconstruction of thin-cut sinus CT demonstrating large supra-agger frontal cell extending along nasal beak onto anterior table of frontal sinus *(single asterisk)*. This patient continued to have symptoms of chronic rhinosinusitis despite aggressive medical management and prior endoscopic sinus surgery. (**b**) Coronal view demonstrating lateral location of residual left supra-agger frontal cell along lamina papyracea *(single asterisk)*. (**c**) Initial intraoperative view of left frontal recess using 45-degree endoscopic showing obstruction of drainage pathway by scarred anterior ethmoid cell *(double asterisk)*. The curette is placed in a palpable tract postero-medial to this bony lamella. (**d**) View of frontal recess using 45-degree endoscope after partial removal of residual supra-agger frontal cell. The cell extends high into the frontal sinus, creating the false appearance of a fully dissected frontal recess *(triple asterisk)*. The curette is placed behind a subtle lamella of bone into the medially displaced frontal outflow tract. (**e**) Endoscopic view of complete frontal recess dissection after removal of medial wall of supra-agger frontal cell. The roof of the supra-agger frontal cell is noted laterally *(triple asterisk)*, with the posterior table of the frontal sinus visible within the frontal outflow tract medially *(quadruple asterisk)*

residual frontoethmoidal cells was noted in one large study [5]. Figure 12.7 illustrates an example of a retained supra-agger frontal cell, Type III frontoethmoidal, removed at the time of revision Draf IIA sinusotomy.

Approach to the Failed Frontal Sinusotomy

Not all patients with endoscopic or radiographic evidence of persistent frontal sinus opacification or frontal outflow tract obstruction are symptomatic [4]. In the absence of extenuating circum-

stances such as immunodeficiency or a history of complicated sinusitis, watchful waiting with topical nasal steroid and saline lavages represents a reasonable approach in asymptomatic patients. Symptomatic patients are typically treated with aggressive medical therapy, with revision surgery offered to those who fail to improve.

Medical Management

Medical management with culture-directed antibiotics, topical and/or oral steroids, and nasal saline lavages is an appropriate first-line treatment for symptomatic failed frontal sinus surgery. Adjuvant therapies including topical antibiotics, leukotriene antagonists, allergy immunotherapy, and aspirin desensitization may also be indicated in certain patients.

Surgical Options

Multiple modalities are available with varying levels of invasiveness, ranging from simple balloon dilation to complete obliteration of the frontal sinus. Current literature regarding revision frontal sinus surgery outcomes relies upon the Draf criteria. Wormald et al. (2016) proposed a novel Classification of the Extent of Frontal Sinus Surgery (EFSS) [12]. This is discussed in detail in Chap. 4. In summary, they propose the following grades:

1. Grade 0: Balloon sinus dilation (no tissue removal)
2. Grade 1: Clearance of cells in frontal recess without surgery within frontal ostium
3. Grade 2: Clearance of cells obstructing frontal sinus ostium
4. Grade 3: Clearance of cells pneumatizing through frontal ostium to frontal sinus
5. Grade 4: Clearance of cell pneumatizing through the frontal ostium with removal of bone of frontal beak
6. Grade 5: Enlargement of the frontal ostium from lamina papyracea to nasal septum (analogous to Draf IIB)
7. Grade 6: Removal of entire floor of frontal sinus, creating common ostium via septal window (analogous to Draf III)

In the future, stratification of surgical options based upon the updated EFSS criteria may improve our understanding of anatomic complexity and surgical outcomes in revision frontal surgery.

Balloon Sinus Dilation

Balloon sinus dilation may be useful in select patients who have undergone restenosis of the frontal outflow tract after traditional endoscopic sinus surgery. Potential advantages include decreased operative time, avoidance of general anesthesia, decreased postoperative pain, and need for fewer debridements. Outcomes data for the use of this technology are incomplete. Further large, well-controlled studies are necessary to determine long-term efficacy, particularly in comparison to revision ESS. Eloy et al. (2011) reported a series of five patients with symptomatic restenosis of the frontal recess following Draf IIA or IIB sinusotomy. All elected to undergo in-office balloon sinus dilation, which was technically successful in 100% of cases. All patients were asymptomatic and demonstrated endoscopically patent frontal outflow tracts at a mean of 5 months after the procedures (see Fig. 12.8) [13].

Revision Draf IIA Surgery

The majority of patients with persistent, symptomatic frontal sinus disease following frontal sinus surgery can be managed with revision Draf IIA surgery. In a subset analysis of 48 patient undergoing revision Draf IIA frontal sinusotomy for chronic rhinosinusitis with and without nasal polyposis, Askar et al. (2015) reported a 92.4% ostial patency rate at 6 months or greater, with a significant improvement in all RSDI domains [2]. Meticulous dissection of residual cells and bony partitions as well as careful mucosal preservation is critical in preventing further surgical failure.

Draf III Frontal Sinusotomy

It involves removal of all frontal sinus cells and frontal beak and the anterior insertion of bilateral middle turbinates, anterior/superior nasal septum, and intersinus septum, thereby opening the floor of the frontal sinus from orbit to orbit. Anderson and Sindwani (2009) performed a review and meta-analysis of 18 studies evaluating Draf III sinusotomy, reporting objective endoscopic frontal sinus patency in 95.9% of 394 patients at 28.5 months. Symptom improvement was noted in 82.2% of 430 patients. Of 612 patients, further surgery was required in 13.9% [14]. More recent studies vary in patency rates; at the high end,

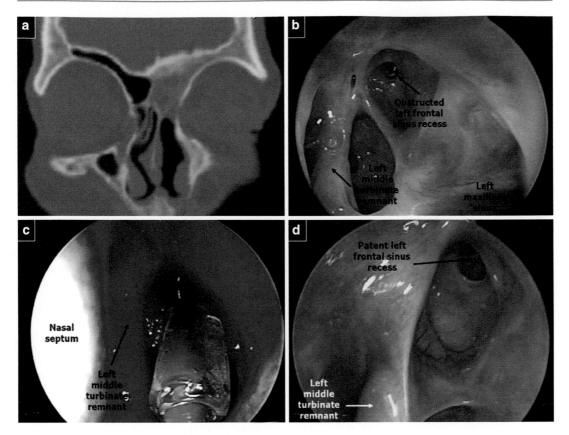

Fig. 12.8 Balloon sinus dilation of stenosed neo-ostium following frontal sinus surgery. (**a**) Coronal computed tomography scan of patient after a failed left Draf IIB. (**b**) Thirty-degree endoscopic view of the scarred frontal recess. (**c**) In-office cannulation and dilation of the left frontal recess. (**d**) Postoperative 70-degree endoscopic view at 5 months. (Used with permission from Eloy et al. [13])

Naidoo et al. (2014) reported 97% Draf III success in 229 patients at 45 months. Restenosis of Draf III neo-ostia was noted to progress for up to 2 years, mandating careful, long-term follow-up [15]. Maximizing neo-ostial size is a critical step toward preventing failure [1].

Mucosal grafting may help with Draf III sinusotomy. Creation of an appropriately large Draf III common frontal drainage pathway necessitates drilling of the bony frontal outflow tract. Animal models have suggested, however, that exposed bone serves as a nidus for osteoneogenesis and inflammation, increasing the risk of postoperative restenosis [16]. Several small, retrospective studies have reported a decreased incidence of restenosis following Draf III surgery with the use of free or pedicled mucosal grafts over areas of exposed bone [16]. In a prospective study of mucosal grafting, Illing et al. (2016)

reported that 65 of 67 (97%) patients maintained >50% of intraoperative anterior-posterior frontal diameter at a mean of 34 months. Despite being considered surgical failures, the remaining two patients nevertheless maintained patent frontal outflow tracts and did not require further surgical intervention [17].

Frontal Sinus Obliteration/ Cranialization

In most situations, a patent frontal sinus outflow tract can be restored surgically, but in select cases the creation of a nonfunctional frontal sinus is clinically indicated. Riedel described an open approach to the frontal sinus in 1889 with removal of the anterior table; this was modified in the mid-twentieth century to involve preservation of a viable anterior osteoplastic bone flap with stripping of the sinus mucosa and obliteration of the sinus space. Success rates of 75–93% have been reported for this procedure [1].

Frontal sinus obliteration carries additional morbidities when compared to endoscopic approaches, including risks of external scarring, forehead numbness, frontal embossment, graft extrusion, and cosmetic deformity. Late mucocele formation may occur in 10% or more of cases with higher numbers being seen with longer follow-up [18].

Summary

With advances in technology and improved surgical technique, frontal sinus surgery failure rates have decreased but still remain an issue for even the most experienced rhinologic surgeon.

Careful preoperative review of CT scans and meticulous surgical technique are necessary to minimize technical failures leading to ostial restenosis. Such technical lapses include overaggressive mucosal removal, excessive bone exposure, and failure to completely remove all cell partitions impinging upon the frontal outflow tract. Ideally, the postsurgical ostial size should be at least 4.5–5.0 mm, in order to minimize the risk of restenosis. Individual patient anatomy may preclude this goal, however, and a high level of suspicion for restenosis should occur in patients with smaller ostia. Ostial size should not be increased at the expense of mucosal sacrifice. In most situations, revision Draf IIA frontal sinus surgery can effectively restore sinus function and patency of the outflow tract. In select cases, a Draf III sinus drill-out procedure has an excellent success rate for salvage of the failed frontal sinusotomy. The concomitant use of mucosal grafts to areas of exposed bone may further enhance surgical outcomes.

Frontal sinus obliteration and cranialization are options when creation of a functioning sinus is not feasible, though long-term complication rates including mucocele formation are high.

References

1. DeConde AS, Smith TL. Outcomes after frontal sinus surgery: an evidence-based review. Otolaryngol Clin N Am. 2016;49(4):1019–33.
2. Askar MH, Gamea A, Tomoum MO, Elsherif HS, Ebert C, Senior BA. Endoscopic management of chronic frontal sinusitis: prospective quality of life analysis. Ann Otol Rhinol Laryngol. 2015;124(8):638–48.
3. Naidoo Y, Wen D, Bassiouni A, Keen M, Wormald PJ. Long-term results after primary frontal sinus surgery. Int Forum Allergy Rhinol. 2012;2(3):185–90.
4. Chandra RK, Palmer JN, Tangsujarittham T, Kennedy DW. Factors associated with failure of frontal sinusotomy in the early follow-up period. Otolaryngol Head Neck Surg. SAGE Publications. 2004;131:514–8.
5. Valdes CJ, Bogado M, Samaha M. Causes of failure in endoscopic frontal sinus surgery in chronic rhinosinusitis patients. Int Forum Allergy Rhinol. 2014;4(6):502–6.
6. Otto KJ, DelGaudio JM. Operative findings in the frontal recess at time of revision surgery. Am J Otolaryngol. 2010;31(3):175–80.
7. Gore MR, Ebert CS, Zanation AM, B A S. Beyond the "central sinus": radiographic findings in patients undergoing revision functional endoscopic sinus surgery. Int Forum Allergy Rhinol. 2013;3(2):139–46.
8. Hosemann W, Kuhnel T, Held P, Wagner W, Felderhoff A. Endonasal frontal sinusotomy in surgical management of chronic sinusitis: a critical evaluation. Am J Rhinol. 1997;11(1):1–9.
9. Bassiouni A, Chen PG, Naidoo Y, Wormald PJ. Clinical significance of middle turbinate lateralization after endoscopic sinus surgery. Laryngoscope. 2015;125(1):36–41.
10. Soler ZM, Hwang PH, Mace J, Smith TL. Outcomes after middle turbinate resection: revisiting a controversial topic. Laryngoscope. 2010;120(4):832–7.
11. Bent JP, Guilty-Siller G, Kuhn FA. The frontal cell as a cause of frontal sinus obstruction. Am J Rhinol. 1994;8(4):185–91.
12. Wormald PJ, Hoseman W, Callejas C, Weber RK, Kennedy DW, Citardi MJ, et al. The international frontal sinus anatomy classification (IFAC) and classification of the extent of endoscopic frontal sinus surgery (EFSS). Int Forum Allergy Rhinol. 2016;6:677–96.
13. Eloy JA, Friedel ME, Eloy JD, Govindaraj S, Folbe AJ. In-office balloon dilation of the failed frontal sinusotomy. Otolaryngol Head Neck Surg. 2012;146(2):320–2.
14. Anderson P, Sindwani R. Safety and efficacy of the endoscopic modified lothrop procedure: a systematic review and meta-analysis. Laryngoscope. 2009;119(9):1828–33.
15. Naidoo Y, Bassiouni A, Keen M, Wormald PJ. Long-term outcomes for the endoscopic modified lothrop/draf III procedure: a 10-year review. Laryngoscope. 2014;124(1):43–9.

16. Wei CC, Sama A. What is the evidence for the use of mucosal flaps in Draf III procedures? Curr Opin Otolaryngol Head Neck Surg. 2014;22(1):63–7.
17. Illing EA, Cho DY, Riley KO, Woodworth BA. Draf III mucosal graft technique: long-term results. Int Forum Allergy Rhinol. 2016;6:514–7.
18. Weber R, Draf W, Keerl R, Kahle G, Schinzel S, Thomann S, et al. Osteoplastic frontal sinus surgery with fat obliteration: technique and long-term results using magnetic resonance imaging in 82 operations. Laryngoscope. 2000;110:1037–44.

Contemporary Management of Frontal Sinus Mucoceles

13

Christopher D. Brook and Benjamin S. Bleier

Clinical Presentation

A mucocele is defined as an epithelial-lined cavity filled with mucus and forms from obstruction of the sinus ostia or local glandular outflow, leading to accumulation of mucus and expansion of the cavity [1, 2]. The frontal sinus is the most common location for paranasal sinus mucoceles, although they can form in other sinuses as well [1–5], and they most commonly occur between the 4th and 7th decades of life [5]. Prolonged expansion of a mucocele can lead to complications such as pain and pressure, eyelid edema, frontal headaches, cranial nerve palsy, and facial deformity from bony remodeling (Fig. 13.1a, b) [1, 2, 6–8]. The most common presenting symptoms are headache, pressure, congestion, and drainage [3], although in one series over 80% of patients presented with orbital manifestations of the mucocele [9]. In these two series, there was an incidence over 40% of skull base erosion and

extension of the mucocele intraorbitally or intracranially [3, 9]. In addition infection of a mucocele leads to formation of a mucopyocele and can lead to serious intracranial infectious complications such as meningitis or intracranial abscess [10].

As mentioned previously, mucoceles develop due to accumulation of physiologic mucus production which has lost an avenue for egress. Development of sinus obstruction leading to this accumulation often occurs after previous surgical intervention, and multiple authors have detailed this relationship. In a large review of 133 mucoceles, Scangas et al. noted that more than 50% had undergone some type of previous sinus surgery [3]. Herndon et al. noted in a series of 13 fronto-orbital-ethmoid mucoceles that 9 had undergone previous sinus procedures, including 4 that had previously had a frontal sinus obliteration [2]. Chiu et al. in a series of ten patients with lateral frontal sinus and supraorbital ethmoid mucoceles noted that nine of the ten had previously had a sinus procedure, including six endoscopic sinus surgeries, two external ethmoidectomies, and a single frontal sinus fracture repair [11]. Mucoceles may also develop after a craniotomy that violates the paranasal sinuses [12] or, infrequently, after skull base reconstruction [13]. Notably, patients undergoing sinus surgery typically have chronic rhinosinusitis and sinus inflammatory disease that may also be a contributory factor in mucocele formation.

Electronic Supplementary Material The online version of this chapter (doi:10.1007/978-3-319-97022-6_13) contains supplementary material, which is available to authorized users.

C. D. Brook
Boston University Medical Center, Department of Otolaryngology, Boston, MA, USA

B. S. Bleier (✉)
Massachusetts Eye and Ear Infirmary, Harvard Medical School, Department of Otolaryngology, Boston, MA, USA

© Springer Nature Switzerland AG 2019
D. Lal, P. H. Hwang (eds.), *Frontal Sinus Surgery*, https://doi.org/10.1007/978-3-319-97022-6_13

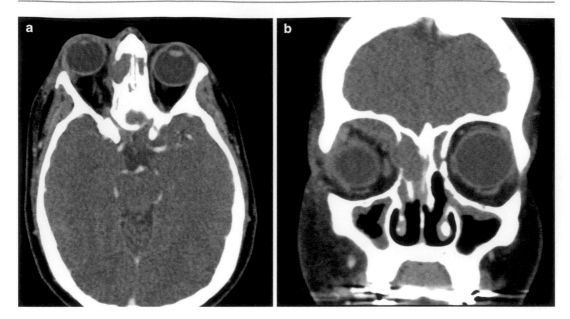

Fig. 13.1 (a) Axial CT scan demonstrating orbital proptosis from a right frontoethmoidal mucocele. (b) Coronal CT view demonstrating right frontoethmoidal mucocele with associated subperiosteal abscess

Unsurprisingly, trauma that disrupts sinus anatomy can also lead to luminal obstruction and later mucocele development in a similar manner to previous surgery (Video 13.1). Scangas et al. noted that approximately 8% of patients in their series of 133 had a history of sinus trauma that preceded the development of a mucocele [3]. In addition, several other papers have cited previous trauma as a risk factor for the development of mucoceles [1, 2, 8, 11]. Traditionally, frontal sinus fractures that involved the frontal sinus recess or frontal sinus outflow tract were treated with removal of the frontal sinus via obliteration or cranialization due to this risk. However, in the contemporary era, management has gravitated toward less invasive monitoring and endoscopic intervention in patients at risk for development of frontal sinus disease after trauma [14, 15]. It is important to note that mucocele formation after trauma can be delayed significantly from the time of the injury and present many years later. Thus suspicion should remain high regardless of how distant in time a traumatic event may have occurred [3, 16].

There are other inherent patient risk factors for mucocele development as well, including cystic fibrosis and immotile cilia syndrome [17–19]. However, at least in cystic fibrosis, the most common location for mucocele formation seems to be the maxillary and ethmoid sinuses as opposed to the frontal sinuses [17, 18]. In these patients, the frontal sinuses are often hypoplastic or underdeveloped, thereby lessening the likelihood of frontal sinus mucocele formation [20, 21].

Mucocele Management

Management of frontal sinus mucoceles involves workup and excision or drainage of the mucocele. Workup generally entails radiologic evaluation with computed tomography (CT) scan to determine the extent of the lesion, associated bony resorption, and the surgical anatomy. MRI can be used as an adjunctive tool to evaluate for neoplasm or meningoencephalocele but provides poor bony anatomic description for surgical planning [22], and the two modalities are often used in a complimentary manner during the workup of skull base and frontal sinus mucocele [23]. After the diagnosis is made, mucoceles require drainage and marsupialization of the mucus-filled cavity. Though rare, patients with complications due to mucocele expansion or infection can require hospital admission, intravenous antibiotics, and multiple specialty involvement, including consultation with neurosurgery or ophthalmology as indicated.

Traditionally drainage of a mucocele was accomplished through open approaches to the sinuses with complete excision of the mucocele. However, mucoceles have increasingly become managed with endoscopic marsupialization techniques since Kennedy et al. described this method in 1989 [22, 24]. It is now recognized that mucocele lining may be adherent to the dura or periorbita in some cases, putting patients at risk or intracranial or orbital complications with complete excision of the mucocele lining, and that endoscopic marsupialization can achieve the same objectives as excision [25]. Interestingly, Stokken et al. noted the persistent idea of the invasiveness of mucoceles in the neurosurgical literature and the idea that these lesions need complete excision. This suggests that, despite recognition in the otolaryngology literature of the success of marsupialization, this knowledge is not disseminated yet in all surgical literature [25]. Drainage can be accomplished with either external or endoscopic techniques. External frontal sinus procedures range from simple trephination to transcaruncular approach to osteoplastic flap with or without frontal sinus obliteration (FSO) [24, 26], while endoscopic techniques range from frontal sinusotomy via Draf IIa to Draf IIb and finally modified endoscopic Lothrop procedure (MELP) or Draf III procedure. Often both endoscopic and external techniques are used in combination approaches for complicated mucoceles [2, 27, 28]. Additionally, some authors have described endoscopic management in the clinic setting under local anesthesia for selected mucoceles without significant neo-osteogenesis or septations [29].

A large meta-analysis published in 2014 examined papers describing management of mucoceles in the historical era compared with the modern era, defined as published after 2002 [24]. This date was chosen by the authors because it represented a time point representing about 10 years of accumulated experience with endoscopic sinus surgery and broad adaptation of the technique within the otolaryngology community. In the historical era, the authors noted that there were large series of patients treated with predominantly external approaches [30], although there were some early adopters of the endoscopic approach [9, 22, 31]. In the modern era, the authors found that the rate of endoscopic approach for frontal mucoceles was much higher than the historical era but that there were still significant numbers of external approaches and combined approaches to the frontal sinus [32, 33]. Other authors in the modern era have demonstrated successful endoscopic frontal sinus procedures for reversal and management of frontal sinus mucoceles associated with previous frontal sinus obliteration [27, 34, 35], erosion of the anterior table of the frontal sinus (Video 13.2) [27], and extensive "giant" frontal mucoceles associated with displacement of the intracranial contents or orbital contents [25, 36] and in the far lateral portion of the frontal sinus [11]. Often the challenge encountered when performing endoscopic approaches for this type of procedures is lateral access to the sinus. In the paper by Chandra et al., the authors noted that laterally based mucoceles recurring after FSO often required the use of a drill to gain access to the mucocele through unilateral or transseptal Draf III approaches [36]. Chiu et al. also commented on the use of modern angle instruments and a thorough knowledge of anatomy often coupled with the use of computer-aided image guidance [11]. Additionally, many contemporary authors have advocated combined endoscopic and external approaches for difficult to reach mucoceles or revision cases depending on the situation [2, 22, 32], and still a subset of authors advocates for frontal sinus obliteration in some cases [33, 37]. In particular, frontal sinus mucoceles which remain entirely lateral to the midportion of the globe will often require an adjunctive external approach. However, access may still be achieved through a cosmetically favorable manner such as employing a trephine, superior lid crease, or transcaruncular approach.

In the meta-analysis comparing the modern era to the historical era, Courson et al. noted that rates of recurrence and complications were different when comparing the endoscopic and open approaches in the historical era [22]. In the historical era, when compared with open surgery, endoscopic drainage was associated with a decreased rate of recurrence and of major complications, which were defined as life-threatening infection or blood loss, CSF leak, or vision loss. In the modern era, however, there were no significant differences between recurrence and major complication rates between the two difference approaches. Minor complications, such as wound breakdown, epistaxis, superficial infection, or temporary vision changes, were significantly higher in the open surgical groups in both eras. When comparing the historical cohort to the endoscopic cohort, the results were similar in both the historical and modern era. They found a rate of recurrence of 4.7% in the historical and 3.1% in the modern era and a rate of major complication of 3.4% and 1.8%, respectively. None of these differences were statistically significant. The paper also examined the results of the senior author's own practice, comparing differences in the historical and modern era. In this analysis again, there were not significant differences between the historical and modern cohorts, suggesting that the evolution from open approaches to the endoscopic approach has not detracted from the treatment of this condition or led to higher rates of complication [22].

While in the meta-analysis there were not significant differences between open and endoscopic approaches in the modern era, there is data that suggests that some open and endoscopic approaches for these conditions have specific advantages and disadvantages. Externally, a Lynch approach or a transcaruncular approach has been employed to approach the frontoethmoidal region for mucoceles; however, they can create the risk of external scar, diplopia, and caruncular scarring [5]. Although early studies did not demonstrate a high rate of complications with FSO in a large series of patients [30], FSO is now known to place patients at risk for development of later mucocele formation years after the initial surgery. In two studies examining MRI findings in patients who had undergone previous FSO, mucoceles were detected within the obliterated sinuses in 5 of 59 cases and 3 of 13 cases,

for a range of mucocele formation of 10–23% [38, 39]. In contrast, articles that have focused on endoscopic techniques for frontal mucocele management have recorded higher rates of restenosis with Draf IIb approaches when compared with Draf IIa procedures [28], while others have found the Draf IIb procedure to be effective and maintain long-term patency rates greater than 90% [40]. Still yet other authors have reported restenosis rates of approximately 10% following Draf III procedure [41, 42]. These findings suggest that the choice of approach should ultimately be dictated by the balance between maximizing the drainage pathway and minimizing the amount of denuded mucosa and raw bone exposure and that long-term follow-up of these patients is critical due to the risk of recurrence of restenosis.

Summary

Contemporary management of frontal sinus mucocele has evolved from more invasive, open attempts at excision to less invasive, endoscopic attempts at marsupialization. Despite this trend, open surgical techniques may still be employed as stand-alone procedures or in combination with endoscopic management, particular for laterally located lesions. Due to the risk of late recurrence or restenosis of the frontal sinus, these patients require long-term follow-up.

References

1. Busaba NY, Salman SD. Ethmoid mucocele as a late complication of endoscopic ethmoidectomy. Otolaryngol Head Neck Surg. 2003;128(4):517–22.
2. Herndon M, McMains KC, Kountakis SE. Presentation and management of extensive fronto-orbital-ethmoid mucoceles. Am J Otolaryngol. 2007;28(3):145–7.
3. Scangas GA, Gudis DA, Kennedy DW. The natural history and clinical characteristics of paranasal sinus mucoceles: a clinical review. Int Forum Allergy Rhinol. 2013;3(9):712–7.
4. Thio D, Phelps PD, Bath AP. Maxillary sinus mucocele presenting as a late complication of a maxillary advancement procedure. J Laryngol Otol. 2003;117(5):402–3.

5. Lai PC, Liao SL, Jou JR, Hou PK. Transcaruncular approach for the management of frontoethmoid mucoceles. Br J Ophthalmol. 2003;87(6):699–703.
6. Lin CJ, Kao CH, Kang BH, Wang HW. Frontal sinus mucocele presenting as oculomotor nerve palsy. Otolaryngol Head Neck Surg. 2002;126(5):588–90.
7. Ehrenpreis SJ, Biedlingmaier JF. Isolated third-nerve palsy associated with frontal sinus mucocele. J Neuroophthalmol. 1995;15(2):105–8.
8. Malhotra R, Wormald PJ, Selva D. Bilateral dynamic proptosis due to frontoethmoidal sinus mucocele. Ophthal Plast Reconstr Surg. 2003;19(2):156–7.
9. Har-El G. Endoscopic management of 108 sinus mucoceles. Laryngoscope. 2001;111(12):2131–4.
10. Cultrera F, Giuffrida M, Mancuso P. Delayed post-traumatic frontal sinus mucopyocoele presenting with meningitis. J Craniomaxillofac Surg. 2006;34(8):502–4. Epub 2006 Dec 6
11. Chiu AG, Vaughan WC. Management of the lateral frontal sinus lesion and the supraorbital cell mucocele. Am J Rhinol. 2004;18(2):83–6.
12. Meetze K, Palmer JN, Schlosser RJ. Frontal sinus complications after frontal craniotomy. Laryngoscope. 2004;114(5):945–8.
13. Bleier BS, Wang EW, Vandergrift WA 3rd, Schlosser RJ. Mucocele rate after endoscopic skull base reconstruction using vascularized pedicled flaps. Am J Rhinol Allergy. 2011;25(3):186–7.
14. Smith TL, Han JK, Loehrl TA, Rhee JS. Endoscopic management of the frontal recess in frontal sinus fractures: a shift in the paradigm? Laryngoscope. 2002;112(5):784–90.
15. Guy WM, Brissett AE. Contemporary management of traumatic fractures of the frontal sinus. Otolaryngol Clin N Am. 2013;46(5):733–48.
16. Koudstaal MJ, van der Wal KG, Bijvoet HW, Vincent AJ, Poublon RM. Post-trauma mucocele formation in the frontal sinus; a rationale of follow-up. Int J Oral Maxillofac Surg. 2004;33(8):751–4.
17. Qureishi A, Lennox P, Bottrill I. Bilateral maxillary mucoceles: an unusual presentation of cystic fibrosis. J Laryngol Otol. 2012;126(3):319–21.
18. Di Cicco M, Costantini D, Padoan R, Colombo C. Paranasal mucoceles in children with cystic fibrosis. Int J Pediatr Otorhinolaryngol. 2005;69(10):1407–13.
19. Berlucchi M, Maroldi R, Aga A, Grazzani L, Padoan R. Ethmoid mucocele: a new feature of primary ciliary dyskinesia. Pediatr Pulmonol. 2010;45(2):197–201.
20. Ferril GR, Nick JA, Getz AE, et al. Comparison of radiographic and clinical characteristics of low-risk and high-risk cystic fibrosis genotypes. Int Forum Allergy Rhinol. 2014;4(11):915–20.
21. Berkhout MC, van Rooden CJ, Rijntjes E, Fokkens WJ, el Bouazzaoui LH, Heijerman HG. Sinonasal manifestations of cystic fibrosis: a correlation between genotype and phenotype? J Cyst Fibros. 2014;13(4):442–8.
22. Kennedy DW, Josephson JS, Zinreich SJ, et al. Endoscopic sinus surgery for mucoceles: a viable alternative. Laryngoscope. 1989;99:885–95.
23. Tsitouridis I, Michaelides M, Bintoudi A, Kyriakou V. Frontoethmoidal Mucoceles: CT and MRI evaluation. Neuroradiol J. 2007;20(5):586–96.
24. Courson AM, Stankiewicz JA, Lal D. Contemporary management of frontal sinus mucoceles: a meta-analysis. Laryngoscope. 2014;124(2):378–86.
25. Stokken J, Wali E, Woodard T, Recinos PF, Sindwani R. Considerations in the management of giant frontal mucoceles with significant intracranial extension: a systematic review. Am J Rhinol Allergy. 2016;30(4):301–5.
26. Schneider JS, Day A, Clavenna M, Russell PT, Duncavage J. Early practice: external sinus surgery and procedures and complications. Otolaryngol Clin N Am. 2015;48(5):839–50.
27. Woodworth BA, Harvey RJ, Neal JG, Palmer JN, Schlosser RJ. Endoscopic management of frontal sinus mucoceles with anterior table erosion. Rhinology. 2008;46:231–7.
28. Dhepnorrarat RC, Subramaniam S, Sethi SS. Endoscopic surgery for fronto-ethmoidal mucoceles: a 15-year experience. Otolaryngol Head Neck Surg. 2012;147:345–50.
29. Barrow EM, DelGaudio JM. In-office drainage of sinus Mucoceles: An alternative to operating-room drainage. Laryngoscope. 2015;125(5):1043–7.
30. Hardy JM, Montgomery WW. Osteoplastic frontal sinusotomy: an analysis of 250 operations. Ann Otol Rhinol Laryngol. 1976;85:523–32.
31. Lund VJ. Endoscopic management of paranasal sinus mucocoeles. J Laryngol Otol. 1998;112:36–40.
32. Bockmühl U, Kratzsch B, Benda K, Draf W. Surgery for paranasal sinus mucocoeles: efficacy of endonasal micro-endoscopic management and long-term results of 185 patients. Rhinology. 2006;44(1):62–7.
33. Kristin J, Betz CS, Stelter K, et al. Frontal sinus obliteration—a successful treatment option in patients with endoscopically inaccessible frontal mucoceles. Rhinology. 2008;46:70–4.
34. Wormald PJ. Salvage frontal sinus surgery: the endoscopic modified Lothrop procedure. Laryngoscope. 2003;113:276–83.
35. Chandra RK, Kennedy DW, Palmer JN. Endoscopic management of failed frontal sinus obliteration. Am J Rhinol. 2004;18(5):279–84.
36. Bozza F, Nisii A, Parziale G, et al. Transnasal endoscopic management of frontal sinus mucopyocele with orbital and frontal lobe displacement as minimally invasive surgery. J Neurosurg Sci. 2010;54:1–5.
37. Silverman JB, Gray ST, Busaba NY. Role of osteoplastic frontal sinus obliteration in the era of endoscopic sinus surgery. Int J Otolaryngol. 2012;2012:501896.
38. Weber R, Draf W, Keerl R, et al. Osteoplastic frontal sinus surgery with fat obliteration: technique and long-term results using magnetic resonance imaging in 82 operations. Laryngoscope. 2000;110:1037–44.
39. Loevner L, Yousem DM, Lanza DC, Kennedy DW. MR evaluation of frontal sinus osteoplastic

flaps with autogenous fat grafts. Am J Neuroradiol. 1995;16:1721–6.

40. Turner JH, Vaezeafshar R, Hwang PH. Indications and outcomes for Draf IIB frontal sinus surgery. Am J Rhinol Allergy. 2016;30(1):70–3.

41. Georgalas C, Hansen F, Videler WJ, Fokkens WJ. Long terms results of Draf type III (modified endoscopic Lothrop) frontal sinus drainage procedure in 122 patients: a single Centre experience. Rhinology. 2011;49(2):195–201.

42. Khong JJ, Malhotra R, Selva D, Wormald PJ. Efficacy of endoscopic sinus surgery for paranasal sinus mucocele including modified endoscopic Lothrop procedure for frontal sinus mucocele. J Laryngol Otol. 2004;118:352–6.

Management of Frontal Sinus Cerebrospinal Fluid Leaks

14

Arjun K. Parasher, Alan D. Workman, and James N. Palmer

Introduction

Frontal sinus cerebrospinal fluid (CSF) leaks, while relatively uncommon, present a surgical challenge. CSF leaks in other areas of the sinonasal cavity are successfully repaired with endoscopic techniques alone, but depending on the location, CSF leaks within the frontal sinus can be difficult to access with a transnasal endoscopic approach. In addition, the frontal sinus CSF leaks create the dual challenge of successful repair of the skull base defect while maintaining patency of the frontal sinus drainage pathway. Historically, collaboration with neurosurgery was often necessary in frontal sinus CSF leak repair. This multidisciplinary approach consisted of an external incision, craniotomy, and flap closure. Advances

A. K. Parasher
Division of Rhinology and Skull Base Surgery, Department of Otolaryngology – Head and Neck Surgery, University of South Florida, Tampa, FL, USA

Department of Health Policy and Management, University of South Florida, Tampa, FL, USA

A. D. Workman
Department of Otolaryngology, Massachusetts Eye and Ear Infirmary, Boston, MA, USA

J. N. Palmer (✉)
Division of Rhinology, Department of Otorhinolaryngology – Head and Neck Surgery, Hospital of the University of Pennsylvania, Philadelphia, PA, USA

in angled instruments, surgical navigation, and endoscopic surgical training have allowed for increased access to the frontal sinus through endoscopic means alone (Fig. 14.1). Figure 14.2 shows the differences in visualization of the frontal sinuses with various angled endoscopes. Repair rates for CSF leaks in favorable locations in or near the frontal sinus are as high as 97%, with repair of defects measuring up to 48 mm by 35 mm [1, 2]. However, anatomic variants, posterior table CSF leaks, and postoperative stenosis create technical challenges that may preclude comprehensive endoscopic management.

Patients with CSF rhinorrhea are at risk for intracranial complications, including meningitis and epidural or subdural abscesses [3]. Clinical management of these leaks must result in cessation of CSF flow and complete repair of the defect to reduce these morbidities. However, it is also critical to consider the patency of the frontal sinus following repair, which can be accomplished by maintaining a wide frontal sinus ostium with maximal preservation of frontal sinus and frontal recess mucosa. In the present chapter, we discuss the anatomy and categorization of frontal sinus CSF leaks, leak etiologies, diagnosis, and surgical approaches.

Anatomy

Frontal sinus CSF leaks are most often categorized by location in relation to the frontal recess. While individual anatomy can be variable, the

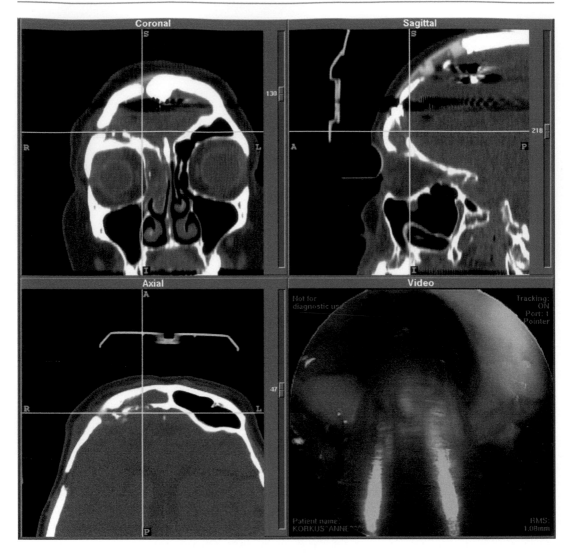

Fig. 14.1 Intraoperative surgical navigation showing posterior table pathology

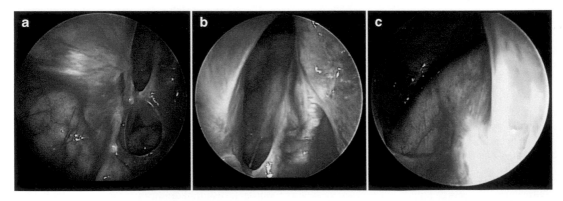

Fig. 14.2 View of the frontal sinus with 30-degree (**a**), 45-degree (**b**), and 70-degree endoscopes (**c**)

frontal recess boundaries are the internal nasofrontal beak anteriorly, the ethmoid roof posteriorly, the orbit laterally, and the middle turbinate attachment medially. Frontal sinus CSF leaks can be in one or more of three areas: adjacent to the frontal recess, involving the frontal recess, or in the frontal sinus proper. Those involving the frontal recess are associated with increased difficulty of maintaining frontal sinus patency. In general, the more superior and lateral extents of the frontal sinus are difficult to reach endoscopically, while the inferior and posterior portions of the frontal sinus are challenging to reach from an external approach such as trephination. In particular, skull base defects lateral to the mid-orbit may require an external approach such as a trephine or osteoplastic flap alone or in combination with the endoscopic approach.

Anatomic frontal sinus variants can affect repair choice for CSF leaks. An endoscopic modified Lothrop procedure (Draf III) allows for visualization of the superior and lateral aspects of the frontal sinus, but passage of instrumentation can still be impeded [4]. The extensive enlargement of the frontal sinus ostium only allows for endoscopic instruments to reach defects in the lateral margin of the frontal sinus only two-thirds of the time [4, 5]. In individuals with very convex posterior walls, access superiorly and laterally can be further inhibited [6]. To determine the feasibility of endoscopic repair of defects on the posterior wall, Sieskiewicz et al. suggested that an imaginary line be drawn between the most anteroinferior point of the frontal sinus ostium and the inferior part of the defect. Instrumentation is likely possible if the line reaches the defect without touching the posterior wall [7].

While classification by anatomical location is most frequently cited, Shi et al. created another system to classify frontal sinus CSF leaks by both site and size. This classification system focuses on surgical approach to be used. Type A leaks are situated on the posterior wall at the level of the frontal recess and are less than 1 cm in greatest dimension. Type B leaks are situated higher on the posterior wall, while type C leaks are either larger than 1 cm, associated with a frontal sinus ostium of <6 mm, associated with a poorly pneumatized

agger nasi, or localized to the posterolateral wall. Shi et al. argue that type C leaks are those that warrant a combined endoscopic and open approach, while type A and B leaks can likely be managed in a purely endoscopic fashion [8].

Etiologies

CSF leaks can result from one of four causes: trauma, neoplastic, congenital, or spontaneous. The cause of the leak often has a substantial influence on appearance and clinical management. In general, all leaks other than those resulting from blunt trauma require surgical attention and repair [1], while 70% of trauma-related CSF leaks close with conservative management with strict bed rest and stool softeners to prevent increased intracranial pressure. Most CSF leaks will present within the first 2 days following high-energy trauma, with 95% appearing within 3 months [9]. However, blunt trauma with associated frontal sinus fracture is often associated with late mucocele formation and potential aesthetic deformity, so informed clinical decision-making is necessary [10]. A conservative approach is more appropriate with injuries limited to the frontal recess or the posterior table.

High-energy trauma-related leaks are distinct from iatrogenic CSF leaks, which do require surgical repair. Complex functional endoscopic sinus surgery (FESS) can be associated with a risk of CSF leak as high as 10% [11]. The posterior table can be significantly thinner than the anterior table, and slight dehiscence from rough instrumentation can cause a leak to occur. Additionally, already-present mucoceles can erode the posterior table further. Neurosurgical frontal craniotomy can also iatrogenically cause CSF leaks as the superior or lateral recesses of the frontal sinuses are approached externally.

Non-traumatic causes of CSF leak also occur. Through slow erosion of the posterior table or frontal recess, sinonasal tumors can create leaks. Additionally, removal of a tumor can create defects that result in a leak, and associated chemotherapy and radiation can result in poor healing or graft failure of a repaired defect. While the frontal sinus is not yet developed at birth, congenital leaks can develop during the first several years of life within or adjacent to the frontal recess. Related posterior table defects and frontal sinus floor anomalies can also contribute to pathology in this case. Finally, spontaneous CSF leaks are often associated with idiopathic intracranial hypertension (IIH), which is most often seen in obese females [12]. These IIH-related leaks are associated with elevated encephalocele formation and can have very high recurrence rates (over 50%) when compared to leaks of other etiologies (10%) [13–15]. If intracranial hypertension is not concurrently managed with leak repair, the increased pressure will put considerable strain on the surgical site and potentially cause re-leaks. These spontaneous leaks are rarely observed occurring through the posterior table and are more likely to present at weaker areas of the skull base adjacent to the frontal recess.

Diagnosis

Diagnosis of a frontal sinus CSF leak can be quite challenging. There is no universally accepted algorithm for evaluation, and sensitivities and specificities of the various tests used can vary depending on leak etiology, demographics, and anatomical factors. Patients experiencing CSF rhinorrhea classically describe a constant or intermittent clear nasal discharge that has a metallic or salty taste. Depending on etiology and complications, patients can also present with nasal obstruction (in the case of a neoplasm) or headache and neck stiffness during intracranial complications of CSF leak. If the CSF leak is spontaneous and associated with IIH, the patient may report nausea, pulsatile tinnitus, and papilledema associated with increased intracranial pressure (ICP) [6].

CSF itself is rarely visible on endoscopy; mucus drainage pathways and the possibility of an intermittent leak obscure definitive evaluation. Several tests are used for more conclusive diagnosis. A beta-2 transferrin test of secretions is very useful for determining if CSF is present and should be used as a first-line test, but it is non-localizing [16]. Radiographically, high-resolution CT scans are appropriate for showing bony dehiscence and preoperative planning, but not all dehiscence is associated with a leak. If beta-2 transferrin testing or CT scan fails to diagnose or localize a suspected CSF leak, MR cisternography should be employed as a second-line test. Radioactive cisternography can be used to detect intermittent leaks but has a high rate of false positives, which limits its utility. The intraoperative use of intrathecal fluorescein can assist in precise localization of CSF leak, particularly when multiple skull base defects are suspected, but this requires skull base exposure. 0.1 ml of fluorescein in 10 cc of CSF is injected over 10 min at the beginning of the case, which aids in both localization and confirmation of a seal at the end of the repair.

A critical evaluation of the size and extent of the CSF leak, dural disruption, intracranial pressure, and presence or absence of meningoencephalocele should accompany diagnosis. Additionally, patient age and presence of associated injury or fracture can inform approach and treatment strategy. In general, patients with severe medical comorbidities and high bleeding risk are best stabilized prior to proceeding with a potential operation.

Surgical Repair

The majority of the literature on CSF leak repair focuses on ethmoid and sphenoid sinus leaks [4]. Many guiding principles from the repair of these leaks apply in the frontal sinus as well. Overall, the objective is to achieve complete separation between the nasal airway and cranial cavity, leave no remaining dead space, preserve vascular and ocular function, and reconstruct a functional tissue barrier [1]. Other factors, which are advisable but not individually mandatory, include mucosal resection, impermeability of the first layer, the use of multiple layers, and utilization of grafts and flaps to facilitate healing [6]. Frontal sinus repairs tend to have a significantly higher failure rate than those in other locations, as a superior and lateral location of the leak on the posterior table can create an obstacle to successful repair [17]. Meningoceles or meningoencephaloceles can further complicate surgical management [18], and these and other factors can be predictive on long-term outcomes.

Maintenance of frontal sinus patency is an additional important principle in frontal sinus CSF leak repair [19]. If the defect is located near the frontal sinus outflow tract, traditionally, the frontal sinus was obliterated by removing all the mucosa via an osteoplastic approach. However, with advances in endoscopic techniques and the late complication rate of frontal sinus obliteration, every effort should be made to preserve patency of the frontal outflow tract with the use of an extended frontal sinusotomy if needed. Defects not near the outflow tract, such as those in the lateral recess, may be treated with more conservative surgery. Fully removing mucosa can lead to an increased failure rate and osteitic bone, so it is only advisable if patency of the outflow tract cannot be maintained. Even in defects that are adjacent to the frontal recess (classification type 1), the frontal recess must be addressed. Grafts in this area can affect outflow, and the frontal recess should be opened to prevent synechiae formation and mucoceles. Figure 14.3 shows a defect just posterior to the frontal sinus recess. Agger nasi and posterior suprabullar air cells should also be removed to ensure patency [1]. In achieving exposure, a standard approach of maxillary antrostomy, ethmoidectomy, and sphenoidotomy is performed, followed by a Draf IIB frontal sinusotomy for unilateral defects and Draf III for bilateral posterior table exposure.

A solely endoscopic approach is most favorable to minimize patient morbidity. Any external techniques used involve incision and the potential for extensive dissection, increased complications, aesthetic asymmetry, and risk for a delayed mucocele [20]. However, an external approach is sometimes necessary to achieve a stable repair. The narrow dimensions of the frontal recess can preclude endoscopic exposure [21]. Becker et al. demonstrated in a cadaveric study that the superior and lateral areas of the frontal sinus could not always be reached endoscopically even following a Draf III procedure [4]. A surgeon who is unsure of the adequacy of endoscopic approach should explore the frontal recess with instrumentation to determine the accessibility of the defect to endonasal techniques. If extracranial repair is necessary, a combined approach using a frontal trephine can provide increased access to superior and lateral portions of a defect. Trephination carries much less morbidity than a craniotomy, and this graduated approach to repair that results in the least external exposure is ideal (Fig. 14.4). In some cases, especially if all frontal sinus mucosa needs to be obliterated to maintain frontal patency, an open approach with an osteoplastic flap is most appropriate (Fig. 14.5). A narrow anterior-posterior frontal recess diameter or a defect located far laterally also make open approaches more favorable. For extensive posterior table defects, such as in the case of severe trauma or tumor obliteration, cranialization of the frontal sinus with a pericranial flap may be required. However, this approach requires retraction on the frontal lobe, which can result in significantly increased morbidity.

Graft sites are best prepared by removing a portion of normal mucosa around the defect both to provide adherent surface for the graft and to elicit the process of bone thickening. Following this, choosing grafting substrate and an appropriate technique is critical. Our preference is for a multilayer closure. When possible, the first layer of a graft should be an intradural underlay, especially in the presence of a large primary defect [22]. If an intradural underlay is not possible, an extradural underlay should be placed between the bone and dura. Finally, an overlay graft with a mucosal flap or other grafts can be used as the final layer, laid extracranially adjacent to the skull base [6]. Grafts are highly variable and are very situation dependent; the choice of cartilage, mucosa, fascia, or alloplastic material should be dictated by the size and stability needed. Free grafts or vascularized flaps including the nasoseptal flap or pericranial flap can be utilized. Gelfoam or fibrin glue is used to buttress the graft to maintain stability during the healing period. A frontal stent left in place for 2 weeks following surgery can buttress the repair and increase the likelihood of frontal patency, especially when paired with weekly debridement to reduce synechiae and crusting.

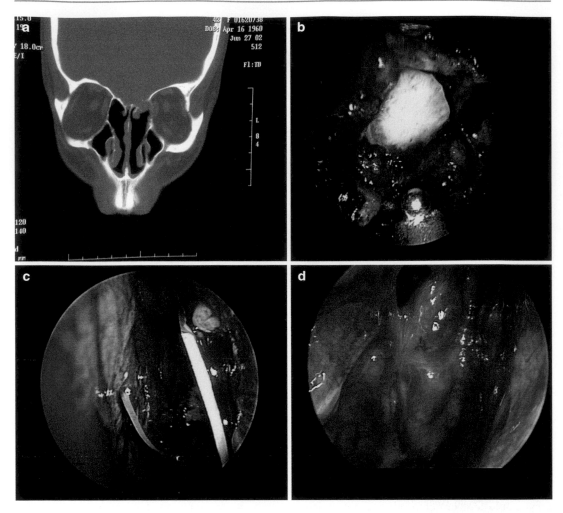

Fig. 14.3 Type 1 frontal sinus defect adjacent to the recess (**a**), repaired with bone graft (**b**). A silastic stent is placed within the frontal sinus recess to maintain patency after the repair (**c**). A 3-month postoperative view of the repair with a patent frontal sinus (**d**)

Bone grafts are most appropriate for large defects (>5 mm) or for spontaneous CSF leaks due to IIH regardless of associated defect size [1]. The structural support provided by a bone graft is invaluable to counteract elevated ICP. Septum or turbinate bone spares external incision and is most often utilized. For larger defects, mastoid or parietal cortex can be utilized, but this is rare. Intranasal packing is used to support the bone graft, with removal of this packing at 2 weeks postoperation. In the case of tumor-associated CSF leak, bone grafts are less acceptable due to the need for postoperative radiation.

Intraoperative and Postoperative Care

A lumbar drain placed preoperatively is not routinely used but can be advantageous in cases of idiopathic intracranial hypertension [23, 24]. It can aid in leak localization with the injection of fluorescein, lower intracranial pressure immediately postoperatively, and attenuate the pressure of increased CSF production against a closed defect in the days following the operation. A lumbar drain that is open during emergence from anesthesia prevents Valsalva- and coughing-induced

Fig. 14.4 Frontal sinus trephination, as an adjunct to endoscopic approach, to address lateral frontal sinus pathology

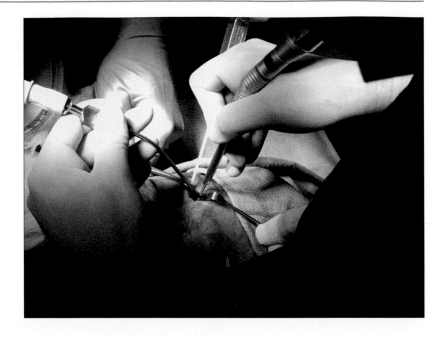

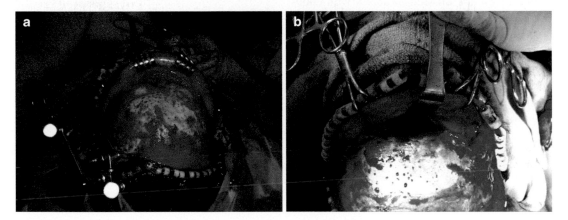

Fig. 14.5 Bicoronal approach (**a**) to the frontal sinus with osteoplastic flap elevated (**b**)

ICP increases as well. Avoidance of positive pressure ventilation by the anesthesia team can also help to prevent pneumocephalus [19]. Acetazolamide can be used adjunctively in spontaneous CSF leak patients to reduce production of CSF by as much as 50% [25], thus decreasing the pressure and lowering the rate of recurrence. Patients should also be on laxatives to prevent straining, avoid carrying heavy loads, and avoid blowing their nose.

To prevent ascending infection, perioperative and postoperative antibiotics with high CSF penetration should be utilized. Ceftriaxone, often in addition to vancomycin, is given preoperatively and for the first 48 h postoperatively. Patients are then transitioned to oral amoxicillin/clavulanate, while intranasal packing remains in place. Intraoperative surgical complications include trauma to the anterior ethmoid or spheno-palatine artery, intraorbital hematoma requiring emergency decompression, or damage to the supraorbital neurovascular bundle from the trephination incision. Care should be taken to avoid these structures in surgical approach. Delayed repair complications include frontal sinus stenosis, recurrent CSF leak, or mucocele formation. The literature shows that most frontal sinus CSF leaks have repair rates that are over 90% [19], although spontaneous CSF leaks are overrepresented in the recurring cohort.

Summary

Frontal sinus leaks are technically challenging to repair, and there are a number of important considerations in evaluation and surgical management. It is critical that special attention be given to maintaining frontal sinus patency, specifically in defects near or involving the frontal sinus outflow tract. The superior and lateral extents of the frontal recess are difficult to access with endoscopic instruments alone and may require an adjunct trephination or open approach. Spontaneous CSF leaks, often due to IIH, require more extensive repair as well as concurrent management of increased ICP. Rhinologists should carefully evaluate demographic factors, leak etiology, and anatomical access as they plan an approach to repair a CSF leak in the frontal sinus.

References

1. Jones V, Virgin F, Riley K, Woodworth BA. Changing paradigms in frontal sinus cerebrospinal fluid leak repair. Int Forum Allergy Rhinol. 2012;2:227–32.
2. Zweig JL, Carrau RL. Celin SE et al. Endoscopic repair of cerebrospinal fluid leaks to the sinonasal tract: predictors of success. Otolaryngol Head Neck Surg. 2000;123:195–201.
3. Bernal-Sprekelsen M, Bleda-Vazquez C, Carrau RL. Ascending meningitis secondary to traumatic cerebrospinal fluid leaks. Am J Rhinol. 2000;14:257–9.
4. Becker SS, Bomeli SR, Gross CW, Han JK. Limits of endoscopic visualization and instrumentation in the frontal sinus. Otolaryngol Head Neck Surg. 2006;135:917–21.
5. Chaaban MR, Conger B, Riley KO, Woodworth BA. Transnasal endoscopic repair of posterior

6. table fractures. Otolaryngol Head Neck Surg. 2012;147:1142–7.
6. Patron V, Roger V, Moreau S, Babin E, Hitier M. State of the art of endoscopic frontal sinus cerebrospinal fluid leak repair. Eur Ann Otorhinolaryngol Head Neck Dis. 2015;132:347–52.
7. Sieskiewicz A, Lyson T, Rogowski M, Rutkowski R, Mariak Z. Endoscopic repair of CSF leaks in the postero-superior wall of the frontal sinus - report of 2 cases. Minim Invasive Neurosurg. 2011;54:260–3.
8. Shi JB, Chen FH, Fu QL, et al. Frontal sinus cerebrospinal fluid leaks: repair in 15 patients using an endoscopic surgical approach. ORL J Otorhinolaryngol Relat Spec. 2010;72:56–62.
9. Zlab MK, Moore GF, Daly DT, Yonkers AJ. Cerebrospinal fluid rhinorrhea: a review of the literature. Ear Nose Throat J. 1992;71:314–7.
10. Guy WM, Brissett AE. Contemporary management of traumatic fractures of the frontal sinus. Otolaryngol Clin N Am. 2013;46:733–48.
11. Schlosser RJ, Zachmann G, Harrison S, Gross CW. The endoscopic modified Lothrop: long-term follow-up on 44 patients. Am J Rhinol. 2002;16:103–8.
12. Schlosser RJ, Bolger WE. Management of multiple spontaneous nasal meningoencephaloceles. Laryngoscope. 2002;112:980–5.
13. Schick B, Ibing R, Brors D, Draf W. Long-term study of endonasal duraplasty and review of the literature. Ann Otol Rhinol Laryngol. 2001;110:142–7.
14. Campbell RG, Farquhar D, Zhao N, Chiu AG, Adappa ND, Palmer JN. Cerebrospinal fluid rhinorrhea secondary to idiopathic intracranial hypertension: long-term outcomes of endoscopic repairs. Am J Rhinol Allergy. 2016;30:294–300.
15. Woodworth BA, Palmer JN. Spontaneous cerebrospinal fluid leaks. Curr Opin Otolaryngol Head Neck Surg. 2009;17:59–65.
16. Bleier BS, Debnath I, O'Connell BP, Vandergrift WA, Palmer JN, Schlosser RJ. Preliminary study on the stability of beta-2 transferrin in extracorporeal cerebrospinal fluid. Otolaryngol Head Neck Surg. 2011;144:101–3.
17. Purkey MT, Woodworth BA, Hahn S, Palmer JN, Chiu AG. Endoscopic repair of supraorbital ethmoid cerebrospinal fluid leaks. ORL J Otorhinolaryngol Relat Spec. 2009;71:93–8.
18. Woodworth BA, Schlosser RJ, Palmer JN. Endoscopic repair of frontal sinus cerebrospinal fluid leaks. J Laryngol Otol. 2005;119:709–13.
19. Illing EA, Woodworth BA. Management of Frontal Sinus Cerebrospinal Fluid Leaks and Encephaloceles. Otolaryngol Clin N Am. 2016;49:1035–50.
20. Kanowitz SJ, Batra PS, Citardi MJ. Comprehensive management of failed frontal sinus obliteration. Am J Rhinol. 2008;22:263–70.
21. Schlosser RJ, Bolger WE. Nasal cerebrospinal fluid leaks: critical review and surgical considerations. Laryngoscope. 2004;114:255–65.

22. Bernal-Sprekelsen M, Rioja E, Ensenat J, et al. Management of anterior skull base defect depending on its size and location. Biomed Res Int. 2014;2014:346873.

23. Ramakrishnan VR, Suh JD, Chiu AG, Palmer JN. Reliability of preoperative assessment of cerebrospinal fluid pressure in the management of spontaneous cerebrospinal fluid leaks and encephaloceles. Int Forum Allergy Rhinol. 2011;1:201–5.

24. Schlosser RJ, Wilensky EM, Grady MS, Palmer JN, Kennedy DW, Bolger WE. Cerebrospinal fluid pressure monitoring after repair of cerebrospinal fluid leaks. Otolaryngol Head Neck Surg. 2004;130:443–8.

25. Blount A, Riley K, Cure J, Woodworth BA. Cerebrospinal fluid volume replacement following large endoscopic anterior cranial base resection. Int Forum Allergy Rhinol. 2012;2:217–21.

Management of Frontal Sinus Trauma

15

Mohamad Raafat Chaaban
and Bradford A. Woodworth

Introduction

The frontal sinus is the last sinus to develop, becomes radiologically detectable at the age of 8, and reaches adult size by 15 years [1, 2]. The sinuses are bilateral but can be unilateral in 15% and absent in 8% of the population [3]. The floor of the frontal sinus forms the orbital roof, while the posterior wall of the sinus creates the anterior limit of the anterior cranial fossa. The frontal sinus drainage pathway (FSDP) has an hourglass shape with its recess located posteriorly and medially on the floor [4]. The anterior table is thicker and the stronger of the two walls of the frontal sinus.

Frontal sinus fractures account for 2–15% of all maxillofacial fractures [1, 5–7]. They most commonly occur as result of high-velocity motor vehicle accidents (MVAs) [8, 9]. The force required to break the frontal bone is 800–2200 pounds [10] which can be reached with a frontal collision at 30 mph [11] in an unrestrained passenger. Mandatory seat belt and airbag laws have

decreased the incidence of frontal sinus fractures secondary to MVAs; however, an increasing incidence is seen with low-velocity impacts such as sports injuries and assault [12]. These fractures are usually the result of blunt anterior facial trauma and are frequently associated with intracranial injuries and fractures of other maxillofacial bones [13].

Traditionally, frontal sinus fractures were classified into two categories – type 1, which includes fronto-orbital fractures that spare the posterior table, and type 2, which involves the anterior and posterior table. Unfortunately, this classification does not consider patients with isolated posterior table fractures; thus an anatomical classification that characterizes anterior and posterior table fractures with/without displacement and with/without frontal sinus outflow tract obstruction is more comprehensive. One third of frontal sinus fractures are isolated anterior table fractures, and two thirds are combined [14]. Combined fractures are almost invariably associated with injuries of the FSDP [12, 15, 16].

Despite being fairly uncommon, fractures of the frontal sinus can be very serious and inadequate, or delayed treatment may result in sequelae that range from aesthetic to life-threatening [17]. Importantly, the treatment paradigm for frontal sinus fractures has evolved over the past decade with a trend toward conservative management and preservation of the FSDP whenever possible.

M. R. Chaaban (✉)
Department of Otolaryngology, University of Texas
Medical Branch, Galveston, TX, USA

B. A. Woodworth
Department of Otolaryngology, University
of Alabama at Birmingham, Gregory Fleming James
Cystic Fibrosis Research Center,
Birmingham, AL, USA

© Springer Nature Switzerland AG 2019
D. Lal, P. H. Hwang (eds.), *Frontal Sinus Surgery*, https://doi.org/10.1007/978-3-319-97022-6_15

Initial Evaluation and Management

Initial evaluation should focus on standard trauma protocol starting with assessment of the airway, breathing, and circulation. When patients are stable, they are evaluated for signs and symptoms that are generally indicative of the extent of injury. For anterior table fractures, the most common signs include soft tissue swelling, forehead laceration, hypoesthesia, inability to lift the eyebrow, and contour irregularities. It is important to document on physical exam the status of the first branch of the trigeminal nerve and the temporal branch of the facial nerve. Extensive injuries involving the cribriform plate may lead to anosmia as a result of shearing injury to the olfactory nerves [18]. Fractures that involve the posterior table may be associated with CSF leak with or without exposure or herniation of intracranial contents [18]. Neurosurgical consultation is warranted in patients with suspected intracranial involvement.

Physical examination is limited when assessing the depth of involvement of frontal sinus fractures, so a high-resolution computed tomography (CT) scan is the gold standard evaluation. Sagittal and coronal reconstructions are particularly helpful in identifying involvement of the FSDP.

The main goals of management are to provide a safe sinus separated from the intracranial contents, restore form and aesthetics, and maintain the FSDP whenever possible. Because there is significant controversy in the management of these fractures, a wide spectrum of options is available ranging from observation for nondisplaced fractures to cranialization for comminuted posterior table fractures.

Observation

The decision on when to manage frontal sinus fractures expectantly depends on the degree of displacement, intracranial involvement, whether or not the FSDP is involved, and patient compliance. Generally, patients with isolated nondisplaced anterior table fractures and displaced anterior table fractures with no injury of the FSDP do not require surgical repair; however, surgery may be needed to restore form and cosmesis.

Traditionally, fractures involving the FSDP were treated with obliteration. However, some studies have shown that fractures involving the FSDP can be managed conservatively provided they are not part of a naso-orbito-ethmoid fracture (NOE) [19]. Patients with a fracture of the drainage pathway can be followed clinically and salvaged with a Draf II or III should symptoms and radiographic sinusitis develop [19]. Jafari et al. [20] showed that anterior and posterior table fractures involving the FSDP (including those associated with NOE fractures) may be managed expectantly without the need of obliteration in 88% of patients [21, 22]. The authors suggested that the main determinant of postoperative reventilation is the absence of medial orbital blowout fracture obstructing the FSDP rather than a mere fracture involving the frontal recess. Due to the lack of high-quality studies on this topic, management of these fractures remains controversial. Current guidelines for the management of posterior table fractures still advocate for cranialization and/or obliteration of the sinus to avoid potential complications such as CSF leaks, brain abscesses, or mucoceles [9, 22, 23]. For patients that are observed for opacified frontal sinuses, CT scan is recommended to check for adequate aeration of the sinuses 6 weeks to 3 months following the trauma.

Surgical Management

The surgical approach to maxillofacial trauma has evolved over the past several decades with the introduction of nasal endoscopes in the management of orbital blowout fractures, zygomaticomaxillary complex fractures, mandible condylar fractures, and frontal sinus fractures [24–31]. Surgical management of frontal sinus fractures ranges from repair of the anterior table to cranialization for posterior table fractures. The complications of the various procedures to address frontal sinus fractures are listed on Table 15.1. There are several considerations for the different approaches used in frontal sinus fractures (Table 15.2); however there are four main goals of surgical repair:

Table 15.1 Complications of frontal sinus fractures

Complications of frontal sinus fractures			
Sinonasal	Intracranial	Ophthalmological	Soft tissue/musculoskeletal
Mucocele	CSF leak	Blindness	Acute and chronic osteomyelitis
Pott's puffy	Meningoencephalocele	Enophthalmos/	Forehead numbness
tumor	Contusion	exophthalmos	Facial nerve injury (frontal branch of
	Pneumatocele	Ophthalmoplegia	facial nerve)
	Brain abscess		Aesthetic

Table 15.2 Advantages and disadvantages of different approaches to the frontal sinus

Surgical approach	Advantages	Disadvantages
External approach: Bitemporal/brow incisions approach with or without obliteration/cranialization	Direct visualization and proximity the fracture site, visualization of the frontal recess from above Ability to obliterate the frontal sinus (if needed)	Hair loss, scar, blood loss, increased length of hospital stay, temporal hallowing of scalp and forehead in bitemporal approach
Endoscopic-assisted external approach	Smaller incisions and dissections, improved visibility, avoid long scars, shorter hospital stay, shorter recovery period, enhanced resident education	Scar, requirement of endoscopic surgical equipment, steep learning curve, variable operative time (dependent on surgeon experience)
Percutaneous reduction without fixation (Anterior table only)	Minimal external trauma, quick	Edema at site of incision, may not have adequate reduction
Transnasal endoscopic approach	No external incision, avoids scar, improved visibility, shorter hospital stay, maintains frontal sinus patency, shorter recovery, enhanced resident education	Requires facile use of 70 degree endoscope and advanced expertise with endoscopic frontal sinus surgery

- Separating the sinuses from the intracranial contents with repair of the CSF leak (if present)
- Maintaining frontal sinus function (whenever possible)
- Avoiding long-term complications such as mucocele formation
- Restoring facial aesthetics

The traditional surgical approach the frontal sinus has been the bitemporal approach or forehead incisions that are used to access the fracture sites. Minimally invasive surgery is appealing to patients with better aesthetic results compared to traditional external approaches. In addition, advances in transnasal endoscopic surgery of the frontal recess [32] have resulted in viable alternative methods to preserve frontal sinus patency. Maintenance of sinus patency is possible in all fractures without significant intracranial injury.

Surgical management of frontal sinus fractures not only depends on the type of fracture (anterior, posterior, or combined) but also on the extent of injury and surgeon's experience. Traditional as well as transnasal endoscopic repair of frontal sinus fractures are discussed below.

Anterior Table Fractures

Traditional Management

Isolated anterior table fractures account for 33% of all frontal sinus fractures [33] and are usually the result of low-velocity injuries [33]. The management of these fractures primarily depends on the extent of injury, which is best assessed following resolution of the soft tissue swelling around 7–10 days from the time of initial insult. Nondisplaced fractures with no injury to the frontal recess do not require surgery as they are generally not associated with sinus mucosal entrapment or mucocele formation. Minimally displaced fractures that result in minor aesthetic abnormalities may only require injectable fillers, and mild or moderately displaced anterior table fractures can be addressed through an external incision.

Repair of displaced anterior table fractures depends on whether or not there is a preexisting forehead laceration. In the absence of a laceration, repair has been described utilizing small incisions or brow incisions with or without endoscopy [33, 34]. Contrary to the bi-coronal incision, these minimally invasive methods avoid the supratrochlear and supraorbital vasculature [35]. Simpler techniques such as applying percutaneous screws were also described to reduce fracture segments without fixation [36]. It has been suggested that the reduced bones are capable of producing an interlocking force between the irregular surfaces further stabilizing the segments [36]. A C-arm or endoscopy may be used to ensure proper fracture reduction since no direct visualization is possible with these small incisions. Chen [37] was the first to describe an endoscopic-assisted technique to repair displaced anterior table fractures, utilizing microplates and bony fragments as free grafts. Endoscopic-assisted approaches to the repair are now performed with either fracture reduction or camouflage. The former method involves actual reduction of the fracture with endoscopic brow lift incisions [30, 38, 39]. A scope is used to visualize the dissection that involves subperiosteal elevation carried down to the level of the fracture. Fixation screws are then applied through small incisions to aid in fracture reduction [33, 40]. In fracture camouflage, the fracture is not reduced, but a porous polyethylene implant is fixated with percutaneously inserted screws over the depressed bony segments. Proponents of minimal incisions without the use of endoscopes suggest that the use of scopes prolongs the surgical operating time [35].

Improved access to anterior table fractures can be through larger external incisions that can be used depending on the location of the fracture and the presence or absence of rhytids or receded hairline. These incisions include the bi-coronal incision, pretrichial, butterfly, and direct incisions. The bi-coronal incision provides the best exposure and access to the entire frontal sinus. The incision is placed 2 cm behind the hairline, and dissection is carried in the subgaleal plane up to the level of the supraorbital ridge. This approach carries risk of injury to the supratrochlear and supraorbital nerves [41]. The butterfly incision extends above the eyebrows on both sides and connects at the glabella. This approach is best suited for medial or low-lying anterior table fractures, with complications similar to the bitemporal approach including scarring and forehead numbness. The direct approach utilizes either a new incision or an existing laceration. This approach is best suited for bald patients or those with high receding hairlines. The bony segments that are encountered are generally reduced with miniplates, and bone grafting is reserved for defects greater than 1 cm [18].

The ideal approach for anterior table fracture depends on the surgeon's experience, extent of injury, and the presence of forehead lacerations that could be used for access to the fracture site. Closed reduction of anterior table fractures may result in improper reduction [42] requiring revision surgery. Although revision for failed closed repair of anterior table fractures may require refracturing, wide exposure, and possible grafting [37], camouflage techniques can usually obviate the need for extensive open reduction/internal fixation.

Transnasal Endoscopic Repair

Transnasal endoscopic reduction of anterior table fractures is a recently described technique that avoids using external incisions altogether and has the additional advantage of maintaining the FSDP (Fig. 15.1). In this approach, facile use of the 70° scope is critical for visualization and dissection of the frontal sinus since many fractures extend laterally [43]. Most transnasal reductions can be accomplished via a Draf IIb frontal sinusotomy on the side of the injury but can be extended to a Draf III if required for visualization or bilateral fractures. Timing of the repair within 10 days is crucial for anterior table fractures

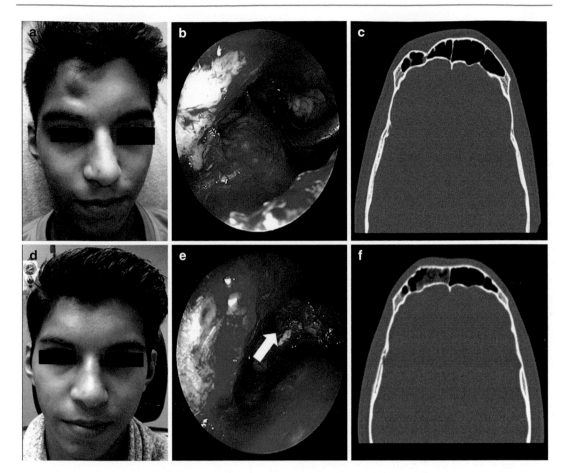

Fig. 15.1 A displaced anterior table fracture after blunt trauma causing a brow divot (**a**). The fracture is reduced using a frontal curette and a 70 degree endoscope after Draf IIb procedure (**b**). The displacement is seen best on axial CT scan (**c**). He had excellent cosmesis (**d**) following reduction (**e** – Arrow) with realignment of the segments on postoperative CT scan (**f**). (Copyright retained by Bradford A. Woodworth, MD)

since fibrosis and healing of the segments in their fractured position may be difficult to manually reduce after this time period. Even comminuted segments can be adequately reduced using this technique in combination with requisite internal support.

Posterior Table Fractures

Traditional Management

Due to the tightly adherent dura and mucosal invaginations in the posterior table, the potential for CSF leak and long-term complications with CSF leak and mucocele formation is high. In addition, fractures involving the posterior table may result in obstruction of the FSDP, orbital injury, and NOE fracture. Most authors have recommended cranialization and/or obliteration of the frontal sinus in patients with a blocked FSDP, CSF leak, or significantly displaced or comminuted fracture with loss of at least 25% of the posterior table [10, 33, 44, 45]. Similar to previous discussion regarding the anterior table, there has been a prominent shift in recommendations to more conservative routes of management, such as intervention only when CSF leak is present or posterior table displacement is severe.

Posterior table fractures are usually associated with anterior table fractures. When both of these fractures are present, the external approach via a bi-coronal incision allows for identification of the anterior table fracture segments allowing for an open reduction/internal fixation. For full exposure, outlining the extent of the frontal sinus preoperatively is an important step. This traditionally has been through the use of a 6-foot Caldwell film, but image guidance systems now provide an additional safety measure to avoid inadvertent entry into the intracranial cavity. A cutting burr or drill is then used to cut through the anterior table. The intersinus septum is removed, and full exposure of the posterior table is obtained. If obliteration is needed, the mucosa of the posterior table is removed under the microscope to ensure complete extirpation of the mucosa. If cranializing, the posterior table is removed along with the mucosa. Obliteration of the sinus has been described using abdominal fat, temporalis muscle, pericranial flap, or other materials such as hydroxyapatite, cartilage chips [45], or demineralized bone matrix [13]. We strongly recommend using the patient's own tissue rather than external substances such as hydroxyapatite or methyl methacrylate if obliteration is performed. The rate of mucocele formation is high with obliteration, and use of hard materials is a setup for infected foreign body material. An "unobliteration" Draf III procedure is also impossible in this setting. Following repair of the fracture, the anterior table or craniotomy flap is replaced and repaired with titanium plates [18, 41].

Transnasal Endoscopic Repair

The advantages of transnasal endoscopic repair include maintenance of the FSDP, a unique opportunity for postoperative surveillance, and lack of scar formation from external incisions. In addition, this technique can be utilized for revision surgeries where a previous open surgical procedure was performed with CSF leak recurrence. In those revision cases, this approach has the advantage of inspecting the entire skull base to assess the integrity of the pericranial flap or other dural repair. Transnasal endoscopic repair is useful only if the patient does not have a traumatic brain injury necessitating neurosurgical intervention, or if a preexisting large laceration overlies the fracture segment (favors direct external approach). This approach has been used for any posterior table fracture whether displaced or comminuted [32].

Additional preoperative counseling and written consent is required if the use of intrathecal fluorescein is considered. Fluorescein is widely utilized for intraoperative localization of dural defects with high sensitivity and specificity of 92.9% and 100%, respectively [46]. However, it is not Food and Drug Administration approved for intrathecal use and has rare but significant risk of neurotoxicity and seizures, although these risks are largely dose dependent and associated with rapid administration [47–51]. We use 0.1 cc of 10% preservative-free fluorescein diluted in 10 cc of the patient's own CSF or normal saline, injected over 10 min. Complications are limited with this technique.

Surgical exposure, usually Draf IIb or III, is influenced by the location of the fracture, degree of comminution, and frontal sinus anteroposterior (AP) diameter (Figs. 15.2, 15.3, and 15.4) [52]. When possible, mucosal grafts placed on the drilled anterior beak decrease long-term stenosis rates [43, 53, 54]. Sinus mucosa in and around the fracture line is removed either manually or with a coblator (Smith and Nephew, London, UK) [55–57], and the fracture segments either reduced or removed when severely comminuted. A porcine small intestinal submucosal graft (Biodesign®, Cook Biomedical, Bloomington, In) or other dural repair graft is placed in an underlay fashion when segments are removed rather than reduced [58]. An overlay graft or nasoseptal flap based on the posterior septal artery [59] may be used for coverage. A nasoseptal flap can reach unilateral defects up to 3 cm of posterior table [60]. In revision cases for failed cranialization or craniotomy when the frontal sinus was ablated, the pericranial flap is evaluated for any tears or defects and covered with an overlay graft. Following repair, silastic stents are placed in the frontal sinus and middle meatal spacers in the ethmoid cavity.

Postoperative Care

Patients should be monitored overnight in an ICU setting with frequent neurological checks following posterior table fracture repair. CSF leak repairs

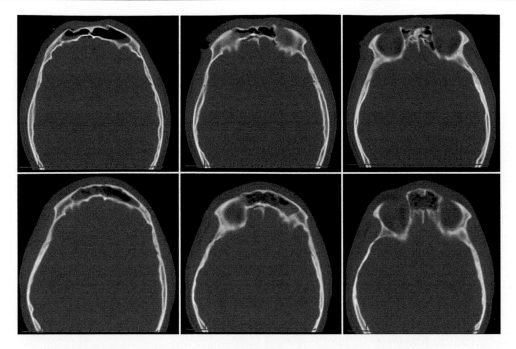

Fig. 15.2 Axial CT scans of a significantly comminuted crush fracture of the anterior and posterior table before (upper panel) and after (lower panel) reduction. (Copyright retained by Bradford A. Woodworth, MD)

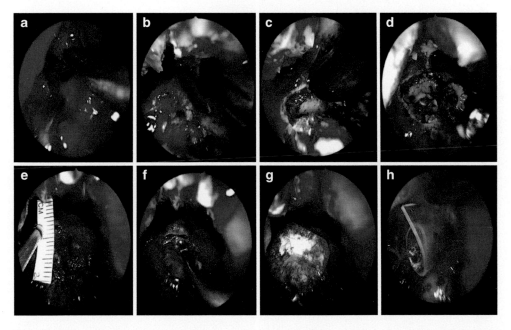

Fig. 15.3 Transnasal 70 degree endoscopic views of sequential surgical steps for the endoscopic repair in Fig. 15.4. After clearing the frontal recess bilaterally and performing upper septectomy, anterior table segments are gradually pushed anteriorly to accommodate exposure (**a**). The Draf III is completed to grant full access to the anterior and posterior tables (**b**). Mucosa is removed from within and around the comminuted posterior table fractures with a coblator (**c, d**). The posterior table fractures are measured in length and diameter (**e**). An underlay porcine SIS graft is placed (**f**) followed by overlay SIS graft (**g**). The entire frontal sinus is filled with gelfoam and silastic stents to support the grafts and the anterior table segments (**h**). (Copyright retained by Bradford A. Woodworth, MD)

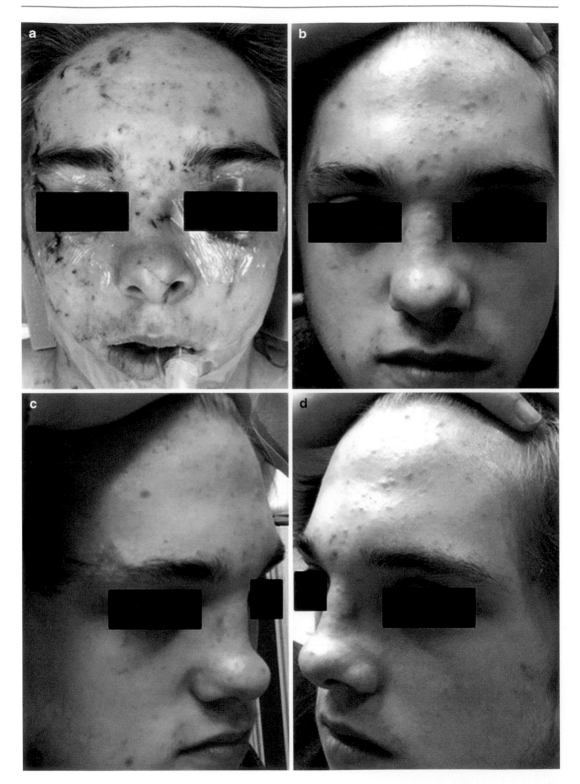

Fig. 15.4 Preoperative A-P view (**a**) demonstrates significant cosmetic deformity of the anterior table. Postoperative A-P (**b**) and oblique (**c** and **d**) views show complete correction of the large depression. (Copyright retained by Bradford A. Woodworth, MD)

are placed on IV ceftriaxone for 24 h and then converted to oral amoxicillin/clavulanate for 3 weeks postoperatively. Disruption of the FSDP is a very important factor for postoperative care and surveillance in patients with frontal sinus fractures. Rolled silastic stents are removed at the first postoperative debridement visit around 9–13 days. Further follow-up visits can be scheduled at 1–4-week intervals, and all patients are instructed to use saline irrigations. Patients are placed on stool softeners and told to avoid strenuous activity and Valsalva. Patients should be educated to recognize symptoms of new CSF leak, as many iatrogenic leaks have a delayed presentation.

Outcomes

The management of posterior table fractures has remained controversial due to the lack of large prospective studies examining the long-term effects of repair. Several complications of posterior table fractures may occur several years following repair making their evaluation with prospective studies difficult. Open reduction/internal fixation with either osteoplastic flap with obliteration or cranialization has traditionally been employed with the premise of preventing early and late complications from the injuries. However, many of the complications from open approaches are infectious or obstructive in nature resulting from the procedures intended to avoid them. Chronic headaches are present in over 50% of frontal sinus trauma patients and overall complication rates for open fracture repair range from 10% to 17% [61]. Sinus cranialization carries significant issues with cosmesis [62], resorption of autologous fat [21, 63], and reepithelialization in 50% of cases increasing risk of postoperative mucocele formation [64, 65]. Furthermore, obliteration has also been plagued with high failure rates and long-term risk of mucocele formation due to inadequate elimination of all mucosa within the ablated cavity. The true incidence of mucocele formation is grossly underestimated since a follow-up of 16 years was required to capture 50% of all post-traumatic mucoceles [66].

Minimally invasive surgery to repair anterior and posterior table fractures through a transnasal endoscopic approach requires careful patient selection, adequate instrumentation, and surgeon experience. The transnasal endoscopic approach to frontal sinus trauma allows for optimal assessment and repair of injuries with true preservation of functional sinus drainage. Steiger [29] was the first to describe the technique of the transnasal approach to the anterior table. In their series, they had five patients treated with four of them required trephination to access the laterally based fractures. Recently, we described completely transnasal endoscopic reduction through Draf IIb or III procedures for lateral and comminuted anterior table fractures with excellent cosmesis [67]. Likewise, transnasal endoscopic management of frontal sinus CSF leaks was first reported in 2006, [68] but advancements in surgical methods permitting closure of multi-centimeter defects of the posterior table of all etiologies were reported several years later [32, 69]. The senior author (BAW) recently reported outcomes on forty-six patients with frontal sinus trauma successfully managed using transnasal endoscopic techniques without major complications (brain abscess, meningitis, or mucoceles) and acceptable cosmesis [67]. The ability to address complicated posterior table fractures and dural lacerations is highlighted by a 0% leak recurrence rate in this study. Overall complication rate was low (4%) and well below the reported outcomes for both cranialization and obliteration of the frontal sinus (range of 6–71%) [5, 7, 21, 22, 44, 65, 70, 71]. Importantly, Draf IIb and III techniques have such high rates of success for maintaining a patent FSDP that the likelihood of frontal sinus closure long term is much lower than the risk of mucocele formation with open procedures [52, 72].

References

1. Kalavrezos N. Current trends in the management of frontal sinus fractures. Injury. 2004;35(4):340–6.
2. Yavuzer R, et al. Management of frontal sinus fractures. Plast Reconstr Surg. 2005;115(6):79e–93e. discussion 94e-95e

3. Danesh-Sani SA, Bavandi R, Esmaili M. Frontal sinus agenesis using computed tomography. J Craniofac Surg. 2011;22(6):e48–51.
4. Stammberger HR, Kennedy DW, G. Anatomic Terminology. Paranasal sinuses:anatomic terminology and nomenclature. Ann Otol Rhinol Laryngol Suppl. 1995;167:7–16.
5. Gerbino G, et al. Analysis of 158 frontal sinus fractures: current surgical management and complications. J Craniomaxillofac Surg. 2000;28(3):133–9.
6. Larrabee WF Jr, Travis LW, Tabb HG. Frontal sinus fractures--their suppurative complications and surgical management. Laryngoscope. 1980;90(11 Pt 1):1810–3.
7. Wilson BC, et al. Comparison of complications following frontal sinus fractures managed with exploration with or without obliteration over 10 years. Laryngoscope. 1988;98(5):516–20.
8. Manolidis S, Hollier LH Jr. Management of frontal sinus fractures. Plast Reconstr Surg. 2007;120(7 Suppl 2):32S–48S.
9. Metzinger SE, Guerra AB, Garcia RE. Frontal sinus fractures: management guidelines. Facial Plast Surg. 2005;21(3):199–206.
10. Lakhani RS, et al. Titanium mesh repair of the severely comminuted frontal sinus fracture. Arch Otolaryngol Head Neck Surg. 2001;127(6):665–9.
11. Nathum AM. The biomechanics of facial bone fracture. Laryngoscope. 1975;85:140.
12. Strong EB, Pahlavan N, Saito D. Frontal sinus fractures: a 28-year retrospective review. Otolaryngol Head Neck Surg. 2006;135(5):774–9.
13. Rodriguez IZ, et al. Posttraumatic frontal sinus obliteration with calvarial bone dust and demineralized bone matrix: a long term prospective study and literature review. Int J Oral Maxillofac Surg. 2013;42(1):71–6.
14. Sataloff RT, et al. Surgical management of the frontal sinus. Neurosurgery. 1984;15(4):593–6.
15. Piccolino P, et al. Frontal bone fractures: new technique of closed reduction. J Craniofac Surg. 2007;18(3):695–8.
16. Stanley RB Jr. Management of severe frontobasilar skull fractures. Otolaryngol Clin N Am. 1991;24(1):139–50.
17. Rohrich RJ, Hollier LH. Management of frontal sinus fractures. Changing concepts. Clin Plast Surg. 1992;19(1):219–32.
18. Enepekides D, Donald P. Frontal sinus trauma. In: Stewart M, editor. Head, face, and neck trauma: comprehensive management. New York: Thieme Medical Publishers; 2005. p. 26–39.
19. Smith TL, et al. Endoscopic management of the frontal recess in frontal sinus fractures: a shift in the paradigm? Laryngoscope. 2002;112(5):784–90.
20. Jafari A, et al. Spontaneous ventilation of the frontal sinus after fractures involving the frontal recess. Am J Otolaryngol. 2015;36(6):837–42.
21. Gonty AA, Marciani RD, Adornato DC. Management of frontal sinus fractures: a review of 33 cases. J Oral Maxillofac Surg. 1999;57(4):372–9. discussion 380-1

22. Gossman DG, Archer SM, Arosarena O. Management of frontal sinus fractures: a review of 96 cases. Laryngoscope. 2006;116(8):1357–62.
23. Carter KB Jr, Poetker DM, Rhee JS. Sinus preservation management for frontal sinus fractures in the endoscopic sinus surgery era: a systematic review. Craniomaxillofac Trauma Reconstr. 2010;3(3):141–9.
24. Farwell DG, Strong EB. Endoscopic repair of orbital floor fractures. Otolaryngol Clin N Am. 2007;40(2):319–28.
25. Kellman RM, Cienfuegos R. Endoscopic approaches to subcondylar fractures of the mandible. Facial Plast Surg. 2009;25(1):23–8.
26. Kim KK, et al. Endoscopic repair of anterior table: frontal sinus fractures with a Medpor implant. Otolaryngol Head Neck Surg. 2007;136(4):568–72.
27. Lee CH, et al. A cadaveric and clinical evaluation of endoscopically assisted zygomatic fracture repair. Plast Reconstr Surg. 1998;101(2):333–45. discussion 346-7
28. Pham AM, Strong EB. Endoscopic management of facial fractures. Curr Opin Otolaryngol Head Neck Surg. 2006;14(4):234–41.
29. Steiger JD, et al. Endoscopic-assisted reduction of anterior table frontal sinus fractures. Laryngoscope. 2006;116(10):1936–9.
30. Strong EB. Endoscopic repair of anterior table frontal sinus fractures. Facial Plast Surg. 2009;25(1):43–8.
31. Strong EB, Kim KK, Diaz RC. Endoscopic approach to orbital blowout fracture repair. Otolaryngol Head Neck Surg. 2004;131(5):683–95.
32. Chaaban MR, et al. Transnasal endoscopic repair of posterior table fractures. Otolaryngol Head Neck Surg. 2012;147(6):1142–7.
33. Lappert PW, Lee JW. Treatment of an isolated outer table frontal sinus fracture using endoscopic reduction and fixation. Plast Reconstr Surg. 1998;102(5):1642–5.
34. Chen DJ, et al. Endoscopically assisted repair of frontal sinus fracture. J Trauma. 2003;55(2):378–82.
35. Kim NH, Kang SJ. A simple aesthetic approach for correction of frontal sinus fracture. J Craniofac Surg. 2014;25(2):544–6.
36. Mavili ME, Canter HI. Closed treatment of frontal sinus fracture with percutaneous screw reduction. J Craniofac Surg. 2007;18(2):415–9.
37. Chen RF, et al. Optimizing closed reduction of nasal and zygomatic arch fractures with a mobile fluoroscan. Plast Reconstr Surg. 2010;126(2):554–63.
38. Forrest CR. Application of minimal-access techniques in lag screw fixation of fractures of the anterior mandible. Plast Reconstr Surg. 1999;104(7):2127–34.
39. Shumrick KA. Endoscopic management of frontal sinus fractures. Facial Plast Surg Clin North Am. 2006;14(1):31–5.
40. Graham HD, Spring P. Endoscopic repair of frontal sinus fracture: case report. J Craniomaxillofac Trauma. 1996;2(4):52–5.
41. Rice DH. Management of frontal sinus fractures. Curr Opin Otolaryngol Head Neck Surg. 2004;12(1):46–8.

42. Verwoerd CD. Present day treatment of nasal fractures: closed versus open reduction. Facial Plast Surg. 1992;8(4):220–3.
43. Conger BT, Riley KO, Woodworth BW. The Draf III mucosal grafting technique: a prospective study. Otolaryngol Head Neck Surg. 2010;146(4):664–8.
44. Chen KT, et al. Frontal sinus fractures: a treatment algorithm and assessment of outcomes based on 78 clinical cases. Plast Reconstr Surg. 2006;118(2):457–68.
45. Sailer HF, Gratz KW, Kalavrezos ND. Frontal sinus fractures: principles of treatment and long-term results after sinus obliteration with the use of lyophilized cartilage. J Craniomaxillofac Surg. 1998;26(4):235–42.
46. Raza SM, et al. Sensitivity and specificity of intrathecal fluorescein and white light excitation for detecting intraoperative cerebrospinal fluid leak in endoscopic skull base surgery: a prospective study. J Neurosurg. 2016;124(3):621–6.
47. Guimaraes RE, et al. Chemical and cytological analysis of cerebral spinal fluid after intrathecal injection of hypodense fluorescein. Braz J Otorhinolaryngol. 2015;81(5):549–53.
48. Placantonakis DG, et al. Safety of low-dose intrathecal fluorescein in endoscopic cranial base surgery. Neurosurgery. 2007;61(3 Suppl):161–5. discussion 165-6
49. Tabaee A, et al. Intrathecal fluorescein in endoscopic skull base surgery. Otolaryngol Head Neck Surg. 2007;137(2):316–20.
50. Seth R, et al. The utility of intrathecal fluorescein in cerebrospinal fluid leak repair. Otolaryngol Head Neck Surg. 2010;143(5):626–32.
51. Banu MA, et al. Low-dose intrathecal fluorescein and etiology-based graft choice in endoscopic endonasal closure of CSF leaks. Clin Neurol Neurosurg. 2014;116:28–34.
52. Illing EA, Woodworth BA. Management of Frontal Sinus Cerebrospinal Fluid Leaks and Encephaloceles. Otolaryngol Clin N Am. 2016;49(4):1035–50.
53. Alexander NS, et al. Treatment strategies for lateral sphenoid sinus recess cerebrospinal fluid leaks. Arch Otolaryngol Head Neck Surg. 2012;138(5):471–8.
54. Illing EA, et al. Draf III mucosal graft technique: long-term results. Int Forum Allergy Rhinol. 2016;6(5):514–7.
55. Kostrzewa JP, et al. Radiofrequency coblation decreases blood loss during endoscopic sinonasal and skull base tumor removal. ORL J Otorhinolaryngol Relat Spec. 2010;72(1):38–43.
56. Smith N, Riley KO, Woodworth BA. Endoscopic Coblator-assisted management of encephaloceles. Laryngoscope. 2010;120(12):2535–9.
57. Virgin FW, Bleier BS, Woodworth BA. Evolving materials and techniques for endoscopic sinus surgery. Otolaryngol Clin N Am. 2010;43(3):653–72. xi

58. Illing E, et al. Porcine small intestine submucosal graft for endoscopic skull base reconstruction. Int Forum Allergy Rhinol. 2013;3(11):928–32.
59. Hadad G, et al. A novel reconstructive technique after endoscopic expanded endonasal approaches: vascular pedicle nasoseptal flap. Laryngoscope. 2006;116(10):1882–6.
60. Virgin F, et al. Frontal sinus skull base defect repair using the pedicled nasoseptal flap. Otolaryngol Head Neck Surg. 2011;145(2):338–40.
61. Adelson RT, Wei C, Palmer JN. Frontal sinus fractures. In: Palmer JN, Chiu AG, Adappa ND, editors. Atlas of endoscopic and Sinonasal skull base surgery. Pennsylvania: Elsevier; 2013. p. 337–56.
62. Emara TA, et al. Frontal sinus fractures with suspected outflow tract obstruction: a new approach for sinus preservation. J Craniomaxillofac Surg. 2015;43(1):1–6.
63. Dolan RW. Facial plastic, reconstructive, and trauma surgery. New York: Marcel Dekker; 2004.
64. Poetker DM, Smith TL. Endoscopic treatment of the frontal sinus outflow tract in frontal sinus trauma. Oper Tech Otolaryngol Head Neck Surg. 2006;17(1):66–72.
65. Rodriguez ED, et al. Twenty-six year experience treating frontal sinus fractures: a novel algorithm based upon anatomical fracture pattern and failure of conventional techniques. Plast Reconstr Surg. 2008;122(6):1850–66.
66. Koudstaal MJ, et al. Post-trauma mucocele formation in the frontal sinus; a rationale of follow-up. Int J Oral Maxillofac Surg. 2004;33(8):751–64.
67. Jessica W, Grayson M, Jeyarajan H, Illing EA, Cho D-Y, Riley KO, Woodworth BA. Changing the surgical dogma in frontal sinus trauma: Transnasal endoscopic repair. Int Forum Allergy Rhinol. 2017;7:441.
68. Woodworth BA, Schlosser RJ, Palmer JN. Endoscopic repair of frontal sinus cerebrospinal fluid leaks. J Laryngol Otol. 2005;119(09):709–13.
69. Jones V, et al. Changing paradigms in frontal sinus cerebrospinal fluid leak repair. Int Forum Allergy Rhinol. 2012;2(3):227–32.
70. Pollock RA, et al. Cranialization in a cohort of 154 consecutive patients with frontal sinus fractures (1987-2007): review and update of a compelling procedure in the selected patient. Ann Plast Surg. 2013;71(1):54–9.
71. Bell RB, et al. A protocol for the management of frontal sinus fractures emphasizing sinus preservation. J Oral Maxillofac Surg. 2007;65(5):825–39.
72. Conger BT, et al. Management of lateral frontal sinus pathology in the endoscopic era. Otolaryngol Head Neck Surg. 2014;15(1):159–63.

Fibro-osseous Lesions of the Frontal Sinus

16

Ben McArdle, Dongho Shin, and Ian Witterick

Osteoma

Osteoma is the most common fibro-osseous lesion encountered in the frontal sinus and its drainage pathway. It was first described by Veiga in 1506, whereas Vallisnieri was credited with detailing their bony origin [1]. Osteomas have been found in 1% of frontal sinus radiographs in symptomatic individuals (Fig. 16.1) [2]. Osteomas present typically in the third and fourth decades of life and have a slight male preponderance. Symptoms on presentation may include headache, pain over the frontal sinus, and infection but often are found incidentally on imaging. Complications, or late presentation, may include cosmetic deformity, visual disturbances, CSF leak, meningitis, seizure, and potentially death. Infection penetrating through the bone anteriorly may also present with Pott's puffy tumor.

While most frontal sinus osteomas are unifocal, the presence of multiple osteomas should lead the clinician to consider Gardner's syndrome (familial colorectal polyposis). This autosomal dominant condition is significant due to the high rate of malignant degeneration of associated colonic polyps, with an increased risk of thyroid cancers, desmoid tumors, fibromas, and dermoid cysts.

Osteomas typically have a slow pattern of growth and may not change in size over the course of a patient's life [3]. Others may grow rapidly and therefore require surveillance in all patients that present with frontal sinus osteoma.

There are multiple hypotheses as to the origin of osteomas. The developmental theory proposes that osteomas tend to arise in areas of fusion between tissues of varying embryologic origin such as the membranous frontal bone and cartilaginous ethmoid bone [4]. This is unsatisfying as many paranasal osteomas arise at sites distant from these junctions. The traumatic theory and the infectious theory both cite an inflammatory process as the inciting force for bony tumor formation. It is, however, difficult to determine if the osteoma or the infection is the primary process, as tumor and infection frequently coexist at the time of diagnosis. The presence of head trauma is almost universal to the human condition, to varying degrees. However, the type of bone in an osteoma differs significantly from the bony hyperplasia expected to characterize reactive osteitis [4].

B. McArdle
Department of Otolaryngology, Sunshine Coast University Hospital, Birtinya, Qld, Australia

D. Shin
University of Toronto, Faculty of Medicine, Toronto, ON, Canada

I. Witterick (✉)
Department of Otolaryngology – Head and Neck Surgery, University of Toronto, Sinai Health System, Toronto, ON, Canada

© Springer Nature Switzerland AG 2019
D. Lal, P. H. Hwang (eds.), *Frontal Sinus Surgery*, https://doi.org/10.1007/978-3-319-97022-6_16

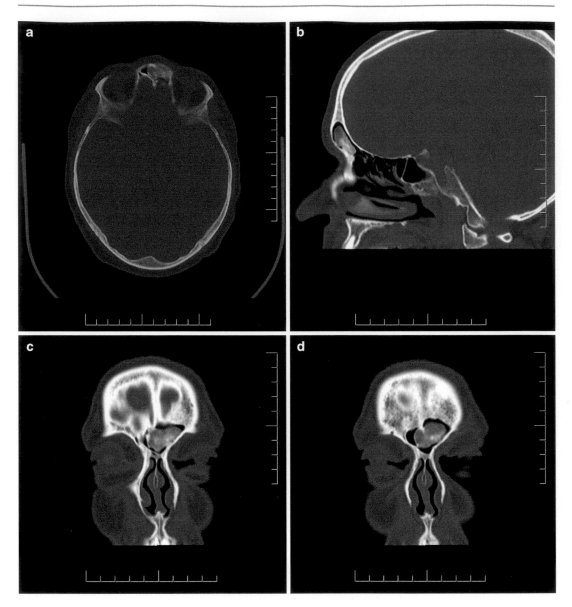

Fig. 16.1 CT sinus scans of (**a**) axial, (**b**) sagittal, and (**c**) and (**d**) coronal views showing osteoma in the left frontal sinus

Ossifying Fibroma

OF is a rare benign fibro-osseous lesion which was first described by Menzel in 1872. First considered a type of osteoma, the term of "ossifying fibroma" was subsequently coined by Montgomery in 1927 [5]. The bone most commonly associated in the head and neck is the mandible, but it can also occur in the paranasal

sinuses including the frontal sinus. In the head and neck, the lesions arise in the mandible in about 62–89% of patients, followed by the maxilla and rarely the orbit, skull base, and calvarium. Women are affected more often than men with a female to male ratio of 2:1.9. Ossifying fibroma of the sinonasal tract occurs at a slightly older age (third to fourth decade of life) and preferentially in black women. There is no evidence of hereditary predominance [5–7]. There is an extremely rare but reported potential for malignant transformation.

While many and sometimes overlapping terms are used to describe OF, including cementifying fibroma, cemento-ossifying fibroma, desmo-osteoblastoma, psammo-osteoid fibroma, psammomatoid ossifying fibroma, juvenile ossifying fibroma, juvenile aggressive ossifying fibroma, or juvenile active ossifying fibroma, it is reasonable from a clinical point of view to divide OF into cemento-ossifying fibroma (COF) and juvenile ossifying fibroma (JOF) [8]. COFs tend to occur in the mandibulo-odontal region in children and respond well to surgery with limited recurrence [9]. JOFs are more common in the paranasal sinus region and often have a more aggressive course with potential for local destruction and complications [10].

Symptoms tend to be similar to those of other fibro-osseous lesions and are related to mass effect, which includes headache, epiphora, proptosis, and blockage of the frontal drainage pathway. OFs manifest typically as painless, slow-growing tumors, but extra-mandibular lesions such as those occurring in the paranasal sinuses and midface tend to display more aggressive behavior and rapid growth [5]. Significant growth and local tissue destruction can mimic FD radiologically and histologically. The primary distinction between OF and FD in regard to histology is the presence of lamellar bone and peripheral osteoblasts in OF and the absence of both in FD [11]. Grossly, an ossifying fibroma is most often grayish-white in color, dry, avascular, and either crumbly, cheesy, or gritty. It has definite boundaries but is not truly encapsulated [12].

Radiologically, OF appears as a well-circumscribed expansile mass with variable bony density in a bony shell. Indeed, this sharply demarcated bony shell is considered the most important radiological sign for distinguishing it from FD, where there is merging of diseased bone with healthy bone [11]. Histologically, OF characteristically shows osteoblastic rimming of the trabeculae, monomorphic stroma with high cell density and sparse collagen fibers [13].

OFs manifest typically as painless slow-growing tumors, but extra-mandibular lesions such as those that occur in the paranasal sinuses and midface tend to display more aggressive behavior and rapid growth [9]. Radical resection of paranasal ossifying fibromas is widely considered the treatment of choice due to their locally aggressive behavior [8]. Endoscopic approaches are viable in some settings [14]. However, the otolaryngologist must be prepared for an open or endoscopic approach depending on the individual characteristics of the patient and pathology concerned. Radiotherapy is ineffective for dealing with OF and may result in malignant transformation [15]. Due to the relatively common rate of recurrence, close follow-up and long-term surveillance is recommended after surgical resection [16].

Fibrous Dysplasia

FD is an uncommon disease of the bone that has a rare but clear potential for malignant transformation [17, 18]. It is typically a benign, idiopathic, slowly progressive lesion where normal bone is replaced by fibrous tissue and immature woven bone [19].

FD exists in monostotic (70–75%) and polyostotic (25–30%) forms, with the monostotic form being more common in the craniofacial bones, ribs, femurs, tibias, and humeri and the polyostotic form more common in the femur, tibia, skull and facial bones, pelvis, rib, humerus, radius and ulna, lumbar spine, clavicle, and cervical spine [18]. Patients with paranasal sinus disease usually present with painless swelling and/or facial deformity, usually by the age of 30. The underlying genetic cause is due to a subunit of G-protein receptors, found on chromosome 20 (20q13). Patients with the monostotic form are frequently asymptomatic and are often diagnosed incidentally during radiographic evaluation for another purpose. Conversely, patients with the polyostotic form have early manifestations including bone pain and/or bone deformity [20]. FD may be associated with other syndromes such as McCune–Albright (precocious puberty, FD and cutaneous pigmentation-café au lait spots) [21]. The risk of malignant transformation for monostotic FD is 0.5%, whereas it is up to 4% for polyostotic disease [22].

Histologically, fibrous dysplasia is composed of highly cellular fibrous tissue with uniform spindle-shaped fibroblasts. Irregular trabeculae of woven bone without lamellar bone or osteoblastic rimming may also be found [23].

CT scanning shows normal bone to be replaced with a more radiolucent, "ground-glass" appearing pattern, with no visible trabecular pattern (Fig. 16.2) [16]. There may be endosteal scalloping of the inner cortex, but the periosteal surface is smooth and nonreactive. On MRI, FD has intermediate signal on T1 and hypointense signal on T2. FD is usually much more irregular or ill-defined on imaging than both osteoma and OF.

FD has an irregular growth pattern and is thought to be active during adolescence and pregnancy, intimating a hormonal association [24]. FD may also stabilize over time, and given this tendency and the overall low risk of malignant transformation, lesions that are asymptomatic may be observed with both clinical and radiological monitoring [25]. Symptomatic, disfiguring, or suspicious lesions may be treated, however the exact approach (open vs endoscopic), and extent of resection depends on individual characteristics of the patient and the disease. Efforts should be made to decompress any affected structures and/ or to restore cosmesis as best as possible. Often, complete resection of these lesions is difficult due to the lack of defined borders of the lesion itself, with added desire to avoid damage to major structures. For these reasons, FD has a relatively high recurrence rate, and it must be monitored closely postoperatively [10].

Investigations/Workup

Patients presenting with symptoms of chronic or recurrent sinusitis should always undergo full history, thorough head and neck examination, and nasal endoscopy. While symptomatology in the paranasal sinuses can be quite diverse and vague, any history of frontal headaches, visual changes, cosmetic changes, or meningitis should lead the judicious physician to entertain the possibility of frontal sinus pathology.

High-resolution computed tomography (CT) is the most useful first-line imaging for conditions of the paranasal sinuses [26]. CT imaging allows for visualization of bony structures of the paranasal sinuses, the skull base, the orbit, and all of the vital structures of the surrounding area. Opacification, hyperostosis, bony dehiscence, and the majority of pathology will be seen on CT imaging. If doubt arises to the underlying pathology, then magnetic

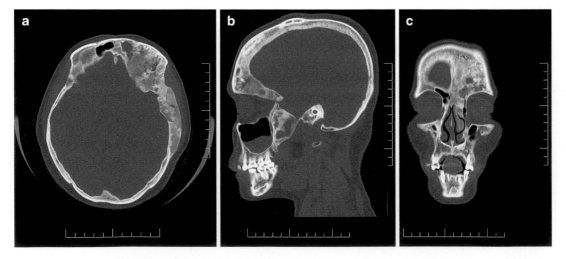

Fig. 16.2 CT sinus scans (**a**) axial, (**b**) sagittal, and (**c**) coronal views showing ground-glass pattern, indicative of fibrous dysplasia in the left frontal sinus and the lateral skull

resonance imaging (MRI) is also useful in delineating fungal debris versus retained secretions, as well as evaluating for intracerebral or other soft tissue complications.

Baseline imaging is also useful in the context of watchful waiting. Serial imaging allows the physician to monitor any change in size of a lesion and permits early intervention to remove any lesion that is growing and likely to cause complications before they happen [10].

Imaging benefits the physician by permitting the planning of any surgical intervention and anticipating any preexisting or likely complications of any surgery and planning for those eventualities. In the modern era, the use of image guidance CT and/or MRI may almost be considered mandatory for treating complicated frontal sinus disease.

Management

Management of frontal sinus tumors now encompasses an endonasal endoscopic approach in addition to the open approaches. Although the open approaches – including trephination, Lynch procedure, and osteoplastic flaps with or without sinus obliteration – used to be the gold standards for surgical management, an endoscopic technique and/or a combination approach is being utilized much more commonly to address different situations [27, 28]. Since most fibro-osseous lesions in the frontal sinus are benign, slow-growing, and asymptomatic, watchful waiting is also a reasonable option with regular imaging to monitor the growth of the lesion (Table 16.1) [29–31].

It is unclear why patients with fibro-osseous lesions have chronic rhinosinusitis-like symptoms such as frontal headache, nasal obstruction, pain, and pressure. In fact, there are questions as to whether the fibro-osseous lesion itself causes symptoms or if the symptoms are due to secondary sinusitis from the obstruction of the sinus drainage pathway [3]. Ooi et al. showed that 27/30 (90%) patients with fibro-osseous lesion remained asymptomatic or had improvements in their symptoms when managed conservatively with serial imaging and medical treatment (saline

Table 16.1 Management consideration for fibro-osseous lesions

Osteoma	Ossifying fibroma	Fibrous dysplasia
Watchful waiting with imaging is recommended for small, asymptomatic lesions. Surgery should be considered for tumors with rapid growth (>1 mm/yr), large tumors that occupy >50% of the frontal sinus, intracranial or intraorbital extension, symptomatic tumors (e.g., chronic rhinosinusitis), and complications (tumor obstruction, headaches, and facial deformity) [30].	Treatment is dependent on the location of the tumor. Observation is recommended for asymptomatic mandible lesions. Surgical resection is recommended for tumors invading midfacial portion and the sinonasal tract, which tend to be more aggressive and have a high chance of recurrence [32].	Patients with monostotic fibrous dysplasia are usually asymptomatic and can be followed with regular imaging [32]. Bisphosphonates have been shown to reduce fractures and bone pain [33]. Octreotide can also be helpful for McCune-Albright syndrome [32]. Surgical resection & recommended based on symptoms, extent of disease, and age [32]. Endonasal endoscopic treatment can be used to decompress optic nerve(s) or for chronic rhinosinusitis [32].

douching, topical and/or systemic corticosteroids, and culture-directed antibiotics as indicated) or with endoscopic sinus surgery without resecting the bony abnormality [3]. Patients with minimal symptoms were followed with serial imaging, and only 2/36 (5.5%) cases showed evidence of interval growth [3]. These results support that the symptoms are due to the obstruction of the sinus pathways and that avoiding major resections of the lesions in patients with minimal symptoms and/or without complications may be beneficial.

Conservative therapy should involve serial imaging to observe potential growth of the lesions. Our patients are observed using annual CT scans for the first 2 years after the diagnosis. If the lesion was stable, then scans were performed at biannual intervals. If they continue to be stable, MRI imaging is preferred for long-term follow-up, if there are no contraindications to this method. This will remove radiation and potential harm to the patients that is present with CT.

Regardless of the type of fibro-osseous lesion, nasal endoscopy and CT are essential in preoperative planning and the management plan. The size of tumor, its location, and attachment site should be considered for operative planning as well [28]. Some features that may be contraindications for an endoscopic approach include anterior-posterior dimension of the frontal and posterior tables <10 mm, increased convexity of the posterior wall of the frontal sinus, large tumor occupying more than 75% of the frontal sinus, tumor located laterally and behind the virtual plane of the lamina papyracea, previous meningitis or CSF leak, extensive intracranial extension, and significant supraorbital component with lateral orbital mucoceles [29, 34]. In the case of uncertainty from radiological and endoscopic evidence, a biopsy or excision may be required to confirm the diagnosis (Fig. 16.3) [3].

Surgical management should be considered when the lesions are large and symptomatic, or causing complications such as obstruction, and intracranial extension (Fig. 16.4) [28–30]. Chiu et al.'s frontal sinus osteoma grading system helps to guide the management plan [35]. It considers the location of the tumor attachment, anterior-posterior dimension of the lesion, and tumor location relative to the virtual sagittal plane through the lamina papyracea [35]. An endoscopic approach is recommended for grade II or lower, and an open surgical or combination approach is recommended for grade III/IV [35]. Ledderose et al. and Rokade and Sama have shown that some patients with grade III/IV can be operated on completely using an endoscopic approach alone with Draf III, although some still required a combination approach [29, 36]. An osteoplastic flap approach is helpful for many fibro-osseous lesions that are large and that extend laterally into the superior orbit or extend intracranially (Fig. 16.5). Intraoperative navigation has shown to improve the endoscopic approach as well [36].

Recurrence of fibro-osseous lesions is uncommon, but postoperative follow-up should still be recommended [27]. Patients are hospitalized for an average of 9.2 days following open approaches and 5.3 days for endoscopic

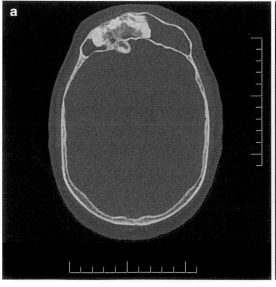 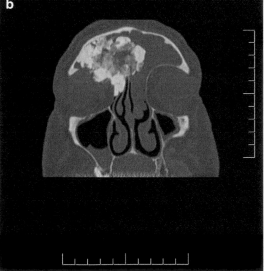

Fig. 16.3 A case of fibro-osseous lesion where radiological diagnosis was uncertain, thus requiring a biopsy. Images (**a** and **b**) show preoperative CT sinus scans in axial and coronal views. The lesion was diagnosed as an osteosarcoma

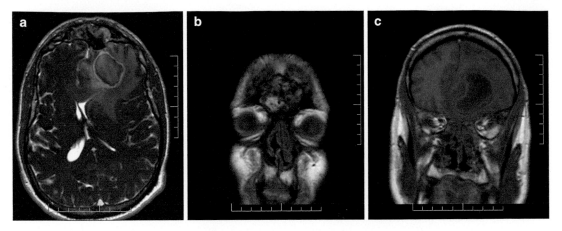

Fig. 16.4 MRI scan (**a**) axial and (**b**) and (**c**) coronal views of osteoma with intracranial abscess, invading into the brain, causing mass effect

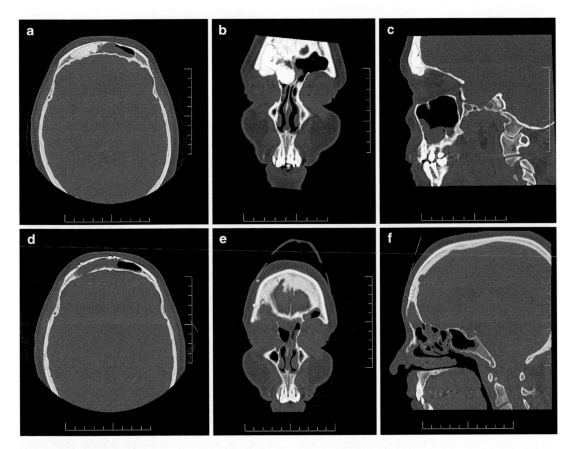

Fig. 16.5 Preoperative (**a–c**) and postoperative (**d–f**) CT sinus scans of treated osteoma in the right frontal sinus. Images showing the removed osteoma in axial (**a** and **d**), sagittal (**b** and **e**), and coronal (**c** and **f**) views

approaches [36]. Postoperative oral antibiotics should be given at the surgeon's discretion and saline irrigation conducted 4–6 times a day. A follow-up endoscopic exam should be done 7–14 days postoperatively to remove crusts and adhesions. Depending on the findings, healing, and surgeon preference, subsequent follow-up should be scheduled at appropriate intervals [37].

Complications of Management

Several key structures must be identified during the surgical procedure to prevent complications [28]:

1. Orbit – prevent injury to the eye, the optic nerve, or the extraocular muscles.
2. Anterior ethmoidal artery – prevent intranasal or intraorbital bleeding which can progress into a retro-orbital hematoma.
3. Skull base – prevent CSF leak and life-threatening central nervous system infection.

The Draf III procedure may stenose postoperatively. Conger et al. have shown that a mucosal graft placed over the exposed anterior and lateral bone may help prevent or minimize the stenosis [37, 38]. Although endoscopic surgery reduces hospital stay and morbidity, complete resection of margins may sometimes prove to be difficult. On the other hand, open surgeries such as osteoplastic flap are associated with cosmetic deformities, dural injury, CSF leakage, forehead numbness, damage to the frontal branch of the facial nerve, orbital or intracranial injury, and headache [39]. However, external surgery provides greater access and is the preferred surgical option for grade III/IV fibro-osseous lesions.

Summary

Fibro-osseous lesions are the most common benign bony abnormalities encountered in the frontal sinus and its drainage pathway. They are often asymptomatic and are identified incidentally on imaging.

The most common is osteoma, followed by ossifying fibroma and fibrous dysplasia.

Patients presenting with symptoms of chronic or recurrent sinusitis should undergo full history, thorough head and neck examination, and nasal endoscopy. CT is the most useful first-line imaging for conditions of the paranasal sinuses.

Asymptomatic lesions should be followed with serial imaging.

Symptomatic and large lesions with complications should be removed surgically. There are three main approaches: open, endoscopic, or combined endoscopic-open.

Disclosure Ian Witterick – Shareholder of Proteocyte Diagnostics Inc.

References

1. Broniatowski M. Osteomas of the frontal sinus. Ear Nose Throat J. 1984;63:267–71.
2. Mehta BS, Grewal GS. Osteoma of the Paranasal Sinuses Along with a Case Report of an Orbito-Ethmoidal Osteoma. J Laryngol Otol. 1963;77:601–10.
3. Ooi EH, Glicksman JT, Vescan AD, Witterick IJ. An alternative management approach to paranasal sinus fibro-osseous lesions. Int Forum Allergy Rhinol. 2011;1:55–63. https://doi.org/10.1002/alr.20004.
4. Kenneth Rodriguez MT, Brent A. Senior. In: The Frontal Sinus Ch. 36. Berlin/Heidelberg: Springer; 2016. p. 495–507.
5. Mohsenifar Z, Nouhi S, Abbas FM, Farhadi S, Abedin B. Ossifying fibroma of the ethmoid sinus: report of a rare case and review of literature. J Res Med Sci. 2011;16:841–7.
6. Sciubba JJ, Younai F. Ossifying fibroma of the mandible and maxilla: review of 18 cases. J Oral Pathol Med. 1989;18:315–21.
7. Saito K, Fukuta K, Takahashi M, Seki Y, Yoshida J. Benign fibroosseous lesions involving the skull base, paranasal sinuses, and nasal cavity. Report of two cases. J Neurosurg. 1998;88:1116–9. https://doi.org/10.3171/jns.1998.88.6.1116.
8. Ledderose GJ, Stelter K, Becker S, Leunig A. Paranasal ossifying fibroma: endoscopic resection or wait and scan? Eur Arch Otorhinolaryngol. 2011;268:999–1004. https://doi.org/10.1007/s00405-011-1503-4.
9. London SD, Schlosser RJ, Gross CW. Endoscopic management of benign sinonasal tumors: a decade of experience. Am J Rhinol. 2002;16:221–7.
10. Eller R, Sillers M. Common fibro-osseous lesions of the paranasal sinuses. Otolaryngol Clin North Am. 2006;39:585–600. https://doi.org/10.1016/j.otc.2006.01.013.
11. Post G, Kountakis SE. Endoscopic resection of large sinonasal ossifying fibroma. Am J Otolaryngol. 2005;26:54–6.

12. Thomas GK, Kasper KA. Ossifying fibroma of the frontal bone. Arch Otolaryngol. 1966;83:43–6.

13. Wenig BM, et al. Aggressive psammomatoid ossifying fibromas of the sinonasal region: a clinicopathologic study of a distinct group of fibro-osseous lesions. Cancer. 1995;76:1155–65.

14. Wang H, Sun X, Liu Q, Wang J, Wang D. Endoscopic resection of sinonasal ossifying fibroma: 31 cases report at an institution. Eur Arch Otorhinolaryngol. 2014;271:2975–82. https://doi.org/10.1007/s00405-014-2972-z.

15. Bertrand B, et al. Juvenile aggressive cemento-ossifying fibroma: case report and review of the literature. Laryngoscope. 1993;103:1385–90. https://doi.org/10.1288/00005537-199,312,000-00013.

16. MacDonald-Jankowski DS. Fibro-osseous lesions of the face and jaws. Clin Radiol. 2004;59:11–25.

17. Ruggieri P, Sim FH, Bond JR, Unni KK. Malignancies in fibrous dysplasia. Cancer. 1994;73:1411–24.

18. Riddle ND, Bui MM. Fibrous dysplasia. Arch Pathol Lab Med. 2013;137:134–8. https://doi.org/10.5858/arpa.2012.0013-RS.

19. Commins DJ, Tolley NS, Milford CA. Fibrous dysplasia and ossifying fibroma of the paranasal sinuses. J Laryngol Otol. 1998;112:964–8.

20. Rojas R, Palacios E, Kaplan J, Wong LK. Fibrous dysplasia of the frontal sinus. Ear Nose Throat J. 2004;83:14–5.

21. Derham C, Bucur S, Russell J, Liddington M, Chumas P. Frontal sinus mucocele in association with fibrous dysplasia: review and report of two cases. Childs Nerv Syst. 2011;27:327–31. https://doi.org/10.1007/s00381-010-1266-z.

22. Mohammadi-Araghi H, Haery C. Fibro-osseous lesions of craniofacial bones. The role of imaging. Radiol Clin North Am. 1993;31:121–34.

23. Senior BA, Dubin MG. In: The Frontal Sinus Ch. 18. Berlin/Heidelberg: Springer; 2005. p. 153–64.

24. Stevens-Simon C, Stewart J, Nakashima II, White M. Exacerbation of fibrous dysplasia associated with an adolescent pregnancy. J Adolesc Health. 1991;12:403–5.

25. Charlett SD, Mackay SG, Sacks R. Endoscopic treatment of fibrous dysplasia confined to the frontal sinus. Otolaryngol Head Neck Surg. 2007;136:S59–61. https://doi.org/10.1016/j.otohns.2006.10.025.

26. Rao VM, Sharma D, Madan A. Imaging of frontal sinus disease: concepts, interpretation, and technology. Otolaryngol Clin North Am. 2001;34:23–39.

27. Turri-Zanoni M, et al. Frontoethmoidal and intraorbital osteomas: exploring the limits of the endoscopic approach. Arch Otolaryngol Head Neck Surg. 2012;138:498–504. https://doi.org/10.1001/archoto.2012.644.

28. Selleck AM, Desai D, Thorp BD, Ebert CS, Zanation AM. Management of Frontal Sinus Tumors. Otolaryngol Clin North Am. 2016;49:1051–65. https://doi.org/10.1016/j.otc.2016.03.026.

29. Rokade A, Sama A. Update on management of frontal sinus osteomas. Curr Opin Otolaryngol Head Neck Surg. 2012;20:40–4. https://doi.org/10.1097/MOO.0b013e32834e9037.

30. Arslan HH, Tasli H, Cebeci S, Gerek M. The Management of the Paranasal Sinus Osteomas. J Craniofac Surg. 2017;28:741–5. https://doi.org/10.1097/SCS.0000000000003397.

31. Senior BA, Lanza DC. Benign lesions of the frontal sinus. Otolaryngol Clin North Am. 2001;34:253–67.

32. Lund VJ, et al. European position paper on endoscopic management of tumours of the nose, paranasal sinuses and skull base. Rhinol Suppl. 2010;22:1–143.

33. Chapurlat RD, Delmas PD, Liens D, Meunier PJ. Long-term effects of intravenous pamidronate in fibrous dysplasia of bone. J Bone Miner Res. 1997;12:1746–52. https://doi.org/10.1359/jbmr.1997.12.10.1746.

34. Sieskiewicz A, Lyson T, Piszczatowski B, Rogowski M. Endoscopic treatment of adversely located osteomas of the frontal sinus. Ann Otol Rhinol Laryngol. 2012;121:503–9.

35. Chiu AG, Schipor I, Cohen NA, Kennedy DW, Palmer JN. Surgical decisions in the management of frontal sinus osteomas. Am J Rhinol. 2005;19:191–7.

36. Ledderose GJ, Betz CS, Stelter K, Leunig A. Surgical management of osteomas of the frontal recess and sinus: extending the limits of the endoscopic approach. Eur Arch Otorhinolaryngol. 2011;268:525–32. https://doi.org/10.1007/s00405-010-1384-y.

37. Seiberling K, Floreani S, Robinson S, Wormald PJ. Endoscopic management of frontal sinus osteomas revisited. Am J Rhinol Allergy. 2009;23:331–6. https://doi.org/10.2500/ajra.2009.23.3321.

38. Conger BT Jr, Riley K, Woodworth BA. The Draf III mucosal grafting technique: a prospective study. Otolaryngol Head Neck Surg. 2012;146:664–8. https://doi.org/10.1177/0194599811432423.

39. Exley RP, Markey A, Rutherford S, Bhalla RK. Rare giant frontal sinus osteoma mimicking fibrous dysplasia. J Laryngol Otol. 2015;129:283–7. https://doi.org/10.1017/S0022215114003211.

Frontal Sinus Inverted Papilloma: Unique Considerations

17

Vidur Bhalla, Alexander Chiu, and D. David Beahm

Background

Schneiderian papillomas are sinonasal, benign neoplasms of the mucosa consisting of squamous or columnar epithelium. Several types of papillomas exist in the sinonasal cavity, most commonly exophytic (fungiform), cylindrical (oncocytic), and inverted. Inverted papillomas (IPs) are named for squamous metaplasia that histologically expands inward toward the stroma. These are rare tumors occurring in 0.7/100,000 individuals [1] representing 0.5–4% of primary sinonasal tumors [2]. Males are more frequently affected than women at a 3.4:1 ratio [3]. The average age of presentation is in the mid-50s. IP is thought to arise from a single progenitor cell [4]. The etiology is unknown. Viruses including EBV [5] and HPV [6] are thought to play a role in all papilloma types, including IP; however, not all specimens demonstrate positivity. HPV is present in approximately 38% of IPs [7]. This low number, however, could be due to limitations of testing methods or degradation of specimens. Other potential causes include industrial exposure [8], smoking (particularly in recurrence) [9], and chronic inflammation [10]. Surgical resection is the treatment of choice.

IP is thought to originate from the frontal sinus in 1–16% of patients [11]. Generally speaking, bilateral disease is also rare in the lower sinuses; however, this is not the case in the frontal sinus as 16% of patients present with bilateral disease [12]. The intersinus septum serves as a poor barrier to contralateral spread (Fig. 17.1). Intracranial extension is rare with around 20 cases in the literature, with the frontal sinus being the most common site of invasion [13]. Aggressive resection of tumor and involved dura is recommended. Radiation can also be considered. Intradural extension has a poor prognosis [14].

There are two major staging systems, Krouse [15] and Cannady [16]. The Krouse staging system stages all frontal sinus IP tumors as at least T3 and up to T4 if involving the spread through the skull base or orbit or associated with carcinoma (Table 17.1). The Cannady system is based on recurrence rates, and all frontal sinus IP tumors are Group B, unless there is extrasinus involvement or malignancy (Table 17.2).

Ultimately, inverted papilloma represents metaplastic changes, not dysplastic changes; however, malignant conversion is estimated to occur in up to 7–10% of patients [17] [18]. Metachronous carcinomas are noted in 4% of patients [18]. There is active research in identifying which patients are at risk for malignant conversion. A recent meta-analysis showed HPV+ tumors were more likely to convert to squamous cell carcinoma (SCCa) [19]. HPV 16 and 18,

V. Bhalla (✉) · A. Chiu · D. David Beahm
University of Kansas Medical Center, Department of Otolaryngology – Head and Neck Surgery, Kansas City, KS, USA

© Springer Nature Switzerland AG 2019
D. Lal, P. H. Hwang (eds.), *Frontal Sinus Surgery*, https://doi.org/10.1007/978-3-319-97022-6_17

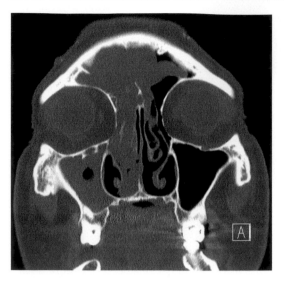

Fig. 17.1 Bilateral extension of a frontal sinus IP through the intersinus septum

Table 17.1 Krouse staging system for inverted papilloma

T1	Tumor totally confined to the nasal cavity, without extension into the sinuses. The tumor can be localized to one wall or region of the nasal cavity, or can be bulky and extensive within the nasal cavity, but must not extend into the sinuses or into any extranasal compartment. There must be no concurrent malignancy
T2	Tumor involving the ostiomeatal complex, and ethmoid sinuses, and/or the medial portion of the maxillary sinus, with or without involvement of the nasal cavity. There must be no concurrent malignancy
T3	Tumor involving the lateral, inferior, superior, anterior, or posterior walls of the maxillary sinus, the sphenoid sinus, and/or the frontal sinus, with or without involvement of the medial portion of the maxillary sinus, the ethmoid sinuses, or the nasal cavity. There must be no concurrent malignancy
T4	All tumors with any extranasal/extrasinus extension to involve adjacent, contiguous structures such as the orbit, the intracranial compartment, or the pterygomaxillary space. All tumors associated with malignancy

high risk variants, demonstrated greater chance of conversion than other subtypes of HPV. HPV genes E6 and E7 produce proteins that bind p53 and pRb, respectively. Inhibition of these tumor suppressor genes is thought to promote cell immortality and growth [6].

Table 17.2 Cannady staging system for inverted papilloma

Group A	Inverted papilloma confined to the nasal cavity, ethmoid sinuses, or medial maxillary wall
Group B	Inverted papilloma with involvement of any maxillary wall (other than the medial wall), or frontal sinus, or sphenoid sinus
Group C	Inverted papilloma with extension beyond the paranasal sinuses

Smoking is also thought to play a role in malignant conversion [20].

Examination and Workup of Inverted Papilloma

Most patients have non-specific symptoms including facial pressure, nasal obstruction, rhinorrhea, and/or epistaxis. Nasal endoscopy aids in assessing sites of attachment, vascularity, involvement of adjacent structures, as well as facilitating biopsy (Fig. 17.2). Computed tomography (CT) is recommended as first-line imaging. Though there are no specific CT features that are diagnostic for IP, imaging allows for gross evaluation of tumor burden, the tumors relationship to bony structures including the orbit, skull base, anterior wall (AW) and posterior wall (PW) of the frontal sinus, and septum.

IP will typically cause bony remodeling. There is rarely destruction; malignant conversion should be considered if this is present. Focal hyperostosis is highly predictive of IP origin; however not all cases present with this finding [21] (Fig. 17.3). Additionally, calcification may exist within the tumor, which may falsely indicate tumor origin [22]. On T1 magnetic resonance imaging (MRI) series, IP appears isointense to hypointense. On T2-weighted MRI images, IP appears hyperintense to muscle and may help further distinguish post-obstruction/inflammatory changes from tumor [22] (Fig. 17.4). While most tumors are unifocal, multifocal tumors are not uncommon. Additionally, a tumor may become multifocal in revision cases as there may be discontinuous areas of tumor growth. Positron emission testing (PET) scan has low utility. Focal areas of SCCa

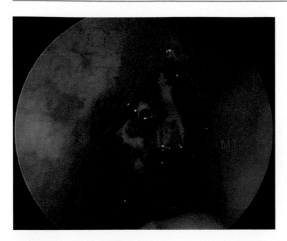

Fig. 17.2 IP originating from the L frontal sinus. *A* axilla, *MT* middle turbinate

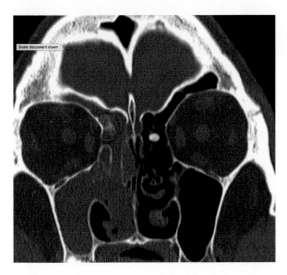

Fig. 17.3 Focal hyperostosis circled in red. The calcification on the left corresponds to an incidental ethmoid osteoma

may be hyperactive on PET, but the test has low utility in detail and is inconsistent in predicting presence of malignancy [23].

Surgical Considerations

Basic surgical principles for tumor resection should be followed. One should be able to obtain necessary surgical exposure while limiting patient morbidity. Specific hallmarks of surgery should be based on three principles:

- Safe clearance of disease with ability to drill origin or origins of the tumor.
- Maintain functional sinus outflow.
- Provide the ability for sinus surveillance.

Clearance of Disease

Surgeon must be able to delineate extent, origin of disease, and obtain clear margins at the time of surgery. Disease burden, anatomy, and exam will dictate which approach is best. If the origin of the tumor cannot be identified, a more aggressive approach should be considered. AP diameter of the frontal sinus at the level of the frontal beak should be assessed in all patients. This will dictate ease and safety of endoscopic approach. Patients with very small AP diameter may be difficult to approach via endoscopic techniques as instruments may not be able to access distal aspects of the frontal sinus. If the disease is superior to this outflow tract, it may be wise to leave the outflow tract intact and access the tumor from an external approach, thus lowering the risk of frontal recess stenosis and subsequent mucocele formation (Fig. 17.5).

General approaches to frontal sinus tumor extirpation include transnasal endoscopic approaches via standard frontal sinusotomy (Draf IIA or IIB) or extended frontal sinusotomy (endoscopic modified Lothrop procedure, or Draf III); or external approaches via an osteoplastic flap or trephine. A combination of approaches can also be used in situations where the outflow tract is obstructed, or the tumor is located high and lateral; using the "above and below" technique, the frontal sinus can be trephined externally to provide access to superior aspects of the frontal sinus, whereas the frontal outflow tract can be established via endoscopic endonasal techniques. Other nontraditional techniques are the endoscopic modified Lothrop (Draf III frontal sinusotomy) and the osteoplastic flap approach, which can be considered for patients with multifocal disease or lateral/anterior disease in which the site of attachment cannot be addressed endoscopically. Attention should be paid to the position of the

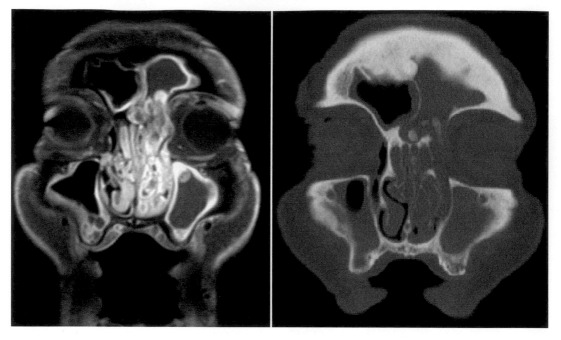

Fig. 17.4 Left: T1 post-contrast MRI image of inverted papilloma extending into the left frontal recess. Note the difference between the tumor and post-obstructive fluid in the frontal and maxillary sinus. Right: Coronal non-contrast CT of the sinuses. While this shows greater detail to bone, there is no discernible difference between fluid and mass

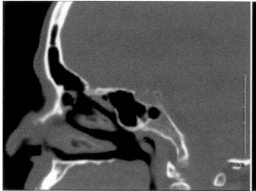
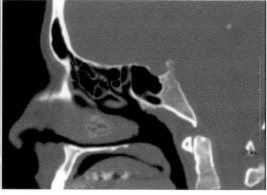

Fig. 17.5 In the picture on the left, the patient has large AP diameter allowing suitable instrumentation of the frontal sinus. In the picture on the right, the patient has a small AP diameter with a relatively prominent beak limiting access to the superior aspect of the frontal sinus

anterior ethmoidal artery in these approaches [24]. Image guidance is recommended for the osteoplastic flap procedure as it assists in delineating the contour of the frontal sinus at the anterior table. If not using image guidance, one may obtain an X-ray of the frontal sinuses with scale and cut out an outline of the frontal sinuses. This should be sterilized and available during the surgery [25]. These procedures are discussed in the specific chapters.

Frozen section biopsy specimens should be sent at the beginning of the case to evaluate for malignancy as this may change management if positive for malignancy. IP is tightly associated with its bony attachment and can invaginate into the underlying bone (Fig. 17.6). Therefore, not

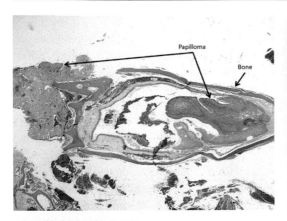

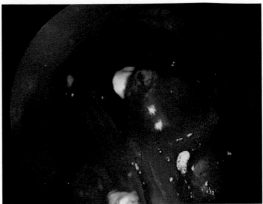

Fig. 17.6 Histologic specimen with hematoxylin and eosin stain of inverted papilloma invaginating into bone. (Courtesy of Sharad Mathur, MD Chief, Pathology and Laboratory Medicine Service, Kansas City VA Medical Center)

Fig. 17.7 IP stalk, visualized via modified Lothrop, noted laterally in right frontal sinus

only does gross disease need to be resected, but the tumor must be systematically followed to its stalk to clear the bony disease (Fig. 17.7). Only stripping mucosa leaves the patient at risk for recurrence. Addressing the underlying bone will often require drilling down the superficial layer of the bone. If IP is adherent to exposed periorbita, then bipolar cautery can be used to cauterize the periorbita in cases without malignancy. If there is malignancy within the IP and it is attached to the periorbita, then the approach should be designed to insure a wide excision of the periorbita and to obtain clean margins.

The lateral and anterior extent is most important in determining the ability for endoscopic approaches to adequately clear disease. Clearing disease lateral to a sagittal plane through the medial wall of the orbit is difficult via endoscopic approach with angled instrumentation (Fig. 17.8). Fulcruming on the posterior wall may be dangerous, as it is 0.1–4 mm thick [26]. Additionally, it may thin out secondary to bulky disease. The Draf III procedure may assist with obtaining a lateral view via the contralateral nostril; however instrumentation may still be limited by the medial wall. It may also help with fully evaluating the posterior wall by obtaining wider exposure and easier access.

While well-aerated sinuses may have bulkier disease, the disease may be easier to clear, particularly if the tumor is attached more infe-

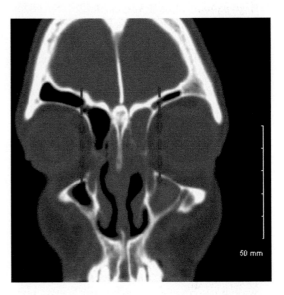

Fig. 17.8 The orbit limits access to the lateral portion of the frontal sinus (beyond the dotted red lines). Diamond burrs can be used to thin the orbit to periorbita to allow greater access. If the tumor extends laterally, but does not attach, it may still be approached endoscopically

riorly and posteriorly. Curved drills should be used to drill the site of attachment. The surgeon should be cognizant of the back side of the burr as unintentional drilling of the posterior wall may occur.

Circumferential mucosal margins should be obtained for frozen specimen to rule out persistent occult disease.

Recurrence rates for endoscopic vs open techniques for all IPs are 12% and 20%, respectively

[27]. A meta-analysis has shown rate of recurrence for frontal sinus disease to be around 22%, and in the frontal sinus, external approaches show lower rates of recurrence than endoscopic techniques [12].

Frontal Sinus Outflow Tract Treatment

While disease clearance is paramount, the sinus must also be left in a functional state. This is difficult given mucosal loss with bony exposure, which places the patient at high risk for stenosis. Iatrogenic mucocele has been shown to occur in 37% of patients after IP resection [28]. Surgeons should avoid cranializing or obliterating the sinus, particularly in benign disease. Radiologic and endoscopic surveillance of recurrence in a post-obliterated or post-cranialized frontal sinus can be very challenging. Recurrences may also be more difficult to treat surgically.

If the mucosa is removed from the outflow tract, several options exist to prevent stenosis. Mucosal grafts can be obtained from the inferior nasal wall, septum, or turbinate and can be placed in the outflow tract to cover exposed bone and prevent stenosis. Alternatively, a frontal sinus rescue flap can be performed to remucosalize the sinus. In a rescue flap, the mucosa on the medial portion of the middle turbinate is rotated into the anterior aspect of the nasofrontal outflow tract to provide bony coverage. Lastly, strip gauze, non-resorbable nasal packing, or silastic implants, either from above or below, can be placed into the outflow tract for a prolonged period of time to prevent stenosis. In addition to the aforementioned techniques, soft tissue stenosis/scar banding can be dilated atraumatically with balloon sinuplasty.

Surveillance

In the absence of evidence-based guidelines on surveillance, one can assume that earlier detection allows for easier resection. Earlier recognition may lower risk of malignant conversion. At the time of initial resection, creating a larger outflow tract or performing a modified Lothrop, even if an external approach is used, may allow easier endoscopic evaluation of the involved areas via nasal endoscopy. Contrasted MRI should be used as surveillance in situations where the site of origin is poorly visualized. MRI helps delineate soft tissue changes with greater accuracy than CT [26]. The majority of recurrences occur within 2 years [27], though 17% occur in 5 years and 6% in 10 years [18]. Given the risk of malignancy, National Comprehensive Cancer Network head and neck oncology screening guidelines [29] offer a good basis for IP surveillance; however screening may be too frequent for benign disease. These guidelines recommend screening every 1–3 months for the first year, every 2–4 months for the second year, and every 4–6 months for years 3–5. For tumor sites that are not visualized, consider imaging at 3 months after resection, 1 year, and then at 2 years, or if there is a change in symptoms. A closer surveillance protocol should be implemented for patients with subtotal resection, HPV + tumors, and recurrent disease.

Alternative strategies for treating IP should be considered in select patients, particularly those that are poor surgical candidates, or those with multifocal/extensive disease. In the past, radiation therapy (RT) was not used for treatment due to its potential for inciting malignant changes within the tumor [30]. Because of advances in radiation delivery and mapping [31], as well as poor correlative data in regard to malignancy [32], RT may be used as treatment for select patients. These patients include poor surgical candidates, multifocal/widespread disease, or patients with concerning histologic features, such as high mitotic index, hyperkeratosis, and squamous epithelial hyperplasia [33]. Radiation therapy should be considered in all patients with SCCA. Chemotherapy should be considered if there is associated malignancy and there are concerns for a positive margin or for presence of distal disease. Antivirals, which have been used with some success in the recurrent respiratory papillomatosis, have been used in isolated case reports and are considered experimental [34, 35].

References

1. Buchwald C, Franzmann M-B, Tos M. Sinonasal papillomas: a report of 82 cases in Copenhagen county, including a longitudinal epidemiological and clinical study. Laryngoscope. 1995;105(1):72–9.
2. Vrabec DP. The inverted Schneiderian papilloma: a clinical and pathological study. Laryngoscope. 1975;85(1):186–220.
3. Lawson W, Patel ZM. The evolution of management for inverted papilloma: an analysis of 200 cases. Otolaryngol Head Neck Surg. 2009;140(3):330–5.
4. Califano J, Koch W, Sidransky D, Westra WH. Inverted Sinonasal Papilloma. Am J Pathol. 2000;156(1):333–7.
5. Macdonald MR, Le KT, Freeman J, Hui MF, Cheung RK, Dosch HM. A majority of inverted sinonasal papillomas carries Epstein-Barr virus genomes. Cancer. 1995;75(9):2307–12.
6. Madkan VK, Cook-Norris RH, Steadman MC, Arora A, Mendoza N, Tyring SK. The oncogenic potential of human papillomaviruses: a review on the role of host genetics and environmental cofactors. Br J Dermatol. 2007;157(2):228–41.
7. Syrjänen K, Syrjänen S. Detection of human papillomavirus in sinonasal papillomas: systematic review and meta-analysis. Laryngoscope. 2013;123(1):181–92.
8. Sham CL, Lee DLY, van Hasselt CA, Tong MCF. A case-control study of the risk factors associated with sinonasal inverted papilloma. Am J Rhinol Allergy. 2010;24(1):e37–40.
9. Roh H-J, Mun SJ, Cho K-S, Hong S-L. Smoking, not human papilloma virus infection, is a risk factor for recurrence of sinonasal inverted papilloma. Am J Rhinol Allergy. 2016;30(2):79–82.
10. Roh H-J, Procop GW, Batra PS, Citardi MJ, Lanza DC. Inflammation and the pathogenesis of inverted papilloma. Am J Rhinol. 2004;18(2):65–74.
11. Shohet JA, Duncavage JA. Management of the frontal sinus with inverted papilloma. Otolaryngol Head Neck Surg. 1996;114(4):649–52.
12. Walgama E, Ahn C, Batra PS. Surgical management of frontal sinus inverted papilloma: a systematic review. Laryngoscope. 2012;122(6):1205–9.
13. Wright EJ, Chernichenko N, Ocal E, Moliterno J, Bulsara KR, Judson BL. Benign inverted papilloma with intracranial extension: prognostic factors and outcomes. Skull Base Rep. 2011;1(2):145–50.
14. Vural E, Suen JY, Hanna E. Intracranial extension of inverted papilloma: an unusual and potentially fatal complication. Head Neck. 1999;21(8):703–6.
15. Krouse JH. Development of a staging system for inverted papilloma. Laryngoscope. 2000;110(6):965–8.
16. Cannady SB, Batra PS, Sautter NB, Roh H-J, Citardi MJ. New staging system for sinonasal inverted papilloma in the endoscopic era. Laryngoscope. 2007;117(7):1283–7.
17. Krouse JH. Endoscopic treatment of inverted papilloma: safety and efficacy. Am J Otolaryngol. 2001;22(2):87–99.
18. Mirza S, Bradley PJ, Acharya A, Stacey M, Jones NS. Sinonasal inverted papillomas: recurrence, and synchronous and metachronous malignancy. J Laryngol Otol. 2007;121(9):857–64.
19. Zhao R-W, Guo Z-Q, Zhang R-X. Human papillomavirus infection and the malignant transformation of sinonasal inverted papilloma: a meta-analysis. J Clin Virol. 2016;79:36–43.
20. Hong S-L, Kim B-H, Lee J-H, Cho K-S, Roh H-J. Smoking and malignancy in sinonasal inverted papilloma. Laryngoscope. 2013;123(5):1087–91.
21. Bhalla RK, Wright ED. Predicting the site of attachment of sinonasal inverted papilloma. Rhinology. 2009;47(4):345–8.
22. Chawla A, Shenoy J, Chokkappan K, Chung R. Imaging features of Sinonasal inverted papilloma: a pictorial review. Curr Probl Diagn Radiol. 2016;45(5):347–53.
23. Jeon TY, Kim H-J, Choi JY, Lee IH, Kim ST, Jeon P, et al. 18F-FDG PET/CT findings of sinonasal inverted papilloma with or without coexistent malignancy: comparison with MR imaging findings in eight patients. Neuroradiology. 2009;51(4):265–71.
24. Joshi AA, Shah KD, Bradoo RA. Radiological correlation between the anterior ethmoidal artery and the supraorbital ethmoid cell. Indian J Otolaryngol Head Neck Surg. 2010;62(3):299–303.
25. Palmer JN, Chiu AG. Atlas of endoscopic sinus and skull base surgery: The Netherlands. Elsevier Health Sciences;2013.416p.https://www.elsevier.com/books/atlas-of-endoscopic-sinus-and-skull-base-surgery/palmer/978-0-323-04408-0
26. Strong EB, Pahlavan N, Saito D. Frontal sinus fractures: a 28-year retrospective review. Otolaryngol Head Neck Surg. 2006;135(5):774–9.
27. Busquets JM, Hwang PH. Endoscopic resection of sinonasal inverted papilloma: a meta-analysis. Otolaryngol Head Neck Surg. 2006;134(3):476–82.
28. Verillaud B, Le Clerc N, Blancal J-P, Guichard J-P, Kania R, Classe M, et al. Mucocele formation after surgical treatment of inverted papilloma of the frontal sinus drainage pathway. Am J Rhinol Allergy. 2016;30(5):181–4.
29. NCCN Clinical Practice Guidelines in Oncology (NCCN Guidelines®) Head and Neck Cancers - NCCN 2014 head-and-neck.pdf [Internet]. [cited 2016 Nov 19]. Available from: http://entcancercare.com/pdf/for_dr/NCCN%202014%20head-and-neck.pdf.
30. Mabery TE, Devine KD, Harrison EG. The problem of malignant transformation in a nasal papilloma: report of a case. Arch Otolaryngol Chic Ill 1960. 1965;82:296–300.
31. Strojan P, Jereb S, Borsos I, But-Hadzic J, Zidar N. Radiotherapy for inverted papilloma: a case

report and review of the literature. Radiol Oncol. 2013;47(1):71.

32. Gomez JA, Mendenhall WM, Tannehill SP, Stringer SP, Cassisi NJ. Radiation therapy in inverted papillomas of the nasal cavity and paranasal sinuses. Am J Otolaryngol. 2000;21(3):174–8.

33. Sauter A, Matharu R, Hörmann K, Naim R. Current advances in the basic research and clinical management of sinonasal inverted papilloma (review). Oncol Rep. 2007;17(3):495–504.

34. Petersen BL, Buchwald C, Gerstoft J, Bretlau P, Lindeberg H. An aggressive and invasive growth of juvenile papillomas involving the total respiratory tract. J Laryngol Otol. 1998;112(11):1101–4.

35. Woodcock M, Mollan SP, Harrison D, Taylor D, Lecuona K. Mitomycin C in the treatment of a Schneiderian (inverted) papilloma of the lacrimal sac. Int Ophthalmol. 2010;30(3):303–5.

Management of Frontal Sinus Malignancy

18

Aykut A. Unsal, Suat Kilic, Peter F. Svider, and Jean Anderson Eloy

Overview

Frontal sinus malignancies are uncommon and are often confused with benign conditions at presentation. According to the Centers for Disease Control and Prevention (CDC), nearly 30 million US adults are diagnosed with sinusitis annually, a figure encompassing both acute and chronic processes. Because many of the initial signs and

A. A. Unsal
Department of Otolaryngology – Head and Neck Surgery, Medical College of Georgia – Augusta University, Augusta, GA, USA

S. Kilic
Department of Otolaryngology – Head and Neck Surgery, Rutgers New Jersey Medical School, Newark, NJ, USA

P. F. Svider
Department of Otolaryngology – Head and Neck Surgery, Wayne State University School of Medicine, Detroit, MI, USA

J. A. Eloy (✉)
Department of Otolaryngology – Head and Neck Surgery, Rutgers New Jersey Medical School, Newark, NJ, USA

Center for Skull Base and Pituitary Surgery, Neurological Institute of New Jersey, Rutgers New Jersey Medical School, Newark, NJ, USA

Department of Neurological Surgery, Rutgers New Jersey Medical School, Newark, NJ, USA

Department of Ophthalmology and Visual Science, Rutgers New Jersey Medical School, Newark, NJ, USA

symptoms of patients with sinusitis are indistinguishable from patients with sinonasal malignancies, identifying individuals in whom further workup is warranted remains a diagnostic dilemma. Particularly, in our contemporary healthcare environment characterized by increasing recognition of the costs associated with pursuing "unnecessary" diagnostic strategies, recognizing individuals with potentially serious etiologies remains an important concern for otolaryngologists, primary care providers, physicians practicing other specialties, and policymakers. In addition to the adverse impact of missing a malignant process and associated healthcare economics, missing a cancer diagnosis also harbors profound potential medicolegal complications, with associated costs passed on to society [1–4].

Although incidence varies by source, sinonasal malignancies occur at an incidence of ten cases per million in the US population [5–8]. Frontal sinus malignancy represents only 1% of these cases [5, 9]. Due to the close proximity of critical intracranial and orbital structures, lesions oftentimes are discovered at advanced stages, necessitating the performance of particularly morbid procedures in many patients with resectable disease. Technological innovations in recent decades have led to the development of more minimally invasive approaches [10, 11]; hence, varying experiences with these approaches combined with the relative rarity of frontal sinus malignancies

© Springer Nature Switzerland AG 2019
D. Lal, P. H. Hwang (eds.), *Frontal Sinus Surgery*, https://doi.org/10.1007/978-3-319-97022-6_18

means that there are few population-based resources allowing for a definitive consensus into optimal management strategies.

There is no American Joint Committee on Cancer (AJCC) staging guideline for malignancies of the frontal sinus [12]. The University of Florida staging system is the most commonly used staging guideline [13]. Stage I includes tumors limited to the site of origin; Stage II includes tumors with extension to adjacent sites such as the orbit, paranasal sinuses, skin, nasopharynx, or pterygo maxillary fossa; and Stage III includes tumors that have eroded the base of the skull or pterygoid plate and/or have intracranial extension [13].

Historically, management of frontal sinus malignancies has involved open surgical approaches with their associated morbidities. Although open frontal sinus surgery has declined markedly in recent years [14], malignancies represent one of the few situations in which these procedures, including frontal sinus obliteration, are still utilized.

Epidemiology

Sinonasal malignancies are considered rare and frontal sinus malignancies even more so [5]. In the USA, frontal sinus malignancies make up approximately 1.2% of all sinonasal malignancies [5] with an incidence of 1.1 cases per ten million people per year [9]. According to recent population studies, patients afflicted by this malignancy are most commonly in their seventh decade of life, with a predominance toward males [9]. Whites are most commonly affected in these studies, but this is likely due to population demographics, as the incidence is not different among different races [9]. Smoking is the principal environmental risk factor for all sinonasal malignancies, as it can lead to a two to threefold increase in developing the disease [15]. Exposure to radium watch dial paint, wood dust, lacquer paints, isopropyl oils, thorium dioxide, and solder and welding materials has also been associated with sinonasal malignancies [15].

Presentation, Diagnosis, and Workup

In general, sinonasal malignancies present in advanced stages, often with nonspecific symptoms [15]. Because the frontal sinus is even more isolated than the rest of the sinonasal cavities, early diagnosis is uncommon. Early symptoms reported in the literature include nasal discharge and sensations of sinus pressure [16]. These vague symptoms seen early on in the disease course allow frontal sinus malignancies to masquerade as more commonly seen benign disorders. The presence of unilateral nasal obstruction, anosmia, and proptosis should raise suspicion for a tumor [16].

As the tumor grows, it can erode through the frontal bone and cause swelling of the forehead or medial aspect of the upper eyelid [16]. In fact, most cases present this way, as localized presentation is uncommon [9]. These patients are often misdiagnosed with frontal sinusitis and concurrent osteomyelitis, especially if there are signs of an infectious process such as fever, cellulitis, or purulent nasal discharge. Infections may develop secondary to the obstruction by the tumor and therefore can also be misleading. If the tumor extends to the orbit, proptosis, blepharoptosis, epiphora, or diplopia may be seen. Since lymphatic drainage of the frontal sinus occurs via the lymphatic channels of the overlying skin and anterior nasal vault, metastasis is rare without involvement of the overlying skin or anterior nasal mucosa.

Computed tomography (CT) and magnetic resonance (MR) imaging are important in confirming suspicion of a tumor. CT is particularly apt for demonstrating bony erosion (Fig. 18.1), whereas MR is superior in differentiating soft tissue characteristics of the lesion. MR imaging is particularly useful in discriminating tumor from adjacent soft tissue structures to determine extent of disease (Fig. 18.2). For example, MR with gadolinium enhancement and fat suppression may differentiate between tumor and thick secretions or demonstrate perineural spread [16]. While clinical examination and

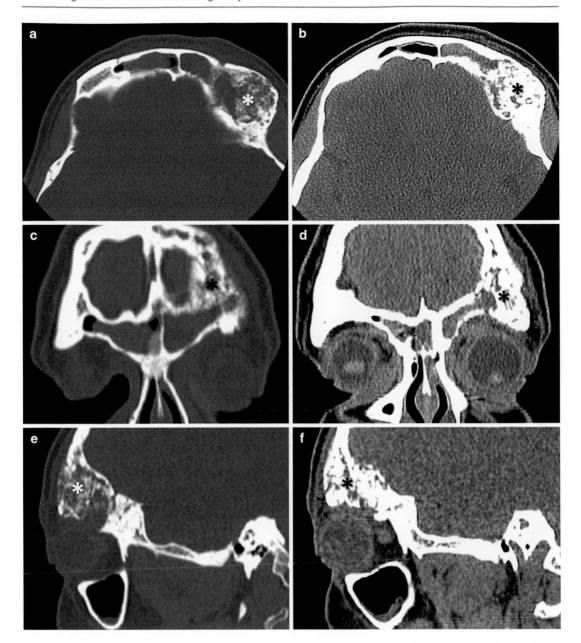

Fig. 18.1 Preoperative axial (**a**) bone window and (**b**) soft tissue window, coronal (**c**) bone window and (**d**) soft tissue window, and sagittal (**e**) bone window and (**f**) soft tissue window computed tomography scan showing opacification of the left frontal sinus with destruction of the posterior table of the sinus and extension into the ethmoid sinuses. Note the lytic destruction of the left lateral frontal sinus (asterisks, **e, f**)

imaging are both important in raising suspicion for frontal sinus malignancies, definitive diagnosis of malignancy can only be made via histopathologic examination. Therefore, biopsy either before or at the time of surgery is essential.

Pathology

In this section, histology-specific epidemiologic information as well as diagnostic and therapeutic considerations are outlined. Only the unique aspects of each histologic subtype are described.

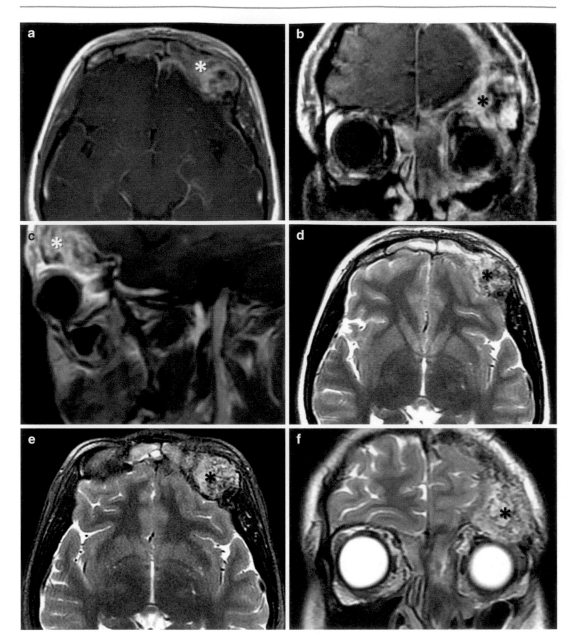

Fig. 18.2 Axial (**a**), coronal (**b**), and sagittal (**c**) T1-weighted gadolinium-enhanced magnetic resonance imaging showing and enhancing lesion of the left frontal sinus extending into the left frontal lobe with significant dural enhancement. Axial (**d**, **e**) and sagittal (**f**) T2-weighted magnetic resonance imaging showing the lesion with the extensive bony destruction (asterisk)

Because frontal sinus malignancies are so rare, much of the discussion applies to sinonasal malignancies in general. However, when available, frontal-sinus-specific information is emphasized.

Squamous Cell Carcinoma (SCC)

As with all subsites of the sinonasal cavities, SCC is the most common malignancy in the frontal sinus (FSSCC) [5]. It comprises almost 40%

of all frontal sinus malignancies in the USA [9]. Smoking is a well-established risk factor, and exposure to nickel, arsenic, chromium, and afla-toxin has also been associated with sinonasal SCC (SNSCC). Individuals that are bakers, pastry cooks, grain millers, textile workers, construction workers, wood-manufacturing workers, and carpenters and joiners are also thought to be at increased risk [17]. Infection from high-risk human papillomavirus (HPV) subtypes 16, 31, and 18 has also been associated with these malignancies [18]. Additionally, 5–10% of inverted sinonasal papillomas will eventually progress to SNSCC [19].

These tumors characteristically demonstrate bone erosion with hyperostosis on CT imaging [20, 21]. Compared to fluid, SNSCC possess intermediate T1 signal intensity and T2 hypointensity. Smaller lesions may appear homogenous on imaging, while larger lesions become more heterogeneous due to necrotic tissue or hemorrhage [22]. Intracranial extension may be seen in advanced cases, and gadolinium-enhanced, fat-suppressed T1 MR imaging is ideal for identifying this extension [22]. Although these imaging characteristics are typically described, oftentimes radiologic findings for SNSCC are nonspecific.

Typically, treatment for SNSCC is with surgery followed by radiotherapy [23]. Radiotherapy of the neck may be considered for locally advanced lesions, and platinum-based chemoradiotherapy may be used when there are positive margins postoperatively or when the malignancy has invaded neural or lymphovascular structures [23]. There are no specific treatment regimens recommended for FSSCC, but one US population-based study has shown that almost 59% of patients are treated with surgery and radiotherapy, with single modality radiotherapy used in about 21% of cases and surgery alone used in only 4% of cases [9].

Variants of Squamous Cell Carcinoma

Variants of SCC are a group of rare malignancies which have unique histologic and clinicopathologic properties. They make up ~7% of SNSCCs

and are comprised of four histologic subtypes: verrucous squamous cell carcinoma (VSCC), papillary squamous cell carcinoma (PSCC), spindle cell (sarcomatoid) carcinoma (SCSC), and basaloid squamous cell carcinoma (BSCC) [24]. However, variants of SCC are extremely rare in the frontal sinus. The largest population-based study of variants of SCC, which captured approximately 28% of the US population, identified just five cases over 40 years [24].

Each of the variants possesses unique properties. For example, BSCC tends to be more aggressive in comparison to the other variants. They may present as multifocal lesions and demonstrate a higher predilection for local invasion and distant metastasis. VSCC on the other hand, has traditionally been described as a lower-grade variant of SCC. Regardless of their pathologic propensities, all variants of SCC should be treated aggressively, especially when found in the frontal sinus.

Adenocarcinoma

Adenocarcinoma is the second or third most common malignancy in the sinonasal cavities overall [5] and the fourth most common in the frontal sinus as per a recent US-based population study [9]. Most sinonasal adenocarcinomas (SNAC) arise from salivary gland tissues, but intestinal-type adenocarcinomas also exist. Working in the leather industry increases the risk of developing SNAC, and this is thought to be from exposure to tannins and chromate. Wood workers, via exposure to formaldehyde-based adhesives, wood dust, and creosote (preservative), also have an increased risk of developing SNAC. These environmental exposures are also thought to be responsible for the multifocal nature of SNAC. Since these occupations have been typically male dominated in the past, some studies have demonstrated discrepancies in gender distribution. A clear male predominance is observed in European studies on SNAC [25, 26], but not in US-based studies (65.0% male in the USA compared to 83.6% male in Europe) [27].

For early-stage low-grade tumors (T1, T2), the treatment is surgical resection of the tumor. Adjuvant radiotherapy is typically added if the tumor presents at an advanced stage, surgical margins are positive, or there is involvement of critical nearby structures such as the dura, brain, or orbit. The role of chemotherapy in SNAC is unclear. A few studies have shown the success of primary chemotherapy in treating intestinal-type adenocarcinomas of the ethmoid sinus with functional TP53 [28–30]. One study has suggested that surgical debulking followed by the administration of topical fluorouracil is effective [31]. Unfortunately, no literature examining frontal sinus-specific adenocarcinomas exists, and thus this discussion is limited to all sinonasal subsites.

Adenoid Cystic Carcinoma

With an incidence of ~0.5 cases per million people per year, sinonasal adenoid cystic carcinoma (SNACC) is also incredibly rare [32]. It is, however, the most common salivary gland malignancy of the sinonasal cavities [32]. Conversely, just 10–25% of adenoid cystic carcinomas are found in the sinonasal cavities. Although these malignancies progress slowly, they are locally destructive with a proclivity for perineural invasion. This is particularly important for the frontal sinus, where destruction of adjacent vital structures can have devastating consequences. Therefore, neural structures of the head and neck deserve special attention on imaging studies. Fortunately, these malignancies are rarely seen in the frontal sinus, with one population-based study on SNACC identifying just five cases (0.7%) in a 40-year period [33].

A recent systematic review identified just two cases in the frontal sinus out of 88 individual patient data [32]. This systematic review also demonstrated that SNACC is most commonly treated with combined surgery and radiotherapy, but single modality surgery and radiotherapy have also been utilized [32]. There have been suggestions that SNACC is less amenable to endoscopic endonasal resection due to its pro-

pensity for perineural spread and that open surgery should be preferred [34]. However, other studies have demonstrated success with the endoscopic method without adverse outcomes [35]. While radiotherapy has been effective in certain cases, it is not considered curative on its own. Its use as a single therapy is mainly reserved for unresectable T4 tumors, to decrease tumor size prior to surgery, or as palliative therapy.

Mucoepidermoid Carcinoma

Mucoepidermoid carcinoma is the most common salivary gland malignancy of the head and neck but is rare in the sinonasal cavities. It has been described as originating from the minor mucoserous glands of the sinonasal cavities. A population-based study of 149 cases of sinonasal mucoepidermoid carcinoma identified only 1 case in the frontal sinus [36]. The majority of cases are treated with surgery and radiotherapy; however, survival outcomes for combined surgery and radiotherapy were not significantly different from surgery alone.

Olfactory Neuroblastoma

Olfactory neuroblastoma (ON), previously known as esthesioneuroblastoma, is a neuroendocrine malignancy which originates from the olfactory epithelium of the sinonasal cavities. However, it is rarely found in the frontal sinus. The overall incidence of ON is approximately 0.5 cases per million people per year, with an unclear gender distribution. While some studies have demonstrated a slight male predominance, others have reported a roughly equal incidence in men and women. Earlier literature had suggested that ON has a bimodal age distribution; however, recent studies have demonstrated the highest frequency of patients aged within the fifth or sixth decade of life. Common presenting symptoms include nasal obstruction, epistaxis, headache, facial pain, and hyposmia/anosmia. Due to its neuroendocrine origins, ON is associated with paraneoplastic syndromes such as syndrome of inappropriate ADH secretion, ectopic ACTH syndrome, humoral hypercalcemia of malignancy, hypertension due to catecholamine secretion, opsoclonus-myoclonus-ataxia, and paraneoplastic cerebellar degeneration [37].

On T1-weighted MR imaging, ON is usually hypointense to gray matter, whereas on T2-weighted MR imaging, it is usually intermediate to hyperintense to gray matter [38]. When there is evidence of intracranial extension, the presence of intracranial cysts is highly suggestive of ON [39]. CT imaging of the neck should be performed to identify potential cervical node metastasis, which is seen in about 20–25% of cases and portends a poorer prognosis [40]. Cervical lymph node involvement also increases the risk of recurrence. While the AJCC staging criteria may be applied in cases of ON of the nasal cavity, maxillary sinus, or ethmoid sinus, its unique clinicopathologic behavior has prompted the development of four different staging systems, proposed by Kadish, Morita, Dulguerov, and Biller [40].

Multimodality treatment is usually necessary for ON. The current, widely accepted treatment regimen is surgical resection of the tumor, either through open or endoscopic means, followed by postoperative radiotherapy. Although single modality treatment with radiotherapy has been utilized in the past, recent studies have demonstrated superior survival outcomes with combined surgery and radiotherapy. The use of irradiation as neoadjuvant therapy prior to surgery has also been described. Elective neck dissection has not shown improve outcomes, but postoperative radiation of the neck is common practice. Recently, IMPBRT (intensity-modulated proton beam radiation therapy) has gained popularity for this lesion due to its ability to minimize the radiation dose to surrounding structures.

Undifferentiated Carcinoma

Sinonasal undifferentiated carcinoma (SNUC) is part of the spectrum of neuroendocrine carcinomas, along with ON and sinonasal neuroendocrine carcinoma (SNEC). SNUC has an incidence

~0.2 per million people per year in the USA and is rarely discovered in the frontal sinus. Patients are typically male and are in their sixth decade of life. Some studies have suggested an association with Epstein-Barr virus (EBV) infection, but this is controversial [41]. Treatment consists of primary surgery excision with adjuvant radiotherapy and/or chemotherapy. A recent population-based analysis of SNUC demonstrated that patients treated with surgery and chemoradiotherapy had better survival outcomes when compared to those treated with surgery and radiotherapy, surgery alone, or radiotherapy alone [42].

Neuroendocrine Carcinoma

Sinonasal neuroendocrine carcinoma is a rare group of neuroendocrine malignancies. It can be classified into three subtypes: typical carcinoid, atypical carcinoid, and small cell carcinoma. The incidence of SNEC is 0.12 cases per million people per year, and it comprises ~5% of all sinonasal malignancies. Only 2% of SNEC is found in the frontal sinus [43]. While there is no consensus on the optimal treatment, in one study, most patients received combined surgery and radiotherapy [43]. Unlike some of the other histologies described, SNEC tend to be chemosensitive, and thus the utilization of induction or adjuvant chemotherapy has also been described.

Mucosal Melanoma

Sinonasal mucosal melanoma (SMM) accounts for just ~1% of all melanomas, and only ~0.4% of SMM are found in the frontal sinus [44]. SMM is an aggressive tumor, and prognosis is generally poor, even more so than cutaneous melanoma. On imaging, there may be evidence of bone remodeling due to pressure effects and may possess a bland margin [22]. Also, certain cases may have enough melanin or undergo hemorrhage to present with T1 hyperintensity; this finding is considered relatively specific, but not sensitive [22].

SMM is associated with higher rates of c-KIT proto-oncogene, and some studies have suggested that imatinib may be helpful in such cases [45]. More recently, ipilimumab, a monoclonal antibody directed against CTLA4, has demonstrated success in patients with stage III or IV mucosal melanoma who have not responded to other treatments [46]. Treatment is primarily surgical resection. Radiotherapy has been shown to improve locoregional control but does not lead to improved survival outcomes.

Rhabdomyosarcoma

Although rare overall, rhabdomyosarcoma (RMS) is the most common sarcoma of the sinonasal cavities [47, 48]. It has an incidence of ~0.34 cases per million people per year [47]. More than half of all patients with sinonasal RMS (SRMS) are under the age of 20 years [47]. There are several different histologic subtypes of RMS; embryonal is the most common type, and alveolar is the second most common. Other types include pleomorphic RMS, mixed-type RMS, and RMS with ganglionic differentiation. In adults, alveolar SRMS is more common [47, 49], whereas the embryonal type is more common in children and adolescents [47]. These are aggressive malignancies, and SRMS has poor prognosis compared to RMS involving other parts of the body.

MR imaging may help differentiate SRMS from sinonasal carcinomas. SRMS may appear isointense when compared to gray matter on T1-weighted MR imaging and hyperintense when compared to gray matter on T2-weighted MR imaging. Sinonasal carcinomas on the other hand are less likely to appear hyperintense on T2-weighted MR imaging [50]. For RMS in general, the Intergroup Rhabdomyosarcoma Study Group has recommended multimodality treatment including surgery, chemotherapy, and radiation [51]. RMS in the frontal sinus is extremely rare; a population-based study of frontal sinus malignancies only identified one case in a 40-year period [9].

Fibrosarcoma

Sinonasal fibrosarcoma (SNFS) is rare. In a recent population-based study, just 51 cases were identified over the span of 39 years. Only two of these (~4%) were found in the frontal sinus. The mean and standard deviation for age at diagnosis are 54.5 and 19.8 years, respectively. These malignancies have a low potential for metastasis, and it is uncommon for patients to have distant metastasis at initial presentation. Hence, compared to other sinonasal malignancies, the prognosis is favorable. Surgery is the primary treatment modality for SNFS, and radiotherapy is only indicated in the case of unresectable disease. Approximately a third of patients receive postoperative radiotherapy.

Angiosarcoma

There are few mentions of sinonasal angiosarcoma (SNAS) in the literature, mostly limited to case reports and single-institution retrospective reviews of a modest number of patients. In one study of ten cases, the mean age of diagnosis was reported as ~47 years. None of these cases involved the frontal sinus, but there have been a few case reports of frontal sinus angiosarcoma in the literature [52–54].

Leiomyosarcoma

Sinonasal leiomyosarcoma is a rare malignancy of smooth muscle origin. At least 63 cases of sinonasal leiomyosarcoma have been reported in the literature [55]. The mean age of diagnosis reported is just over 46 years of age, with a roughly equal gender distribution. It may be associated with a history of radiation therapy, chemotherapy, or retinoblastoma [55]. Most cases are treated with surgical resection of the tumor followed by radiotherapy. Chemotherapy is mainly indicated for palliative therapy [55].

Chondrosarcoma

Sinonasal chondrosarcomas (SCS) are malignancies which arise from hyaline cartilage. One systematic review identified 161 cases, 69 of which were in the nasal septum. The average age at diagnosis was reported to be about 42 years of age [56]. Almost 75% of the cases presented in the study were treated primarily with surgery, while 20% of cases were treated with surgery and radiotherapy. On CT imaging, SCS usually demonstrates intense enhancement. As opposed to osteosarcoma, which is associated with the "sunburst" appearance, SCS tends to be associated with suture margins and curvilinear calcifications on imaging [22]. There is a low potential for metastasis but a high rate of local recurrence. In a single-institutional retrospective review, 28 chondrosarcomas of the head and neck were reported, 1 of which was in the frontal sinus.

Diffuse Large B-Cell Lymphoma

Sinonasal non-Hodgkin's lymphoma (NHL) makes up just 0.2–2.0% of all NHL in the western world [57]. The most common histologic subtype is diffuse large B-cell lymphoma (DLBCL). The mean age at diagnosis is approximately 66 years of age, and there seems to be no difference in gender distribution [58]. DLBCL is the second most common malignancy of the frontal sinus [9]. The frontal sinus is the least common sinonasal location in the sinonasal tract for DLBCL, but DLBCL is the second most common malignancy in the frontal sinus. Imaging of sinonasal lymphomas tends to demonstrate bone remodeling. On T1 MR imaging, sinonasal lymphomas tend to be isointense to muscle, and post-contrast they typically have at least moderate enhancement [22]. On T2 MR imaging, they tend to be hyperintense to muscle and hypointense to mucosa [22]. Treatment is primarily with radiotherapy, but chemoradiotherapy is used in cases with advanced stage. Per one study, only about 20% of cases of frontal sinus DLBCL received surgery alone. Prognosis for DLBCL of the frontal sinus is excellent when compared to other frontal sinus malignancies [9].

Extranodal NK/T-Cell Lymphoma

Sinonasal extranodal natural killer/T-cell lymphoma (SN-ENKTL) is a type of NHL which arises from natural killer cells or T-cells. It was previously known as "lethal midline granuloma" due to its invasive nature in the bone, cartilage, and soft tissues. SN-ENKTL is believed to develop after EBV infection, and studies have shown that higher EBV titers are associated with worse outcomes. The mean age at diagnosis is about 50 years, which is considerably younger than both sinonasal DLBCL and sinonasal malignancies overall. It rarely occurs in the frontal sinus, with only two cases identified over the span of 40 years in a population study. SN-ENKTL is endemic to many Asian countries and thus may be underrepresented in the US population. On imaging, SN-ENKTL is more likely to show lytic destruction than DLBCL [22]. Prognosis for SN-ENKTL is much worse than that for sinonasal DLBCL.

Hemangiopericytoma

Sinonasal hemangiopericytoma (SN-HPC) is a rare vascular malignancy that makes up ~1/5 of all head and neck hemangiopericytomas [59]. These malignancies tend to originate around small blood vessels. High recurrence rates have been reported [60–63]. The frequency of hemangiopericytomas in the frontal sinus is unclear; however, at least one such case has been reported in the literature [64].

Plasmacytoma

Plasmacytomas are monoclonal B-cell malignancies. They can be divided into three categories: extramedullary plasmacytoma (EMP), solitary bone plasmacytoma, and multiple myeloma. Despite being a rare malignancy overall, EMPs have a high predilection for the head and neck, especially the sinonasal cavities. There is a strong male predominance, over 2:1 compared to females, although incidence is roughly the same between different races. Combined surgery and adjuvant radiotherapy are the most common treatment employed [65], but radiotherapy alone may be utilized in a large number of cases due to the highly radiosensitive nature of these tumors [66]. Prognosis seems to be excellent regardless of the treatment strategy chosen. However, because only ~1.4% of sinonasal EMPs are seen in the frontal sinus, these results may not be generalizable to frontal sinus EMPs [65]. It is important to note that these malignancies may progress to multiple myeloma, and thus appropriate workup should be included in their evaluation.

Therapy

Due to the rarity of sinonasal cancers, currently no treatment algorithms based on evidence from randomized trials are in existence. Most of the recommendations are based on single-institution retrospective review studies which have a wide range of site, histology, and treatment modality distributions. One population-based study on frontal sinus malignancies suggests that about 49% of cases are treated with surgery and radiotherapy, 13% of cases receive surgery alone, and 20% of cases receive radiotherapy alone [9].

In several of the histologies discussed, surgical therapy with or without chemoradiotherapy is essential for the treatment for primary tumors of the frontal sinuses. For common histologies such as SCC, surgical extirpation alone with negative margins may be adequate for small, early-stage malignancies with no evidence of local invasion. Unfortunately, most frontal sinus tumors will present at advanced stages and thus warrant adjuvant radiotherapy. There is general consensus that local control is paramount in improving long-term outcomes [9]. The role of single modality radiotherapy treatment demonstrates overall lower 5-year disease-specific survival and thus is generally discouraged unless certain particular histologies (i.e., lymphomas) are encountered [9, 16]. Additionally, radiotherapy has been associated with a relatively high complication rate of optic neuritis in the past (8%), leading to blindness [67, 68]. However, its

utilization may always be considered for palliation of late-stage disease.

Due to the low likelihood of spread to cervical lymph nodes, elective neck dissections for the treatment of frontal sinus tumors have not been shown to improve survival and consequently are often not recommended. There is inadequate evidence examining the role of adjuvant chemotherapy in the treatment of paranasal tumors, and therefore this modality is not routinely utilized [67].

Preoperative Planning and Approach Considerations

Before proceeding with surgical planning, it is important to first assess the patient's candidacy for resection. Contraindications to surgery include evidence of distant metastasis and medical comorbidities that render a patient unfit to tolerate general anesthesia. It is additionally important to recognize the patient's age, prognosis, and the tumor's invasion into vital surrounding structures. Extension of the primary tumor into the frontal lobes is not a direct contraindication for surgery.

Once the decision has been made to take a patient to the operating room, it is critical to consider the approach of the procedure, whether it be endoscopic, open (craniofacial approaches), or combined. Typically, solely endoscopic approaches to the frontal sinus are reserved for benign tumor processes since their efficacy for malignant disease has not been well studied. Recently, endoscopic-only resections of frontal sinus SCCs and olfactory neuroblastomas have been described in the literature with excellent outcomes [69]. However, these studies are sparse, and the inclusion of craniofacial approaches significantly improves survival by allowing for better control of local disease [9, 16]. Consequently, this discussion focuses on external approaches. Ultimately, the approach utilized in actual practice will depend on the extent of resection required. For any endoscopic-based approaches, appropriate navigation-focused imaging studies for anatomical tracking should be obtained prior to surgery. A 6-foot occipitofrontal Caldwell view X-ray of the frontal sinuses can also be obtained if an external approach is to be utilized. This will determine the surgeon's anatomic limits to prevent accidental entry into the anterior cranial fossa, although the use of CT-based navigation has largely supplanted the reliance on plain film imaging.

Surgical Technique

A Lynch-type frontoethmoidectomy with osteoplastic flap elevation may be utilized in the rare setting of early-stage frontal sinus tumors that possess no bony wall, dural, or periorbital involvement [70]. Typically, a 2–3 cm curvilinear incision is made beginning at the medial brow, extending inferomedially midway between the nasal bridge and medial canthus, along the nasofacial groove. Care should be taken to stay medial to avoid injury to the supraorbital neurovascular bundle. Many advocate interruption of the linear incision with a "W" shape when adjacent to the medial canthus, to avoid producing an epicanthal "bowstring" scar deformity. The incision is carried down to the periosteum which is then subsequently raised. The floor of the frontal sinus may then be accessed with a cutting burr. Tumors that invade the frontal intersinus septum require greater exposure, best accomplished by creating two contralateral Lynch incisions, connected with a horizontal incision over the glabella in an "H" fashion [16, 67, 68, 70]. This approach, unfortunately, involves severing of both supraorbital nerves resulting in bilateral forehead anesthesia. Inferiorly based lateralized tumors can also be accessed by using a Lynch-type incision. However, these incisions will require extension inferiorly to the brow and out laterally for forehead degloving.

Tumors that are larger, more laterally based, or involve bony walls require a bicoronal approach. This allows for the optimal exposure of the entire frontal sinus. The incision is initiated at the midline vertex of the scalp, just above the hairline. The incisions are then carried horizontally bilaterally within the hairline to the lateral limit of the tragus. It is important to keep this incision near the level of the vertex of the scalp to avoid inadvertent injury to the anterior branch of the superficial temporal artery. The vertical limbs of the incisions are then carried bilaterally inferiorly toward the level of the zygoma, along the hairline, and optimally hidden within the preauricular rhytids anterior to the tragus [16, 67, 70]. The depth of the incision within the scalp should be carried down to the pericranium, allowing for elevation of the periosteum and superficial contents within the avascular plane. Care should be taken when manipulating the supraorbital and supratrochlear vessels within the flap, as a robust blood flow is useful in reconstruction efforts following tumor extirpation. The lateral, vertical incisions are carried deep to the deep temporal fascia, thereby avoiding injury to the more superficial temporal arteries and temporal branches of the facial nerve within the temporoparietal fascia and superficial muscular aponeurotic system (SMAS), respectively [16]. The flap is then elevated inferiorly and widely toward the supraorbital rim, where the periosteum is left attached to the bone.

Once the flap is elevated to the supraorbital rim, the frontal sinus osteotomy with an osteoplastic flap may be performed if the tumor is isolated to the sinuses. If the tumor, however, involves the posterior wall of the sinus, the frontal lobe, or its associated dura, a unilateral or bilateral craniotomy should be utilized to facilitate optimal exposure. Involved bony, dural, and frontal lobe tissue requires removal to ensure complete resection [67, 70].

Preservation of the orbit in cases of tumor invasion has been extensively debated in the literature. Traditionally, orbital exenteration was recommended with any evidence of periorbital involvement [71]. The literature does generally recommend this when periorbital penetration or ocular content involvement is observed, especially given the poorer prognosis these patients exhibit compared to others with no orbital invasion [72, 73]. However, other studies have demonstrated no deficits in survival when only the affected periorbital was excised and confirmed with negative margins from frozen section, suggesting that the orbit may be preserved in such cases [71, 74].

Reconstruction Options

Reconstruction of the defects post-extirpation will be determined based on the extent of resection. If skin was excised, defects 2 cm or under can easily be reconstructed utilizing rotation advancement flaps [16, 67, 68]. Larger defects, however, may require free-flap reconstruction with anastomosis to the superficial temporal artery, given the poor laxity of scalp tissue [67]. Managing defects of the anterior table can be achieved from bone harvested during the frontal craniotomy or with split-thickness calvarial bone grafts and fixated using metallic or absorbable plates [16]. Use of hydroxyapatite bone cement and methyl methacrylate overlying a metal mesh has also been described in the literature [68]. Posterior table defects require cranialization of the remaining sinus, along with complete obliteration of the frontonasal outflow pathway (with stripping of mucosa) to prevent mucocele development and cerebrospinal fluid leakage. Dural reconstruction can be accomplished via pericranial flap, which can be separated from the scalp flap and rotated into position. Usually, preservation of a single supraorbital pedicle is sufficient for flap survival [67]. In the scenarios where pericranial tissue is unable to be utilized, dural reconstruction can be accomplished with cadaveric dura, temporalis fascia, or tensor fascia lata [16]. Reconstruction of the orbit after exenteration often requires use of the pericranial flap with overlying split-thickness skin grafts. A systematic approach to reconstructive options that support oncologic resection is critical [75].

Surgical Complications

Complications commonly encountered by surgical resection of frontal sinus malignancies include wound dehiscence and cerebrospinal spinal fluid leaks [69, 70]. Previous studies have cited an approximate 20% risk of complications, although the extent of resection and the patient's comorbidity status ultimately dictate these risks [67]. Additionally, scar tissue from previous procedures/radiation treatment undoubtedly compli-cates wound healing and can increase the overall complication rate. Tumors requiring intracranial resection increase the risk of developing meningitis postoperatively. Additionally, it is important to note that resection of frontal lobe tissue or any aggressive manipulation of the brain may result in mental status changes.

Postoperative Treatment and Care

Given the advanced stages that frontal sinus tumors present, some advocate routine utilization of adjuvant radiotherapy [9]. Others recommend postoperative irradiation only for frontal sinus tumors that possessed invasion beyond the confines of the frontal sinus walls (i.e., Stage II or Stage III), tumors with aggressive histologies, or those with inadequate surgical margins [67]. There is no general consensus on the role of adjuvant chemotherapy, as response to treatment will depend on the histology encountered.

Post-therapeutic surveillance of frontal sinus malignancies should be initially accomplished 3–4 months following the completion of surgery or adjuvant irradiation. MR imaging with gadolinium is the preferred scan of choice. Annual follow-up imaging is recommended up to 4 years or longer for more indolent histologies (i.e., adenoid cystic carcinoma) [67].

Outcomes

Outcomes data evaluating treatment of frontal sinus malignancy are sparse due to the relative infrequency of this location as a primary site. Nonetheless, population-based resources, such as the SEER database, have allowed for compilation of relevant data and provide several important insights. Squamous cell carcinomas represent approximately half of malignancies in this location, a more modest proportion than sinonasal malignancies in other locations [5]. Although disease-specific survival is at 41.5% at 5 years, it is important to note that this does not stabilize; 10-year DSS figures decrease to 23.3%. There have been no widespread analyses critically evaluating

open management versus endoscopic resection of
these lesions, although several groups have reported
their experience with the latter in recent years [69].

References

1. Rayess HM, Gupta A, Svider PF, et al. A critical analysis of melanoma malpractice litigation: should we
   biopsy everything? Laryngoscope. 2017;127:134–9.
2. Epstein JB, Kish RV, Hallajian L, Sciubba J. Head
   and neck, oral, and oropharyngeal cancer: a review of
   medicolegal cases. Oral Surg Oral Med Oral Pathol
   Oral Radiol. 2015;119:177–86.
3. Lydiatt DD, Sewell RK. Medical malpractice and
   sinonasal disease. Otolaryngol Head Neck Surg.
   2008;139:677–81.
4. Svider PF, Husain Q, Kovalerchik O, et al.
   Determining legal responsibility in otolaryngology:
   a review of 44 trials since 2008. Am J Otolaryngol.
   2013;34:699–705.
5. Dutta R, Dubal PM, Svider PF, Liu JK, Baredes S,
   Eloy JA. Sinonasal malignancies: a population-
   based analysis of site-specific incidence and survival.
   Laryngoscope. 2015;125:2491–7.
6. Turner JH, Reh DD. Incidence and survival
   in patients with sinonasal cancer: a historical
   analysis of population-based data. Head Neck.
   2012;34:877–85.
7. Kuijpens JH, Louwman MW, Peters R, Janssens GO,
   Burdorf AL, Coebergh JW. Trends in sinonasal cancer in the Netherlands: more squamous cell cancer,
   less adenocarcinoma. A population-based study 1973-
   2009. Eur J Cancer. 2012;48:2369–74.
8. Youlden DR, Cramb SM, Peters S, et al. International
   comparisons of the incidence and mortality of sinonasal cancer. Cancer Epidemiol. 2013;37:770–9.
9. Bhojwani A, Unsal A, Dubal PM, et al. Frontal sinus
   malignancies: a population-based analysis of incidence and survival. Otolaryngol Head Neck Surg.
   2016;154:735–41.
10. Eloy JA, Svider PF, Setzen M. Preventing and manag-
    ing complications in frontal sinus surgery. Otolaryngol
    Clin N Am. 2016;49:951–64.
11. Folbe AJ, Svider PF, Eloy JA. Anatomic consider-
    ations in frontal sinus surgery. Otolaryngol Clin N
    Am. 2016;49:935–43.
12. Frederick L, Page DL, Fleming ID et al. AJCC can-
    cer staging manual. New York: Springer Science &
    Business Media, 2002.
13. Katz TS, Mendenhall WM, Morris CG, Amdur RJ,
    Hinerman RW, Villaret DB. Malignant tumors of
    the nasal cavity and paranasal sinuses. Head Neck.
    2002;24:821–9.
14. Svider PF, Sekhsaria V, Cohen DS, Eloy JA, Setzen
    M, Folbe AJ. Geographic and temporal trends in
    frontal sinus surgery. Int Forum Allergy Rhinol.
    2015;5:46–54.
15. Kilic S, Shukla PA, Marchiano EJ, et al. Malignant
    primary neoplasms of the nasal cavity and paranasal
    sinus. Curr Otorhinolaryngol Rep. 2016:1–10.
16. Gourin CG, Terris DJ. Frontal sinus malignancies. In:
    The frontal sinus. Berlin/Heidelberg: Springer; 2005.
    p. 165–78.
17. Luce D, Leclerc A, Morcet JF, et al. Occupational risk
    factors for sinonasal cancer: a case-control study in
    France. Am J Ind Med. 1992;21:163–75.
18. Bishop JA, Guo TW, Smith DF, et al. Human
    papillomavirus-related carcinomas of the sinonasal
    tract. Am J Surg Pathol. 2013;37:185–92.
19. Karligkiotis A, Lepera D, Volpi L, et al. Survival out-
    comes after endoscopic resection for sinonasal squa-
    mous cell carcinoma arising on inverted papilloma.
    Head Neck. 2016;38:1604–14.
20. Zhang H-Z, Li Y-P, LEI S, et al. Primary carcinoma of
    the frontal sinus with extensive intracranial invasion:
    a case report and review of the literature. Oncol Lett.
    2014;7:1915–8.
21. Brownson RJ, Ogura JH. Primary carcinoma of the
    frontal sinus. Laryngoscope. 1971;81:71–89.
22. Koeller KK. Radiologic features of sinonasal tumors.
    Head Neck Pathol. 2016;10:1–12.
23. Lund VJ, Stammberger H, Nicolai P, et al. European
    position paper on endoscopic management of tumours
    of the nose, paranasal sinuses and skull base. Rhinol
    Suppl. 2010:1–143.
24. Vazquez A, Khan MN, Blake DM, Patel TD, Baredes
    S, Eloy JA. Sinonasal squamous cell carcinoma and
    the prognostic implications of its histologic variants:
    a population-based study. Int Forum Allergy Rhinol.
    2015;5:85–91. Wiley Online Library
25. Bernardo T, Ferreira E, Silva JC, Monteiro
    E. Sinonasal adenocarcinoma—experience of an
    oncology center. Int J Otolaryngol Head Neck Surg.
    2013;2(1):13–6.
26. Cantu G, Solero CL, Mariani L, et al. Intestinal type
    adenocarcinoma of the ethmoid sinus in wood and
    leather workers: a retrospective study of 153 cases.
    Head Neck. 2011;33:535–42.
27. D'Aguillo CM, Kanumuri VV, Khan MN, et al.
    Demographics and survival trends of sinonasal ade-
    nocarcinoma from 1973 to 2009. Int Forum Allergy
    Rhinol. 2014;4:771–6. Wiley Online Library
28. Licitra L, Suardi S, Bossi P, et al. Prediction of TP53
    status for primary cisplatin, fluorouracil, and leucovo-
    rin chemotherapy in ethmoid sinus intestinal-type
    adenocarcinoma. J Clin Oncol. 2004;22:4901–6.
29. Bossi P, Perrone F, Miceli R, et al. Tp53 status as
    guide for the management of ethmoid sinus intestinal-
    type adenocarcinoma. Oral Oncol. 2013;49:413–9.
30. Kang JH, Cho SH, Kim JP, et al. Treatment out-
    comes between concurrent chemoradiotherapy and
    combination of surgery, radiotherapy, and/or che-
    motherapy in stage III and IV maxillary sinus can-
    cer: multi-institutional retrospective analysis. J Oral
    Maxillofac Surg. 2012;70:1717–23.
31. Knegt PP, Ah-See KW, vd Velden L-A, Kerrebijn
    J. Adenocarcinoma of the ethmoidal sinus complex:

surgical debulking and topical fluorouracil may be the optimal treatment. Arch Otolaryngol Head Neck Surg. 2001;127:141–6.

32. Husain Q, Kanumuri VV, Svider PF, et al. Sinonasal adenoid cystic carcinoma systematic review of survival and treatment strategies. Otolaryngol Head Neck Surg. 2013;148:29–39.

33. Unsal AA, Chung SY, Zhou AH, Baredes S, Eloy JA. Sinonasal adenoid cystic carcinoma: a population-based analysis of 694 cases. Int Forum Allergy Rhinol. 2017;7(3):312–20.

34. Poetker DM, Toohill RJ, Loehrl TA, Smith TL. Endoscopic management of sinonasal tumors: a preliminary report. Am J Rhinol. 2005;19:307–15.

35. Nicolai P, Battaglia P, Bignami M, et al. Endoscopic surgery for malignant tumors of the sinonasal tract and adjacent skull base: a 10-year experience. Am J Rhinol. 2008;22:308–16.

36. Patel TD, Vázquez A, Patel DM, Baredes S, Eloy JA. A comparative analysis of sinonasal and salivary gland mucoepidermoid carcinoma using population-based data. Int Forum Allergy Rhinol. 2015;5:78–84. Wiley Online Library

37. Kunc M, Gabrych A, Czapiewski P, Sworczak K. Paraneoplastic syndromes in olfactory neuroblastoma. Contemp Oncol (Pozn). 2015;19:6–16.

38. Dublin AB, Bobinski M. Imaging characteristics of olfactory neuroblastoma (esthesioneuroblastoma). J Neurol Surg B Skull Base. 2016;77:001–5.

39. Som PM, Lidov M, Brandwein M, Catalano P, Biller HF. Sinonasal esthesioneuroblastoma with intracranial extension: marginal tumor cysts as a diagnostic MR finding. AJNR Am J Neuroradiol. 1994;15:1259–62.

40. Ow TJ, Bell D, Kupferman ME, DeMonte F, Hanna EY. Esthesioneuroblastoma. Neurosurg Clin N Am. 2013;24:51–65.

41. Cerilli LA, Holst VA, Brandwein MS, Stoler MH, Mills SE. Sinonasal undifferentiated carcinoma: immunohistochemical profile and lack of EBV association. Am J Surg Pathol. 2001;25:156–63.

42. Kuo P, Manes RP, Schwam ZG, Judson BL. Survival outcomes for combined modality therapy for sinonasal undifferentiated carcinoma. Otolaryngol Head Neck Surg. 2016;0194599816670146

43. Patel TD, Vazquez A, Dubal PM, Baredes S, Liu JK, Eloy JA. Sinonasal neuroendocrine carcinoma: a population-based analysis of incidence and survival. Int Forum Allergy Rhinol. 2015;5:448–53.

44. Khan MN, Kanumuri VV, Raikundalia MD, et al. Sinonasal melanoma: survival and prognostic implications based on site of involvement. Int Forum Allergy Rhinol. 2014;4:151–5.

45. Hodi FS, Corless CL, Giobbie-Harder A, et al. Imatinib for melanomas harboring mutationally activated or amplified KIT arising on mucosal, acral, and chronically sun-damaged skin. J Clin Oncol. 2013;31:3182–90.

46. Del Vecchio M, Di Guardo L, Ascierto PA, et al. Efficacy and safety of ipilimumab 3 mg/kg in patients with pretreated, metastatic, mucosal melanoma. Eur J Cancer. 2014;50:121–7.

47. Sanghvi S, Misra P, Patel NR, Kalyoussef E, Baredes S, Eloy JA. Incidence trends and long-term survival analysis of sinonasal rhabdomyosarcoma. Am J Otolaryngol. 2013;34:682–9.

48. Unsal AA, Chung SY, Unsal AB, Baredes S, Eloy JA. Sinonasal rhabdomyosarcoma: a population-based analysis. Otolaryngol Head Neck Surg. 2017;157(1):142–9.

49. Szablewski V, Neuville A, Terrier P, et al. Adult sinonasal soft tissue sarcoma: analysis of 48 cases from the French Sarcoma Group database. Laryngoscope. 2015;125:615–23.

50. Wang X, Song L, Chong V, Wang Y, Li J, Xian J. Multiparametric MRI findings of sinonasal rhabdomyosarcoma in adults with comparison to carcinoma. J Magn Reson Imaging. 2017;45:998–1004.

51. Raney RB, Maurer HM, Anderson JR, et al. The Intergroup Rhabdomyosarcoma Study Group (IRSG): major lessons from the IRS-I through IRS-IV studies as background for the current IRS-V treatment protocols. Sarcoma. 2001;5:9–15.

52. Tomovic S, Kalyoussef E, Mirani NM, Baredes S, Eloy JA. Angiosarcoma arising from the frontal sinus. Am J Otolaryngol. 2014;35:806–9.

53. Haferkamp C, Pressler H, Koitschev A. Angiosarcoma of the frontal sinus. Case report and review of the literature. HNO. 2000;48:684–8.

54. Smith MT, Latella PD, Schnee I. Angio-fibrosarcoma of the ethmoid and frontal sinuses complicated by osteomyelitis of the frontal bone and epidural abscess. Ann Otol Rhinol Laryngol. 1950;59:650–6.

55. Ulrich CT, Feiz-Erfan I, Spetzler RF, et al. Sinonasal leiomyosarcoma: review of literature and case report. Laryngoscope. 2005;115:2242–8.

56. Khan MN, Husain Q, Kanumuri VV, et al. Management of sinonasal chondrosarcoma: a systematic review of 161 patients. Int Forum Allergy Rhinol. 2013;3:670–7.

57. Quraishi MS, Bessell EM, Clark D, Jones NS, Bradley PJ. Non-Hodgkin's lymphoma of the sinonasal tract. Laryngoscope. 2000;110:1489–92.

58. Kanumuri VV, Khan MN, Vazquez A, Govindaraj S, Baredes S, Eloy JA. Diffuse large B-cell lymphoma of the sinonasal tract: analysis of survival in 852 cases. Am J Otolaryngol. 2014;35:154–8.

59. Dahodwala MQ, Husain Q, Kanumuri VV, Choudhry OJ, Liu JK, Eloy JA. Management of sinonasal hemangiopericytomas: a systematic review. Int Forum Allergy Rhinol. 2013;3:581–7.

60. Compagno J, Hyams VJ. Hemangiopericytoma-like intranasal tumors. A clinicopathologic study of 23 cases. Am J Clin Pathol. 1976;66:672–83.

61. Fletcher CD. Distinctive soft tissue tumors of the head and neck. Mod Pathol. 2002;15:324–30.

62. Eichhorn JH, Dickersin GR, Bhan AK, Goodman ML. Sinonasal hemangiopericytoma. A reassessment with electron microscopy, immunohistochemistry, and long-term follow-up. Am J Surg Pathol. 1990;14:856–66.

63. Tessema B, Eloy JA, Folbe AJ, et al. Endoscopic management of sinonasal hemangiopericytoma. Otolaryngol Head Neck Surg. 2012;146:483–6.

64. Koscielny S, Bräuer B, Förster G. Hemangiopericytoma: a rare head and neck tumor. Eur Arch Otorhinolaryngol. 2003;260:450–3.

65. Patel TD, Vázquez A, Choudhary MM, Kam D, Baredes S, Eloy JA. Sinonasal extramedullary plasmacytoma: a population-based incidence and survival analysis. Int Forum Allergy Rhinol. 2015;5:862–9. Wiley Online Library

66. D'Aguillo C, Soni RS, Gordhan C, Liu JK, Baredes S, Eloy JA. Sinonasal extramedullary plasmacytoma: a systematic review of 175 patients. Int Forum Allergy Rhinol. 2014;4:156–63. Wiley Online Library

67. Osguthorpe JD, Richardson M. Frontal sinus malignancies. Otolaryngol Clin N Am. 2001;34:269–81.

68. Balikian RV, Smith RV. Frontal sinus malignancies. Oper Tech Otolaryngol Head Neck Surg. 2004;15:42–9.

69. Selleck AM, Desai D, Thorp BD, Ebert CS, Zanation AM. Management of frontal sinus tumors. Otolaryngol Clin N Am. 2016;49:1051–65.

70. Catalano PJ, Sen C. Management of anterior ethmoid and frontal sinus tumors. Otolaryngol Clin N Am. 1995;28:1157–74.

71. Imola MJ, Schramm VL Jr. Orbital preservation in surgical management of sinonasal malignancy. Laryngoscope. 2002;112:1357–65.

72. Neel GS, Nagel TH, Hoxworth JM, Lal D. Management of orbital involvement in sinonasal and ventral skull base malignancies. Otolaryngol Clin N Am. 2017;50(2):347–64.

73. Carrau RL, Segas J, Nuss DW, et al. Squamous cell carcinoma of the sinonasal tract invading the orbit. Laryngoscope. 1999;109:230–5.

74. McCary WS, Levine PA, Cantrell RW. Preservation of the eye in the treatment of sinonasal malignant neoplasms with orbital involvement. A confirmation of the original treatise. Arch Otolaryngol Head Neck Surg. 1996;122:657–9.

75. Lal D, Cain RB. Updates in reconstruction of skull base defects. Curr Opin Otolaryngol Head Neck Surg. 2014;22(5):419–28.

Managing Frontal Sinusitis from Systemic Inflammatory Disease

19

Lester E. Mertz, Rohit Divekar, and Matthew A. Rank

Abbreviations

ACE	Angiotensin-converting enzyme
ACR	American College of Rheumatology
AERD	Aspirin-exacerbated respiratory disease
AFS	Allergic fungal sinusitis
ANCA	Anti-neutrophil cytoplasmic antibody
Anti-MPO ab	Anti-myeloperoxidase antibody
Anti-PR3 ab	Anti-proteinase 3 antibody
BVAS	Birmingham Vasculitis Activity Score
BVAS/WG	BVAS for Wegener's granulomatosis (GPA)
C-ANCA	Cytoplasmic anti-neutrophil cytoplasmic antibody
CF	Cystic fibrosis
CHCC	Chapel Hill Consensus Conference
CIMDL	Cocaine-induced midline destructive lesions syndrome
CRP	C-reactive protein
CRS	Chronic rhinosinusitis
CRSsNP	Chronic rhinosinusitis without (*sans*) nasal polyps
CRSwNP	Chronic rhinosinusitis with nasal polyps
CVID	Common variable immune deficiency
EGPA	Eosinophilic granulomatosis with polyangiitis (Churg-Strauss syndrome)
EMA	European Medical Agency
ENT	Ear, nose, and throat
ESR	Erythrocyte sedimentation rate
EULAR	European League Against Rheumatism
GPA	Granulomatosis with polyangiitis (Wegener's granulomatosis)
HEENT	Head, eye, ear, nose, and throat
HIV	Human immunodeficiency virus
Ig	Immunoglobulin
IgG4-RD	IgG4-related disease
MPA	Microscopic polyangiitis
P-ANCA	Perinuclear anti-neutrophil cytoplasmic antibody
PCD	Primary ciliary dyskinesia
TMP/SMX	Trimethoprim/sulfamethoxazole
VDI	Vasculitis damage index

L. E. Mertz (✉)
Division of Rheumatology, Department of Medicine, Mayo Clinic, Scottsdale, AZ, USA

R. Divekar
Division of Allergic Diseases, Mayo Clinic, Rochester, MN, USA

M. A. Rank
Division of Allergy, Asthma, and Clinical Immunology, Mayo Clinic, Scottsdale, AZ, USA

© Springer Nature Switzerland AG 2019
D. Lal, P. H. Hwang (eds.), *Frontal Sinus Surgery*, https://doi.org/10.1007/978-3-319-97022-6_19

Introduction

Optimizing medical management of chronic rhinosinusitis (CRS) should be preceded by a careful approach to diagnosing the cause or type of CRS. In this chapter, we will focus on CRS that can manifest as chronic frontal sinusitis with a special focus on autoimmune and granulomatous diseases. Maintaining a broad differential diagnosis while keeping in mind that the most common causes of frontal sinusitis are localized CRS [with or without nasal polyposis (CRSwNP/CRSsNP)], we propose an evaluation that starts with an assessment of symptoms beyond the upper airway, a review of endoscopic and imaging findings, a review of response to previous interventions, and a routine physical examination. Not all patients presenting with CRS need an exhaustive evaluation. For example, a patient with local symptoms of nasal congestion and hyposmia only, pansinusitis on imaging, and nasal polyps on exam who is improved following endoscopic sinus surgery and topical corticosteroids is less likely to benefit from an exhaustive evaluation for systemic disease beyond the usual history and physical examination. In fact, the majority of patients presenting with CRS will not have a systemic disease related to the CRS. Learning the common and distinguishing features of systemic diseases that can present with CRS will help determine when to perform additional diagnostic evaluations.

Diagnosis of CRS

The first step is confirming the diagnosis of CRS. Headache disorders can commonly mimic CRS, and therefore reviewing all previous CT and MRI scans of the frontal sinuses, including those prior to any surgical intervention, is very helpful to confirm diagnosis [1]. In addition to confirming the diagnosis, the patterns seen on imaging can help begin the diagnostic process. We present Fig. 19.1 as an algorithmic, initial approach to abnormal imaging findings of the frontal sinuses. Additional laboratory tests should be considered in medically and surgically recalcitrant disease. Patients with osteitis on imaging without any prior history of surgery should also be investigated. Tests that are helpful include complete blood count with differential CBC/diff; C-reactive protein (CRP); sedimentation rate (ESR); immunoglobulins A, G, E, and M; angiotensin-converting enzyme (ACE); antineutrophil cytoplasmic antibodies (ANCA); vitamin D; specific antibody responses for tetanus, diphtheria, and pneumococcus; human immunodeficiency virus (HIV) screen; T and B cell quantitation; cystic fibrosis (CF) testing (sweat chloride and/or genetic); and IgE to staphylococcal enterotoxins. Strong consideration should be given to performing aeroallergen testing in recalcitrant disease. Cultures should be taken with endoscopic guidance when purulence is noted and during surgical procedures. These can be sent for aerobic, anaerobic, and fungal growth. Biopsies can be obtained from the sinonasal mucosa to rule out features of vasculitis. It is important to note that frank vasculitis is often not seen on mucosal biopsy even in patients with documented systemic vasculitis so that absence of vasculitis on biopsy is not proof of absence of a systemic vasculitic disorder. A structured histopathology report of ethmoid tissue removed at surgery can be very helpful to characterize the severity and features of inflammation [2].

Recognizing Patterns of Systemic Diseases Associated with Chronic Frontal Sinusitis

Autoimmune and Granulomatous Diseases

Background

The syndromes of eosinophilic granulomatosis with polyangiitis (EGPA, formerly Churg-Strauss syndrome), granulomatosis with polyangiitis (GPA, formerly Wegener's granulomatosis), IgG4-related disease (IgG4-RD), sarcoidosis, and cocaine-induced midline destructive lesions (CIMDL) include prominent otolaryngologic features. Otorhinolaryngologists should be familiar with these pathologies, as patients may ini-

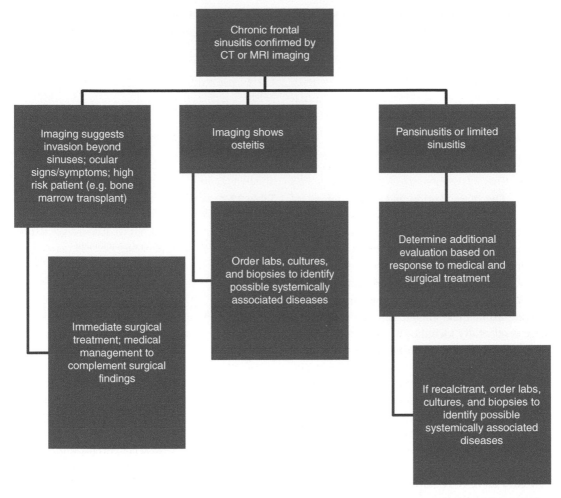

Fig. 19.1 The slide presents an algorithmic, initial approach to abnormal imaging findings of the frontal sinuses. Tests should be considered appropriate to the clinical context

tially present to them prior to a formal diagnosis. Additional ENT symptoms commonly develop later in the clinical course. Serious multisite and systemic manifestations of these syndromes may occur coincident or subsequent to the ENT features. Among the otolaryngologic manifestations of these syndromes, CRS is common.

Recognition of these disease entities can be difficult as these conditions are rare and uncommonly encountered in a routine ENT practice. Table 19.1 summarizes recent incidence and prevalence estimates of these conditions in the general population. Although sarcoidosis is more common than EGPA or GPA, CRS is more often a feature of GPA and EGPA than sarcoidosis.

IgG4-RD is a recently identified systemic fibro-inflammatory disorder with rough prevalence estimates available only from Japan. CIMDL is encountered only in the population of cocaine users. The volume of literature addressing the ENT manifestations of EGPA and GPA greatly exceeds that of CIMDL, sarcoidosis, and IgG4-RD and is reflected in the relative extent of coverage below.

Pathogenesis

EGPA

ANCA-associated vasculitis conditions include GPA, MPA (microscopic polyangiitis), and

Table 19.1 Epidemiology of immune-mediated and granulomatous causes of CRS

Disorder	Incidence[a]		Prevalence[a]	
EGPA	1.5	UK[b]	10.7	France[c]
GPA	8.2	UK[b]	23.7	France[c]
CIMDL	Rare (cocaine users)		Rare	
Sarcoidosis	178	USA Black[d]	1414	USA Black[d]
	81	USA White[d]	217	USA White[d]
	100	USA[e]		
IgG4-RD	Unknown		2.8–10.8	Japan[f]

[a]Per 1,000,000 population, [b][3], [c][4], [d][5], [e][6], [f][7]

EGPA. The classification and epidemiology of these disorders have recently been summarized [8]. The manifestations of EGPA are preceded by asthma and allergic rhinitis in 90–100% of patients, representing the first stage of this disorder [9]. Although rare in the general population, the incidence is much higher in patients with pre-existing asthma and allergic rhinitis. The second stage is generally identified by progressive eosinophilia associated with eosinophilic tissue infiltration that may affect the lungs and heart and may lead to cardiomyopathy. Patients may progress to a third stage, inconsistently associated with the appearance of an ANCA, when vasculitis most often affects the skin, peripheral nerves, and kidneys. Not all patients with ANCA have clinical vasculitis, and not all patients with vasculitis have an ANCA although in one study of 31 patients with EGPA-associated renal disease, and all 16 patients with crescentic necrotizing GN (renal vasculitis) were ANCA positive [10]. The pathogenesis and mechanism of EGPA evolution are unknown but are likely analogous to GPA (below) with the vasculitic and eosinophilic components distinct aspects of one pathologic process [11]. Eosinophil extracellular trap cell death (ETosis) may be involved in eosinophilic disorders in general [12] but has not been directly implicated in the pathogenesis of EGPA [13]. All vasculitis disorders, including EGPA and GPA, manifest both active inflammation and irreversible damage that are quantitated by the BVAS (Birmingham Vasculitis Activity Score) [14] and VDI (Vasculitis Damage Index) [15], respectively, which both include ENT specific sub-scores (Table 19.2). A specific BVAS exists for GPA (BVAS/WG), but there is no EGPA-specific

Table 19.2 ANCA-associated vasculitis ENT activity and damage sub-scores

BVAS version 3 ENT sub-score[a]	(a) Bloody nasal discharge/crusts/ulcers/granulomata
	(b) Paranasal sinus involvement
	(c) Subglottic stenosis
	(d) Conductive hearing loss
	(e) Sensorineural hearing loss
BVAS/WG ENT sub-score[b]	(a) Bloody nasal discharge/nasal crusting or ulcer
	(b) Sinus involvement
	(c) Swollen salivary gland
	(d) Subglottic inflammation
	(e) Conductive deafness
	(f) Sensorineural deafness
VDI ENT sub-score[c]	1. Hearing loss
	2. Nasal blockage or discharge or crusting
	3. Nasal bridge collapse or septal perforation
	4. Chronic sinusitis or radiologic evidence of bone destruction
	5. Subglottic stenosis without surgery
	6. Subglottic stenosis with surgery

[a][14], [b][16], [c][15]

BVAS. The Five-Factor Score developed in earlier EGPA studies [18, 19] is predictive of mortality in some studies but not all [20–22]. Interestingly, ENT involvement in EGPA predicts less morbidity and mortality.

GPA

A more frequent disorder, GPA, has been more thoroughly studied than EGPA. Unlike EGPA, GPA is not preceded by a well-defined clinical prodrome although approximately 75% of patients manifest head and neck symptoms at initial diagnosis, including rhinosinusitis in approximate one-half [23, 24]. Chronic sinonasal carriage and infection with *Staphylococcus aureus* have been associated with a more frequent initial sinonasal presentation of GPA, increased sinonasal GPA activity, and increased risk of systemic relapses [25–30]. A role for staphylococcal toxic shock syndrome toxin-1 has been suggested [31], and this superantigen or other staphylococcal antigens may contribute to the pathogenesis when detected by mucosal antigen-presenting cells subsequently leading to immune system stimulation and both B cell (ANCA) and T cell (granuloma) responses [32]. Peculiarly, however, patients with GPA demonstrate a lower anti-staphylococcal antibody response than healthy controls [33]. Furthermore, transcriptional profiling of genes associated with antimicrobial defense mechanisms and epithelial barrier function performed on nasal biopsy specimens was found to be independent of nasal *Staphylococcus aureus* colonization, suggesting that such colonization may be the consequence rather than the cause of the disturbed nasal mucosal barrier function [34]. The exact role of *Staphylococcus aureus* in the pathogenesis of GPA remains uncertain, and the mechanism of TMP/SMX in preventing relapses of GPA in remission remains unclear [29]. Importantly, TMP/SMX alone or with prednisone was found to be inferior to methotrexate in maintaining remission [35].

Anti-neutrophil cytoplasmic antibodies, the defining feature of ANCA-associated vasculitides, are considered directly pathogenic in MPA (anti-MPO ab predominantly) and possibly EGPA but less clearly so in GPA (anti-PR3 ab predominantly) where both B cell and T cell inflammatory responses are characteristic [36]. Anti-MPO-positive and anti-PR3-positive patients with vasculitis differ not only in genetic background but also response to treatment, suggesting a different pathogenesis for patients in these two autoantibody groups [37]. Importantly, the serum concentration of ANCA is not always a reliable predictor of disease severity nor risk of relapse, and the benefit of plasma exchange, a logical treatment for an antibody-mediated disorder, is unproven and remains the subject of ongoing research [38].

Interpreting the clinical features of GPA is further complicated by the coexistence of both inflammatory activity that responds to immune suppression and also chronic postinflammatory damage and secondary infection that do not respond to immune suppression [14, 15, 38, 39]. Inflammatory activity may be either vasculitic or granulomatous in nature, and these two inflammatory components may not respond identically to treatment, the granulomatous component appearing more refractory to treatment in some but not all reports [40–43]. As for EGPA, GPA vasculitis activity is summarized by the Birmingham Vasculitis Activity Score, modified for GPA (BVAS/WG) [16], and damage is summarized by the VDI. Neutrophil extracellular trap cell death (NETosis) may be involved in both the initial ANCA immune response and subsequent pathogenesis [44, 45]. Similar to EGPA, ENT involvement in GPA predicts a less severe disease course and longer survival possibly due to earlier disease diagnosis in patients with ENT symptoms or the granulomatous nature of ENT involvement predicting less serious vasculitic manifestations affecting the lungs and kidneys [46].

CIMDL

Sinonasal and systemic inflammatory complications arise from chronic nasal insufflation of cocaine and may be exacerbated by the presence of levamisole used as an adulterant. Both local and widespread tissue destruction is common. The diagnosis of CIMDL is relatively straightforward in a patient known to use cocaine, but when use is concealed, CIMDL may be confused with GPA due to the similar sinonasal destructive lesions and presence of ANCA [47–49]. Levamisole, an antihelminthic but also an immune system stimulator and antineoplastic agent, contributes agranulocytosis to the clinical picture. Cocaine itself has vasoconstrictive and immune-stimulating effects [49, 50]. Hypothetically, nasal mucosal damage initially induced by cocaine may lead to ANCA production in genetically susceptible individuals, exacerbated by the immune-stimulating effect of levamisole and further modulated by local *Staphylococcus aureus* infection.

Sarcoidosis

Identification of noncaseating (almost exclusively non-necrotizing) granulomatous inflammation on a tissue biopsy specimen in the setting of typical multi-organ involvement without credible evidence of an alternative granulomatous disorder verifies a diagnosis of sarcoidosis with the highest certainty [51]. Lacking a truly specific diagnostic test, the diagnosis of sarcoidosis may be highly probable, probable, possible, or unlikely [52, 53]. The proposed pathogenesis of sarcoidosis is suspected to resemble that of other granulomatous disorders such as tuberculosis, and although an antigenic stimulus for sarcoidosis is highly suspected, no microorganism or environmental antigen has been clearly identified [54]. Formation of granulomas requires the influence of the innate and adaptive immune systems and involves T lymphocytes, dendritic cells, macrophages, fibroblasts, B lymphocytes, and cytokines [55]. ENT involvement is presumed to follow the same pathogenesis as that hypothesized to occur in other anatomic locations. A secure diagnosis of isolated sinonasal involvement is difficult since many patients with sarcoidosis are asymptomatic, and such localized disease would not constitute the multi-organ involvement typical of sarcoidosis. The identification of noncaseating granulomatous inflammation on sinonasal biopsy should initiate an investigation for additional organ involvement supportive of the diagnosis of sarcoidosis or perhaps an alternative granulomatous disorder [56]. Identifying patients with sarcoidosis may be difficult since many are clinically asymptomatic, the diagnosis made during evaluation of incidentally identified pulmonary adenopathy.

IgG4-RD

Relatively recently identified, IgG4-RD was first described in 2003 on the background of autoimmune pancreatitis type 1 with widespread organ involvement subsequently identified [57–59]. IgG4-RD may affect one or more organs simultaneously or sequentially, and similar to sarcoidosis, a secure diagnosis of IgG4-RD is based on histopathology, specifically biopsy evidence of dense lymphoplasmacytic inflammation, storiform fibrosis, obliterative phlebitis, and eosinophilic infiltrates in association with typical clinical manifestations and after exclusion of clinically similar disorders. Histopathology varies to some extent as a function of the anatomic biopsy site and age of the lesion, fibrosis more often identified in chronic lesions. The diagnosis is often supported by identifying eosinophilia, elevated serum IgE and IgG4, and circulating IgG4-positive plasmablasts. However, a recent report suggested that only histopathology distinguished patients experiencing ENT symptoms from GPA, CIMDL, and IgG4-RD [60]. Diagnostic criteria for IgG4-RD have been proposed but not verified [7]. Head and neck features are very common and characteristic [61]. In contrast, sinonasal IgG4-RD has only recently received attention and appears to be an uncommon disorder sharing similarities with eosinophilic chronic rhinosinusitis (ECRS) and is the subject of case reports and diagnostic uncertainty [62–65]. Genetic, microbiological, and autoimmune contributors to the etiology and pathogenesis of IgG4-RD have been proposed but not confirmed [66].

Suspecting Immune-Mediated and Granulomatous Causes of CRS

Algorithms for diagnosing and treating CRS recommend an assessment for an underlying granulomatous disorder such as GPA and EGPA in treatment-resistant patients with CRSsNP but not treatment-resistant CRSwNP [67]. However, many patients with EGPA have nasal polyps, and therefore we do not use the presence or absence of nasal polyps to determine further evaluation for immune-mediated and granulomatous causes of CRS in our practice. Instead, we use disease recalcitrance to usual CRS treatments as the primary factor when deciding on further workup for immune-mediated and granulomatous causes of CRS. The differential diagnosis of sinonasal granulomatous disorders has been reviewed and includes trauma, substance abuse, infections, neoplasms, and inflammatory and autoimmune disorders [68, 69].

Recently, a population-based case-control study was reported assessing the 5-year incidence of additional new disease diagnoses subsequent to the initial diagnosis of CRSsNP and CRSwNP. The study protocol included a specific search for autoimmune disorders [70]. The much larger group of patients with CRSsNP were at greater risk than the smaller group of patients with CRSwNP for upper airway diseases including adenotonsillitis, lower aerodigestive tract diseases including asthma, and also epithelial conditions including atopic dermatitis and hypertension. Crohn's disease, ulcerative colitis, rheumatoid arthritis, and systemic lupus erythematosus were identified in patients with CRSsNP at the same rate as controls, but no cases of GPA, EGPA, sarcoidosis, or other systemic conditions were found.

Patients presenting to a university ENT department with CRS are more likely to be diagnosed with a granulomatous disorder such as GPA, EGPA, or sarcoidosis. Of 49 consecutive patients with refractory CRS and indications for sinonasal surgery, 10% tested positive for ANCA, one was diagnosed with GPA, and a second appeared to be evolving EGPA [71]. One hundred eighty patients with CRSsNP and 200 patients with CRSwNP undergoing endoscopic sinus surgery were analyzed to determine the correlation of the preoperative clinical diagnosis and the postoperative histopathologic diagnosis. Sarcoidosis was identified in two patients with CRSsNP and in one patient with CRSwNP [72].

Clinical Manifestations of EGPA, GPA, CIMDL, Sarcoidosis, and IgG4-RD

Initial and cumulative head and neck and initial and cumulative sinonasal features are summarized in Table 19.3. These manifestations were not uniformly recorded in each report and some

values are calculated or estimated from the data presented. EGPA and GPA are frequently heralded by head, neck, and specifically sinonasal manifestations. Nearly all patients with CIMDL present with sinonasal features and many with additional head and neck manifestations. Sarcoidosis uncommonly leads to head and neck manifestations with wide estimates of involvement from different authors. In contrast, IgG4-RD commonly presents with head and neck involvement, but sinonasal involvement is only recently being reported.

A suspicion that one of these disorders may explain a patient's sinonasal symptoms will come to mind when correlating the specific nature of the sinonasal symptoms with typical abnormalities on examination, the presence of other HEENT manifestations, and possibly a history of an existing or suspicion of an undiagnosed systemic disorder. Table 19.4 presents a comparison of the sinonasal, HEENT, and systemic features of each disorder. Sinonasal features are similar for EGPA, GPA, CIMDL, sarcoidosis, and IgG4-RD with notable exceptions that may be helpful in the clinical diagnostic evaluation of patients with these manifestations. EGPA rarely leads to sinonasal destructive lesions which occur in descending order of severity in CIMDL, GPA, sarcoidosis, and IgG4-RD. GPA and CIMDL are associated with nasal septal perforation and "saddle nose" deformity (Fig. 19.2), while this occurs rarely in EGPA and sarcoidosis and never in IgG4-RD. Both EGPA and IgG4-RD often include symptoms of allergic rhinosinusitis preceding or coincident with other manifestations. Neo-osteogenesis occurs only with chronic inflammation associated with GPA (see Fig. 19.3). Polyps are commonly identified in EGPA (see Fig. 19.4 for an endoscopic image from a patient with EGPA), occasionally in sarcoidosis, and rarely in IgG4-RD. Sialoadenitis, dacryoadenitis, retro-orbital inflammation and masses as well as lower airway and pulmonary masses are features of GPA, sarcoidosis, and IgG4-RD. Lymphadenopathy is uncommon in

Table 19.3 Initial and cumulative head, neck, and sinonasal manifestations of EGPA, GPA, CIMDL, sarcoidosis, and IgG4-RD

Disorder	Head and neck initial (% cases)	Head and neck cumulative (% cases)	Sinonasal initial (% cases)	Sinonasal cumulative (% cases)
EGPA	46.4%[a]	75%[a]	46.4%[a]	75%[a]
GPA	90%[d]	95%[d]		
	63%[b]		41%[b]	
	82%[c]		68%[c]	
	73%[e]	92%[e]	50%[e]	85%[e]
CIMDL	Unknown	44%[f]	100%[g]	Unknown
Sarcoidosis	Uncommon	1%–6%[h] 10%[i] 30%[j] 38%[k]	Uncommon	Uncommon
IgG4-RD	Common[m,n,o]	Common[m,n,o]	Unknown	55.7%[l]

Refs [a][17], [b][73], [c][74], [d][75], [e][23], [f][48], [g][47], [h][76], [i][77], [j][78], [k][79], [l][63], [m][80], [n][57], [o][61]

EGPA, GPA, and CIMDL but common in sarcoidosis and IgG4-RD. Features of vasculitis are seen in EGPA, GPA, and CIMDL. Significant gastrointestinal involvement is highly suggestive of IgG4-RD but rarely occurs in EGPA.

Radiographic Features of EGPA, GPA, CIMDL, Sarcoidosis, and IgG4-RD

Radiographic imaging of sinuses confirms the clinical and endoscopic features and accurately displays the extent of sinus inflammation and mucosal thickening as well as nasal and paranasal sinus destruction if present. Neo-osteogenesis is specific to GPA. Computed tomography accurately demonstrates lower airway and pulmonary features for all systemic disorders under discussion. Sarcoidosis may be associated with subtle lytic or sclerotic lesions of the skull bones, including the nasal bones (Fig. 19.5), in addition to the characteristic "dactylitis" of the fingers. Both a ^{67}Ga-citrate scan and an ^{18}F-FDG PET/CT scan may identify inflammation involving the lacrimal glands, salivary glands, and intrathoracic lymph nodes that may accompany sarcoidosis or IgG4-RD although the appearance is not specific for either of these disorders (see Table 19.5). Polypoid lesions that are contrast enhancing with CT or MR imaging should raise suspicion for tumors as well as IgG4-RD, which is characterized by tumefactive lesions (Fig. 19.6).

Laboratory Features of EGPA, GPA, CIMDL, Sarcoidosis, and IgG4-RD

The estimated sensitivity and specificity for the laboratory diagnosis of these systemic disorders vary significantly depending on the population under study (community versus referral center patients, varying ethnic distribution), study case finding definition, disease extent (limited versus extensive), and treatment history (pre- and post-treatment). CIMDL is uncommon enough that a large body of data for analysis is nonexistent, and IgG4-RD is new enough that reliable data are just being published. Table 19.6 presents a list of laboratory tests commonly used for the diagnosis of these disorders with sensitivity estimates. Typical of all systemic disorders that demonstrate variable manifestations in different organs over time or possibly multiple simultaneous symptoms at presentation, the diagnosis often ultimately relies on synthesis of the clinical, laboratory, radiographic, and histopathologic data in total.

The erythrocyte sedimentation rate and C-reactive protein are often elevated in all conditions depending on severity but nonspecifically indicate an inflammatory condition. ANCA testing is usually positive in GPA and CIMDL, less often in EGPA, and rarely if ever in sarcoidosis and IgG4-RD. Eosinophilia is usually present in EGPA and frequently in IgG4-RD. Serum IgE and IgG4 are often elevated in EGPA and IgG4-RD. Complement proteins are normal or

Table 19.4 Sinonasal, ENT and systemic manifestations of Common Autoimmune Pathology

Disorder	Sinonasal	HEENT	Systemic
EGPA[a, b, c, d, e, f, g]	Rhinorrhea, hyposmia, allergic rhinosinusitis, mucosal edema and crusting, nasal obstruction and polyps, synechia, nasal septal perforation (rare) Secondary infection	Mastoiditis, episcleritis, ischemic optic neuropathy, otitis media, conductive hearing loss, sensorineural hearing loss, laryngitis (rare)	*Common*: fever, weight loss, asthma, vasculitic cranial and peripheral neuropathy, cutaneous vasculitis, pauci-immune glomerulonephritis, arthralgia, arthritis *Less common*: pericarditis, endocarditis, myocarditis, alveolar hemorrhage, eosinophilic gastroenteritis, GI vasculitis *Rare*: lymphadenopathy, extravascular necrotizing granuloma, CVA, CNS hemorrhage
GPA[i, j, k, l]	Rhinorrhea, hyposmia, rhinosinusitis, mucosal edema and crusting, nasal obstruction, friable and granular mucosal erosions, purulent nasal mucosal ulcers, epistaxis, nasal chondritis, nasal septal perforation, nasal bridge collapse("saddle"), osseous paranasal sinus erosion, paranasal sinus neo-osteogenesis Secondary infection	Mastoiditis, sialoadenitis, dacryocystitis, epiphora, scleritis, episcleritis, retinal vasculitis, ischemic optic neuropathy, retro-orbital mass, proptosis, diplopia, otitis media, otorrhea, auricular chondritis, conductive hearing loss, sensorineural hearing loss, gingivitis, laryngitis, cough, dyspnea, glottitis, subglottic mass, subglottic stenosis Secondary infection	*Common*: cutaneous vasculitis, pauci-immune glomerulonephritis, alveolar hemorrhage; pulmonary infiltrates, fibrosis, nodules or masses; vasculitic cranial and peripheral neuropathy *Less common*: fever, weight loss, granulomatous masses (any site), tracheal and bronchial mass and stenosis; mediastinal and hilar lymphadenopathy, pericarditis, myocarditis, arthralgia, arthritis *Rare*: peripheral lymphadenopathy, meningitis, CNS mass lesions, hypophysitis, diabetes insipidus, CVA, GI vasculitis
CIMDL[m, n, o]	Rhinorrhea, hyposmia, rhinosinusitis, nasal obstruction, epistaxis, mucosal ulcers, crusting and scabs, nasal septal perforation, nasal bridge collapse ("saddle"), centrifugal osseous paranasal sinus destruction Secondary infection	Facial pain, dacryocystitis, hard and soft palate erosion and perforation, orbital destruction, central facial purpura, ecchymosis of nose and ears, oropharyngeal ulcers Secondary infection	*Common*: facial, truncal and extremity cutaneous retiform ecchymosis and ulcers; thrombotic and vasculitic purpura, fevers, sweats *Less common*: weight loss, arthralgia, myalgia *Rare*: alveolar hemorrhage, glomerulonephritis

(continued)

Table 19.4 (continued)

Disorder	Sinonasal	HEENT	Systemic
Sarcoidosis[h, p, q, r, s]	Lupus pernio, rhinorrhea, hyposmia, rhinosinusitis, nasal obstruction, epistaxis, mucosal crusting and friability, mucosal plaques, nodules and polyps, nasal septal perforation (rare), nasal bridge collapse(rare) Secondary infection	Sialoadenitis, dacryoadenitis, epiphora, keratoconjunctivitis, uveitis, retro-orbital mass, proptosis, otitis media, sensorineural hearing loss (rare), oral erosions and fistula (rare), dysphagia, laryngitis, cough, dyspnea, recurrent laryngeal nerve compression, tracheal stenosis (rare)	*Common*: fatigue, granulomatous inflammation (any site), Lofgren's syndrome, lymphadenopathy (any site), erythema nodosum, cutaneous plaques, nodules and papules; hilar adenopathy, granulomatous bronchitis, nodules and masses; pulmonary interstitial fibrosis *Less common*: lupus pernio, small airway obstruction, reactive airway disease, bronchiectasis, post-obstructive atelectasis, pulmonary bullae, cardiac arrhythmia, cardiomyopathy *Rare*: fever, Heerfordt's syndrome (uveoparotid fever), hepatomegaly, splenomegaly, nephritis, nephrolithiasis, arthritis, myositis, vasculitis, osteolytic cysts, meningitis, cranial and peripheral neuropathy, hypophysitis
IgG4-RD[t, u, v, w, x, y, z]	Allergic rhinosinusitis, mucosal crusting and erosion, nasal polyps, nasal mucosal mass (rare), osseous paranasal sinus destruction (rare)	"Mikulicz's disease," "Küttner's tumor," sialoadenitis, dacryoadenitis, labial salivary gland involvement, retro-orbital mass, orbital myositis, nasopharyngitis, nasopharyngeal mass, laryngeal mass, tracheobronchial mass	*Common*: lymphoplasmacytic mass (any site), lymphadenopathy (any site), pancreatitis, allergies, reactive airway disease, cutaneous plaques, papules and nodules; pleuritis, pleural and pulmonary masses, interstitial fibrosis, retroperitoneal mass and fibrosis, periaortitis, aortitis *Less common*: fever, cholangitis, mesenteritis, interstitial nephritis *Rare*: weight loss, arthritis, pericarditis, meningitis, Riedel and Hashimoto's thyroiditis, hypophysitis

elevated (due to inflammation) in patients with EGPA, GPA, and sarcoidosis but are occasionally low in CIMDL and IgG4-RD. Typical of other drug-induced syndromes, patients with CIMDL may display a variety of autoantibodies. Patients with sarcoidosis present unique laboratory abnormalities considered consequences of activation of histiocytes and macrophages.

Each disorder is associated with typical histopathologic features that are clearly evident in a sufficiently large biopsy specimen from typical anatomic sites, but such features are less often present on the small biopsy specimens obtained from the nasal or sinus mucosa. However, a nasal mucosal biopsy suggestive of one of these disorders may be crucial in making a diagnosis even if all typical pathologic features are not present.

Occasionally, repeated biopsies over time eventually demonstrate helpful pathologic features. Necrotizing granulomatous inflammation is typical of EGPA and GPA, but non-necrotizing/non-caseating granulomatous inflammation is characteristic of sarcoidosis. GPA and CIMDL may be difficult to distinguish histopathologically on nasal or sinus biopsy since both demonstrate necrosis, and the additional features typical of GPA including granulomatous inflammation and vasculitis are often not seen simultaneously in a single biopsy specimen. Eosinophils are common histopathologic findings in EGPA and IgG4-RD and less often in GPA. IgG4 plasma cells in large number are typical of IgG4-RD but also visualized in EGPA and GPA in numbers similar to that seen in chronic sinusitis with eosinophilia.

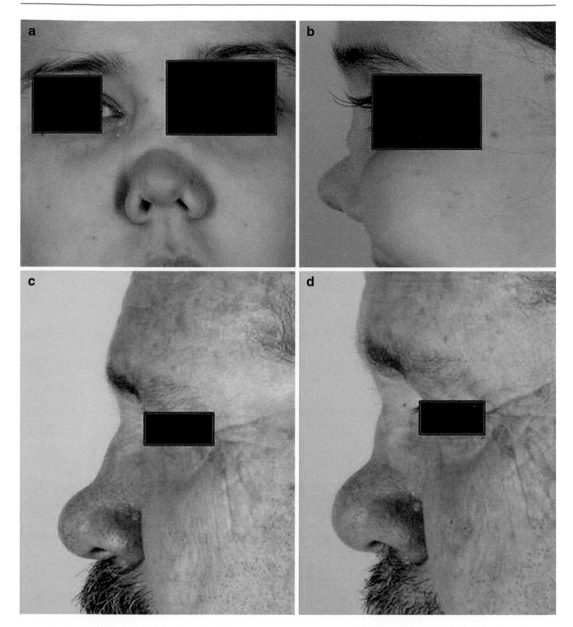

Fig. 19.2 Patients with granulomatosis with polyangiitis showing sequelae: (**a**) Right chronic dacryocystitis with tearing and drainage with anterior view of a saddle nose deformity. (**b**) Lateral view of a saddle nose deformity. (**c**, **d**) Worsening of saddle nose over a 10-month period in a middle-aged male patient

Diagnosing EGPA, GPA, CIMDL, Sarcoidosis, and IgG4-RD

Disease definitions, classification criteria, and diagnostic criteria distill the clinical manifestations along with the radiographic, laboratory, and histopathology features into functional summaries. These exist for EGPA and GPA, are preliminary for IgG4-RD, and are not formalized for sarcoidosis and CIMDL. References to these definitions and criteria are organized in Table 19.7. Definitions provide a conceptual but not clinically pragmatic framework that summarizes critical epidemiologic, clinical, laboratory, histopathologic, and pathogenic knowledge that

Fig. 19.3 Plain sinus CT coronal images depicting extensive osteitis which is a hallmark of granulomatosis with polyangiitis. This patient had several sinus surgery a decade ago prior to presenting work management of acute dacryocystitis

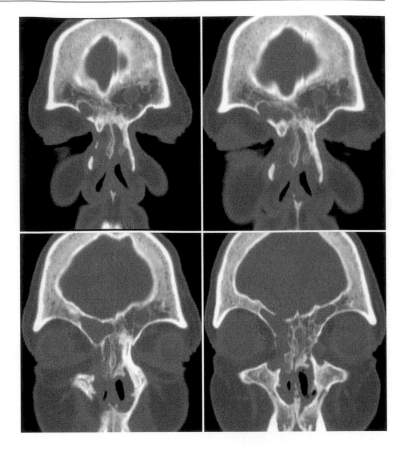

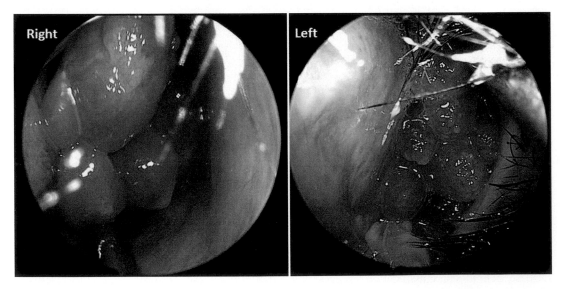

Fig. 19.4 Endoscopic image showing bilateral florid nasal polyposis in a patient with eosinophilic granulomatous polyangiitis. The patient was noted to have eosinophilia and asthma; subsequent testing was positive for pANCA

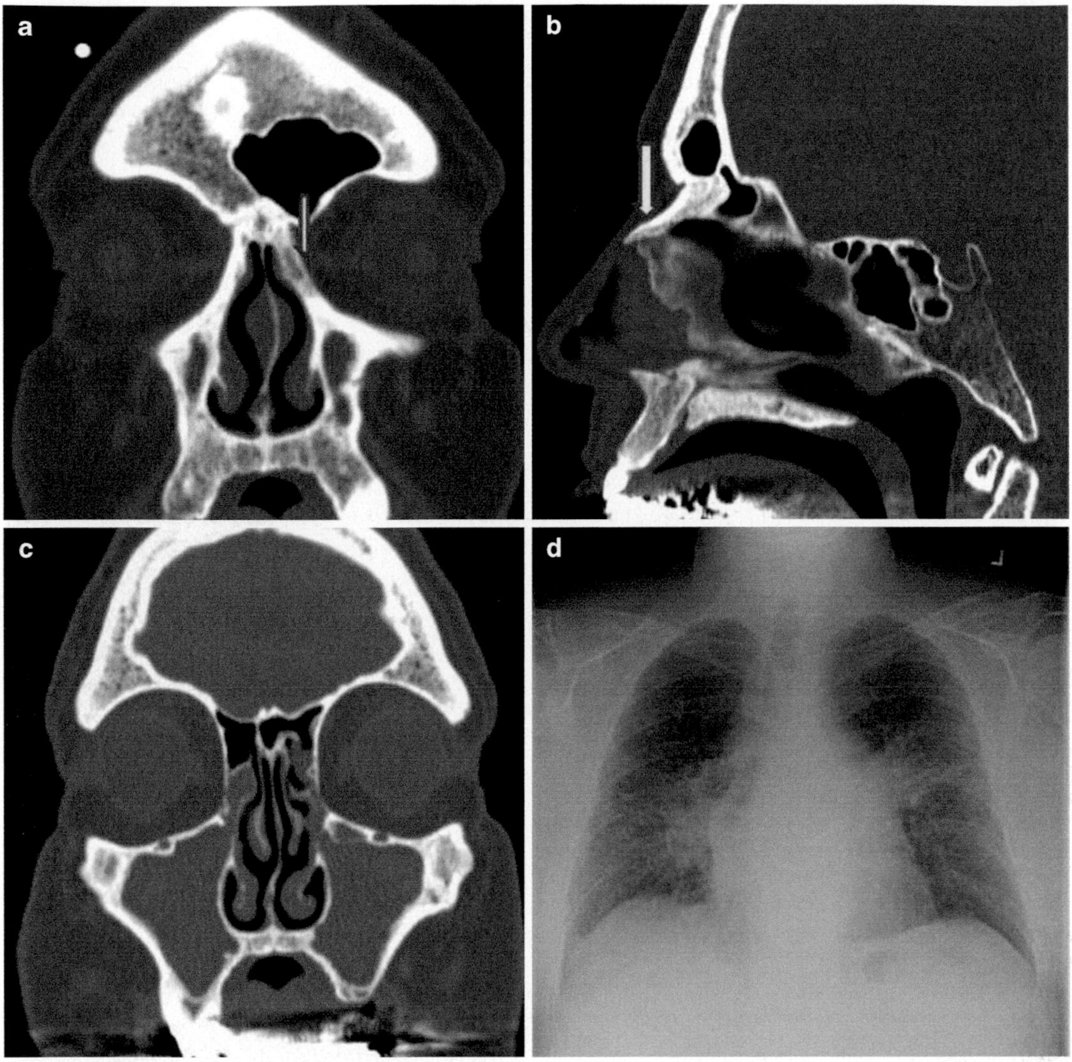

Fig. 19.5 Sinus CT imaging in a patient with known sarcoidosis. (**a**, **b**) Sarcoidosis may be associated with asymmetrical, asymptomatic lytic lesion of the skull bones, including the nasal bone (arrows). Sclerotic lesions (dotted white arrow) of variable size. (**c**) CT imaging of sinuses shows opacification; there are no imaging characteristics specific to sarcoidosis. (**d**) Bilateral hilar lymphadenopathy with right paratracheal nodal enlargement in the chest X-ray of the same patient

define typical features of the disorder that distinguish it from similar disorders. Classification criteria incorporate these definitions but are designed to select a highly homogenous group of patients from among similar disorders for clinical study purposes and are usually too restrictive for clinical use. Diagnostic criteria are the most difficult to construct for systemic illnesses since these illnesses often present dissimilar sets of manifestations in different patients all with the same diagnosis. Diagnostic criteria must account for permutations of all of the clinical, radiographic, and laboratory data that may support the diagnosis in a specific patient [115]. Practically, since diagnostic criteria are not defined for these disorders, classification criteria are often used as a surrogate, recognizing that classification criteria exclude patients with early disease or with an incomplete presentation. For example, the Chapel Hill Consensus Conference (CHCC) definition of

Table 19.5 Radiographic features of EGPA, GPA, CIMDL, sarcoidosis, and IgG4-RD

Disease	Sinus CT/MRI	General radiology
EGPA	Mucosal thickening all sinuses. Middle ear opacification. Mastoid opacification. Nasal septal or paranasal sinus destruction (rare)[a,b]	*Pulmonary*: Bilateral interstitial and alveolar infiltrates and nodules, pleural effusion[c] *Angiography*: Medium vessel stenosis, microaneurysm[d]
GPA	Mucosal thickening, paranasal sinus osteitis, bone erosion and destruction, paranasal neo-osteogenesis, nasal septal or paranasal sinus destruction[e]	*Pulmonary*: Infiltrates/nodules/cavities, mediastinal and hilar adenopathy, pleural effusion[f,g,h] *Upper airway*: Circumferential airway mucosal thickening, subglottic stenosis, airway mass *Head* Orbital mass, basilar meningitis, mastoiditis, otitis *Brain*: Cerebral vasculitis[e]
CIMDL	Rhinosinusitis with centrifugal nasal and sinus cartilage and bone destruction, tonsillar enlargement, otitis media[i]	*Pulmonary*: Infiltrates suggesting alveolar hemorrhage (rare)
Sarcoidosis	Mucosal thickening, nasal septum and turbinate nodules, sinus opacification, nasal and paranasal sinus destruction, osteosclerosis[j,k]	*Pulmonary*: Endobronchial cobble stone lesions, atelectasis, bullae, fibrosis, bronchiectasis, air trapping, hilar adenopathy *Upper airway*: Laryngeal or tracheal stenosis *Gallium scan* Panda sign *18F-FDG PET/CT* Lambda sign[l,m]
IgG4-RD	Nasal polyp (rare), mucosal thickening, nasal and paranasal bone destruction (rare)[o]	*Pulmonary*: Nodules, bronchovascular infiltrates, interstitial infiltrates, ground glass opacities *Head*: Lacrimal gland enlargement, salivary gland enlargement, EOM enlargement, thyromegaly *Abdomen*: Retroperitoneal mass, aortic wall thickening, pancreatic enlargement *Brain*: Dural thickening, pituitary enlargement[n]

[a][93], [b][94], [c][20], [d][81], [e][95], [f][96], [g][97], [h][98], [i][86], [j][76], [k][99], [l][100], [m][101], [n][66]

GPA is "necrotizing granulomatous inflammation usually involving the upper and lower respiratory tract, and necrotizing vasculitis affecting predominantly small to medium vessels (e.g., capillaries, venules, arterioles, arteries and veins). Necrotizing glomerulonephritis is common." This definition is not as clinically helpful as the four American College of Rheumatology (ACR) classification (not diagnostic) criteria for Wegener's granulomatosis (GPA) which are:

1. Nasal or oral inflammation defined as development of painful or painless oral ulcers or purulent or bloody nasal discharge

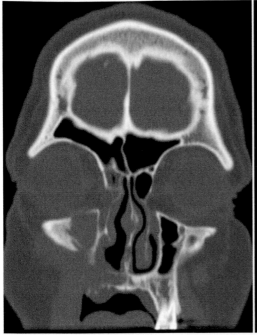

| CT without contrast | T1-weighted MRI with Gadolinium |

Fig. 19.6 These images belong to a patient that had multiple sinus surgeries for early and recurrent nasal "polyps." The CT image shows predominant right-sided ethmoid and maxillary disease. The MRI image on the right shows uptake of gadolinium contrast in the mass on the right side; biopsy of this mass was positive for IgG4-RD. Tumefactive lesions are characteristic of IgG4-RD, and these often are misdiagnosed as tumors as they can also be PET avid. Biopsy and serum IgG4 levels are helpful for differential diagnosis. The presence of uncharacteristic features and orbital invasion or mass should raise suspicion of this entity. Inflammatory polyps do not enhance with contrast on imaging

2. Abnormal chest radiograph defined as a chest radiograph showing the presence of nodules, fixed infiltrates, or cavities
3. Urinary sediment defined as microhematuria (>5 RBCs/HPF) or red cell casts in urine sediment
4. Granulomatous inflammation on biopsy defined as histologic changes showing granulomatous inflammation within the wall of an artery or in the perivascular or extravascular area (artery or arteriole)

The patient is classified with Wegener's granulomatosis (GPA) if at least two criteria are present. More closely approaching diagnostic criteria is the European Medicines Agency (EMA) consensus classification algorithm for diagnosing ANCA-associated vasculitides (EGPA, GPA, and MPA) for epidemiologic studies. Unfortunately, the algorithm can only be used when a clinical diagnosis of primary systemic vasculitis has already been present for at least 3 months. The algorithm design does specify inclusion criteria incorporating CHCC nomenclature, ACR classification criteria, as well as exclusion criteria and surrogate markers for vasculitis. The ACR/EULAR study to develop Diagnostic and Classification Criteria for Vasculitis (DCVAS) aims to develop a process suitable for both the clinician and researcher but is yet to be completed and reported. Consequently, the diagnosis of these conditions continues to require significant clinical experience and judgment. Table 19.8 is a practical guide to features suggesting that a

Table 19.6 Laboratory and histopathology features of EGPA, GPA, CIMDL, sarcoidosis, and IgG4-RD

Disease	Laboratory	Histopathology: common sites
EGPA	+C-ANCA/anti-PR3 ab: 5–10% +P-ANCA/anti-MPO ab: 30–40% -C-ANCA/P-ANCA: 60–70%[a, b] Eosinophilia >1500 80–90%[c, d] Elevated IgE: 90% Elevated IgG4: 100%[e] Elevated ESR and CRP Complement: Normal or elevated Other abnormalities depending on specific organ involvement	*Typical histopathology* Necrotizing eosinophilic granulomatous vasculitis *Bronchial* Normal *Nasal* Eosinophilic infiltrates without vasculitis or extravascular granulomas[f] Ig4 plasma cells: ECRS > GPA = CSS = CRS[e] *Neuromuscular* Necrotizing vasculitis[a,b] *Renal* Necrotizing, crescentic pauci-immune glomerulonephritis, interstitial eosinophilic infiltrates, vasculitis (rare)[g] *Cutaneous* Leukocytoclastic vasculitis, necrotizing vasculitis, extravascular necrotizing granulomas *Pulmonary* Typical histopathology
GPA	+C-ANCA/anti-PR3 ab: 70% +P-ANCA/anti-MPO ab: 15% -C-ANCA/P-ANCA: 15%[h,i,j] (% variable related to disease extent and activity) Anemia of chronic disease Elevated ESR and CRP Elevated creatinine Proteinuria/hematuria Complement: Normal or elevated Other abnormalities depending on specific organ involvement	*Typical histopathology* Necrotizing granulomatous vasculitis, giant cells, eosinophils *Nasal* Granulomatosis +/− necrosis +/− vasculitis (sensitivity: 50%[k], 53%[l], 16–23%[m] with % related to definition), IgG4+ plasma cells[n] *Renal* Necrotizing, crescentic pauci-immune glomerulonephritis *Cutaneous* Leukocytoclastic vasculitis *Pulmonary* Typical histopathology
CIMDL	C-ANCA: 8% P-ANCA: 68% -C-ANCA/P-ANCA: 24% Anti-PR3 ab: 48% Anti-MPO ab: Negative Anti-HNE ab: 68% Mixed or unusual results common (HNE = antihuman neutrophil elastase) Neutropenia ESR and CRP: Mild elevation Antiphospholipid antibodies Hypocomplementemia Positive ANA and anti-DNA[o,p,q,r]	*Typical histopathology* Mixed inflammatory infiltrate, vascular wall microabscesses, microvascular thrombosis and vasculitis, fibrinoid necrosis *Nasal* Typical histopathology *Cutaneous* Leukocytoclastic vasculitis, microvascular thrombosis, panniculitis, necrosis *Renal* Pauci-immune glomerulonephritis[p,q,r]
Sarcoidosis	P-ANCA: Rare Elevated ACE: 40–60%[s,t] (ACE = angiotensin-converting enzyme) Elevated 1, 25 OH vitamin D Hypercalciuria >hypercalcemia Hypergammaglobulinemia Elevated soluble IL-2 receptor Complement: Normal RF: Occasional positive	*Typical histopathology* Noncaseating (non-necrotizing) compact granulomas, asteroid bodies, Schaumann bodies, crystalline inclusions (not entirely specific) *Sinus* Granulomas, mixed inflammatory infiltrate, giant cells, intracellular inclusions[u] *Cutaneous* Typical histopathology, erythema nodosum (septal panniculitis)

Table 19.6 (continued)

Disease	Laboratory	Histopathology: common sites
IgG4-RD	C-ANCA/P-ANCA: Negative Anti-PR3 ab/anti-MPO ab: Negative Elevated serum IgG4: 50–80% Elevated IgE: 58% Eosinophilia: 34% Hypocomplementemia: 25% Elevated blood IgG4 plasmablasts ANA: 32% RF: 20%[v,w]	*Typical histopathology* Dense lymphoplasmacytic infiltrate, storiform pattern of fibrosis, obliterative phlebitis, often eosinophils, IgG4+ cells >10/HPF[x,y] (features dependent on anatomic site of biopsy) *Head and neck mass lesions* Typical histopathology *Lacrimal, salivary glands* Typical histopathology but usually without storiform fibrosis *Labial salivary glands*: IgG4 infiltrate only[z] *Nasal* Nonspecific IgG4 plasma cell infiltrate with or without fibrosis, without phlebitis[aa,bb] *Lymph nodes* Typical histopathology without storiform fibrosis *Renal* IgG4 tubulointerstitial nephritis with fibrosis Membranous nephropathy *Cutaneous, pulmonary, pancreatic* Typical histopathology

[a][21], [b][22], [c][81], [d][20], [e][102], [f][17], [g][10], [h][103], [i][104], [j][105], [k][106], [l][107] [m][108], [n][109], [o][110], [p][48][q][47], [r][49], [s][111], [t][6][u][56], [v][92], [w][59], [x][112], [y][113], [z][114], [aa][64], [bb][63]

Table 19.7 Formal definitions, classification, and diagnostic criteria for EGPA, GPA, CIMDL, sarcoidosis, and IgG4-RD

Disorder	Formal definition	Classification criteria	Diagnostic and classification criteria
EGPA	2012 Revised International CHCC Nomenclature of Vasculitides[a]	The ACR 1990 Criteria for the Classification of Churg-Strauss Syndrome[b] EMA ANCA-associated vasculitis and PAN Classification Criteria[c]	Diagnostic and Classification Criteria for Vasculitis (DCVAS)[d] (in process)
GPA	2012 Revised International CHCC Nomenclature of Vasculitides[a]	The ACR 1990 Criteria for the Classification of Wegener's Granulomatosis[e] EMA ANCA-associated vasculitis and PAN Classification Criteria[c]	Diagnostic and Classification Criteria for Vasculitis (DCVAS)[d] (in process)
CIMDL	None	None	Clinical only[f]
Sarcoidosis	None	None	Clinical only[h]
IgG4-RD	Pathologic only[g]	None	Diagnostic[i]

[a][115], [b][116], [c][117], [d][118], [e][119], [f][49], [g][112], [h][53], [i][7]

systemic or autoimmune condition may be the cause of CRS, requiring additional testing and consultation.

Differential Diagnostic Considerations

Infections

The degree of inflammation, purulent ulceration, and mucosal damage created by these disorders may suggest an infectious process, excluded confidently only by biopsy and culture. Damage done to the sinonasal mucosa from EGPA, GPA, or CIMDL and less likely sarcoidosis or IgG4-RD may impair normal immune barrier function resulting in a superimposed superficial mucosal infection or may lead to sinus ostial obstruction and infectious sinusitis. Sinonasal staphylococcal infection has specifically been identified as a likely

Table 19.8 Summary of important ENT features suggesting EGPA, GPA, CIMDL, sarcoidosis, and IgG4-RD

Disorder	History	ENT examination	Sinus CT	Nasal biopsy	Laboratory
EGPA	Asthma, allergic rhinosinusitis, hearing loss, eye inflammation. Systemic illness (common)	Crusting, ulcers, synechia, nasal polyps, nasal septal perforation (rare)	Diffuse mucosal thickening, mastoiditis	Nonspecific eosinophilic inflammation	Eosinophilia, elevated ESR or CRP, elevated creatinine, hematuria, proteinuria, positive ANCA
GPA	Rhinosinusitis, epistaxis, nasal or auricular chondritis, eye inflammation, epiphora, otorrhea, hearing loss, hoarseness, stridor, dyspnea. Systemic illness (common)	Crusting, friable or granular mucosa, purulent ulcers, polyps absent, nasal septal perforation, paranasal sinus erosion, nasal chondritis or "saddle nose," sialoadenitis, proptosis, upper airway inflammation or mass	Diffuse mucosal thickening, mastoiditis, nasal septal perforation, paranasal sinus destruction, paranasal neo-osteogenesis, retro-orbital mass	Granulomatosis +/− necrosis +/− vasculitis	Elevated ESR or CRP, elevated creatinine, hematuria, proteinuria, positive ANCA
CIMDL	Cocaine use, rhinosinusitis, epistaxis, facial pain. Systemic illness (rare)	Crusting, ulcers, nasal septal perforation, paranasal sinus erosion/destruction, hard and soft palate perforation, "saddle nose," facial and periauricular purpura, and ecchymoses	Centrifugal pattern of mucosal thickening, paranasal sinus and orbital destruction, nasal septal perforation, retro-orbital mass	Nonspecific inflammatory infiltrate, vascular wall microabscesses, microvascular thrombosis and vasculitis, fibrinoid necrosis	Positive ANCA with unusual pattern, neutropenia (levamisole)
Sarcoidosis	Rhinosinusitis, epistaxis, eye inflammation, hoarseness, cough, dyspnea. Systemic illness (frequent)	Crusting or friable mucosa, mucosal plaques, nodules and polyps, septal perforation (rare), nasal bridge collapse (rare). Lupus pernio, sialoadenitis, dacryoadenitis, proptosis, vocal cord paralysis, upper airway inflammation and mass	Mucosal thickening and nodules, sinus opacification, nasal and paranasal sinus destruction, osteosclerosis, retro-orbital mass, sialoadenitis	Mixed inflammatory infiltrate, granulomas, giant cells, intracellular inclusions	Elevated ACE, elevated 1,25 OH vitamin D, hypercalciuria, hypercalcemia
IgG4-RD	Allergic rhinosinusitis. Systemic illness (frequent)	Crusting, erosion, polyps, nasal mass (rare), paranasal sinus erosion (rare), sialoadenitis, dacryoadenitis, proptosis, nasopharyngeal, laryngeal and tracheal mass	Mucosal thickening, nasal polyps, paranasal sinus bone destruction (rare), retro-orbital mass, sialoadenitis	Nonspecific IgG4 plasma cell infiltrate with or without fibrosis, without phlebitis	Elevated serum IgG4, elevated IgE, eosinophilia, elevated circulating IgG4 plasmablasts

contributor to both the initiation and maintenance of the immunopathogenic process of GPA (above).

Malignancy

The Epstein-Barr virus-associated NK/T cell lymphoma may also produce significant nasal obstruction, mucosal erosion, and epistaxis. Centrifugal extension into the paranasal sinuses, retro-orbital region, and contiguous areas resembles that encountered in CIMDL or very aggressive GPA. IgG4-RD may be suggested when lymphadenopathy occurs along with the nasal manifestations [120, 121]. In 60–70% of NK/T cell lymphoma cases, sinus CT scanning demonstrates an infiltrative pattern without a prominent mass, suggesting a nonmalignant process and obscuring the suspicion for lymphoma [122].

Hypereosinophilic Syndrome (HES)

Hypereosinophilia is characteristic of EGPA but may occur in reactive, neoplastic, and idiopathic disorders. The presence of asthma, chronic allergic rhinosinusitis, and nasal polyps along with a positive ANCA or biopsy evidence of vasculitis will validate the diagnosis of EGPA. Unfortunately, in many patients suspected with EGPA, the ANCA is negative, and tissue confirmation of vasculitis is impossible. In such cases, lymphocyte immunophenotyping, clonal T cell studies, and molecular analysis for neoplastic causes of HES may be helpful [123, 124].

AFS, AERD, CRSwNP, CRSsNP, CF, and PCD

EGPA, GPA, CIMDL, sarcoidosis, and IgG4-RD resemble common disorders initially and evolve in severity and extent both locally and systemically. Crusting of the nasal mucosa, mucosal ulcers, and a purulent discharge, commonly identified in these disorders, can occur in AFS, AERD, CF, PCD, and odontogenic sinusitis, but are usually not as severe as can be seen in GPA and CIMDL (see Figs. 19.7 and 19.8). Nasal polyps are often visualized in EGPA, IgG4-RD, CF, and AERD but rarely in GPA and PCD. CT evidence of pansinusitis is common to all of the disorders under discussion except odontogenic sinusitis (typically unilateral and maxillary), but CT evidence of destructive rhinosinusitis should immediately raise the suspicion of CIMDL, GPA, and much less often EGPA and sarcoidosis. Treatment resistance, presence of other head and neck symptoms, or other body organ involvement would suggest the possible diagnoses of EGPA, GPA, sarcoidosis, and IgG4-RD and complicated CIMDL. A nasal or sinus mucosal biopsy demonstrating granulomas, giant cells, or vasculitis is consistent with EGPA, GPA, CIMDL, and sarcoidosis. Additional content specific to AERD, AFS, CRSwNP, CF, and PCD is discussed in later parts of the chapter and will help further differentiate these conditions for the autoimmune and granulomatous causes of CRS.

Infection-Related CRS

Background

Infection-related chronic frontal sinusitis can overlap significantly with underlying systemic inflammatory disorders. For example, staphylococcus colonization may be more frequent in patients who have GPA or who have various types of eosinophilic sinusitis, thought to be related to staphylococcal enterotoxins [125]. Infectious manifestations can occur in patients who are predisposed to infections due to primary or secondary immune deficiencies. In this section, we will describe the most common infection-related disorders manifesting as chronic frontal sinusitis: primary immune deficiency, HIV, CF, primary ciliary dyskinesia (PCD), and invasive fungal sinusitis.

Primary and Acquired Immune Deficiency (Including HIV)

Primary immune deficiency is identified in a small percentage of patients with recalcitrant frontal sinusitis. Approximately 12% of patients with HIV have CRS, though the prevalence of CRS in HIV prior to a known HIV diagnosis is unknown, and so therefore, is the utility in screening for HIV in patients with CRS [126]. HIV screening, given its high sensitivity and specificity and disease prevalence in the general population, may be considered in even general, low-risk populations in patients without CRS.

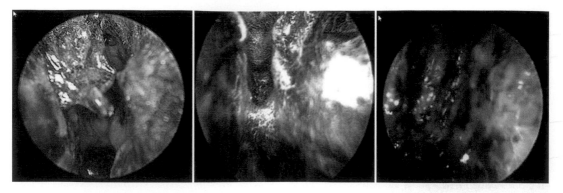

Fig. 19.7 The presence of extensive mucosal erosion and crusting in the nasal mucosa should raise suspicion of Wegener's granulomatosis. The middle image belongs to a patient who was treated for 6 months with antibiotics for presumed injuries from his occupation as a sandblaster

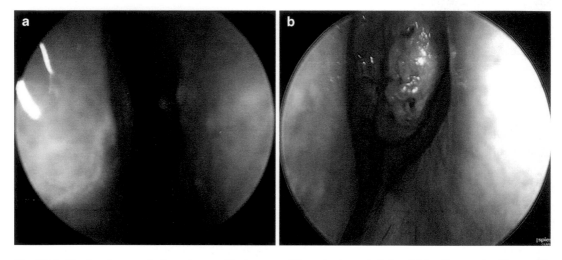

Fig. 19.8 Nasal endoscopy findings in sarcoidosis may be subtle or normal. The classic "strawberry" or "nodular appearance" is not always present. Panel (**a**) shows nasal endoscopy findings of the right nasal cavity with a nodular appearance to the mucosa of the nasal septum (arrow). The patient was tested and later diagnosed with sarcoidosis. Panel (**b**) shows right nasal endoscopic findings in a patient with a known history of sarcoidosis and sinusitis. Only crusting (arrow) on the middle turbinate is noted, a nonspecific finding on nasal dryness

Common variable immune deficiency (CVID) has been diagnosed in 10% and selective IgA deficiency in 6% of a difficult-to-treat CRS population [127]. Sinusitis is usually pansinusitis without nasal polyps in patients with CVID (see Fig. 19.9, A-endoscopic image from a patient with CVID and B-CT image from same patient). The same group performed another more recent study and found low immunoglobulins (IgG 9%, IgA 3%, and IgM 12%) and that 67% of patients failed to increase pneumococcal titers fourfold in <7/14 tested serotypes and were considered to have functional antibody deficiency [128].

A different group identified 245 patients with CRS not responding to prolonged antibiotics and found low immunoglobulins in 22(9%) and CVID in 5(2%) patients. There were 17 with IgG subclass deficiency, 3 of which had poor response to pneumococcal vaccine [129]. In another report of 307 subjects with refractory rhinosinusitis, only 2.2% had IgA deficiency and none had CVID (IgG subclass deficiency was noted in 19.9% of subjects) [130]. In a meta-analysis of 11 studies from a systematic review of 13 studies and 1418 patients, the authors concluded that pooled deficiencies of IgG, IgA, and IgM were

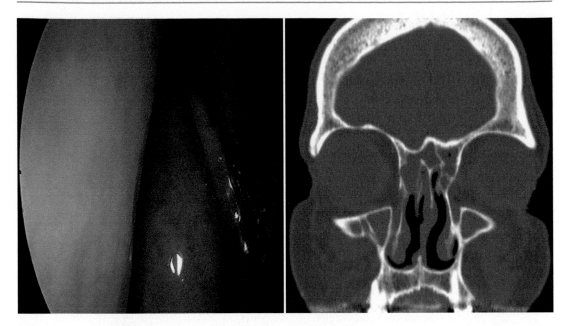

Fig. 19.9 Purulent secretions may be seen in patients with immunodeficiency as in the endoscopic image of the left middle meatus of the patient whose CT image is presented alongside

13% in recurrent sinusitis and 23% in difficult-to-treat CRS [131]. However, with the exception of one study, the definitions of CVID were unclear in these studies, and therefore estimating the CVID prevalence was challenging. In summary, HIV and primary immune deficiency should be strongly considered in patients with recurrent or recalcitrant frontal sinusitis.

Immune deficiency tests to consider include HIV, immunoglobulins (IgG, IgA, and IgM), B and T cell quantitation, and specific antibody testing (tetanus, diphtheria, and pneumococcal). Though CVID and specific antibody deficiency can be identified in a subset of patients with recalcitrant frontal sinusitis, interventions such as replacement of gamma globulin can have uncertain benefit for sinusitis but have more clear benefits for preventing pneumonia and extending longevity [132, 133]. This will be discussed later in the chapter when treatments are considered in more detail. Primary immune deficiency disorders have a myriad of systemic symptoms beyond sinuses. The most commonly associated immune deficiency syndrome, common variable immune deficiency (CVID), can involve lung disease like recurrent pneumonia, bronchiectasis, granuloma-

tous lymphocytic interstitial lung disease (GLILD), bacteremia/sepsis, hemolytic autoimmune anemia, benign lymphoid hyperplasia of intestines, and cancers such as lymphomas [132]. HIV can present with complications in nearly every body organ (CNS, kidney, heart, blood, skin, etc.). Please see Table 19.9 for details and comparisons of systemic manifestations of immune deficiencies.

Odontogenic Sinusitis

Patients can have infection-related CRS from contiguous spread from dental infections (odontogenic infections), which are most commonly suspected in chronic or recurrent unilateral maxillary sinusitis with foul-smelling drainage [134]. Odontogenic sinusitis accounts for 10–40% of chronic maxillary sinusitis cases [135]. About 50% may extend to anterior ethmoid [136], but descriptions of extending to frontal sinuses could not be found in the literature. However, cerebral abscess, subdural empyema, and epidural abscess have been reported to be associated with odontogenic sinusitis. Plain dental films may not detect maxillary dental infection and therefore CT imaging may be needed [135]. Microbiology

Table 19.9 Concise summary of the local and systemic manifestations of diseases associated with CRS

Disease	Local sinus manifestations	Systemic manifestations
Allergic fungal sinusitis (AFS)	Pressure effects, local erosions, sinusitis, nearly always nasal polyps	Asthma, allergic manifestations to inhaled mold
Aspirin-exacerbated respiratory disease (AERD)	Pansinusitis with nasal polyps	Asthma, difficult-to-control asthma, potentially fatal aspirin reactions
Common variable immune deficiency (CVID)	Purulent, neutrophilic localized or pansinusitis	Recurrent pneumonias, bronchiectasis, granulomatous lymphocytic interstitial lung disease (GLILD), benign lymphoid hyperplasia, recurrent giardiasis, neoplasm (especially lymphoma), autoimmune cytopenias
Eosinophilic granulomatosis with polyangiitis (EGPA)	Pansinusitis, nasal polyps, obstruction, crusting and rarely nasal septal perforation	Asthma, alveolar hemorrhage, fever, weight loss, extravascular necrotizing granulomas, vasculitis of skin, CNS, cranial and peripheral nervous system and rarely GI tract. Pericarditis, myocarditis, endocarditis, pauci-immune glomerulonephritis, arthralgia, arthritis
Granulomatosis with polyangiitis (GPA)	Pansinusitis, mucosal crusting with friable, granular mucosal erosions and purulent ulcers, epistaxis, nasal chondritis, septal perforation, nasal bridge collapse ("saddle nose") Osseous paranasal sinus erosion and destruction, neo-osteogenesis Secondary infections	Granulomatous masses of any anatomic site, fever, weight loss, lymphadenopathy (uncommon), vasculitis of skin, CNS, cranial and peripheral nervous system Tracheal and bronchial mass and stenosis, pulmonary infiltrates, fibrosis, nodules and masses, alveolar hemorrhage Pericarditis, myocarditis Pauci-immune glomerulonephritis, arthralgia, arthritis Meningitis, CNS mass lesions, hypophysis, diabetes insipidus
Human immunodeficiency virus (HIV)	Purulent sinusitis	Acute retroviral syndrome, fever, malaise/fatigue, lymphadenopathy, nausea/diarrhea/weight loss, opportunistic infections including candidiasis, *Pneumocystis jiroveci* pneumonia, mycobacterium avium, Kaposi sarcoma
IgG4-related disease (IgG4-RD)	Pansinusitis with nasal polyps, nasal mucosal crusting and erosion. Rarely nasal mucosal mass and osseous paranasal sinus destruction	Lymphoplasmacytic mass of any anatomic site, fever, weight loss (rare) Lymphadenopathy, any site Allergies (common), reactive airway disease Cutaneous plaques, papules, nodules Pleural and pulmonary masses, pleuritis, interstitial fibrosis Aortitis, periaortitis, pericarditis (rare) Pancreatitis, cholangitis, mesenteritis Retroperitoneal mass, fibrosis Interstitial nephritis Arthritis (rare) Meningitis Riedel's and Hashimoto's thyroiditis, hypophysitis
Odontogenic sinusitis	Usually unilateral maxillary sinusitis	Oral dental disease

Table 19.9 (continued)

Disease	Local sinus manifestations	Systemic manifestations
Cystic fibrosis (CF)	Pansinusitis, about 30% also have nasal polyps (Ramsey B, Richardson MA, Impact of sinusitis in cystic fibrosis. *J Allergy Clin Immunol* 1992;90(3 Pt 2):547)	Pneumonia/bronchiectasis, pancreatic insufficiency with steatorrhea, distal ileal obstruction, progressive liver disease (fibrosis/cirrhosis), male infertility
Primary ciliary dyskinesia (PCD)	Purulent sinusitis	Kartagener's: Bronchiectasis, situs inversus, male infertility
Sarcoidosis	Chronic rhinosinusitis, lupus pernio, mucosal friability with crusting and epistaxis, mucosal plaques and nodules Rarely nasal septal perforation, nasal bridge collapse ("saddle nose") Secondary infection	Granulomatous inflammation of any anatomic site Lofgren's syndrome, Heerfordt's syndrome Fever (rare), fatigue Lymphadenopathy, any site Lupus pernio, erythema nodosum, cutaneous plaques, nodules, papules Granulomatous bronchitis, nodules, mass Small airway obstruction, reactive airway disease, bronchiectasis, post-obstructive atelectasis, pulmonary bullae, interstitial fibrosis Cardiac arrhythmia, cardiomyopathy Hepatomegaly, splenomegaly Nephritis, nephrolithiasis Arthritis, myositis, osteolytic cysts, vasculitis Meningitis, cranial and peripheral neuropathy Hypophysitis
Cocaine-induced midline destructive lesions (CIMDL)	Chronic rhinosinusitis, severe mucosal crusting, ulcers, scabs and epistaxis Nasal septal perforation, nasal bridge collapse ("saddle nose") Centrifugal osseous paranasal sinus destruction Secondary infection	Fevers, sweats, weight loss Facial, truncal, and extremity cutaneous retiform ecchymosis and ulcers, thrombotic and vasculitic purpura Alveolar hemorrhage (rare) Arthralgia, myalgia Pauci-immune glomerulonephritis (rare)

reveals anaerobic and aerobic bacteria, with the most common isolates being anaerobic streptococci, gram-negative bacilli, and *Enterobacteriaceae* [137]. In summary, bilateral chronic frontal sinusitis is less likely odontogenic; unilateral disease involving maxillary, ethmoid, and possibly frontal may represent odontogenic sinusitis.

Cystic Fibrosis

Cystic fibrosis (CF) is an autosomal recessive disorder of anion channel function that affects approximately 1 in 3500 births in the USA. A mutation in the CF transmembrane conductance gene (CFTR) is responsible for the pathology related to CF. CF newborn screening is now the standard of care across the USA and is how most new diagnoses are made. However, children and adults not screened or those screened

but still presenting with systemic symptoms including severe sinus disease still should have investigations for CF. CF affects the sinuses (nasal polyps, neutrophilic inflammation), lungs (bronchiectasis, pseudomonas, and other infections), intestines, and liver. Treatment of sinuses may be important for managing lung disease [138].

Primary Ciliary Dyskinesia (PCD)

PCD is a disorder of ciliary motility usually inherited in an autosomal recessive pattern, and patients with this disorder almost always have CRS [139]. The prevalence of PCD in a population presenting with CRS is unknown, and the estimated prevalence of PCD is 1 in 10,000 individuals [139]. Nasal nitric oxide appears to be a sensitive screen for PCD-associated CRS [140, 141] with the gold standard diagnosis being mucosal biopsy with light and electron microscopy to evaluate for ciliary ultrastructural defects [20]. Systemic manifestations of PCD includes Kartagener's syndrome, defined as the triad of sinusitis, bronchiectasis, and situs inversus. In addition, males with PCD are infertile due to immotile spermatozoa. In PCD, the maxillary and ethmoid sinuses are most commonly affected, with the frontal and sphenoid sinuses often failing to develop.

Non-bacterial Infections

Invasive fungal sinusitis usually occurs in patients who are immunocompromised secondarily, such as in bone marrow transplant, cancer and chemotherapy treatment, diabetes, and systemic corticosteroid treatment. Diagnosis depends on a high index of suspicion and expert otolaryngology examination and treatment, which includes surgical debridement and systemic antifungal therapy. Systemic manifestations include other infections more likely to occur in immunocompromised hosts.

Atypical mycobacterial or fungal infection may present as difficult-to-treat CRS, though the prevalence of these infections in CRS is not established. Cultures for fungal and acid-fast bacilli may be helpful for patients not responding to treatment.

The role of viruses in triggering and perpetuating chronic frontal sinusitis is mostly unknown. While epidemiological patterns suggest a possible relationship [142], measurement of viruses has not been undertaken in a large-scale study, nor are specific antiviral therapies currently available.

Neoplasm-Related CRS

Upper airway neoplasms can manifest as CRS symptoms. Therefore, patients not responding to treatment should have sinus CT scans and rhinoscopy, and suspicious findings should be referred to an otorhinolaryngology specialist for biopsy and management. Unilateral findings (such as unilateral polyp) are indications for referral and consideration for biopsy. The estimated incidence of inverted papillomas (the most common sinonasal neoplasm) is 1.5 cases per 100,000

individuals per year [143]. In a study of 380 patients undergoing endoscopic sinus surgery that all had multiple biopsy samples, 5 were diagnosed with inverted papilloma (1% of CRS surgical cases) [72].

Th2-Inflammation-Related CRS

Aspirin-Exacerbated Respiratory Disease (AERD)

Aspirin-exacerbated respiratory disease (AERD) is the condition that has been eponymously called Samter-Widal syndrome. AERD is a chronic unrelenting condition characterized by persistent upper airway inflammation leading to chronic rhinosinusitis CRS with nasal polyposis, persistent lower airway inflammation manifesting as asthma, and aspirin sensitivity. It has been estimated that approximately 13% of the population suffers from CRS, and 15% of those patients with CRS with nasal polyposis have AERD [144]. Suspicion for the presence of AERD depends on recognition of the tetrad of symptoms (sinusitis, nasal polyposis, asthma, and history of reaction to aspirin). Clinical challenge with supervised exposure to NSAID or aspirin with manifestation of classical signs confirms the aspirin sensitivity. Noninvasive diagnostic tests are being investigated and could potentially assist in correct assessment of the presence of AERD [145–147].

Allergic Fungal Sinusitis (AFS)

While invasive fungal infections can certainly manifest with systemic symptoms, local fungal infection as in the form of AFS may be associated with concurrent difficult-to-treat asthma. Local extension into orbit or intracranial structures due to pressure effects and necrosis prompt urgent surgical intervention with medical therapy. A number of fungal organisms including dematiaceous (brown-pigmented) fungi have been identified in AFS tissue samples. Diagnosis can be clinically made based on the presence of "classic allergic" mucin in the sinus cavity (see Fig. 19.6, endoscopic image of allergic mucin), presence of fungal hyphal elements in the mucin, and presence of sensitization to mold [148, 149]. Data suggest that there may not be a predilection for AFS to affect any one group of paranasal sinuses more than others including frontal sinuses [150] although unilateral involvement may be commonly seen as is nasal polyposis (see Fig. 19.10). Involvement of frontal sinuses is not uncommon [151–153].

Other Eosinophilic Sinus Diseases Including Chronic Rhinosinusitis with Nasal Polyps

Eosinophils play an important role in the development of inflammation in chronic sinusitis. Some systemic eosinophilic diseases such as hypereosinophilic syndrome (HES) can manifest with chronic sinusitis. A large multicenter analysis of patients with idiopathic HES reported sinusitis as clinical manifestation on initial presentation in nine instances of 188 (~4.8%) [154]. EGPA, which also can manifest with sinusitis, asthma, and peripheral eosinophilia, is discussed elsewhere in this chapter. Interestingly, chronic sinus disease by itself can have symptoms that may suggest systemic consequences of local inflammation. Patients with CRS reported cognitive dysfunction and fatigue [155]. Furthermore, management of sinus disease was shown to also improve sleep-related disturbances and psychological dysfunction [156, 157].

Summary of Systemic Disease Pattern Recognition

Table 19.9 provides a concise summary of the local and systemic patterns of diseases frequently encountered in patients with CRS. Figure 19.8 represents a diagram of frontal sinus disease types and how they relate to one another. Using the table and figure together may assist in creating a differential diagnosis and planning a more detailed laboratory, radiographic, and tissue-level evaluation.

Management of Systemic Diseases Associated with Chronic Frontal Sinusitis

Management of Autoimmune and Granulomatous-Related CRS

EGPA and GPA

EGPA and GPA will be optimally diagnosed and treated in centers specializing in vasculitis conditions where a standardized, comprehensive, multisystem evaluation is possible and treatment guidelines can be developed, tested, and implemented [20, 158, 159]. Recommendations for the management of ANCA-associated vasculitis conditions (EGPA, GPA, and MPA) have been recently published [38].

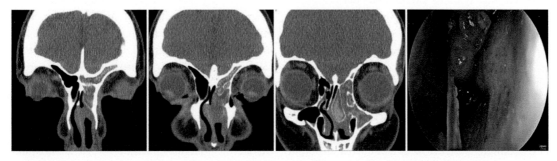

Fig. 19.10 CT scan and nasal endoscopy of patient with unilateral (left-sided) allergic fungal sinusitis. Allergic fungal sinusitis is usually characterized by the presence of bilateral nasal polyps and opacification on CT imaging. The opacification has a characteristic heterogeneous appearance due to the presence of mineralized debris. However, allergic fungal sinusitis may often present as a unilateral disease. Endoscopic image shows the presence of polyps and the characteristic allergic mucin. Tumor should be considered in the differential diagnosis of such patients, even if the characteristic heterogeneous opacification is noted on CT. Further workup with MRI or biopsy should be considered to rule out tumor

When reviewing literature regarding vasculitis treatment trials and outcomes, it is important to recognize that many trials for statistical reasons combine patients with GPA and MPA into an "ANCA-associated vasculitis" treatment group. EGPA is excluded from most of these trials and fewer trials have been conducted exclusively enrolling patients with GPA. Patients with EGPA are, however, included in studies performed by French Vasculitis Study Group reported by [18, 19] which employ the Five-Factor Score as a predictor of mortality. Clinical studies of patients specifically diagnosed with EGPA include [10, 20–22, 81, 82]. Trials that largely or exclusively enrolled patients with GPA include those reported by [16, 24, 104, 160–166]. Treatment experience focused on patients with ENT manifestations of GPA has been reported by [42, 75, 84, 167–170] and recently reviewed by [171].

The data explicitly delineating the ENT involvement and response to treatment may be difficult to identify in "ANCA-associated vasculitis" treatment studies. Many GPA treatment studies appropriately focus on disease complications contributing to organ failure and premature mortality, summarizing outcomes using the BVAS and VDI, and generally recording ENT and sinonasal manifestations, but treatment outcomes for specific ENT manifestation are often not presented individually or with enough detail to permit conclusions useful for clinical treatment decisions. However, the BVAS and BVAS/WG scoring systems do include ENT specific activity sub-scores (above) which are separately analyzed in some studies with an ENT focus. Notably, a number of well-recognized ENT features of GPA are not included in either the BVAS or VDI. Further complicating a review of the literature, the definitions of disease stage vary among studies so that systemic disease, generalized disease, localized disease, and limited disease connote patients with somewhat different involvement depending on the study [85, 172, 173]. For example, the European Vasculitis Study Group (EUVAS) defines the different disease stages of GPA as localized, early systemic, generalized, severe, and refractory, whereas the Vasculitis Clinical Research Consortium (VCRC)

defines disease stages as limited and severe only. In particular, neither the EUVAS nor VCRC GPA disease states define a stage where manifestations are limited to the ENT region alone ("ENT-limited GPA"). The EUVAS localized disease stage includes patients with ENT and lung involvement but not beyond, whereas the VCRC limited disease stage includes patients with manifestation even beyond the ENT and lung regions. The disease stage often changes over the disease duration and localized disease remains so in only 3.2% of patients [174]. Patients defined with localized disease, most of whom have ENT manifestations, rarely develop systemic, vasculitic features but often present with high levels of local damage, accrue more damage, and develop new involvement over time [175]. Taylor [75] evaluated 24 patients referred to a university tertiary care ENT department who were treated primarily with prednisone, methotrexate, and cyclophosphamide and over the course of 6.8 years of follow-up reported that most had progressive organ involvement with the percent of patients with sinusitis increasing from approximately 65% to 75%.

Except for recent studies assessing the effect of rituximab on ENT manifestations of GPA, no study has specifically analyzed the response of individual ENT manifestations of GPA to any systemic treatment. Unfortunately, immunosuppression given for vasculitic manifestations generally leads to poor response of ENT manifestations. Robson [39] summarized treatment responses from six EUVAS vasculitis studies at 6 months after initiation of treatment and at long-term follow-up and demonstrated that in patients with GPA, nasal blockage and crusting increased from approximately 30% to 45% and hearing loss from 22% to 32%. de Groot analyzed 100 patients with early systemic disease (organ- and life-threatening disease excluded) treated with either methotrexate or cyclophosphamide for 18 months and concluded that methotrexate was less effective than cyclophosphamide and resulted in more frequent relapses [160]. Methotrexate reduced the number of patients with ENT manifestations from 90% to approximately 70% and cyclophosphamide from 90% to approximately 55% over the treatment period. Rituximab, the newest available treatment for GPA, has been analyzed in several studies. Aries [40] did not find that a single course of rituximab was efficacious in eight patients with refractory granulomatous manifestations when given with prednisolone and either cyclophosphamide, methotrexate, or mycophenolate mofetil. A retrospective analysis of 11 patients with GPA failing other treatments and subsequently treated with one or more doses of rituximab was reported by Malm [169] who noted persistent and increasing ENT manifestations. In contrast, Seo [170] found that one or more courses of rituximab were effective in refractory granulomatous manifestations in their eight patients manifesting orbital pseudotumor or subglottic stenosis. Lally [167] reported on 99 patients with GPA treated over 10 years, 51 of which received rituximab at least once and found that these patients demonstrated no ENT manifestations during 92% of the observation period compared to 53.7% of those patients who never received rituximab. Thirty-four patients with refractory head and neck involvement from GPA were treated with repeated doses of rituximab in a study reported by [42] who found improvement in all ENT manifestations including patients with retro-orbital pseudotumor and subglottic stenosis. Possible reasons for failing to respond to rituximab included the presence of fibrotic rather than inflammatory disease and failure to repeat rituximab treatment over a sufficiently long period of time especially for large inflammatory lesions.

Systemic GPA is initially treated with induction therapy including a high dose of an intravenous or oral glucocorticoid and either rituximab or cyclophosphamide and rarely plasma exchange until remission is induced and then maintenance therapy with decremental doses of a glucocorticoid and replacement of rituximab or cyclophosphamide with azathioprine, methotrexate, or mycophenolate mofetil. Maintenance therapy with intermittent courses of rituximab is also an option. The duration of maintenance therapy is uncertain and a small subset of patients will enjoy medication-free disease remission. For localized, non-organ-threatening disease, a glucocorticoid along with methotrexate or mycophenolate mofetil is often sufficient.

Concomitant treatment with trimethoprim 160 mg plus sulfamethoxazole 800 mg twice daily may reduce the frequency of disease relapse and provides prophylaxis against *Pneumocystis jiroveci* pneumonitis. Intravenous gamma globulin and leflunomide are nonstandard options in special circumstances. Treatment of local rhinosinusitis may include nasal saline, antibiotic or glucocorticoid irrigations, topical mupirocin, systemic antibiotics for superimposed infectious sinusitis, as well as debridement and judicious surgical intervention as needed. No clinical trials assessing the efficacy of topical therapy in treating GPA-associated rhinosinusitis have been performed. When optimal medical therapy is initiated early in the course of the disease, surgical intervention is rarely needed.

Management and treatment of EGPA generally follow that outlined for GPA with recommendations limited by the absence of any controlled clinical treatment trials for EGPA [38]. Groh [159] published EGPA specific evaluation and management recommendations derived largely on the basis of observational studies supporting the use of glucocorticoids and cyclophosphamide for severe disease and azathioprine or methotrexate for less severe disease and for maintenance therapy. Rituximab, plasma exchange, and IVIG were of undocumented value for routine treatment, and mepolizumab (anti-interleukin-5 monoclonal antibody) and omalizumab (anti-IgE monoclonal antibody) are investigational. A repeated theme is the need to continue therapy long term, including low-dose glucocorticoids, to prevent relapses. The ENT and specifically the rhinosinusitis involvement in patients with EGPA is generally much less severe than in patients with GPA and most commonly resolve with glucocorticoid and immune suppression given for systemic manifestations. Local treatment of rhinosinusitis is similar to that described for GPA [17, 176].

CIMDL

As expected for any drug-induced syndrome, elimination of cocaine and levamisole exposure is crucial to treatment success. Treatment of local rhinosinusitis and soft tissue or bone destruction includes saline irrigation, debridement, and topical or systemic antibiotics. Glucocorticoid treatment may improve early, mild disease manifestations. Surgical procedures may be needed including closure of nasal septal, nasal cutaneous, palatal and skull-based defects, rhinoplasty, reconstruction, and prostheses [49, 86]. Patients with systemic and vasculitic features may require glucocorticoids and immunosuppression, especially when complicated by pulmonary hemorrhage or glomerulonephritis [50, 87]. Patients with severe systemic disease and vasculitis may achieve benefit from immune suppression even if total cocaine abstinence is not achieved.

Sarcoidosis

There are few controlled treatment trials for patients with systemic sarcoidosis and none for ENT and sinonasal sarcoidosis. Treatment recommendations are predominantly based on retrospective case series. Of 1774 patients with sarcoidosis seen over a 12-year period of time and followed for an average of 42 months, approximately 40% did not require any treatment with 60% receiving treatment primarily for pulmonary, neurologic, cardiac, skin, eye, and ENT involvement [77]. Typical of the response of sarcoidosis to glucocorticoids in general, sinonasal and ENT involvement often responds to topical, intralesional, or systemic glucocorticoids which are often sufficient treatment. Nasal saline irrigation and emollients provide symptomatic improvement in nasal crusting. Surgery is generally only indicated for obstructive rhinosinusitis. Recalcitrant or more severe sinonasal disease may respond to medications usually administered for systemic disease including chloroquine, hydroxychloroquine, methotrexate, azathioprine, or TNFα antagonists [76, 78, 79, 89, 177, 178]. A recent review of treatment options for systemic sarcoidosis affirmed the value of glucocorticoids for symptomatic involvement at any anatomic site, and for severe, organ-threatening, or persistent disease, methotrexate, azathioprine, leflunomide, mycophenolate mofetil, TNFα antagonists, rituximab, or Acthar gel are effective in many patients. Double-blind placebo-controlled randomized trials suggest benefit for methotrexate, TNFα antagonists, and pentoxifylline [179].

IgG4-RD

Literature regarding the relatively recently described IgG4-RD is focused primarily on recognition and proper diagnosis of the disorder with case series reports on evolving treatment experience but no controlled clinical studies. Of 79 patients diagnosed with IgG4-RD, 41 were found to have CT evidence of associated rhinosinusitis with histopathology consistent with IgG4-RD identified in 4 patients. Oral prednisolone administration improved rhinosinusitis symptoms in 14 of the 41 patients [63]. An ENT oriented literature review of 43 articles which included a total of 484 patients concluded that surgery was rarely needed except for biopsy to diagnose ENT related IgG4-RD mass lesions and that of 129 patients for which treatment results were available, 90% had disease remission with medical therapy alone only occasionally requiring one or more immunosuppressive medications [80]. Treatment of autoimmune pancreatitis type 1, the first and most widely described manifestation of IgG4-RD, forms the basis of treatment recommendations of most systemic manifestations. However, a summary of treatment results in 125 patients with widespread organ involvement revealed an 86% response rate to initial glucocorticoids alone but only 23% achieving stable disease remission, the remaining 77% requiring further treatment with immunomodulators, stents, or radiation therapy [92]. Consensus guidelines have been published that suggest observation and no additional treatment for patients with only asymptomatic lymphadenopathy or mild submandibular gland involvement but recommend early treatment for patients likely to develop irreversible fibrotic complications including those with autoimmune pancreatitis and more widespread salivary gland involvement [180]. These guidelines also recommend urgent treatment for patients manifesting aortitis, retroperitoneal fibrosis, proximal biliary strictures, tubulointerstitial nephritis, pachymeningitis, pancreatic enlargement, and pericarditis as well as patients experiencing organ dysfunction or significant cosmetic complications. An important goal of therapy is to avoid development of end-stage and large fibrotic lesions which may not respond to medical therapy and require surgical intervention. Medical treatment of symptomatic involvement always includes initial moderate-dose glucocorticoid medication with many patients requiring maintenance treatment on low-dose glucocorticoid with or without immunosuppressive medications such as azathioprine, mycophenolate mofetil, 6-mercaptopurine, tacrolimus, cyclophosphamide, or rituximab. Depending on initial treatment, disease relapses may be treated with an increase in glucocorticoid therapy alone or with the addition of an immunosuppressive medication or rituximab. The treatment efficacy of rituximab 1000 mg given twice over 15 days with or without glucocorticoids was assessed in an open-label study of 30 patients which demonstrated disease response in 97% of patients with 40% incomplete remission after 12 months [181]. Additional controlled clinical treatment trials will be needed to develop reliable recommendations for the administration of glucocorticoids, immunosuppressive and immunomodulating medications.

Management of Infection-Related CRS

Primary Immune Deficiency and HIV

Management of infectious-related chronic frontal sinusitis may vary depending on whether an underlying systemic disease was identified. For HIV, treatment of the underlying disease using evidence-based antiviral regimens, along with antibiotics when purulent secretions are present, is the best approach. For CVID, most patients should start replacement gamma globulin infusions (either intravenously or subcutaneously), and some may be considered for chronic or rotating antibiotic courses. Adjusting replacement gamma globulin dosing to achieve adequate trough levels and reductions in lower respiratory tract infections is key for chronic management of CVID [182, 183]. While the evidence that gamma globulin treatment can reduce lower respiratory infections is strong, the impact on sinusitis is less certain. We recommend culture-directed antibiotics when purulent secretions are identified for patients with CVID, similar to non-CVID patients.

PCD and CF

For PCD and CF, treatment will include endoscopic sinus surgery to facilitate gravity-dependent drainage of the sinuses, irrigation treatment meant to compensate for poor ciliary function, and antibiotics directed at organisms identified by culture. In a systematic review of 12 studies and 701 patients, dornase alfa and topical steroids demonstrated benefit for CRS in patients with CF [184]. The benefit of antibiotics for sinusitis in CF patients is uncertain based on existing medical evidence [184]. However, antibiotics are generally recommended for lower respiratory disease exacerbations based on lower respiratory culture results. In addition, for CF patients with specific genotypes, ivacaftor may lead to improved sinus outcomes [185].

Odontogenic

Odontogenic sinusitis is best treated by dental specialists who remove infected teeth along with antibiotics and endoscopic sinus surgery. Odontogenic sinusitis is rarely associated with frontal sinusitis so we will not discuss its treatment in more detail in this chapter.

Infection-Related Complications

If no specific underlying diagnosis is made, and the patient is classified as CRSsNP, infection-related complications should be addressed. A positive culture does not equal clinical disease, and interpretation of culture results can be challenging. In general, we recommend performing cultures only when purulent material is visible. Results from previous culture studies of patients with CRS have been described and provide an overall estimation of the different types of bacteria that can be isolated from sinuses [186]. In patients not responding to treatment, one may consider a bacterial culture, carefully sampled from the middle meatus. Such culture results appear to influence antibiotic choice, changing antibiotic selection in 52% of patients in one study [187]. Studies suggest that endoscopically obtained cultures correlate highly with culture results from antral taps [188, 189]. Guidelines for CRS management suggest that long-term use of macrolide antibiotics for patients with low total serum IgE may be effective [190].

Bacterial culture for diagnosis and to direct management may be helpful in patients with CRS, though data supporting this approach are limited. We were unable to identify any high-quality clinical trials comparing culture-directed and empiric use of antibiotics in CRS. A recent case series found that the most common microbes grown in culture from endoscopically guided cultures were *Staphylococcus aureus* and *Pseudomonas aeruginosa* and that most patients treated using cultures as guides had improved patient-reported outcomes [2]. Previous studies also identified frequent growth of coagulase-negative staphylococci [191]. Despite the limited prospective, controlled data for the use of culture-directed antibiotics, we still recommend this approach when purulent secretions are seen on examination.

Management of Th2-Inflammation-Related CRS

Th2-inflammation-related CRS tends to have an eosinophilic component to inflammation which is reflected both in local tissue and systemically with elevated blood eosinophil counts. Though attractive, such generalizations may seem too simplistic and may not be applicable in all clinical scenarios. A key to identifying a Th2-related inflammation in CRS is the response to systemic and local corticosteroid. This therapy has been the mainstay of the treatment for CRS for several years. However, recent recognition of different endotypes that drive the phenotypic differences [192] has led to efforts for identification of specific pathways that can be modulated for control of disease. Thus specific cytokine blockade has been shown to be effective in clinical studies including IL-5 antagonists such as mepolizumab [193] and reslizumab [194] or with the recent trial with dupilumab (combined IL-4 and IL-13 blockade via a shared heteroreceptor) [195]. Case series and one clinical trial have also been published that demonstrate effectiveness of anti-IgE therapy (omalizumab) in CRS [196, 197]. We recommend consideration of these therapies if sinus disease is recalcitrant

or if the concurrent comorbid illness such as asthma is difficult-to-control. Though biologicals mepolizumab, reslizumab, dupilumab and omalizumab may be effective in controlling sinus symptoms in clinical trials, as of 2019, they are FDA approved only for difficult-to-control asthma and not CRSwNP.

In addition to conventional approaches for therapy which include topical saline irrigations with or without added corticosteroids, topical intranasal corticosteroids, antihistamine medications, systemic corticosteroids, and surgical management, specific disease phenotypes do yield themselves to specific therapies. For example, AERD is known to be driven at least in part by an exaggerated and dysregulated arachidonic acid metabolic pathway with increased production of leukotriene and prostaglandin metabolites [198]. Thus leukotriene receptor antagonists (CysLT1) such as montelukast and zafirlukast or 5-lipoxygenase inhibitors (zileuton) are essential in symptomatic treatment of sinus disease, asthma, and aspirin reaction in these patients [199]. Aspirin desensitization has been shown to be useful in reducing recurrence of nasal polyposis and improve the management of symptoms in AERD [200].

Summary of the Approach to Diagnosis and Management of Systemic Diseases Associated with Chronic Frontal Sinusitis

A stepwise approach to patients presenting with recalcitrant chronic frontal sinusitis will improve the care we provide. Making an accurate diagnosis of diseases that may extend beyond the sinus cavities will lead to consideration of broader treatment options, especially as concomitant lower airway diseases are considered. Using the tables and figures from this chapter can assist in recognizing patterns of systemic disease related to chronic frontal sinusitis. Applying treatment specific to the underlying systemic disease diagnosis is likely to lead to globally improved outcomes for the patient and may also enhance the local management typically employed for chronic frontal sinusitis (Fig. 19.11).

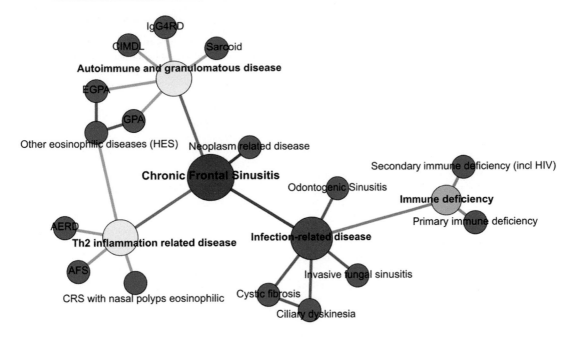

Fig. 19.11 Relationship between types of chronic frontal sinusitis

Acknowledgments We thank Drs. Rodrigo Cartin-Ceba and Devyani Lal, both from Mayo Clinic Arizona, for their input on this chapter.

References

1. Rank MA, Hoxworth JM, Lal D. Sorting out "sinus headache". J Allergy Clin Immunol Pract. 2016;4(5):1013–4.

2. Snidvongs K, McLachlan R, Sacks R, Earls P, Harvey RJ. Correlation of the Kennedy Osteitis Score to clinico-histologic features of chronic rhinosinusitis. Int Forum Allergy Rhinol. 2013;3(5):369–75.

3. Pearce FA, Lanyon PC, Grainge MJ, Shaunak R, Mahr A, Hubbard RB, et al. Incidence of ANCA-associated vasculitis in a UK mixed ethnicity population. Rheumatology (Oxford). 2016;55(9):1656–63.

4. Mahr A, Guillevin L, Poissonnet M, Ayme S. Prevalences of polyarteritis nodosa, microscopic polyangiitis, Wegener's granulomatosis, and Churg-Strauss syndrome in a French urban multiethnic population in 2000: a capture-recapture estimate. Arthritis Rheum. 2004;51(1):92–9.

5. Baughman RP, Field S, Costabel U, Crystal RG, Culver DA, Drent M, et al. Sarcoidosis in America. Analysis based on health care use. Ann Am Thorac Soc. 2016;13(8):1244–52.

6. Ungprasert P, Carmona EM, Crowson CS, Matteson EL. Diagnostic utility of angiotensin-converting enzyme in sarcoidosis: a population-based study. Lung. 2016;194(1):91–5.

7. Umehara H, Okazaki K, Masaki Y, Kawano M, Yamamoto M, Saeki T, et al. Comprehensive diagnostic criteria for IgG4-related disease (IgG4-RD), 2011. Mod Rheumatol. 2012;22(1):21–30.

8. Watts RA, Mahr A, Mohammad AJ, Gatenby P, Basu N, Flores-Suarez LF. Classification, epidemiology and clinical subgrouping of antineutrophil cytoplasmic antibody (ANCA)-associated vasculitides. Nephrol Dial Transplant. 2015;30(Suppl 1):i14–22.

9. Lanham JG, Elkon KB, Pusey CD, Hughes GR. Systemic vasculitis with asthma and eosinophilia: a clinical approach to the Churg-Strauss syndrome. Medicine. 1984;63(2):65–81.

10. Sinico RA, Di Toma L, Maggiore U, Tosoni C, Bottero P, Sabadini E, et al. Renal involvement in Churg-Strauss syndrome. Am J Kidney Dis. 2006;47(5):770–9.

11. Chaigne B, Terrier B, Thieblemont N, Witko-Sarsat V, Mouthon L. Dividing the Janus vasculitis? Pathophysiology of eosinophilic granulomatosis with polyangiitis. Autoimmun Rev. 2016;15(2):139–45.

12. Ueki S, Tokunaga T, Fujieda S, Honda K, Hirokawa M, Spencer LA, et al. Eosinophil ETosis and DNA traps: a new look at eosinophilic inflammation. Curr Allergy Asthma Rep. 2016;16(8):54.

13. Khoury P, Grayson PC, Klion AD. Eosinophils in vasculitis: characteristics and roles in pathogenesis. Nat Rev Rheumatol. 2014;10(8):474–83.

14. Mukhtyar C, Lee R, Brown D, Carruthers D, Dasgupta B, Dubey S, et al. Modification and validation of the Birmingham Vasculitis Activity Score (version 3). Ann Rheum Dis. 2009;68(12):1827–32.

15. Exley AR, Bacon PA, Luqmani RA, Kitas GD, Gordon C, Savage CO, et al. Development and initial validation of the Vasculitis Damage Index for the standardized clinical assessment of damage in the systemic vasculitides. Arthritis Rheum. 1997;40(2):371–80.

16. Stone JH, Hoffman GS, Merkel PA, Min YI, Uhlfelder ML, Hellmann DB, et al. A disease-specific activity index for Wegener's granulomatosis: modification of the Birmingham Vasculitis Activity Score. International Network for the Study of the Systemic Vasculitides (INSSYS). Arthritis Rheum. 2001;44(4):912–20.

17. Bacciu A, Bacciu S, Mercante G, Ingegnoli F, Grasselli C, Vaglio A, et al. Ear, nose and throat manifestations of Churg-Strauss syndrome. Acta Otolaryngol. 2006;126(5):503–9.

18. Guillevin L, Lhote F, Gayraud M, Cohen P, Jarrousse B, Lortholary O, et al. Prognostic factors in polyarteritis nodosa and Churg-Strauss syndrome. A prospective study in 342 patients. Medicine. 1996;75(1):17–28.

19. Guillevin L, Pagnoux C, Seror R, Mahr A, Mouthon L, Le Toumelin P. The Five-Factor Score revisited: assessment of prognoses of systemic necrotizing vasculitides based on the French Vasculitis Study Group (FVSG) cohort. Medicine. 2011;90(1):19–27.

20. Moosig F, Bremer JP, Hellmich B, Holle JU, Holl-Ulrich K, Laudien M, et al. A vasculitis centre based management strategy leads to improved outcome in eosinophilic granulomatosis and polyangiitis (Churg-Strauss, EGPA): monocentric experiences in 150 patients. Ann Rheum Dis. 2013;72(6):1011–7.

21. Comarmond C, Pagnoux C, Khellaf M, Cordier JF, Hamidou M, Viallard JF, et al. Eosinophilic granulomatosis with polyangiitis (Churg-Strauss): clinical characteristics and long-term followup of the 383 patients enrolled in the French Vasculitis Study Group cohort. Arthritis Rheum. 2013;65(1):270–81.

22. Durel CA, Berthiller J, Caboni S, Jayne D, Ninet J, Hot A. Long-term followup of a multicenter cohort of 101 patients with eosinophilic granulomatosis with polyangiitis (Churg-Strauss). Arthritis Care Res. 2016;68(3):374–87.

23. Hoffman GS, Kerr GS, Leavitt RY, Hallahan CW, Lebovics RS, Travis WD, et al. Wegener granulomatosis: an analysis of 158 patients. Ann Intern Med. 1992;116(6):488–98.

24. Villa-Forte A, Clark TM, Gomes M, Carey J, Mascha E, Karafa MT, et al. Substitution of methotrexate for cyclophosphamide in Wegener granulomatosis: a 12-year single-practice experience. Medicine. 2007;86(5):269–77.

25. DeRemee RA. The treatment of Wegener's granulomatosis with trimethoprim/sulfamethoxazole: illusion or vision? Arthritis Rheum. 1988;31(8):1068–74.

26. Leavitt RY, Hoffman GS, Fauci AS. The role of trimethoprim/sulfamethoxazole in the treatment of Wegener's granulomatosis. Arthritis Rheum. 1988;31(8):1073–4.

27. Rasmussen N, Petersen J, Remvig L, Andersen V. Treatment of Wegener's granulomatosis with trimethoprim-sulfamethoxazole. APMIS Suppl. 1990;19:61–2.

28. Stegeman CA, Tervaert JW, Sluiter WJ, Manson WL, de Jong PE, Kallenberg CG. Association of chronic nasal carriage of Staphylococcus aureus and higher relapse rates in Wegener granulomatosis. Ann Intern Med. 1994;120(1):12–7.

29. Stegeman CA, Tervaert JW, de Jong PE, Kallenberg CG. Trimethoprim-sulfamethoxazole (co-trimoxazole) for the prevention of relapses of Wegener's granulomatosis. Dutch Co-Trimoxazole Wegener Study Group. N Engl J Med. 1996;335(1):16–20.

30. Laudien M, Gadola SD, Podschun R, Hedderich J, Paulsen J, Reinhold-Keller E, et al. Nasal carriage of Staphylococcus aureus and endonasal activity in Wegener s granulomatosis as compared to rheumatoid arthritis and chronic rhinosinusitis with nasal polyps. Clin Exp Rheumatol. 2010;28(1 Suppl 57):51–5.

31. Popa ER, Stegeman CA, Abdulahad WH, van der Meer B, Arends J, Manson WM, et al. Staphylococcal toxic-shock-syndrome-toxin-1 as a risk factor for disease relapse in Wegener's granulomatosis. Rheumatology. 2007;46(6):1029–33.

32. Lepse N, Abdulahad WH, Kallenberg CG, Heeringa P. Immune regulatory mechanisms in ANCA-associated vasculitides. Autoimmun Rev. 2011;11(2):77–83.

33. Glasner C, van Timmeren MM, Stobernack T, Omansen TF, Raangs EC, Rossen JW, et al. Low anti-staphylococcal IgG responses in granulomatosis with polyangiitis patients despite long-term Staphylococcus aureus exposure. Sci Rep. 2015;5:8188.

34. Laudien M, Hasler R, Wohlers J, Bock J, Lipinski S, Bremer L, et al. Molecular signatures of a disturbed nasal barrier function in the primary tissue of Wegener's granulomatosis. Mucosal Immunol. 2011;4(5):564–73.

35. de Groot K, Reinhold-Keller E, Tatsis E, Paulsen J, Heller M, Nolle B, et al. Therapy for the maintenance of remission in sixty-five patients with generalized Wegener's granulomatosis. Methotrexate versus trimethoprim/sulfamethoxazole. Arthritis Rheum. 1996;39(12):2052–61.

36. Kallenberg CG. Pathogenesis and treatment of ANCA-associated vasculitides. Clin Exp Rheumatol. 2015;33(4 Suppl 92):S11–4.

37. Cornec D, Cornec-Le Gall E, Fervenza FC, Specks U. ANCA-associated vasculitis – clinical utility of using ANCA specificity to classify patients. Nat Rev Rheumatol. 2016;12(10):570–9.

38. Yates M, Watts RA, Bajema IM, Cid MC, Crestani B, Hauser T, et al. EULAR/ERA-EDTA recommendations for the management of ANCA-associated vasculitis. Ann Rheum Dis. 2016;75(9):1583–94.

39. Robson J, Doll H, Suppiah R, Flossmann O, Harper L, Hoglund P, et al. Damage in the anca-associated vasculitides: long-term data from the European vasculitis study group (EUVAS) therapeutic trials. Ann Rheum Dis. 2015;74(1):177–84.

40. Aries PM, Hellmich B, Voswinkel J, Both M, Nolle B, Holl-Ulrich K, et al. Lack of efficacy of rituximab in Wegener's granulomatosis with refractory granulomatous manifestations. Ann Rheum Dis. 2006;65(7):853–8.
41. Holle JU, Dubrau C, Herlyn K, Heller M, Ambrosch P, Noelle B, et al. Rituximab for refractory granulomatosis with polyangiitis (Wegener's granulomatosis): comparison of efficacy in granulomatous versus vasculitic manifestations. Ann Rheum Dis. 2012;71(3):327–33.
42. Martinez Del Pero M, Chaudhry A, Jones RB, Sivasothy P, Jani P, Jayne D. B-cell depletion with rituximab for refractory head and neck Wegener's granulomatosis: a cohort study. Clin Otolaryngol. 2009;34(4):328–35.
43. Taylor SR, Salama AD, Joshi L, Pusey CD, Lightman SL. Rituximab is effective in the treatment of refractory ophthalmic Wegener's granulomatosis. Arthritis Rheum. 2009;60(5):1540–7.
44. Kessenbrock K, Krumbholz M, Schonermarck U, Back W, Gross WL, Werb Z, et al. Netting neutrophils in autoimmune small-vessel vasculitis. Nat Med. 2009;15(6):623–5.
45. Surmiak M, Hubalewska-Mazgaj M, Wawrzycka-Adamczyk K, Szczeklik W, Musial J, Brzozowski T, et al. Neutrophil-related and serum biomarkers in granulomatosis with polyangiitis support extracellular traps mechanism of the disease. Clin Exp Rheumatol. 2016;34(3 Suppl 97):S98–104.
46. Bligny D, Mahr A, Toumelin PL, Mouthon L, Guillevin L. Predicting mortality in systemic Wegener's granulomatosis: a survival analysis based on 93 patients. Arthritis Rheum. 2004;51(1):83–91.
47. Trimarchi M, Gregorini G, Facchetti F, Morassi ML, Manfredini C, Maroldi R, et al. Cocaine-induced midline destructive lesions: clinical, radiographic, histopathologic, and serologic features and their differentiation from Wegener granulomatosis. Medicine. 2001;80(6):391–404.
48. McGrath MM, Isakova T, Rennke HG, Mottola AM, Laliberte KA, Niles JL. Contaminated cocaine and antineutrophil cytoplasmic antibody-associated disease. Clin J Am Soc Nephrol. 2011;6(12):2799–805.
49. Trimarchi M, Sinico RA, Teggi R, Bussi M, Specks U, Meroni PL. Otorhinolaryngological manifestations in granulomatosis with polyangiitis (Wegener's). Autoimmun Rev. 2013;12(4):501–5.
50. Ullrich K, Koval R, Koval E, Bapoje S, Hirsh JM. Five consecutive cases of a cutaneous vasculopathy in users of levamisole-adulterated cocaine. J Clin Rheumatol. 2011;17(4):193–6.
51. Govender P, Berman JS. The diagnosis of sarcoidosis. Clin Chest Med. 2015;36(4):585–602.
52. Judson MA, Baughman RP, Teirstein AS, Terrin ML, Yeager H Jr. Defining organ involvement in sarcoidosis: the ACCESS proposed instrument. ACCESS Research Group. A Case Control Etiologic Study of Sarcoidosis. Sarcoidosis Vasc Diffuse Lung Dis. 1999;16(1):75–86.
53. Judson MA, Baughman RP. How many organs need to be involved to diagnose sarcoidosis?: an unanswered question that, hopefully, will become irrelevant. Sarcoidosis Vasc Diffuse Lung Dis. 2014;31(1):6–7.
54. Lazarus A. Sarcoidosis: epidemiology, etiology, pathogenesis, and genetics. Dis Mon. 2009;55(11):649–60.
55. Zissel G, Muller-Quernheim J. Cellular players in the immunopathogenesis of sarcoidosis. Clin Chest Med. 2015;36(4):549–60.
56. deShazo RD, O'Brien MM, Justice WK, Pitcock J. Diagnostic criteria for sarcoidosis of the sinuses. J Allergy Clin Immunol. 1999;103(5 Pt 1):789–95.
57. Inoue D, Yoshida K, Yoneda N, Ozaki K, Matsubara T, Nagai K, et al. IgG4-related disease: dataset of 235 consecutive patients. Medicine. 2015;94(15):e680.
58. Yamamoto M, Takahashi H. IgG4-related disease in organs other than the hepatobiliary-pancreatic system. Semin Liver Dis. 2016;36(3):274–82.
59. Stone JH, Brito-Zeron P, Bosch X, Ramos-Casals M. Diagnostic approach to the complexity of IgG4-related disease. Mayo Clin Proc. 2015;90(7):927–39.
60. Lanzillotta M, Campochiaro C, Trimarchi M, Arrigoni G, Gerevini S, Milani R, et al. Deconstructing IgG4-related disease involvement of midline structures: comparison to common mimickers. Mod Rheumatol. 2016:1–8.
61. Deshpande V. IgG4 related disease of the head and neck. Head Neck Pathol. 2015;9(1):24–31.
62. Takano K, Yamamoto M, Kondo A, Himi T. A case of reversible hyposmia associated with Mikulicz's disease. Otolaryngol Head Neck Surg. 2009;141(3):430–1.
63. Takano K, Abe A, Yajima R, Kakuki T, Jitsukawa S, Nomura K, et al. Clinical evaluation of cinonasal lesions in patients with immunoglobulin G4-related disease. Ann Otol Rhinol Laryngol. 2015;124(12):965–71.
64. Ohno K, Matsuda Y, Arai T, Kimura Y. Nasal manifestations of IgG4-related disease: a report of two cases. Auris Nasus Larynx. 2015;42(6):483–7.
65. Cain RB, Colby TV, Balan V, Patel NP, Lal D. Perplexing lesions of the sinonasal cavity and skull base: IgG4-related and similar inflammatory diseases. Otolaryngol Head Neck Surg. 2014;151(3):496–502.
66. Stone JH, Zen Y, Deshpande V. IgG4-related disease. N Engl J Med. 2012;366(6):539–51.
67. Peters AT, Spector S, Hsu J, Hamilos DL, Baroody FM, Chandra RK, et al. Diagnosis and management of rhinosinusitis: a practice parameter update. Ann Allergy Asthma Immunol. 2014;113(4):347–85.
68. Fuchs HA, Tanner SB. Granulomatous disorders of the nose and paranasal sinuses. Curr Opin Otolaryngol Head Neck Surg. 2009;17(1):23–7.
69. Kohanski MA, Reh DD. Chapter 11: Granulomatous diseases and chronic sinusitis. Am J Rhinol Allergy. 2013;27(Suppl 1):S39–41.
70. Hirsch AG, Yan XS, Sundaresan AS, Tan BK, Schleimer RP, Kern RC, et al. Five-year risk of incident disease following a diagnosis of chronic rhinosinusitis. Allergy. 2015;70(12):1613–21.

71. Goncalves C, Pinaffi JV, Carvalho JF, Pinna FR, Constantino GT, Voegels RL, et al. Antineutrophil cytoplasmic antibodies in chronic rhinosinusitis may be a marker of undisclosed vasculitis. Am J Rhinol. 2007;21(6):691–4.

72. Busaba NY, de Oliveira LV, Kieff DL. Correlation between preoperative clinical diagnosis and histopathological findings in patients with rhinosinusitis. Am J Rhinol. 2005;19(2):153–7.

73. Srouji IA, Andrews P, Edwards C, Lund VJ. Patterns of presentation and diagnosis of patients with Wegener's granulomatosis: ENT aspects. J Laryngol Otol. 2007;121(7):653–8.

74. Sproson EL, Jones NS, Al-Deiri M, Lanyon P. Lessons learnt in the management of Wegener's granulomatosis: long-term follow-up of 60 patients. Rhinology. 2007;45(1):63–7.

75. Taylor SC, Clayburgh DR, Rosenbaum JT, Schindler JS. Progression and management of Wegener's granulomatosis in the head and neck. Laryngoscope. 2012;122(8):1695–700.

76. Morgenthau AS, Teirstein AS. Sarcoidosis of the upper and lower airways. Expert Rev Respir Med. 2011;5(6):823–33.

77. Judson MA, Boan AD, Lackland DT. The clinical course of sarcoidosis: presentation, diagnosis, and treatment in a large white and black cohort in the United States. Sarcoidosis Vasc Diffuse Lung Dis. 2012;29(2):119–27.

78. Aloulah M, Manes RP, Ng YH, Fitzgerald JE, Glazer CS, Ryan MW, et al. Sinonasal manifestations of sarcoidosis: a single institution experience with 38 cases. Int Forum Allergy Rhinol. 2013;3(7):567–72.

79. Zeitlin JF, Tami TA, Baughman R, Winget D. Nasal and sinus manifestations of sarcoidosis. Am J Rhinol. 2000;14(3):157–61.

80. Mulholland GB, Jeffery CC, Satija P, Cote DW. Immunoglobulin G4-related diseases in the head and neck: a systematic review. J Otolaryngol Head Neck Surg. 2015;44:24.

81. Guillevin L, Cohen P, Gayraud M, Lhote F, Jarrousse B, Casassus P. Churg-Strauss syndrome. Clinical study and long-term follow-up of 96 patients. Medicine. 1999;78(1):26–37.

82. Samson M, Puechal X, Devilliers H, Ribi C, Cohen P, Stern M, et al. Long-term outcomes of 118 patients with eosinophilic granulomatosis with polyangiitis (Churg-Strauss syndrome) enrolled in two prospective trials. J Autoimmun. 2013;43:60–9.

83. Seccia V, Fortunato S, Cristofani-Mencacci L, Dallan I, Casani AP, Latorre M, Paggiaro P, Bartoli ML, Sellari-Franceschini S, Baldini C. Focus on audiologic impairment in eosinophilic granulomatosis with polyangiitis. Laryngoscope. 2016;126(12):2792–7. https://doi.org/10.1002/lary.25964. Epub 2016 Apr 14.

84. Cannady SB, Batra PS, Koening C, Lorenz RR, Citardi MJ, Langford C, et al. Sinonasal Wegener granulomatosis: a single-institution experience with 120 cases. Laryngoscope. 2009;119(4):757–61.

85. Stone JH. Limited versus severe Wegener's granulomatosis: baseline data on patients in the Wegener's granulomatosis etanercept trial. Arthritis Rheum. 2003;48(8):2299–309.

86. Trimarchi M, Bertazzoni G, Bussi M. Cocaine induced midline destructive lesions. Rhinology. 2014;52(2):104–11.

87. Carlson AQ, Tuot DS, Jen KY, Butcher B, Graf J, Sam R, et al. Pauci-immune glomerulonephritis in individuals with disease associated with levamisole-adulterated cocaine: a series of 4 cases. Medicine. 2014;93(17):290–7.

88. Lawson W, Jiang N, Cheng J. Sinonasal sarcoidosis: a new system of classification acting as a guide to diagnosis and treatment. Am J Rhinol Allergy. 2014;28(4):317–22.

89. Badhey AK, Kadakia S, Carrau RL, Iacob C, Khorsandi A. Sarcoidosis of the head and neck. Head Neck Pathol. 2015;9(2):260–8.

90. Culver DA. Sarcoidosis. Immunol Allergy Clin N Am. 2012;32(4):487–511.

91. Song BH, Baiyee D, Liang J. A rare and emerging entity: sinonasal IgG4-related sclerosing disease. Allergy Rhinol (Providence). 2015;6(3):151–7.

92. Wallace ZS, Deshpande V, Mattoo H, Mahajan VS, Kulikova M, Pillai S, et al. IgG4-related disease: clinical and laboratory features in one hundred twenty-five patients. Arthritis Rheumatol. 2015;67(9):2466–75.

93. Petersen H, Gotz P, Both M, Hey M, Ambrosch P, Bremer JP, et al. Manifestation of eosinophilic granulomatosis with polyangiitis in head and neck. Rhinology. 2015;53(3):277–85.

94. Nakamaru Y, Takagi D, Suzuki M, Homma A, Morita S, Homma A, et al. Otologic and rhinologic manifestations of eosinophilic granulomatosis with polyangiitis. Audiol Neurootol. 2016;21(1):45–53.

95. Pakalniskis MG, Berg AD, Policeni BA, Gentry LR, Sato Y, Moritani T, et al. The many faces of granulomatosis with polyangiitis: a review of the head and neck imaging manifestations. AJR Am J Roentgenol. 2015;205(6):W619–29.

96. Cordier JF, Valeyre D, Guillevin L, Loire R, Brechot JM. Pulmonary Wegener's granulomatosis. A clinical and imaging study of 77 cases. Chest. 1990;97(4):906–12.

97. Anderson G, Coles ET, Crane M, Douglas AC, Gibbs AR, Geddes DM, et al. Wegener's granuloma. A series of 265 British cases seen between 1975 and 1985. A report by a sub-committee of the British Thoracic Society Research Committee. Q J Med. 1992;83(302):427–38.

98. Ikeda S, Arita M, Misaki K, Kashiwagi Y, Ito Y, Yamada H, et al. Comparative investigation of respiratory tract involvement in granulomatosis with polyangiitis between PR3-ANCA positive and MPO-ANCA positive cases: a retrospective cohort study. BMC Pulm Med. 2015;15:78.

99. Braun JJ, Imperiale A, Riehm S, Veillon F. Imaging in sinonasal sarcoidosis: CT, MRI, 67Gallium scintigraphy and 18F-FDG PET/CT features. J Neuroradiol. 2010;37(3):172–81.

100. Palmucci S, Torrisi SE, Caltabiano DC, Puglisi S, Lentini V, Grassedonio E, et al. Clinical and radiological features of extra-pulmonary sarcoidosis: a pictorial essay. Insights Imaging. 2016;7(4):571–87.
101. Oksuz MO, Werner MK, Aschoff P, Pfannenberg C. 18F-FDG PET/CT for the diagnosis of sarcoidosis in a patient with bilateral inflammatory involvement of the parotid and lacrimal glands (panda sign) and bilateral hilar and mediastinal lymphadenopathy (lambda sign). Eur J Nucl Med Mol Imaging. 2011;38(3):603.
102. Vaglio A, Strehl JD, Manger B, Maritati F, Alberici F, Beyer C, et al. IgG4 immune response in Churg-Strauss syndrome. Ann Rheum Dis. 2012;71(3):390–3.
103. Hagen EC, Daha MR, Hermans J, Andrassy K, Csernok E, Gaskin G, et al. Diagnostic value of standardized assays for anti-neutrophil cytoplasmic antibodies in idiopathic systemic vasculitis. EC/BCR Project for ANCA Assay Standardization. Kidney Int. 1998;53(3):743–53.
104. Wegener's Granulomatosis Etanercept Trial (WGET) Research Group. Etanercept plus standard therapy for Wegener's granulomatosis. N Engl J Med. 2005;352(4):351–61.
105. Finkielman JD, Lee AS, Hummel AM, Viss MA, Jacob GL, Homburger HA, et al. ANCA are detectable in nearly all patients with active severe Wegener's granulomatosis. Am J Med. 2007;120(7):643.e9–14.
106. Borner U, Landis BN, Banz Y, Villiger P, Ballinari P, Caversaccio M, et al. Diagnostic value of biopsies in identifying cytoplasmic antineutrophil cytoplasmic antibody-negative localized Wegener's granulomatosis presenting primarily with sinonasal disease. Am J Rhinol Allergy. 2012;26(6):475–80.
107. Del Buono EA, Flint A. Diagnostic usefulness of nasal biopsy in Wegener's granulomatosis. Hum Pathol. 1991;22(2):107–10.
108. Devaney KO, Travis WD, Hoffman G, Leavitt R, Lebovics R, Fauci AS. Interpretation of head and neck biopsies in Wegener's granulomatosis. A pathologic study of 126 biopsies in 70 patients. Am J Surg Pathol. 1990;14(6):555–64.
109. Chang SY, Keogh KA, Lewis JE, Ryu JH, Cornell LD, Garrity JA, et al. IgG4-positive plasma cells in granulomatosis with polyangiitis (Wegener's): a clinicopathologic and immunohistochemical study on 43 granulomatosis with polyangiitis and 20 control cases. Hum Pathol. 2013;44(11):2432–7.
110. Wiesner O, Russell KA, Lee AS, Jenne DE, Trimarchi M, Gregorini G, et al. Antineutrophil cytoplasmic antibodies reacting with human neutrophil elastase as a diagnostic marker for cocaine-induced midline destructive lesions but not autoimmune vasculitis. Arthritis Rheum. 2004;50(9):2954–65.
111. Consensus conference: activity of sarcoidosis. Third WASOG meeting, Los Angeles, USA, September 8-11, 1993. Eur Respir J. 1994;7(3):624–7.
112. Deshpande V, Zen Y, Chan JK, Yi EE, Sato Y, Yoshino T, et al. Consensus statement on the pathology of IgG4-related disease. Mod Pathol. 2012;25(9):1181–92.
113. Kamisawa T, Zen Y, Pillai S, Stone JH. IgG4-related disease. Lancet. 2015;385(9976):1460–71.
114. Akiyama M, Kaneko Y, Hayashi Y, Takeuchi T. IgG4-related disease involving vital organs diagnosed with lip biopsy: a case report and literature review. Medicine. 2016;95(24):e3970.
115. Jennette JC, Falk RJ, Bacon PA, Basu N, Cid MC, Ferrario F, et al. 2012 revised international Chapel Hill consensus conference nomenclature of vasculitides. Arthritis Rheum. 2013;65(1):1–11.
116. Masi AT, Hunder GG, Lie JT, Michel BA, Bloch DA, Arend WP, et al. The American College of Rheumatology 1990 criteria for the classification of Churg-Strauss syndrome (allergic granulomatosis and angiitis). Arthritis Rheum. 1990;33(8):1094–100.
117. Watts R, Lane S, Hanslik T, Hauser T, Hellmich B, Koldingsnes W, et al. Development and validation of a consensus methodology for the classification of the ANCA-associated vasculitides and polyarteritis nodosa for epidemiological studies. Ann Rheum Dis. 2007;66(2):222–7.
118. Craven A, Robson J, Ponte C, Grayson PC, Suppiah R, Judge A, et al. ACR/EULAR-endorsed study to develop Diagnostic and Classification Criteria for Vasculitis (DCVAS). Clin Exp Nephrol. 2013;17(5):619–21.
119. Leavitt RY, Fauci AS, Bloch DA, Michel BA, Hunder GG, Arend WP, et al. The American College of Rheumatology 1990 criteria for the classification of Wegener's granulomatosis. Arthritis Rheum. 1990;33(8):1101–7.
120. Beasley MJ. Lymphoma of the thyroid and head and neck. Clin Oncol. 2012;24(5):345–51.
121. Laudien M. Orphan diseases of the nose and paranasal sinuses: pathogenesis – clinic – therapy. GMS Curr Top Otorhinolaryngol Head Neck Surg 2015;14:Doc04.
122. Hsu YP, Chang PH, Lee TJ, Hung LY, Huang CC. Extranodal natural killer/T-cell lymphoma nasal type: detection by computed tomography features. Laryngoscope. 2014;124(12):2670–5.
123. Valent P, Gleich GJ, Reiter A, Roufosse F, Weller PF, Hellmann A, et al. Pathogenesis and classification of eosinophil disorders: a review of recent developments in the field. Expert Rev Hematol. 2012;5(2):157–76.
124. Mouthon L, Dunogue B, Guillevin L. Diagnosis and classification of eosinophilic granulomatosis with polyangiitis (formerly named Churg-Strauss syndrome). J Autoimmun. 2014;48-49:99–103.
125. Bachert C, van Steen K, Zhang N, Holtappels G, Cattaert T, Maus B, et al. Specific IgE against Staphylococcus aureus enterotoxins: an independent risk factor for asthma. J Allergy Clin Immunol. 2012;130(2):376–81.e8.

126. Miziara ID, Araujo Filho BC, La Cortina RC, Romano FR, Lima AS. Chronic rhinosinusitis in HIV-infected patients: radiological and clinical evaluation. Braz J Otorhinolaryngol. 2005;71(5):604–8.
127. Chee L, Graham SM, Carothers DG, Ballas ZK. Immune dysfunction in refractory sinusitis in a tertiary care setting. Laryngoscope. 2001;111(2):233–5.
128. Alqudah M, Graham SM, Ballas ZK. High prevalence of humoral immunodeficiency patients with refractory chronic rhinosinusitis. Am J Rhinol Allergy. 2010;24(6):409–12.
129. May A, Zielen S, von Ilberg C, Weber A. Immunoglobulin deficiency and determination of pneumococcal antibody titers in patients with therapy-refractory recurrent rhinosinusitis. Eur Arch Otorhinolaryngol. 1999;256(9):445–9.
130. Vanlerberghe L, Joniau S, Jorissen M. The prevalence of humoral immunodeficiency in refractory rhinosinusitis: a retrospective analysis. B-ENT. 2006;2(4):161–6.
131. Schwitzguebel AJ, Jandus P, Lacroix JS, Seebach JD, Harr T. Immunoglobulin deficiency in patients with chronic rhinosinusitis: systematic review of the literature and meta-analysis. J Allergy Clin Immunol. 2015;136(6):1523–31.
132. Park MA, Li JT, Hagan JB, Maddox DE, Abraham RS. Common variable immunodeficiency: a new look at an old disease. Lancet. 2008;372(9637):489–502.
133. Quinti I, Soresina A, Spadaro G, Martino S, Donnanno S, Agostini C, et al. Long-term follow-up and outcome of a large cohort of patients with common variable immunodeficiency. J Clin Immunol. 2007;27(3):308–16.
134. Wang KL, Nichols BG, Poetker DM, Loehrl TA. Odontogenic sinusitis: a case series studying diagnosis and management. Int Forum Allergy Rhinol. 2015;5(7):597–601.
135. Patel NA, Ferguson BJ. Odontogenic sinusitis: an ancient but under-appreciated cause of maxillary sinusitis. Curr Opin Otolaryngol Head Neck Surg. 2012;20(1):24–8.
136. Crovetto-Martinez R, Martin-Arregui FJ, Zabala-Lopez-de-Maturana A, Tudela-Cabello K, Crovetto-de la Torre MA. Frequency of the odontogenic maxillary sinusitis extended to the anterior ethmoid sinus and response to surgical treatment. Med Oral Patol Oral Cir Bucal. 2014;19(4):e409–13.
137. Brook I. Sinusitis of odontogenic origin. Otolaryngol Head Neck Surg. 2006;135(3):349–55.
138. Chang EH. New insights into the pathogenesis of cystic fibrosis sinusitis. Int Forum Allergy Rhinol. 2014;4(2):132–7.
139. Barbato A, Frischer T, Kuehni CE, Snijders D, Azevedo I, Baktai G, et al. Primary ciliary dyskinesia: a consensus statement on diagnostic and treatment approaches in children. Eur Respir J. 2009;34(6):1264–76.
140. Marthin JK, Nielsen KG. Choice of nasal nitric oxide technique as first-line test for primary ciliary dyskinesia. Eur Respir J. 2011;37(3):559–65.
141. Mateos-Corral D, Coombs R, Grasemann H, Ratjen F, Dell SD. Diagnostic value of nasal nitric oxide measured with non-velum closure techniques for children with primary ciliary dyskinesia. J Pediatr. 2011;159(3):420–4.
142. Rank MA, Wollan P, Kita H, Yawn BP. Acute exacerbations of chronic rhinosinusitis occur in a distinct seasonal pattern. J Allergy Clin Immunol. 2010;126(1):168–9.
143. Outzen KE, Grontveld A, Jorgensen K, Clausen PP, Ladefoged C. Inverted papilloma: incidence and late results of surgical treatment. Rhinology. 1996;34(2):114–8.
144. Chang JE, White A, Simon RA, Stevenson DD. Aspirin-exacerbated respiratory disease: burden of disease. Allergy Asthma Proc. 2012;33(2):117–21.
145. Divekar R, Hagan J, Rank M, Park M, Volcheck G, O'Brien E, et al. Diagnostic utility of urinary LTE4 in asthma, allergic rhinitis, chronic rhinosinusitis, nasal polyps, and aspirin sensitivity. J Allergy Clin Immunol Pract. 2016;4(4):665–70.
146. Laidlaw TM, Boyce JA. Platelets in patients with aspirin-exacerbated respiratory disease. J Allergy Clin Immunol. 2015;135(6):1407–14. quiz 15.
147. Kowalski ML, Ptasinska A, Jedrzejczak M, Bienkiewicz B, Cieslak M, Grzegorczyk J, et al. Aspirin-triggered 15-HETE generation in peripheral blood leukocytes is a specific and sensitive Aspirin-Sensitive Patients Identification Test (ASPITest). Allergy. 2005;60(9):1139–45.
148. Bent JP 3rd, Kuhn FA. Diagnosis of allergic fungal sinusitis. Otolaryngol Head Neck Surg. 1994;111(5):580–8.
149. deShazo RD, Swain RE. Diagnostic criteria for allergic fungal sinusitis. J Allergy Clin Immunol. 1995;96(1):24–35.
150. Wise SK, Rogers GA, Ghegan MD, Harvey RJ, Delgaudio JM, Schlosser RJ. Radiologic staging system for allergic fungal rhinosinusitis (AFRS). Otolaryngol Head Neck Surg. 2009;140(5):735–40.
151. Chen IH, Chen TM. Isolated frontal sinus aspergillosis. Otolaryngol Head Neck Surg. 2000;122(3):460–1.
152. Panda NK, Ekambar Eshwara Reddy C. Primary frontal sinus aspergillosis: an uncommon occurrence. Mycoses. 2005;48(4):235–7.
153. Gupta AK, Ghosh S. Sinonasal aspergillosis in immunocompetent Indian children: an eight-year experience. Mycoses. 2003;46(11–12):455–61.
154. Ogbogu PU, Bochner BS, Butterfield JH, Gleich GJ, Huss-Marp J, Kahn JE, et al. Hypereosinophilic syndrome: a multicenter, retrospective analysis of clinical characteristics and response to therapy. J Allergy Clin Immunol. 2009;124(6):1319–25.e3.
155. Soler ZM, Eckert MA, Storck K, Schlosser RJ. Cognitive function in chronic rhinosinusitis: a controlled clinical study. Int Forum Allergy Rhinol. 2015;5(11):1010–7.
156. Levy JM, Mace JC, DeConde AS, Steele TO, Smith TL. Improvements in psychological dysfunction after endoscopic sinus surgery for patients with

chronic rhinosinusitis. Int Forum Allergy Rhinol. 2016;6(9):906–13.

157. El Rassi E, Mace JC, Steele TO, Alt JA, Smith TL. Improvements in sleep-related symptoms after endoscopic sinus surgery in patients with chronic rhinosinusitis. Int Forum Allergy Rhinol. 2016;6(4):414–22.

158. Reinhold-Keller E, Beuge N, Latza U, de Groot K, Rudert H, Nolle B, et al. An interdisciplinary approach to the care of patients with Wegener's granulomatosis: long-term outcome in 155 patients. Arthritis Rheum. 2000;43(5):1021–32.

159. Groh M, Pagnoux C, Baldini C, Bel E, Bottero P, Cottin V, et al. Eosinophilic granulomatosis with polyangiitis (Churg-Strauss) (EGPA) Consensus Task Force recommendations for evaluation and management. Eur J Intern Med. 2015;26(7):545–53.

160. De Groot K, Rasmussen N, Bacon PA, Tervaert JW, Feighery C, Gregorini G, et al. Randomized trial of cyclophosphamide versus methotrexate for induction of remission in early systemic antineutrophil cytoplasmic antibody-associated vasculitis. Arthritis Rheum. 2005;52(8):2461–9.

161. Langford CA, Monach PA, Specks U, Seo P, Cuthbertson D, McAlear CA, et al. An open-label trial of abatacept (CTLA4-IG) in non-severe relapsing granulomatosis with polyangiitis (Wegener's). Ann Rheum Dis. 2014;73(7):1376–9.

162. Azar L, Springer J, Langford CA, Hoffman GS. Rituximab with or without a conventional maintenance agent in the treatment of relapsing granulomatosis with polyangiitis (Wegener's): a retrospective single-center study. Arthritis Rheumatol. 2014;66(10):2862–70.

163. Hoffman GS. Immunosuppressive therapy is always required for the treatment of limited Wegener's granulomatosis. Sarcoidosis Vasc Diffuse Lung Dis. 1996;13(3):249–52.

164. Cartin-Ceba R, Golbin JM, Keogh KA, Peikert T, Sanchez-Menendez M, Ytterberg SR, et al. Rituximab for remission induction and maintenance in refractory granulomatosis with polyangiitis (Wegener's): ten-year experience at a single center. Arthritis Rheum. 2012;64(11):3770–8.

165. Stone JH, Tun W, Hellman DB. Treatment of non-life threatening Wegener's granulomatosis with methotrexate and daily prednisone as the initial therapy of choice. J Rheumatol. 1999;26(5):1134–9.

166. Metzler C, Miehle N, Manger K, Iking-Konert C, de Groot K, Hellmich B, et al. Elevated relapse rate under oral methotrexate versus leflunomide for maintenance of remission in Wegener's granulomatosis. Rheumatology (Oxford). 2007;46(7):1087–91.

167. Lally L, Lebovics RS, Huang WT, Spiera RF. Effectiveness of rituximab for the otolaryngologic manifestations of granulomatosis with polyangiitis (Wegener's). Arthritis Care Res. 2014;66(9):1403–9.

168. Harabuchi Y, Kishibe K, Tateyama K, Morita Y, Yoshida N, Kunimoto Y, et al. Clinical features and treatment outcomes of otitis media with antineutrophil cytoplasmic antibody (ANCA)-associated vasculitis (OMAAV): a retrospective analysis of 235 patients from a nationwide survey in Japan. Mod Rheumatol. 2016:1–8.

169. Malm IJ, Mener DJ, Kim J, Seo P, Kim YJ. Otolaryngological progression of granulomatosis with polyangiitis after systemic treatment with rituximab. Otolaryngol Head Neck Surg. 2014;150(1):68–72.

170. Seo P, Specks U, Keogh KA. Efficacy of rituximab in limited Wegener's granulomatosis with refractory granulomatous manifestations. J Rheumatol. 2008;35(10):2017–23.

171. Wojciechowska J, Krajewski W, Krajewski P, Krecicki T. Granulomatosis with polyangiitis in otolaryngologist practice: a review of current knowledge. Clin Exp Otorhinolaryngol. 2016;9(1):8–13.

172. Mueller A, Holl-Ulrich K, Feller AC, Gross WL, Lamprecht P. Immune phenomena in localized and generalized Wegener's granulomatosis. Clin Exp Rheumatol. 2003;21(6 Suppl 32):S49–54.

173. Hellmich B, Flossmann O, Gross WL, Bacon P, Cohen-Tervaert JW, Guillevin L, et al. EULAR recommendations for conducting clinical studies and/or clinical trials in systemic vasculitis: focus on antineutrophil cytoplasm antibody-associated vasculitis. Ann Rheum Dis. 2007;66(5):605–17.

174. Pagnoux C, Stubbe M, Lifermann F, Decaux O, Pavic M, Berezne A, et al. Wegener's granulomatosis strictly and persistently localized to one organ is rare: assessment of 16 patients from the French Vasculitis Study Group database. J Rheumatol. 2011;38(3):475–8.

175. Holle JU, Gross WL, Holl-Ulrich K, Ambrosch P, Noelle B, Both M, et al. Prospective long-term follow-up of patients with localised Wegener's granulomatosis: does it occur as persistent disease stage? Ann Rheum Dis. 2010;69(11):1934–9.

176. Goldfarb JM, Rabinowitz MR, Basnyat S, Nyquist GG, Rosen MR. Head and neck manifestations of eosinophilic granulomatosis with polyangiitis: a systematic review. Otolaryngol Head Neck Surg. 2016;155(5):771–8.

177. Gulati S, Krossnes B, Olofsson J, Danielsen A. Sinonasal involvement in sarcoidosis: a report of seven cases and review of literature. Eur Arch Otorhinolaryngol. 2012;269(3):891–6.

178. Knopf A, Lahmer T, Chaker A, Stark T, Hofauer B, Pickhard A, et al. Head and neck sarcoidosis, from wait and see to tumor necrosis factor alpha therapy: a pilot study. Head Neck. 2013;35(5):715–9.

179. Baughman RP, Lower EE. Treatment of sarcoidosis. Clin Rev Allergy Immunol. 2015;49(1):79–92.

180. Khosroshahi A, Wallace ZS, Crowe JL, Akamizu T, Azumi A, Carruthers MN, et al. International consensus guidance statement on the management and treatment of IgG4-related disease. Arthritis Rheumatol. 2015;67(7):1688–99.

181. Carruthers MN, Topazian MD, Khosroshahi A, Witzig TE, Wallace ZS, Hart PA, et al. Rituximab

for IgG4-related disease: a prospective, open-label trial. Ann Rheum Dis. 2015;74(6):1171–7.

182. Orange JS, Belohradsky BH, Berger M, Borte M, Hagan J, Jolles S, et al. Evaluation of correlation between dose and clinical outcomes in subcutaneous immunoglobulin replacement therapy. Clin Exp Immunol. 2012;169(2):172–81.

183. Orange JS, Grossman WJ, Navickis RJ, Wilkes MM. Impact of trough IgG on pneumonia incidence in primary immunodeficiency: a meta-analysis of clinical studies. Clin Immunol. 2010;137(1):21–30.

184. Liang J, Higgins T, Ishman SL, Boss EF, Benke JR, Lin SY. Medical management of chronic rhinosinusitis in cystic fibrosis: a systematic review. Laryngoscope. 2014;124(6):1308–13.

185. Chang EH, Tang XX, Shah VS, Launspach JL, Ernst SE, Hilkin B, et al. Medical reversal of chronic sinusitis in a cystic fibrosis patient with ivacaftor. Int Forum Allergy Rhinol. 2015;5(2):178–81.

186. Brook I. The role of anaerobic bacteria in sinusitis. Anaerobe. 2006;12(1):5–12.

187. Cincik H, Ferguson BJ. The impact of endoscopic cultures on care in rhinosinusitis. Laryngoscope. 2006;116(9):1562–8.

188. Casiano RR, Cohn S, Villasuso E 3rd, Brown M, Memari F, Barquist E, et al. Comparison of antral tap with endoscopically directed nasal culture. Laryngoscope. 2001;111(8):1333–7.

189. Gold SM, Tami TA. Role of middle meatus aspiration culture in the diagnosis of chronic sinusitis. Laryngoscope. 1997;107(12 Pt 1):1586–9.

190. Fokkens WJ, Lund VJ, Mullol J, Bachert C, Alobid I, Baroody F, et al. EPOS 2012: European position paper on rhinosinusitis and nasal polyps 2012. A summary for otorhinolaryngologists. Rhinology. 2012;50(1):1–12.

191. Nadel DM, Lanza DC, Kennedy DW. Endoscopically guided cultures in chronic sinusitis. Am J Rhinol. 1998;12(4):233–41.

192. Bachert C, Akdis CA. Phenotypes and emerging endotypes of chronic rhinosinusitis. J Allergy Clin Immunol Pract. 2016;4(4):621–8.

193. Gevaert P, Van Bruaene N, Cattaert T, Van Steen K, Van Zele T, Acke F, et al. Mepolizumab, a humanized anti-IL-5 mAb, as a treatment option for severe nasal polyposis. J Allergy Clin Immunol. 2011;128(5):989–95. e1–8.

194. Gevaert P, Lang-Loidolt D, Lackner A, Stammberger H, Staudinger H, Van Zele T, et al. Nasal IL-5 levels determine the response to anti-IL-5 treatment in patients with nasal polyps. J Allergy Clin Immunol. 2006;118(5):1133–41.

195. Bachert C, Mannent L, Naclerio RM, Mullol J, Ferguson BJ, Gevaert P, et al. Effect of subcutaneous dupilumab on nasal polyp burden in patients with chronic sinusitis and nasal polyposis: a randomized clinical trial. JAMA. 2016;315(5):469–79.

196. Bachert C, Zhang L, Gevaert P. Current and future treatment options for adult chronic rhinosinusitis: focus on nasal polyposis. J Allergy Clin Immunol. 2015;136(6):1431–40. quiz 41

197. Gevaert P, Calus L, Van Zele T, Blomme K, De Ruyck N, Bauters W, et al. Omalizumab is effective in allergic and nonallergic patients with nasal polyps and asthma. J Allergy Clin Immunol. 2013;131(1):110–6.e1.

198. Laidlaw TM, Boyce JA. Aspirin-exacerbated respiratory disease – new prime suspects. N Engl J Med. 2016;374(5):484–8.

199. Lee RU, Stevenson DD. Aspirin-exacerbated respiratory disease: evaluation and management. Allergy, Asthma Immunol Res. 2011;3(1):3–10.

200. Simon RA, Dazy KM, Waldram JD. Update on aspirin desensitization for chronic rhinosinusitis with polyps in aspirin-exacerbated respiratory disease (AERD). Curr Allergy Asthma Rep. 2015;15(3):508.

Postoperative Care of the Frontal Sinus

20

Jose Luis Mattos and Zachary M. Soler

Introduction

Endoscopic surgery of the frontal sinus can prove challenging even for the most experienced rhinologic surgeon. The narrow confines of the frontal recess and the critical structures that surround it make surgery in this region technically unforgiving. Additionally, the anatomic location of the frontal recess often requires the use of angled endoscopes and specialized instrumentation, which further adds to the level of difficulty. Despite a patent sinus at the conclusion of surgery, dissection in the tight confines of the frontal recess can cause mucosal edema and apposition of damaged epithelial surfaces, leading to granulation tissue, adhesions, neo-osteogenesis, and ultimately obstruction of the frontal sinus outflow tract in the postoperative setting [1]. Iatrogenic obstruction of the frontal outflow tract is particularly problematic in patients with a narrow frontal recess or in the setting of significant inflammation [1, 2].

Given the technical and anatomic challenges in frontal sinus surgery, it is not surprising that reported success rates are variable. Outcomes after frontal sinus surgery are typically reported in terms of maintenance of postoperative sinus patency and symptom resolution. For Draf II frontal sinusotomies, the overall patency after primary surgery has been reported to be between 69% and 92% [3–8], but follow-up in these studies is variable. The largest series with the longest follow-up period was published in 2012, showing frontal sinus patency at 17 months to be 92%, with 78% of patients experiencing complete symptom resolution [8]. The final size of the intraoperative ostium correlated with the rate of restenosis, and re-stenosis of the frontal sinus correlated with persistence of symptoms [8]. Clearly, maintaining a patent and functional frontal sinus outflow tract postoperatively is of utmost importance to the frontal sinus surgeon.

Successful outcomes for the Draf III are similarly defined in the literature, with primary outcome measures being neo-ostial patency and symptom resolution. A recent meta-analysis has reported long-term outcomes after Draf III [9]. On average, 19% of patients suffer from significant restenosis, and 14% of Draf III patients require revision frontal sinusotomy; this equates to a long-term success rate of 86% [9]. However, reports of successful long-term outcomes after Draf III vary between 70% and 95% [10, 11]. The majority of patients who fail Draf III usually do so within the first 2 years, but failures can be seen up to a decade postoperatively [12]. Tran et al. report that an intraoperative ostium with an area

J. L. Mattos · Z. M. Soler (✉)
Division of Rhinology and Sinus Surgery,
Department of Otolaryngology – Head and Neck
Surgery, Medical University of South Carolina,
Charleston, SC, USA

© Springer Nature Switzerland AG 2019
D. Lal, P. H. Hwang (eds.), *Frontal Sinus Surgery*, https://doi.org/10.1007/978-3-319-97022-6_20

of greater than 300 mm² has a 76% chance of patency at 1 year and an area larger than 394 mm² had a 100% chance of patency [13]. While there is a correlation between maintained adequate frontal sinus patency and symptomatic improvement, there are reports of patients with complete ostial restenosis without recurrence of symptoms [9, 12, 14, 15]. Similar to type II frontal sinusotomies, it appears that the size of the intraoperative neo-ostium and the maximal long-term maintenance of this size are the most important factors in outcomes after Draf III.

Given the challenge of maintaining patency of the frontal sinus after surgery, postoperative care is critical to long-term success. Each section of this chapter will begin with a discussion of general postoperative care after sinus surgery, as there are overarching themes and concepts that apply to all of the paranasal sinuses, including the frontal. Approaches that are specific to frontal sinus will then be examined. Since the postoperative care of the Draf II sinusotomy and Draf III differ, postoperative care specific to these procedures will be discussed separately when appropriate. To the extent possible, the highest-level evidence will be reviewed for specific techniques. However, where there is lack of controlled, clinical trials specifically related to post-operative frontal care, recommendations will be made as they apply to postoperative care in endoscopic sinus surgery.

General Postoperative Care

In the vast majority of instances, frontal sinus surgery is performed as part of more extensive sinus surgery. The same general principles that apply to general postoperative sinus care usually apply after frontal sinus surgery. In 2011, Rudmik et al. performed an evidence-based review and recommendation analysis of available literature in postoperative sinus surgery care [16]. This study recommended the use of topical steroids, nasal saline irrigations, and postoperative debridement in the immediate postoperative period. A recent international consensus statement on the treatment of chronic rhinosinusitis supported

these findings [17]. While other medical therapies like oral corticosteroids and oral or topical antibiotics are options for postoperative care, the three aforementioned interventions (topical steroids, nasal saline irrigations, and postoperative debridement) are considered to be the gold standard of postoperative sinus care.

Topical Corticosteroids

Topical corticosteroids are supported by grade A level of evidence, with improved symptomatology, endoscopy appearance, and polyp recurrence when administered after sinus surgery [16, 17]. There are different methods of delivery of topical corticosteroids including nasal sprays, nebulizers, irrigations, and drops. A recent Cochrane review of intranasal steroids in CRS found insufficient evidence to suggest that one type of intranasal steroid is more effective than another [18]. However, cadaver studies suggest that the use of high-volume delivery mechanisms like squeeze bottles or gravity-dependent irrigations (i.e., Neti Pot) has improved topical delivery to the sinuses than sprays [19, 20]. In our practice, most patients are also placed on postoperative irrigations. Therefore, we often combine their topical corticosteroids with their saline rinses; this is begun on postoperative day 1 (see the irrigation section below for a more detailed discussion on sino-nasal irrigations).

Topical steroid drops have been advocated for use after frontal sinus surgery. Theoretically, these deliver a more concentrated steroid solution and might be able to be anatomically directed to the frontal sinus via different head positions like "vertex to floor" and hanging the head off the edge of a bed. Case reports and clinical trials of steroid drops have shown success rates in maintaining frontal sinus patency postoperatively as high as 80% and may be superior to other forms of steroid delivery [21, 22]. There is one prospective, randomized study of frontal steroid drops vs. nasal steroid sprays which suggested that drops might have superior patency rates, but the findings did not reach statistical significance [16, 17].

Sino-nasal Irrigations

Saline irrigations have been shown to improve symptoms and endoscopic appearance of the sinuses, as well as to decrease the rate of synechiae formation after surgery [16, 17]. Overall they have a grade B level of evidence. Several special considerations apply to postoperative irrigation of the frontal sinus. Sino-nasal irrigations and topical medications may have difficulty reaching the frontal sinus outflow tract due to gravity. In the unoperated state, the frontal sinus appears to have the worst penetration of topical medications of all sinuses, and topical access significantly improves in the operated state [19]. A recent study analyzed factors contributing to the penetration of irrigation fluid into the frontal sinus postoperatively [23]. The authors concluded that the most important factor was the extent of surgery, with Draf III achieving significantly better access than Draf IIa [23]. Regardless of surgical approach, vertex down head position (see Fig. 20.1) seems to be associated with improved topical access, and high-volume irrigations appear to reach the sinus cavities with greater success than low-volume techniques [20, 23, 24]. In our practice, patients begin saline irrigations immediately postoperatively twice daily, often with the addition of topical cortico-

steroids in the irrigation solution. For those felt to be at high risk for postoperative frontal stenosis, head position during irrigation can be adjusted to maximize frontal penetration. It should be noted that the frequency and timing of irrigations postoperatively has not been thoroughly studied.

Postoperative Debridement

Postoperative debridement of the frontal sinus has been given a grade B level of evidence, with studies showing that it can decrease the rate of synechiae and middle meatal adhesions after surgery [16, 25]. Frontal sinus care differs from the standard sinus surgery debridement in that angled endoscopes and curved instruments are usually required in the office to achieve successful debridement (see Fig. 20.2). There is a paucity of high-quality evidence to guide clinicians in the optimal timing, frequency, duration, and extent of postoperative debridement [16]. Some authors suggest multiple debridements within the first week to achieve optimal results [26], while others show a single debridement within the first week postoperatively to be equally efficacious, with a greater likelihood of patient follow-up and adherence [27]. No such studies have been undertaken for the frontal sinus specifically. It is

Fig. 20.1 Vertex to floor sino-nasal irrigation head positioning vertex to floor head position maximizes penetration of sino-nasal irrigations to the frontal sinus. (Images are property of MUSC Rhinology)

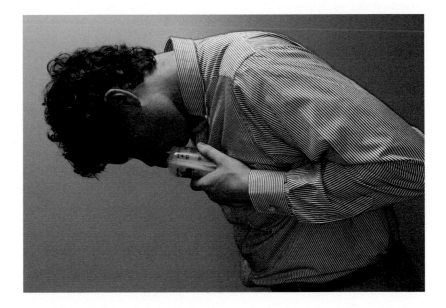

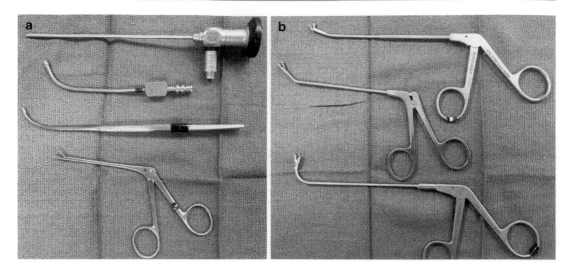

Fig. 20.2 Equipment for in-office frontal sinus debridement. (**a**) Basic instrumentation for frontal sinus debridement, from top to bottom – angled endoscope, curved suction, frontal probe, straight grasper. (**b**) Additional instrumentation for frontal sinus debridement. While not routinely used, angled graspers and cutting instruments are occasionally required for more thorough debridement, lysing of synechiae, etc. (Images are property of MUSC Rhinology)

our practice to see patients 5–7 days postoperatively for their initial debridement and postoperative check following Draf II frontal sinusotomy. Those patients at highest risk of stenosis may be seen weekly until mucosal healing has occurred, whereas others are typically seen 2–4 weeks later for further debridement and reassessment. Ideally, one should visually confirm that the frontal sinus ostium is patent at each visit. In instances where edema or blood obscures visualization, at minimum we would hope to pass a small curved suction or probe with no resistance into the sinus. While we recognize this approach is not necessarily evidence-based, there is no current body of evidence to guide these decisions.

Biomaterials

Although biomaterials are often placed at the time of surgery and thus are not "postoperative" per se, they are usually present in the postoperative period, and decisions must be made regarding the extent and nature of their use. For that reason, biomaterials will be discussed as a component of postoperative care. A multitude of biomaterials has been proposed for use after endoscopic sinus surgery. The only intervention other than topical corticosteroids with grade A evidence is the use of drug-eluting spacers and stents, which are discussed in detail below in the stenting section. Recently, a comprehensive review of controlled randomized trials of biomaterials in rhinology was performed, which focused primarily on middle meatal dressings [28]. This review focused on a material's ability to provide hemostasis and improve wound healing. Of all reviewed biomaterials, chitosan, fibrin glue, and polyvinyl acetate in a latex glove finger proved to have "mostly positive" effects in both of the studied domains. Few clinical trials have focused solely on the frontal sinus when evaluating these materials, although one randomized trial of chitosan did show improvement in frontal ostia patency postoperatively [29]. The ideal indications when or for whom the biomaterials can be best used in have not been definitively studied. In our practice, most patients receive a chitosan middle meatal dressing often impregnated with corticosteroids (see Fig. 20.4). This dressing is not necessarily placed within the frontal recess. Anecdotally, we find this material to significantly improve postoperative healing; the material can easily be suctioned out in the clinic with minimal patient discomfort.

Frontal Sinus Stenting

In addition to the general postoperative care concepts detailed above, frontal sinus stenting has often been described as a technique to maintain long-term patency. In this section, "stenting" is used in a broad fashion to mean any foreign material placed into the frontal recess to augment its patency. The approach and philosophy of stenting differs between Draf IIA or Draf IIB sinusotomies and Draf III procedures. There are no clear or absolute indications for stenting, and the use of stents for these procedures varies widely. Many authors believe that some type of stenting is indicated for Draf III procedures given the significant amount of exposed bone and mucosal trauma. Furthermore, the type and duration of stenting can vary widely, from drug-eluding absorbable stents to synthetic sheeting that is usually left in place for days to weeks or more rigid stents that can be left in place indefinitely. Table 20.1 summarizes commonly used stenting strategies.

Stenting of Draf II Frontal Procedures

Indications

There is no consensus on the indications for postoperative frontal sinus stenting in Draf II A or IIB procedures. The decision to stent the frontal sinus is typically based on individual patient anatomy and disease process, combined with individual surgeon preference. However, there are factors that might increase risk of restenosis like size of the outflow tract, extensive polyposis/inflammation, significant osteitis, demucosalization with circumferential bone exposure, an unstable mid-

dle turbinate, and traumatic fracture of the frontal sinus outflow tract [1, 30]. Weber has shown that a neo-ostium diameter less than 5 mm doubles the rate of stenosis, while a diameter of 2 mm increases the rate to 50% [2]. Rains has indicated that a neo-ostium of less than 5 mm may be an indication for stenting [1, 30]. The exact incidence of frontal sinus stenting is unknown; however, a single-center study of 462 patients undergoing frontal sinus surgery reported that only 2.2% of their patients required stenting, using criteria similar to the ones presented above [31]. However, other surgeons routinely use stenting materials on all cases and evidence to support any specific practice is weak. Weber et al. prospectively studied long-term results of frontal sinus stenting, and patients with stents had 80% chance of long-term patency compared to 33% in un-stented patients. However, these results are hard to interpret as most case series show frontal patency to be much higher than 33%.

Materials

A variety of materials have been used to prevent postoperative stenosis of the frontal sinus, ranging from early attempts at using metals like gold and tantalum [32, 33] to synthetics like Dacron, silicone, and Silastic [2, 30, 34–37] and to modern drug-eluting mechanisms. The Rains silicone stent is widely known and consists of a compressible basket at the distal end which can re-expand to maintain the stent position; it can serve as an irrigation port, can be inserted endoscopically, and can be maintained in place long term [1, 30]. This stent has been reported to have 94% patency at 46 months [1, 30]. Another common practice is to use thin Silastic sheeting, which

Table 20.1 Frontal sinus stenting options

Stent type	Material	Situation for use	Duration
Soft	Silastic sheeting	High risk of restenosis, bone exposure after Draf III	Short term (weeks to months)
Rigid	Silicone (most common), Dacron, tantalum, etc.	High risk of restenosis	Long term (months to years)
Drug-eluting	Bio-absorbable, corticosteroid releasing	High risk of restenosis, sino-nasal polyposis	Short term, dissolves in weeks but may need to be debrided postoperatively
Mucosal graft	Septum or nasal floor mucosa	Bone exposure after Draf III	Permanent, integrates into sino-nasal cavity

can be rolled in a cylindrical shape and placed into the frontal sinus; this is removed in the early postoperative period. In our practice, when stenting is indicated, we utilize a "dart"-shaped soft Silastic sheeting stent (see Figs. 20.3 and 20.4).

The choice of rigid vs. soft stent remains controversial, but some animal studies have shown that softer materials promote re-epithelialization and decrease scar formation compared to rigid stents [1, 35, 38]. Clinical studies in humans have also shown good success with soft sheeting stents, leading to improved re-mucosalization, decreased fibrosis, less neo-osteogenesis, and superior postoperative patency rates compared to no stenting [1, 35, 36].

Duration of Stent Placement

There is wide variability in the literature regarding appropriate duration of frontal sinus stenting, and the appropriate length of stenting is unknown. It does appear that long-term stenting of the frontal sinus can be pursued without significant adverse effect. Several authors have reported good success rates with stenting duration of anywhere from 5 weeks to 6 years postoperatively [2, 31, 39–42]. While complications due to frontal sinus stenting are extremely rare even in the setting of prolonged use, there has been a case report of toxic shock syndrome, a potentially fatal condition, attributed to frontal sinus stents

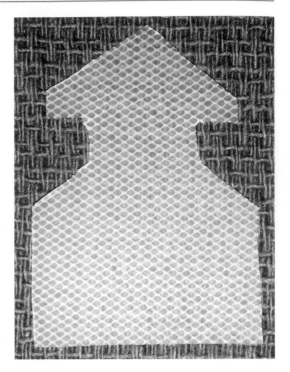

Fig. 20.3 Silastic "dart" for stenting of frontal sinus. Silastic "dart" used for frontal sinus stenting. This is an example of a soft Silastic stent that can be used in the frontal sinus; it is the preferred method of the chapter's authors. The tip of the dart is inserted into the frontal sinus proper, and the tapered shape helps to hold it in place. The neck of the dart ideally rests within the frontal sinus outflow tract; the body of the dart allows for greater surface coverage if needed and allows for removal in the clinic. The size and shape of the different components of the dart can be modified to accommodate for anatomical variations

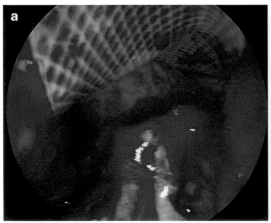

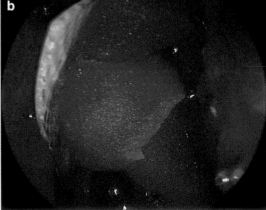

Fig. 20.4 Intraoperative view of Draf III cavity with Silastic stent. (**a**) Intraoperative view of Silastic sheeting after Draf III sinusotomy. Notice Silastic goes into frontal sinus and covers areas of the exposed bone anteriorly. (**b**) Chitosan or other absorbable material can be used both to bolster the Silastic sheeting internally and to serve as a frontal recess and middle meatal dressing material (Images are property of MUSC Rhinology.)

[43]. Prolonged stenting (i.e., months to years) does not seem to be a common current practice. Most surgeons who employ stenting usually do so during the immediate healing phase, usually one week or up to several weeks, before removing, and in these cases stents are often used to aid in debridement of clot and crust when the stents are removed. Those patients who would require long-term stenting to maintain patency are probably more likely to undergo a Draf III procedure rather than have a stent in perpetuity.

Drug-Eluting Stents

Steroids, both topical and oral, have long been used in the treatment of CRS, and topical steroids are considered part of the gold standard in postoperative sinus surgery care as discussed above. As such, several steroid-eluting stents have been devised. Animal models have demonstrated that dexamethasone-releasing stents decrease the amount of osteoneogenesis in operated sinuses and lead to less granulation tissue with decreased stromal thickening and preserved re-epithelialization [44, 45]. Several human trials on the subject have been performed, including ones that are prospective, randomized, double-blinded, and multi-institutional in nature [46–48]. Universally, these studies show a decrease in postoperative inflammation, polyp formation, adhesions, need for postoperative intervention, and middle turbinate lateralization in sinuses where a corticosteroid eluting stent is used, compared to control sinuses without any major observable side effects [46–49]. Furthermore, it appears that patient-reported disease-specific outcomes are also improved in patients who received corticosteroid-eluting stents [47].

Few studies of drug-eluting stent studies have targeted solely the frontal sinus. A recent prospective, multicenter, randomized, blinded trial has been published examining the effect of steroid-releasing implants with a focus on postoperative frontal sinus patency [50]. This study demonstrated a reduction in postoperative restenosis, interventions, inflammation, and oral steroid administration [50]. While most studies focus on the intraoperative placement of these stents, some authors have even reported suc-

cessful in-office steroid-eluting implant placement in the frontal sinuses [51]. Of note, other drugs have been trialed for use with stents, like doxycycline, which may show promise in improving postoperative healing but require further study [52].

Stenting After Endoscopic Draf III Frontal Sinusotomy

The Draf III requires aggressive bone removal and drilling to ensure the largest possible neo-ostium. This results in a significant amount of exposed bone that could predispose the newly created cavity to restenosis. The use of some sort of packing or "stenting" material is often advocated by those authors who describe Draf III procedures. Additionally, while not exactly a stenting procedure, mucosal grafting has been advocated in Draf III cavities due improved postoperative healing and decreased restenosis, and these mucosal grafts are usually bolstered with some type of stent or packing.

Given the degree of exposed bone after Draf III, stenting to prevent restenosis is a rational therapeutic approach. There is, unfortunately, a paucity of high-level evidence regarding packing or stenting after Draf III. Packing with a gloved polyvinyl acetate sponge as described by Toffel for 7 days has been advocated as a useful technique delivering good results [53]. Soft Silastic sheeting is one of the most commonly utilized materials to stent a Draf III cavity (see Figs. 20.3 and 20.4). In a retrospective review of 72 patients, there was no advantage to using soft Silastic stents for long-term frontal ostium patency [14], and this may be due to the already high success rate for Draf III without stenting. In fact, the largest series of 229 patients on the long-term outcomes after Draf III report a success rate of 95% with no packing or stenting used whatsoever [54]. Stents may facilitate postoperative wound care and seem to have no negative impact on the postoperative course [14]. There is also no accepted length of stenting should it be utilized, but one series reports good success with a 2-month duration [14]. There are no studies on drug-eluting stents after Draf III; however, these would be expected to have similar effects as they do in the less extensive frontal sinusotomies as detailed above. Generally, we stent our Draf III cavities with Silastic sheeting that is secured in place with chitosan that is impregnated with corticosteroids, and the sheeting is left in place for approximately 3 weeks. The reality is that many surgeons have different stenting/packing practices, and to date none has been conclusively proved superior to others.

Mucosal Grafting of Frontal Neo-Ostium After Draf III

Covering exposed bone after Draf III with free mucosal grafts has also been used to reduce the rate of ostial stenosis. Exposed bone can lead to osteitis and act as a source of mucosal edema and hypertrophy, scarring, and ultimately surgical failure [12]. Mucosal grafts are usually harvested from the mucosa from the planned nasal septectomy site [12]. However if septal mucosa is not adequate, either because the surgeon is undertaking a revision Draf III or the septum is compromised by tumor, turbinate mucosa can also be used [12]. The mucosal grafts can be thinned if necessary for better adherence and are usually bolstered with stenting materials like Silastic sheeting. Fibrin glue can also be used to promote mucosal adherence [12].

One study of 96 patients undergoing Draf III with mucosal grafting, with a mean follow of 34 months, demonstrated a 97% success rate at maintaining an anterior-posterior diameter > 50% of intraoperative measurement [12]. In this study, the two patients who had greater than 50% restenosis remained patent and had no clinical consequence to their ostial narrowing. No patients in this study required revision due to cavity stenosis. Other studies have shown similar success rates with mucosal grafting [55, 56]. While the data on this technique are limited, compared to traditional Draf III outcomes, the addition of mucosal grafting might significantly improve long-term restenosis and revision rates.

Other Techniques for Frontal Sinus Postoperative Care

Trephination

The use of external procedures in frontal sinus surgery dates back over 100 years to the original descriptions by Lynch. However, the advent of endoscopic surgery has largely replaced external approaches in most circumstances. There remain certain situations where external approaches like trephination are indicated. Trephination involves making a small opening in the anterior table of the frontal sinus, usually through a medial brow incision, in order to gain further lateral and superior access into the frontal sinus. While the indications and technique for trephination in order to successfully complete a surgical procedure are beyond the scope of this chapter, trephination can be useful in the postoperative setting [57]. A catheter through the trephine can be secured to the forehead. Through this catheter, one can irrigate the frontal sinus or apply topical antibiotics in the setting of infection. If there is significant edema of the frontal sinus outflow tract, topical instillation of decongestant or corticosteroid drops can be a useful tool to maintain postoperative patency and allow for adequate drainage.

Summary

Postoperative care of the frontal sinus is critical to maintaining long-term sinus patency. In addition to standard postoperative sinus surgery care consisting of topical steroids, saline irrigations, and debridement, there are special considerations for the frontal sinus. The successful delivery of topical medicine and irrigation to the frontal sinus might be improved by "vertex to floor" head positions, and successful in-office debridement will require angled endoscopies and curved instruments. The use of biomaterials and stents may improve long-term outcomes in select patients. Steroid-eluting stenting mechanisms are a recent development and show promise in improving postoperative outcomes. In the post Draf III setting, mucosal grafting may also improve ostial patency and patient symptomatology.

Conflict of Interest Zachary M. Soler is supported by grants from Entellus, Intersect, and Optinose, none of which is affiliated with this manuscript. Dr. Soler is a consultant for Olympus, which is not affiliated with this manuscript. There are no disclosures for Jose L. Mattos.

References

1. Hunter B, Silva S, Youngs R, Saeed A, Varadarajan V. Long-term stenting for chronic frontal sinus disease: case series and literature review. J Laryngol Otol. 2010;124(11):1216–22. https://doi.org/10.1017/S0022215110001052.
2. Weber R, Mai R, Hosemann W, Draf W, Toffel P. The success of 6-month stenting in endonasal frontal sinus surgery. Ear Nose Throat J. 2000;79(12):930–2. 934, 937–8 passim. http://www.ncbi.nlm.nih.gov/pubmed/11191431.
3. Chandra RK, Palmer JN, Tangsujarittham T, Kennedy DW. Factors associated with failure of frontal sinusotomy in the early follow-up period. Otolaryngol Head Neck Surg. 2004;131(4):514–8. https://doi.org/10.1016/j.otohns.2004.03.022.
4. Friedman M, Landsberg R, Schults RA, Tanyeri H, Caldarelli DD. Frontal sinus surgery: endoscopic technique and preliminary results. Am J Rhinol. 2000;14(6):393–403. http://www.ncbi.nlm.nih.gov/pubmed/11197116.
5. Hosemann W, Kuhnel T, Held P, Wagner W, Felderhoff A. Endonasal frontal sinusotomy in surgical management of chronic sinusitis: a critical evaluation. Am J Rhinol. 1997;11(1):1–9.
6. Friedman M, Bliznikas D, Vidyasagar R, Joseph NJ, Landsberg R. Long-term results after endoscopic sinus surgery involving frontal recess dissection. Laryngoscope. 2006;116(4):573–9. https://doi.org/10.1097/01.MLG.0000202086.18206.C8.
7. Chan Y, Melroy CT, Kuhn CA, Kuhn FL, Daniel WT, Kuhn FA. Long-term frontal sinus patency after endoscopic frontal sinusotomy. Laryngoscope. 2009;119(6):1229–32. https://doi.org/10.1002/lary.20168.
8. Naidoo Y, Wen D, Bassiouni A, Keen M, Wormald PJ. Long-term results after primary frontal sinus surgery. Int Forum Allergy Rhinol. 2012;2(3):185–90. https://doi.org/10.1002/alr.21015.
9. Anderson P, Sindwani R. Safety and efficacy of the endoscopic modified lothrop procedure: a systematic review and meta-analysis. Laryngoscope. 2009;119(9):1828–33. https://doi.org/10.1002/lary.20565.
10. Ting JY, Wu A, Metson R. Frontal sinus drillout (modified Lothrop procedure): long-term results in 204 patients. Laryngoscope. 2014;124(5):1066–70. https://doi.org/10.1002/lary.24422.
11. Naidoo A, Naidoo K, Yende-zuma N, Gengiah TN. Changes to antiretroviral drug regimens during integrated TB-HIV treatment: results of the SAPiT trial. Antivir Ther. 2015;19(2):161–9. https://doi.org/10.3851/IMP2701.Changes.
12. Illing EA, Cho DY, Riley KO, Woodworth BA. Draf III mucosal graft technique: long-term results. Int Forum Allergy Rhinol. 2016;6(5):514–7. https://doi.org/10.1002/alr.21708.
13. Tran KKN, Beule AAG, Singal D, Wormald P-J. Frontal ostium restenosis after the endoscopic modified Lothrop procedure. Laryngoscope. 2007;117(8):1457–62. https://doi.org/10.1097/MLG.0b013e31806865be.
14. Casiano R, Banhiran W, Sargi Z, Collins W, Kaza S. Long-term effect of stenting after an endoscopic modified Lothrop procedure. Am J Rhinol. 2006;20(6):595–9. https://doi.org/10.2500/ajr.2006.20.2912.
15. Wei CC, Sama A. What is the evidence for the use of mucosal flaps in Draf III procedures? Curr Opin Otolaryngol Head Neck Surg. 2014;22(1):63–7. https://doi.org/10.1097/MOO.0000000000000023.
16. Rudmik L, Soler ZM, Orlandi RR, et al. Early postoperative care following endoscopic sinus surgery: an evidence-based review with recommendations. Int Forum Allergy Rhinol. 2011;1(6):417–30. https://doi.org/10.1002/alr.20072.
17. Orlandi RR, Kingdom TT, Hwang PH, et al. International consensus statement on allergy and rhinology: rhinosinusitis. Int Forum Allergy Rhinol. 2016;6:S22–S209. https://doi.org/10.1002/alr.21695.
18. Chong LY, Head K, Hopkins C, Philpott C, Burton MJ, Schilder AGM. Different types of intranasal steroids for chronic rhinosinusitis. Cochrane Database Syst Rev. 2016;2016(4) https://doi.org/10.1002/14651858.CD011993.pub2.
19. Harvey RJ, Goddard JC, Wise SK, Schlosser RJ. Effects of endoscopic sinus surgery and delivery device on cadaver sinus irrigation. 2008;139:137–42. https://doi.org/10.1016/j.otohns.2008.04.020.
20. Thomas WW, Harvey RJ, Rudmik L, Hwang PH, Schlosser RJ. Distribution of topical agents to the paranasal sinuses : an evidence-based review with recommendations. 2013;3(9):691–703. https://doi.org/10.1002/alr.21172.
21. DelGaudio JM, Wise SK. Topical steroid drops for the treatment of sinus ostia stenosis in the postoperative period. Am J Rhinol. 2006;20(6):563–7. http://www.ncbi.nlm.nih.gov/pubmed/17181093.
22. Hong SD, Jang JY, Kim JH, et al. The effect of anatomically directed topical steroid drops on frontal recess patency after endoscopic sinus surgery: a prospective randomized single blind study. Am J Rhinol Allergy. 2012;26(3):209–12. https://doi.org/10.2500/ajra.2012.26.3758.
23. Barham HP, Ramakrishnan VR, Knisely A, et al. Frontal sinus surgery and sinus distribution of nasal

irrigation. 2016;6(3):238–42. https://doi.org/10.1002/alr.21686.

24. Beule A, Athanasiadis T, Athanasiadis E, Field J, Wormald PJ. Efficacy of different techniques of sinonasal irrigation after modified Lothrop procedure. Am J Rhinol Allergy. 2009;23(1):85–90. https://doi.org/10.2500/ajra.2009.23.3265.

25. Bugten V, Nordgård S, Steinsvåg S. The effects of debridement after endoscopic sinus surgery. Laryngoscope. 2006;116(11):2037–43. https://doi.org/10.1097/01.mlg.0000241362.06072.83.

26. Kemppainen T, Seppä J, Tuomilehto H, Kokki H, Nuutinen J. Repeated early debridement does not provide significant symptomatic benefit after ESS. Rhinology. 2008;46(3):238–42.

27. Lee JY, Byun JY. Relationship between the frequency of postoperative debridement and patient discomfort, healing period, surgical outcomes, and compliance after endoscopic sinus surgery. Laryngoscope. 2008;118:1868–72. https://doi.org/10.1097/MLG.0b013e31817f93d3.

28. Massey CJ, Suh JD, Tessema B, Gray ST, Singh A. Biomaterials in rhinology. Otolaryngol Head Neck Surg. 2016;154:606. https://doi.org/10.1177/0194599815627782.

29. Ngoc Ha T, Valentine R, Moratti S, Robinson S, Hanton L, Wormald PJ. A blinded randomized controlled trial evaluating the efficacy of chitosan gel on ostial stenosis following endoscopic sinus surgery. Int Forum Allergy Rhinol. 2013;3:573–80. https://doi.org/10.1002/alr.21136.

30. Rains B. Frontal sinus stenting. Otolaryngol Clin N Am. 2001;34(1):101–10.

31. Orlandi RR, Knight J. Prolonged stenting of the frontal sinus. Laryngoscope. 2009;119(1):190–2. https://doi.org/10.1002/lary.20081.

32. Ingals E. New operation and instruments for draining the frontal sinus. Tr Am Laryng Rhino Otol Soc. 1905;11:183–9.

33. RL G. Ten years' experience in the use of tantalum in frontal sinus surgery. Laryngoscope. 1954;64(2):65–72. https://doi.org/10.1288/00005537-195402000-00001.

34. Barton R. Dacron prosthesis in frontal sinus surgery. Laryngoscope. 1972;82(10):799–805.

35. Neel HB, Whicker JH, Lake CF. Thin rubber sheeting in frontal sinus surgery: animal and clinical studies. Laryngoscope. 1976;86(4):524–36. https://doi.org/10.1288/00005537-197604000-00008.

36. Amble FR, Kern EB, Neel B, Facer GW, McDonald TJ, Czaja JM. Nasofrontal duct reconstruction with silicone rubber sheeting for inflammatory frontal sinus disease: analysis of 164 cases. Laryngoscope. 1996;106(7):809–15. http://www.ncbi.nlm.nih.gov/pubmed/8667974.

37. Dubin MG, Kuhn FA. Preservation of natural frontal sinus outflow in the management of frontal sinus osteomas. Otolaryngol Head Neck Surg. 2006;134(1):18–24. https://doi.org/10.1016/j.otohns.2005.09.020.

38. Hosemann W, Schindler E, Wiegrebe E, Göpferich A. Innovative frontal sinus stent acting as a local drug-releasing system. Eur Arch Otorhinolaryngol. 2003;260(3):131–4. https://doi.org/10.1007/s00405-002-0534-2.

39. Lin D, Witterick IJ. Frontal sinus stents: how long can they be kept in? J Otolaryngol Head Neck Surg. 2008;37(1):119–23. https://doi.org/10.2310/7070.2008.0017.

40. Weber R, Hosemann W, Draf W, Keerl R, Schick B, Schinzel S. Endonasal frontal sinus surgery with permanent implantation of a place holder. Laryngorhinootologie. 1997;76(12):728–34. https://doi.org/10.1055/s-2007-997515.

41. Yamasoba T, Kikuchi S, Higo R. Transient positioning of a silicone T tube in frontal sinus surgery. Otolaryngol Head Neck Surg. 1994;111(6):776–80. http://www.ncbi.nlm.nih.gov/pubmed/7991258.

42. Schneider JS, Archilla A, J a D. Five "nontraditional" techniques for use in patients with recalcitrant sinusitis. Curr Opin Otolaryngol Head Neck Surg. 2013;21(1):39–44. https://doi.org/10.1097/MOO.0b013e32835bf65b.

43. Chadwell JS, Gustafson LM, Tami TA. Toxic shock syndrome associated with frontal sinus stents. Otolaryngol Head Neck Surg. 2001;124(5):573–4. doi:S0194599801603760 [pii].

44. Beule AG, Steinmeier E, Kaftan H, et al. Effects of a dexamethasone-releasing stent on osteoneogenesis in a rabbit model. Am J Rhinol Allergy. 2009;23(4):433–6. https://doi.org/10.2500/ajra.2009.23.3331.

45. Beule AG, Scharf C, Biebler K-E, et al. Effects of topically applied dexamethasone on mucosal wound healing using a drug-releasing stent. Laryngoscope. 2008;118(11):2073–7. https://doi.org/10.1097/MLG.0b013e3181820896.

46. Han JK, Marple BF, Smith TL, et al. Effect of steroid-releasing sinus implants on postoperative medical and surgical interventions: an efficacy meta-analysis. Int Forum Allergy Rhinol. 2012;2(4):271–9. https://doi.org/10.1002/alr.21044.

47. Forwith KD, Chandra RK, Yun PT, Miller SK, Jampel HD. ADVANCE: a multisite trial of bioabsorbable steroid-eluting sinus implants. Laryngoscope. 2011;121(11):2473–80. https://doi.org/10.1002/lary.22228.

48. Marple BF, Smith TL, Han JK, et al. Advance II: a prospective, randomized study assessing safety and efficacy of bioabsorbable steroid-releasing sinus implants. Otolaryngol Head Neck Surg. 2012;146(6):1004–11. https://doi.org/10.1177/0194599811435968.

49. Murr AH, Smith TL, Hwang PH, et al. Safety and efficacy of a novel bioabsorbable, steroid-eluting sinus stent. Int Forum Allergy Rhinol. 2011;1(1):23–32. https://doi.org/10.1002/alr.20020.

50. Smith TL, Singh A, Luong A, et al. Randomized controlled trial of a bioabsorbable steroid-releasing implant in the frontal sinus opening. Laryngoscope. 2016;126:1–6. https://doi.org/10.1002/lary.26140.

51. Janisiewicz A, Lee JT. In-office use of a steroid-eluting implant for maintenance of frontal ostial

patency after revision sinus surgery. Allergy Rhinol (Providence). 2015;6(1):68–75. https://doi.org/10.2500/ar.2015.6.0104.

52. Huvenne W, Zhang N, Tijsma E, et al. Pilot study using doxycycline-releasing stents to ameliorate postoperative healing quality after sinus surgery. Wound Repair Regen. 2008;16(6):757–67. https://doi.org/10.1111/j.1524-475X.2008.00429.x.

53. Toffel PH. Secure endoscopic sinus surgery with middle meatal stenting. Oper Tech Otolaryngol Head Neck Surg. 1995;6(3):157–62. https://doi.org/10.1016/S1043-1810(06)80006-0.

54. Naidoo Y, Bassiouni A, Keen M, Wormald PJ. Long-term outcomes for the endoscopic modified lothrop/draf III procedure: a 10-year review. Laryngoscope. 2014;124(1):43–9. https://doi.org/10.1002/lary.24258.

55. Hildenbrand T, Wormald PJ, Weber RK. Endoscopic frontal sinus drainage Draf type III with mucosal transplants. Am J Rhinol Allergy. 2012;26(2):148–51. https://doi.org/10.2500/ajra.2012.26.3731.

56. Seyedhadi S, Mojtaba MA, Shahin B, Hoseinali K. The Draf III septal flap technique: a preliminary report. Am J Otolaryngol - Head Neck Med Surg. 2013;34(5):399–402. https://doi.org/10.1016/j.amjoto.2013.01.019.

57. Seiberling K, Jardeleza C, Wormald PJ. Mini-trephination of the frontal sinus: indications and uses in today's era of sinus surgery. Am J Rhinol Allergy. 2009;23(2):229–31. https://doi.org/10.2500/ajra.2009.23.3298.

Frontal Sinus Stenting: Intraoperative and Postoperative Use

21

Erin K. O'Brien

Introduction

Frontal sinus surgery can be complicated by post-operative stenosis or obstruction of the frontal outflow tract, leading to what Dr. RC Lynch described as "many a heartaches over the results which were so far removed from my ideal" [1]. In order to maintain the patency of the frontal recess after surgery on the frontal sinus, the use of frontal sinus stents has been frequently described in the literature since Dr. Lynch's publication on his approach to the frontal sinus in 1921. In this chapter, historical use of stents with open or external frontal sinus surgery will be reviewed as well as descriptions and evidence on the use of stents in conjunction with endoscopic sinus surgery, both intraoperatively and in the postoperative period.

Historical Use of Frontal Sinus Stents

Dr. Lynch described his external approach to the frontal sinus with the removal of the orbital wall including the frontal process of the superior maxilla, the lower lateral edge of the nasal bone, the lacrimal bone, and the lamina papyracea [1]. He

E. K. O'Brien (✉)
Department of Otorhinolaryngology, Mayo Clinic
Rochester, Rochester, MN, USA

inserted a rubber drainage tube (3/8 inch diameter) into the frontal recess and removed the tube 5 days later. Postoperative care included passing a large dilator or sound into the sinus daily for 10 days. The tubing helped prevent obstruction of the frontal recess by prolapsed orbital contents, as the bony wall of the lamina and superior maxilla had been removed.

Additional early reports of the use of stents in frontal sinus surgery also include the Ingalls gold tube first described in 1905 and later reported in 1940 by Dr. Anthony, who felt that the gold tube prevented the foreign body reaction associated with the use of rubber tubing utilized by other surgeons [2, 3]. Another option for stenting the frontal recess after a Lynch approach was the use of a Dacron woven arterial stent, described by Dr. Barton in his series from 1972 [4]. The stent was secured with wires and left in place indefinitely, although some patients developed episodes of crusting, odor, or drainage necessitating treatment with antibiotics.

Dr. Neel and colleagues at the Mayo Clinic modified the Lynch approach to preserve the frontal process of the superior maxilla, preventing collapse of the orbital contents into the lateral portion of the frontal sinus and outflow tract [5, 6]. They also described the use of thin Silastic sheeting rolled into a tube, inserted via the external incision into the sinus through the nasofrontal communication and sutured to the septum. The Silastic sheet was removed 6 weeks postoperatively or

© Springer Nature Switzerland AG 2019
D. Lal, P. H. Hwang (eds.), *Frontal Sinus Surgery*, https://doi.org/10.1007/978-3-319-97022-6_21

later. They compared the thin Silastic sheet stents versus fairly rigid 3/8 inch silicone rubber tubing in a dog model of the external modified Lynch approach with the creation of a large nasofrontal opening [6]. The stents and tubes were removed at 2 months, and the animals were sacrificed at 4 months. On histologic examination, the rigid tubes were associated with only minimal epithelium and increased fibrosis and osteoblastic activity with new bone growth along with fibrin within the sinus. The sinuses stented with thin Silastic sheets had a lining of normal mucosa in the "nasofrontal duct," less fibrosis, and little to no osteoblastic activity, and the diameter of the ducts was larger than in the sinuses with rigid tubing. In patients, they also found superior results with the use of a thin Silastic sheet rolled into a tube rather than thicker, more rigid rubber tubing. They hypothesized that the more rigid tube led to local ischemia of the mucosa, obstruction and infection, and therefore poor wound healing. They also advocated preservation of mucosa within the frontal recess and sinus when possible, challenging the notion of removal of diseased mucosa. In 1996, they reviewed their results from 1972 to 1992 using the external modified Lynch approach and 6–8 weeks of stenting with a roll of thin Silastic sheeting [7]. Although the revision rate was 18%, the eventual success of this approach using the thin stent was reported to be 96%.

Frontal Sinus Stents During Endoscopic Sinus Surgery

Indications

Stenosis and obstruction of the frontal sinus may develop due to iatrogenic injury to the mucosa, the underlying disease process or infection, or the size and anatomy of the frontal sinus outflow tract. Examination of the CT scan prior to surgery is necessary to understand the anatomy of the frontal recess and ethmoid cells including the agger nasi cells, frontal cells above the agger nasi or intersinus septal cells, supraorbital ethmoid cells, and suprabullar cells. Removal of the septations of these cells may be necessary to identify

and provide the optimal diameter opening to the frontal sinus. However, the mucosa of the frontal recess should be preserved when possible. Circumferential removal of mucosa within the frontal recess increases the risk of stenosis.

The size of the frontal neo-ostium created with the endoscopic frontal sinusotomy is associated with the rate of stenosis of the frontal recess after surgery. Hosemann reported an average diameter of the neo-ostium of 5.6 mm at the time of surgery, but the size decreased to an average diameter of 3.5 mm postoperatively [8]. Neo-ostia greater than 5 mm in diameter were associated with a 16% rate of stenosis, but openings less than 5 mm in diameter had a 33% rate of stenosis, with only 50% patency for neo-ostia less than 2 mm at the time of surgery. Naidoo found long-term patency was associated with a minimum dimension of >4.8 mm, while stenosis was associated with a dimension of less than 3.7 mm [9].

Frontal sinus stents may help prevent stenosis of the frontal sinus neo-ostium after endoscopic sinus surgery, although no studies to date have compared stenting versus no stent in the frontal recess to prove efficacy. Indications for the use of a frontal sinus stent may include diameter of the opening of less than 5 mm, based on increased rates of stenosis for smaller opening, purulence or osteitic bone, granulomatous inflammation from vasculitis, stenosis from previous failed sinus surgery, middle turbinate lateralization, or denuded mucosa within the frontal recess.

Non-dissolvable Frontal Sinus Stents: Materials and Duration

The literature includes reports on a variety of materials for stenting as well as a range in the recommended duration for the stent. A review by Schaefer and Close in 1990 on 36 patients with unilateral or bilateral frontal sinusotomy included a description on the use of a 4 mm Silastic tube for stenting the frontal sinus [10]. The authors inserted the Silastic tube into the frontal sinus opening in four patients in whom the frontal sinusotomy was only 4–6 mm in diameter. The tube was sutured to the septum and left in place for 6 weeks. The frontal sinus opening remained patent in only two of the four patients. In 1992, Metson also described the use of a 4 mm Silastic drainage catheter after frontal sinusotomy; the catheter was sutured to the septum or lateral nasal wall and left in place for 1–8 weeks (average 3.2 weeks) [11]. After removal of the stent, the ostium decreased in size but stabilized at a 2–4 mm diameter.

Another option for stenting which does not require a suture to keep the tubing in place is the Rains stent, patented in 1996 [12]. The 4 mm or 6 mm stent is made of silicone rubber with a tapered collapsible tip that is self-retaining within the frontal sinus (Fig. 21.1). A frontal probe or sinus is inserted into the stent, and the tapered bulb tip is advanced into the frontal sinus. The probe is removed, and the end of the stent can be trimmed to a level above the inferior border of the middle turbinate. Rains reported on 102 stents of which 5 were left in long term; a majority of stents were removed at 6–130 days (average 35 days). He reported a 94% patency at a follow-up of 8–48 months [12]. The Rains stent was also used by Orlandi in 10 of 462 patients who underwent frontal sinusotomy from 2000 to 2006 [13]. The stent was used when the frontal ostium had circumferential mucosal defects and a diameter of less than 5 mm or a long narrow outflow tract. Nine were left in place long term; of these, one was removed at 11 months for discomfort, and another removed at 61 months for ongoing infec-

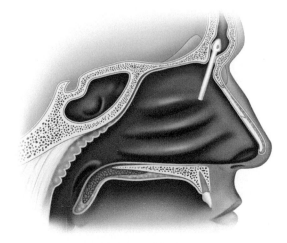

Fig. 21.1 Rains stent. The soft Silastic tube has a larger, basket-like opening to be placed into the frontal sinus. The tube can be left in place to allow for drainage

tion. The remaining seven were still in place at the time of publication. The authors commented that the optimal length of stent duration to prevent stenosis is unknown. Lin and Witterick reported on the use of the Parell frontal sinus T-stent (Medtronic ENT, Jacksonville, FL) for long-term stenting of the frontal sinus (greater than 3 months) [14]. Twenty-one stents placed in 10 patients, with 11 removed or dislodged at an average of 16.3 months and 10 left in place. Complication or failure rates were less than 20%. Patients required suctioning every 2–6 months with daily saline irrigation but overall good tolerance. Weber et al. recommended a duration of 6 months for stent duration, reporting a decreased rate of restenosis compared to stents removed earlier [15]. Perloff and Palmer however found evidence of biofilm formation on the Silastic stents removed from six patients, 1–4 weeks after sinus surgery [16]. The possible effects of biofilm formation on stents for healing and the long-term patency of the frontal sinus ostium are unknown.

Silastic sheeting was initially utilized by Neel et al. via an external approach to stent the frontal sinus and sutured in place [5, 6]. A modification for endoscopic sinus surgery involves cutting the Silastic sheet in a T-shape, with the wider flanges placed using a frontal sinus giraffe forceps into the frontal sinus to retain it without sutures (Fig. 21.2). A larger sheet of Silastic sheeting can be used to line the cavity after a Draf III or modified endoscopic Lothrop procedure, in which the intersinus septum, upper nasal septum, and frontal beak have been removed, creating a large cavity with exposed bone. However, Banhiran et al. did not find a difference after Draf III procedures in the patency of the common ostium or symptoms in the 25 patients stented with Silastic for 8 weeks versus the 72 patients without stenting [17].

Foreign material placed within the sinuses can be a source of complications after surgery, either serving as a nidus for infection or becoming dislodged and then aspirated or swallowed. Biofilm can be found on Silastic stents in the frontal sinus as early as 1 week after insertion [16]. While Neel et al. sutured Silastic sheeting to the septum after placement following an external fronto-ethmoidectomy, most Silastic or silicone stents, although designed to be retained

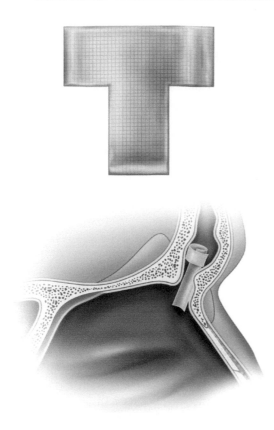

Fig. 21.2 Silastic sheeting. By cutting the pliable Silastic into a T-shape, the larger flanges can be placed into the frontal sinus to retain the temporary stent. Softer Silastic has been associated with better healing than more rigid stents

within in the frontal sinus, are not as definitively secured within the nose [5–7]. While there are no reports of aspiration of unsecured sinus stents, caution must be observed in ensuring that the stent is not loose and easily dislodged and advising the patient of the possibility of aspiration of the foreign body.

Dissolvable Frontal Sinus Stents

While some evidence exists for supporting the use of stents such as Silastic or silicone to preserve the patency of the frontal ostium after sinus surgery, these stents typically require removal, although the timing of removal is debatable. Dissolvable stents placed at the time of surgery

would potentially provide a barrier to synechiae formation and allow drainage of blood and mucus from the sinus during healing while eliminating the need for removal by the surgeon at a later date. One stent with US Food and Drug Administration approval for use in the frontal sinus is a mometasone-eluting implant made of a bioabsorbable polylactide-co-glycolide polymer (PROPEL Mini sinus implants, Intersect ENT, Menlo Park, CA). One study to date has examined the efficacy of the mometasone implant for frontal sinus patency after frontal sinus surgery by either traditional endoscopic techniques or with a balloon dilation of the frontal recess [18]. Patients with bilateral frontal sinus surgery had one implant placed in a randomized fashion on one side, while the other side had no implant (control). The implants were removed at 21 days, and the frontal sinus openings were graded for granulation and scarring, polypoid edema, and patency at 30 and 90 days by the clinicians and an independent reviewer. At 30 days, interventions were reduced in the implanted side versus controls (38.8% versus 62.7%) with decreased inflammation and occlusion or restenosis and increased diameter also in the implanted side. The included 90-day data was limited to reporting of decreased postoperative intervention in the implanted side. Mometasone-eluting stents have also been placed in the frontal outflow tract in the office after dilation of the frontal ostium to maintain patency after revision frontal sinus endoscopic sinus surgery [19].

Magnesium-neodymium alloy (MgNd$_2$) stents have been tested in animal models after sinus surgery with good evidence of biodegradation and patency of the sinuses up to 180 days [20–23]. No human trials have been reported to date, but temporary magnesium stents would potentially allow stenting of the frontal sinus outflow tract after surgery.

Summary

Stenting of the frontal recess and outflow tract after either open or endoscopic sinus surgery may help prevent scarring and narrowing of the opening to the frontal sinus. Both animal and human studies have demonstrated that soft materials such as Silastic may be superior in terms of prevention of scarring and improved patency. While a number of removal frontal sinus stents have been developed and utilized with good success, more recently developed dissolvable stents, some with impregnated medications, may prove to be even more beneficial in improving outcomes after frontal sinus surgery.

Conflict of Interest No commercial or financial conflicts of interest or funding sources

References

1. Lynch RC. The technique of a radical frontal sinus operation which has given me the best results. (original communications are received with the understanding) that they are contributed exclusively to the laryngoscope.). Laryngoscope. 1921;31(1):1–5.
2. Anthony DH. Use of Ingalls gold tube in frontal sinus operations. South Med J. 1940;33:949–55.
3. Ingals EF. XXXII. New operation and instruments for draining the frontal sinus. Ann Otol Rhinol Laryngol. 1905;14(3):513–9.
4. Barton RT. Dacron prosthesis in frontal sinus surgery. Laryngoscope. 1972;82(10):1799–805.
5. Neel HB 3rd, McDonald TJ, Facer GW. Modified Lynch procedure for chronic frontal sinus diseases: rationale, technique, and long-term results. Laryngoscope. 1987;97(11):1274–9.
6. Neel HB, Whicker JH, Lake CF. Thin rubber sheeting in frontal sinus surgery: animal and clinical studies. Laryngoscope. 1976;86(4):524–36.
7. Amble FR, et al. Nasofrontal duct reconstruction with silicone rubber sheeting for inflammatory frontal sinus disease: analysis of 164 cases. Laryngoscope. 1996;106(7):809–15.
8. Hosemann W, et al. Endonasal frontal sinusotomy in surgical management of chronic sinusitis: a critical evaluation. Am J Rhinol. 1997;11(1):1–9.
9. Naidoo Y, et al. Long-term results after primary frontal sinus surgery. Int Forum Allergy Rhinol. 2012;2(3):185–90.
10. Schaefer SD, Close LG. Endoscopic management of frontal sinus disease. Laryngoscope. 1990;100(2 Pt 1):155–60.
11. Metson R. Endoscopic treatment of frontal sinusitis. Laryngoscope. 1992;102(6):712–6.
12. Rains BM 3rd. Frontal sinus stenting. Otolaryngol Clin N Am. 2001;34(1):101–10.
13. Orlandi RR, Knight J. Prolonged stenting of the frontal sinus. Laryngoscope. 2009;119(1):190–2.
14. Lin D, Witterick IJ. Frontal sinus stents: how long can they be kept in? J Otolaryngol Head Neck Surg. 2008;37(1):119–23.
15. Weber R, et al. The success of 6-month stenting in endonasal frontal sinus surgery. Ear Nose Throat J. 2000;79(12):930–2. 934, 937–8 passim.
16. Perloff JR, Palmer JN. Evidence of bacterial biofilms on frontal recess stents in patients with chronic rhinosinusitis. Am J Rhinol. 2004;18(6):377–80.
17. Banhiran W, et al. Long-term effect of stenting after an endoscopic modified Lothrop procedure. Am J Rhinol. 2006;20(6):595–9.
18. Smith TL, et al. Randomized controlled trial of a bioabsorbable steroid-releasing implant in the frontal sinus opening. Laryngoscope. 2016;126:2659.
19. Janisiewicz A, Lee JT. In-office use of a steroid-eluting implant for maintenance of frontal ostial patency after revision sinus surgery. Allergy Rhinol (Providence). 2015;6(1):68–75.
20. Durisin M, et al. Biodegradable nasal stents (MgF2-coated Mg-2 wt %Nd alloy)-A long-term in vivo study. J Biomed Mater Res B Appl Biomater. 2017;105(2):350–65.
21. Eifler R, et al. MgNd2 alloy in contact with nasal mucosa: an in vivo and in vitro approach. J Mater Sci Mater Med. 2016;27(2):25.
22. Durisin M, et al. A novel biodegradable frontal sinus stent (MgNd2): a long-term animal study. Eur Arch Otorhinolaryngol. 2016;273(6):1455–67.
23. Weber CM, et al. Biocompatibility of MgF2-coated MgNd2 specimens in contact with mucosa of the nasal sinus – a long term study. Acta Biomater. 2015;18:249–61.

Shiayin F. Yang, Chirag Rajan Patel,
and James A. Stankiewicz

Bony Complications

Mucocele

Mucoceles are epithelial-lined sacs that contain trapped inspissated mucus. The majority of cases are idiopathic, but mucoceles can also occur secondary to sinus surgery, trauma, or chronic sinus disease [1, 2]. In chronic sinusitis, continued inflammation results in scarring and obstruction of sinus ostia. Inadequate sinus drainage leads to sinus fluid opacification, which over time can cause sinus wall thinning and expansion. Mucoceles can be classified as primary or secondary. Primary mucoceles are mucous retention cysts, and secondary mucoceles occur secondary to ostia obstruction [3]. The frontal sinus is the most commonly affected sinus, followed by the ethmoid sinus [1, 2]. Mucoceles can expand over time and cause thinning and remodeling of the neighboring bone. The most common presenting signs and symptoms are ophthalmologic such as proptosis, periorbital swelling, ptosis, and diplopia. This is due to the mucocele extending through the lamina papyracea or superior orbital rim and causing compression of the orbit. Mucoceles can also extend intracranially via erosion of the skull base (Fig. 22.1) [2, 4]. CT imaging should be obtained to assess the size and location of the mucocele. On CT, mucoceles appear as homogeneous isodense lesions that do not enhance with contrast, unless infected [3]. If there is concern of intraorbital or intracranial extension, MRI can be useful. Early management of mucoceles advocated for complete removal of the mucocele and its epithelial lining. However, recent studies have shown good outcomes and low recurrence rates with endoscopic endonasal marsupialization. This has become the preferred method of management given good outcomes and relatively low morbidity. The goal of endoscopic surgery is to marsupialize the cyst by creating a wide drainage pathway to prevent recurrence and decrease the risk of stenosis [1, 2, 4]. Routine follow-up is recommended to monitor for recurrence.

Osteomyelitis

Osteomyelitis is an infection of the frontal bone due to direct extension or by thrombophlebitis of diploic veins. Headache is the most common presenting symptom. Diagnosis can be obtained with 99-m pertechnetate and gallium-67 citrate bone scans. Treatment consists of a prolonged course of intravenous antibiotics (typically 6 weeks)

S. F. Yang · C. R. Patel (✉) · J. A. Stankiewicz
Department of Otolaryngology – Head and Neck
Surgery, Loyola University Medical Center,
Maywood, IL, USA

© Springer Nature Switzerland AG 2019
D. Lal, P. H. Hwang (eds.), *Frontal Sinus Surgery*, https://doi.org/10.1007/978-3-319-97022-6_22

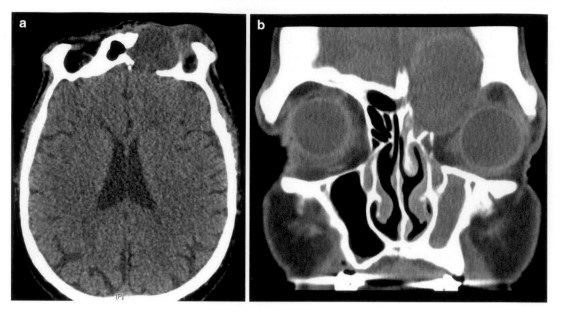

Fig. 22.1 (a) Axial and (b) coronal cuts of CT scan demonstrating frontal mucopyocele that has eroded through the orbit and the posterior table with intracranial exten-sion. The mucopyocele appears as a homogeneous isodense lesion on imaging

and debridement of necrotic bone. Gallium scans can be used to monitor for response to treatment [5]. Persistent infection or scarring may require extensive frontal sinus surgery, either endoscopic or osteoplastic flap.

Pott's Puffy Tumor

Pott's puffy tumor is a characterized by forma-tion of a subperiosteal abscess due to underlying osteomyelitis of the frontal bone. This is typi-cally the result of complicated frontal sinusitis but can also be seen with head trauma. It is most commonly seen in adolescents [6]. Presenting symptoms include headache, fever, nasal drain-age, and forehead swelling. Forehead swelling is the result of the fluctuant subperiosteal abscess, which gives the "puffy" appearance. Pott's puffy tumor is rare but has a high risk of intracranial complications including subdural empyema, intracranial abscess, venous sinus thrombosis, and epidural abscess. These complications occur as a result of infection spreading through the

diploic veins of the frontal sinus or direct exten-sion through the bone. Intracranial complications due to Pott's puffy tumor have been observed in 29–85% of patients [7, 8]. Given the risk of intracranial complications, immediate diagno-sis and treatment are critical. Work-up includes neurologic exam, sinonasal endoscopy, CT scan with intravenous contrast, and MRI to evaluate for intracranial pathology (Figs. 22.2 and 22.3). Treatment includes both surgical and medical therapy. Surgery, whether endoscopic or exter-nal, is targeted at draining the abscess and frontal sinuses as well as removing infected bone and tis-sue. A 6-week course of intravenous antibiotics is recommended postoperatively. Most infections are polymicrobial with the most common organ-isms cultured being streptococci, staphylococci, and anaerobic bacteria. Thus, antibiotic cover-age should initially be broad and subsequently narrowed based on culture susceptibilities [7]. Repeat imaging can be used to evaluate effective-ness of treatment and to monitor for intracranial complications as these can present in asymptom-atic patients, even after initiating treatment.

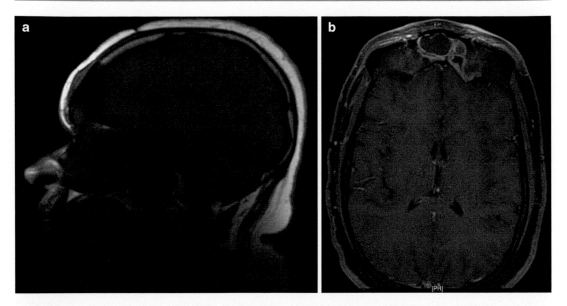

Fig. 22.2 (**a**) Sagittal and (**b**) axial MRI T1 images demonstrating Pott's Puffy tumor with extension from frontal sinus through the anterior table. The lesion appears as a hypodense lesion with enhancing rim

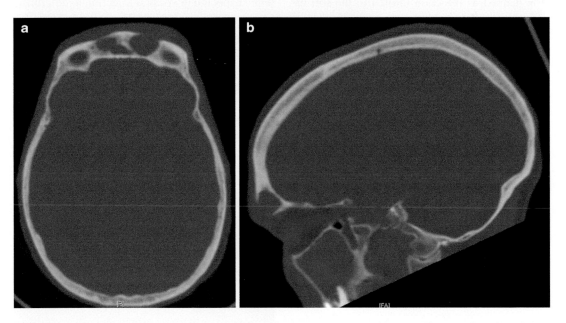

Fig. 22.3 (**a**) Axial and (**b**) sagittal CT images of Pott's Puffy tumor, demonstrating opacification of the frontal sinus with erosion of anterior table and extension of frontal disease into the soft tissue

Orbital Complications

Orbital complications are the most common type of complication related to acute pansinusitis. Sixty to eighty percent of orbital complications are related to sinusitis [9, 10]. The most common sinus of origin is the ethmoid sinus, followed by the frontal sinus. This is due to their close proximity to the orbit. Spread of infection from the sinuses can occur through direct extension via bony dehiscences of the lamina papyracea or through retrograde thrombophlebitis through valveless ophthalmic veins. The severity of the complication varies based on the anatomical site of involvement. The orbital septum is a layer of connective tissue that arises from the periosteum of the orbital rim and acts as a barrier to the spread of infection from the superficial tissue of the eyelid into the orbit. Infection of tissue anterior to the orbital septum is classified as preseptal, and infection posterior is classified as postseptal. Chandler's classification is commonly used to describe orbital complications based on anatomical involvement and increasing severity (Table 22.1) [11].

Preseptal Cellulitis

Preseptal cellulitis (Chandler class I) accounts for 70–80% of all orbital complications [9, 10]. It is defined as infection limited to the soft tissue anterior to the orbital septum. It manifests as eyelid edema and erythema without impairment of extraocular movement or vision [11]. Work-up should include history and physical exam with nasal endoscopy, as well as an ophthalmology consult for evaluation of ocular integrity and visual acuity. CT with contrast should be obtained if there is concern for postseptal involvement or failure of medical therapy after 48 h. Findings on CT demonstrate thickening and increased density of the lid and conjunctiva. Most cases are successfully treated with IV antibiotics, nasal decongestant, and saline irrigations. Antibiotics should cover *Staphylococcus aureus* and *Streptococcus pyogenes* [12]. In cases that fail to respond to antibiotic therapy after 24–48 h or with worsening vision, surgical intervention should be considered [10].

Orbital Cellulitis

Orbital cellulitis (Chandler class II) is a postseptal infection that develops when infection spreads posterior to the orbital septum. Symptoms include periorbital swelling and edema, proptosis, orbital pain, and chemosis. Patients may have some impairment of extraocular movement but have normal vision [9]. Worsening of visual acuity or ophthalmoplegia is indicative of disease progression and possible development of an orbital abscess. Patients with suspected postseptal infection should have a thorough history and physical exam, which include a nasal endoscopy and an ophthalmologic exam to assess visual acuity, extraocular movement, and pupillary reflex. Imaging of the orbits and sinuses with contrast-enhanced CT is recommended at presentation in patients with suspected postseptal infection to determine extent of disease [12]. MRI may be indicated if there is concern for intracranial complications (Fig. 22.4). Initial treatment is similar to that of preseptal cellulitis with intravenous antibiotics, nasal decongestants, and saline irrigations. Surgery is recommended if there is evidence of abscess, 20/60 visual acuity, worsening visual acuity or extraocular movement, or lack of symptom resolution in 48–72 h [10, 13].

Table 22.1 Chandler classification of orbital infection

Class I	Preseptal cellulitis
Class II	Orbital cellulitis
Class III	Subperiosteal abscess
Class IV	Orbital abscess
Class V	Cavernous sinus thrombosis

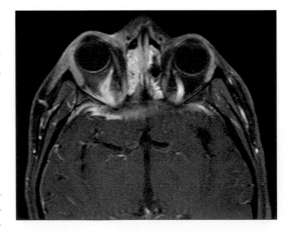

Fig. 22.4 Orbital cellulitis on an axial MRI T1 postcontrast image as characterized by intraconal fat enhancement

Subperiosteal Abscess

Subperiosteal abscess (Chandler class III) is a collection of pus between the orbital periosteum and the bony orbital wall. Most commonly it is found medially between the periorbita and lamina papyracea [13]. It is characterized by periorbital edema, proptosis, impaired extraocular movement, and vision changes. Work-up is similar to that of postseptal infection as discussed for orbital cellulitis. Findings on CT imaging typically demonstrate a hypodense area with rim enhancement adjacent to the lamina papyracea with displacement of orbital contents (Fig. 22.5) [14]. Recommended treatment is IV antibiotics with surgical drainage of the abscess. For smaller-sized abscesses, some authors have recommended initial treatment with IV antibiotics alone, with surgery being done only in patients who do not respond [13, 15]. Surgery can be performed externally through a Lynch incision or through transnasal endoscopic drainage.

Orbital Abscess

Orbital abscess (Chandler class IV) is a collection of pus within the orbital tissue that develops from the progression of orbital cellulitis or the spread of infection from subperiosteal abscess. Presenting symptoms include exophthalmos, chemosis, ophthalmoplegia, and vision impairment. CT imaging demonstrates low-attenuation material surrounded by an enhancing rim within the orbit. Treatment includes both intravenous antibiotics and surgical drainage.

Cavernous Sinus Thrombosis

Cavernous sinus thrombosis (Chandler class V) develops when infection spreads retrograde through valveless veins into the cavernous sinus. Presenting signs and symptoms include fever, headache, orbital pain, chemosis, proptosis, and ophthalmoplegia. In addition, involvement of the cavernous sinus can result in deficits of cranial nerves III, IV, V1, V2, and VI [16]. Early on, only unilateral ocular symptoms may be present, but as the disease progresses, symptoms can occur in the contralateral eye. This is the hallmark of cavernous sinus thrombosis. Diagnosis is made by MRI (Fig. 22.6) [5]. Treatment consists of intravenous antibiotics that cross the blood-brain barrier. Use of anticoagulation to prevent spread of thrombosis is controversial. Infected sinuses should be drained, but timing of surgery is controversial [16].

Intracranial Complications

Intracranial complications of frontal sinusitis are the most severe [17, 18]. Pathogenesis of intracranial complications occurs via two mechanisms. The first is direct extension, which can

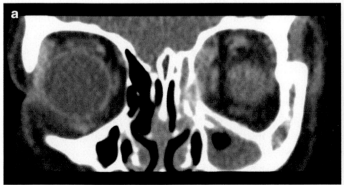 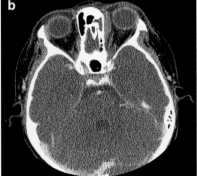

Fig. 22.5 (**a**) Coronal and (**b**) axial CT images of left subperiosteal abscess characterized by hypodense area with enhancement adjacent to the lamina papyracea with displacement of the orbital contents

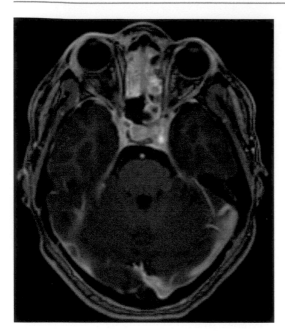

Fig. 22.6 Axial MRI image of cavernous sinus thrombosis can be seen by the relative lack of enhancement in the right cavernous sinus compared to the left

occur through bony dehiscences of the skull, neurovascular foramina, or erosion of the posterior table by osteomyelitis. The second pathway is hematogenous spread via retrograde thrombophlebitis of the valveless diploic veins that drain the sinuses and intracranial structures [19].

Types of intracranial complications include epidural abscess, subdural empyema, intraparenchymal abscess, venous sinus thrombosis, and meningitis. The most common type of intracranial complication varies in the literature [15, 17, 18]. It is not uncommon for patients to present with more than one intracranial complication, with more than one-third of patients having two or more intracranial complications [15, 17]. The incidence of intracranial complications is highest in adolescent males. The high incidence in this population is thought to be a consequence of the rapid growth of the frontal sinuses at this age and the rich network of diploic veins [15, 17, 18, 20].

The clinical presentation and disease course vary based on type of intracranial complication [17]. Patients may or may not report a history of recent sinus infection. It is more common for children to have recent acute sinusitis and for

adults to have history of chronic sinusitis [17, 20]. Symptoms are often vague and nonspecific. Headache and fever are the two most common presenting symptoms [17, 18, 20, 21]. Physical exam findings differ based on the type of intracranial complication. Patients may present with neurologic symptoms such as lethargy, altered mental status, seizures, and cranial nerve palsies [17, 18]. However, many patients often have normal neurologic exams at presentation, which can make the diagnosis difficult [18]. Thus, it is important to have a high index of suspicion of intracranial complications even in the absence of neurologic symptoms. There is also a high incidence of coexisting orbital complications in this population, so they may also present with ophthalmologic complaints including periorbital edema, proptosis, decreased visual acuity, and ophthalmoplegia.

Prompt diagnosis is critical given these complications can rapidly progress and have significant morbidity and mortality. Permanent neurologic sequelae can occur in 25–38% of cases [15, 21, 22]. Reported permanent neurologic deficits from intracranial complications of sinusitis include visual deficits, hearing loss, cranial nerve palsies, aphasia, seizures, cognitive deficits, hydrocephalus, and hemiparesis. Mortality can be as high as 4% and occurs from elevated intracranial pressure, transtentorial herniation, infarction, and sepsis [17].

Work-up with appropriate imaging is essential for accurate diagnosis. CT with contrast is often obtained in patients with suspected sinusitis or history of sinusitis as it defines the bony anatomy and is important in surgical planning. However, CT scans are not as sensitive as MRI in diagnosing intracranial pathology [15]. MRI is better at delineating soft tissue structures and detecting meningeal inflammation when compared to CT. Furthermore, MRI is as accurate in diagnosing sinusitis as CT [17, 23]. Thus, MRI is the imaging modality of choice if there is concern of intracranial involvement. CT may still be necessary if endoscopic sinus surgery is planned as part of the treatment.

Once an intracranial complication of sinusitis has been diagnosed, patients should be started immediately on intravenous antibiotics with CSF penetration [17]. Antibiotics can then be tailored to culture results, which are typically polymicrobial. The most common organisms isolated are *Streptococcus* species and *Staphylococcus* species [15, 17]. Consultation with infectious disease can be beneficial in regard to appropriate type and duration of antibiotic therapy.

In addition to medical therapy, surgical intervention has an important role in treatment of these complications. Neurosurgery consultation should be obtained immediately to assist in management. Type and timing of surgical intervention depends on the type of intracranial complication and are discussed below. If surgery is planned for the intracranial complication, it can be prudent to address the infected sinuses at the same time. Delay in surgical treatment of the paranasal sinuses can result in prolonged hospitalization [18].

Epidural Abscess

Epidural abscess is the coalescence of purulence between the dura mater and skull. The frontal sinus is the most common source of infection [24]. Epidural abscesses tend to expand slowly due to the tight adherence of dura to bone. This slow expansion results in vague symptoms such as forehead swelling, headache, fever, or orbital inflammation. Patients typically have normal neurologic exams [17, 24]. There is a high prevalence of concurrent orbital complications. If the abscess grows large enough, it can result in focal neurologic deficits, seizures, and elevated intracranial pressure [17]. On imaging, an epidural abscess appears as an extra-axial, biconvex mass with low attenuation (Fig. 22.7) [25]. Treatment includes intravenous antibiotics and abscess drainage by neurosurgery via craniotomy [5]. Drainage of the infected sinus should also be considered at the same time. Epidural abscess tends to have a more favorable outcome compared to other intracranial complications.

Subdural Empyema

Subdural empyema is when infection spreads to the subdural space. The propagation of infection in the subdural space occurs more rapidly

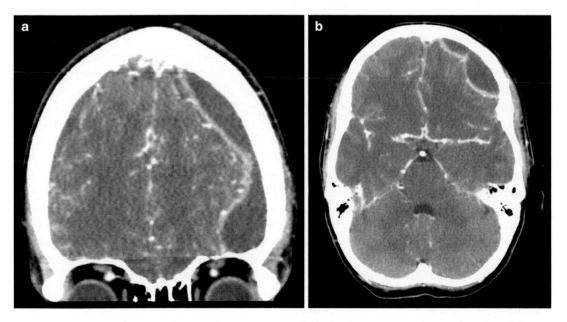

Fig. 22.7 (a) Axial and (b) coronal CT images of epidural empyema characterized by hypodense rim-enhancing fluid collection resulting in midline shift

compared to an epidural abscess due to lack of anatomic barriers in this space. Rapid progression of disease is the hallmark of subdural empyemas. Presenting symptoms include high fever, headache, neck stiffness, seizures, papilledema, hemiparesis, and cranial nerve palsies [24]. Symptoms can progress rapidly, beginning as depressed consciousness and resulting in coma. T1-weighted MRI imaging demonstrates hypointense areas in the subdural space with mass effect and hyperintense areas on T2-weighted images [23]. Prompt diagnosis and immediate intervention are critical in treating this intracranial complication. Treatment consists of neurosurgical evacuation of the subdural empyema and drainage of the infected sinuses. Intravenous antibiotics with CSF penetration should be administered as soon as possible and then tailored to cultures obtained in the operating room. Subdural empyema is considered a neurosurgical emergency and can be associated with significant morbidity and mortality [17, 21, 25].

Intraparenchymal Abscess

Intraparenchymal abscess is a collection of purulence within the brain parenchyma. The most commonly involved site is the frontal lobe due to its close proximity to the frontal sinuses [21, 24]. Patients may be completely asymptomatic in the initial abscess formation. As the abscess develops, patients can develop symptoms such as headache, lethargy, and altered mental status [21]. Large abscesses can result in increased intracranial pressure, seizures, and focal neurologic deficits. If left untreated, the abscess may rupture into the ventricular system, which quickly results in death. Intraparenchymal abscess appears as a hypointense lesion with an enhancing capsule on T2-weighted MRI images (Fig. 22.8). Treatment depends on the patient's condition as well as the size and location of the abscess. Small abscesses have been reported to resolve with medical therapy alone [17, 18]. Larger abscesses require stereotactic aspiration or craniotomy and complete excision [17].

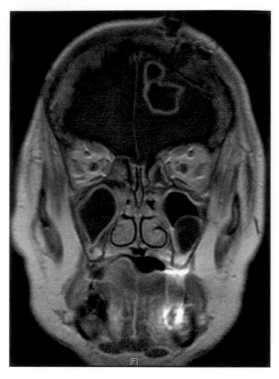

Fig. 22.8 Coronal MRI T1 post-contrast image demonstrating hypodense lesion with surrounding ring enhancement representative of left frontal lobe abscess. There is near complete opacification of the right maxillary sinus and mucus retention cyst in the left maxillary sinus

Meningitis

Meningitis occurs when infection spreads intracranially from the sinuses, resulting in inflammation of the meninges. Patients present with severe headache, fever, neck pain, photophobia, and altered mental status. Diagnosis is made with lumbar puncture. CSF findings from lumbar puncture reveal elevated protein, low glucose, and positive bacterial culture [15]. Imaging of the head must be obtained prior to lumbar puncture to rule out elevated intracranial pressure and prevent herniation. Aggressive medical therapy with intravenous antibiotics is the mainstay of treatment. Anticonvulsants can be used as an adjunct. The use of steroids to help with cerebral edema is controversial. Surgical drainage of the sinuses can be considered if there is no improvement after 24–48 hours of medical therapy [21].

Venous Sinus Thrombosis

Venous sinus thrombosis is the formation of acute thrombus in one of the dural sinuses. It is the result of retrograde thrombophlebitis. The sagittal sinus is the most commonly affected dural sinus in patients with frontal sinusitis. Venous sinus thrombosis is often found in combination with another intracranial complication [26]. Presentation can be variable. Patients often complain of headache, high fevers, and nausea. They can also appear very toxic and have focal neurologic deficits [16]. Imaging studies such as MRI and MR venogram are sensitive in detecting thrombosis and absence of flow voids in the venous sinus [5]. Treatment is with medical therapy including intravenous antibiotics and anticoagulation as indicated.

Summary

- Presenting signs and symptoms of frontal sinusitis complications can be vague and nonspecific such as headache, fever, and forehead swelling.
- CT with contrast is the imaging modality of choice to evaluate complications of the orbit.
- MRI with contrast is the imaging modality of choice to evaluate intracranial complications.
- There should be a low threshold to obtain imaging of the orbits or brain in patients with persistent symptoms not improving with medical therapy.
- Preseptal cellulitis and orbital cellulitis are often managed successfully with intravenous antibiotics, whereas subperiosteal abscess and orbital abscess require surgical drainage.
- Orbital complications frequently coexist with intracranial complications.
- Epidural abscess, subdural empyema, and intraparenchymal abscess require immediate treatment with intravenous antibiotics and neurosurgical intervention.
- Intracranial complications of sinusitis are associated with high morbidity and mortality. Permanent neurologic sequelae occur in 25–38% of cases.

References

1. Dhepnorrarat RC, Subramaniam S, Sethi DS. Endoscopic surgery for frontoethmoidal mucoceles: a 15-year experience. Otolaryngol Head Neck Surg. 2012;47:345–35.
2. Har-El G. Endoscopic management of 108 sinus mucoceles. Laryngoscope. 2001;111(12):2131–4.
3. Stankiewicz JA, Park AA, Newell DJ. Complications of sinusitis. Curr Opin Otolaryngol. 1996;4:17–20.
4. Lee TJ, Li SP, Fu CH, et al. Extensive paranasal sinus mucoceles: a 15-year review of 82 cases. Am J Otolaryngol. 2009;30(4):234–8.
5. Goldberg AN, Oroszlan G, Anderson TD. Complications of frontal sinusitis and their management. Otolaryngol Clin N Am. 2001;34:211–25.
6. Karaman E, Hacizade Y, Isildak H, et al. Pott's puffy tumor. J Craniofac Surg. 2008;19:1694–7.
7. Akiyama K, Karaki M, Mori N. Evaluation of adult Pott's puffy tumor: our five cases and 27 literature cases. Laryngoscope. 2012;122:2382–8.
8. Ketenci I, Unlu Y, Tucer B, et al. The Pott's puffy tumor: a dangerous sign for intracranial complications. Eur Arch Otorhinolaryngol. 2011;268:1755–63.
9. Jackson K, Baker SR. Clinical implications of orbital cellulitis. Laryngoscope. 1986;96(5):568–74.
10. Schramm VL, Myers EN, Kennerdell JS. Orbital complications of acute sinusitis: evaluation, management, and outcome. Otolaryngology. 1978;86(2):ORL221–30.
11. Chandler JR, Langenbrunner DJ, Stevens ER. The pathogenesis of orbital complications in acute sinusitis. Laryngoscope. 1970;80:1414.
12. Botting AM, McIntosh D, Mahadevan M. Paediatric pre- and post-septal peri-orbital infections are different diseases: a retrospective review of 262 cases. Int J Pediatr Otorhinolaryngol. 2007;72:377–83.
13. Oxford LE, McClay J. Medical and surgical management of subperiosteal orbital abscess secondary to acute sinusitis in children. Int J Pediatr Otorhinolaryngol. 2006;70:1853–61.
14. Blumfield E, Misra M. Pott's puffy tumor, intracranial, and orbital complications as the initial presentation of sinusitis in healthy adolescents, a case series. Emerg Radiol. 2011;18(3):203–10.
15. Herrmann BW, Chung JC, Eisenbeis JF, et al. Intracranial complications of pediatric frontal rhinosinusitis. Am J Rhinol. 2006;c20(3):320–4.
16. Morgan PR, Morrison WV. Complications of frontal and ethmoid sinusitis. Laryngoscope. 1980;90:661–6.
17. Germiller JA, Monin DL, Sparano AM, et al. Intracranial complications of sinusitis in children and adolescents and their outcomes. Arch Otolaryngol Head Neck Surg. 2006;132(9):969–76.
18. Clayman GL, Adams GL, Paugh DR, et al. Intracranial complications of paranasal sinusitis: a combined institutional review. Laryngoscope. 1991;101:234–9.
19. Weing BL, Goldstein MN, Abramson AL. Frontal sinusitis and its intracranial complications. Int J Pediatr Otorhinolaryngol. 1983;5:285.

20. Hicks CW, Wever JG, Reid JR, et al. Identifying and managing intracranial complication of sinusitis in children: a retrospective series. Pediatr Infect Dis J. 2011;30(3):222–6.

21. Giannoni CM, Stewart MG, Alford EL. Intracranial complications of sinusitis. Laryngoscope. 1997;107:863–7.

22. DelGaudio JM, Evans SH, Sobol SE, et al. Intracranial complications of sinusitis: what is the role of endoscopic sinus surgery in the acute setting. Am J Otolaryngol. 2010;31(1):25–8.

23. Mafee MF, Tran BH, Chapa AR. Imaging of rhinosinusitis and its complications: plain film, CT, and MRI. Clin Rev Allergy Immunol. 2006;30(3):165–86.

24. Singh B, Dellen Van J, Ramjettan S, et al. Sinogenic intracranial complications. J Laryngol Otol. 1995;109:945.

25. Brook I, Friedman EM, Rodriguez WJ, et al. Complications of sinusitis in children. Pediatrics. 1980;66:568–72.

26. Remmler D, Boles R. Intracranial complications of frontal sinusitis. Laryngoscope. 1980;90:1814–24.

Complications of Frontal Sinus Surgery

Conner J. Massey and Vijay R. Ramakrishnan

Preoperative Assessment

Patient Factors

Performing safe and successful frontal sinus surgery starts with a thorough review of pertinent patient factors, both medical and anatomic, that may impact surgical outcomes. For most patients with frontal sinus disease, medical options should be attempted prior to considering surgical management. A thorough review of the patient's past medical and surgical history is important. Close attention should be paid to conditions that may predispose to hemorrhage, such as clotting disorders or conditions requiring therapeutic anticoagulation, as well as instances of prior postoperative bleeding. A medical history that may associated with aberrant anatomy, like facial trauma, prior sinus surgery, or thyroid eye disease, should be noted [1–3].

Nasal endoscopy is another important part of the preoperative assessment. In surgically naïve patients, direct visualization of the frontal recess may be difficult or impossible. Despite this limitation, important aspects can be gleaned from endoscopy in these patients, such as the presence of polypoid disease and

significant nasal septal deviation. For patients undergoing revision procedures, it is important to note the degree of frontal recess patency, evidence of middle turbinate resection or lateralization, and distortion of other surgical landmarks.

Preoperative Imaging

One of the most critical aspects in performing safe dissection of the frontal sinus is undertaken prior to surgery with a review of appropriate preoperative imaging studies. Among the various imaging modalities, high-resolution computed tomography (CT) of the sinuses is the preferred study as it gives excellent anatomic resolution and discrimination. CT is also good for demonstrating certain osseous alterations that can result from secondary to long-standing sinusitis, namely, bony erosion and/or neo-osteogenesis (Fig. 23.1). Significant bony narrowing of the frontal recess may require implementation of complex intraoperative maneuvers for bony removal and is a risk factor for surgical failure.

In planning for frontal sinus surgery, a number of critical structures should be assessed on preoperative CT. With regard to the frontal sinus itself, surgeons should note the presence of intrasinus septations, which, if not surgically addressed, may result in continued disease

C. J. Massey · V. R. Ramakrishnan (✉)
University of Colorado School of Medicine,
Department of Otolaryngology, Aurora, CO, USA

© Springer Nature Switzerland AG 2019
D. Lal, P. H. Hwang (eds.), *Frontal Sinus Surgery*, https://doi.org/10.1007/978-3-319-97022-6_23

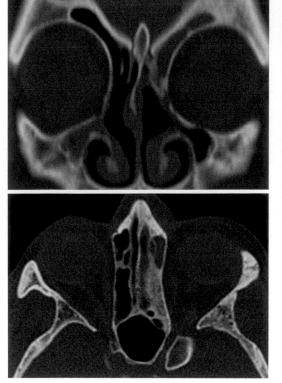

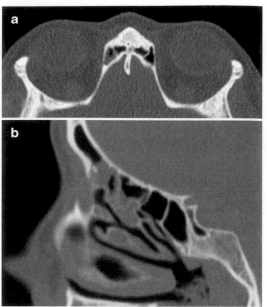

Fig. 23.2 Axial (**a**) and sagittal (**b**) noncontrast sinus CT scans from the same patient demonstrate a narrow frontal recess. The anterior-posterior dimension is limited by a prominent nasofrontal beak anteriorly and location of the anterior cribriform posteriorly

Fig. 23.1 Neo-osteogenesis of the frontal sinus and outflow tract can occur from chronic infection and inflammation or from prior attempts at surgery. This can be challenging to deal with during surgery and is a risk factor for surgical failure that ought to be recognized preoperatively

postoperatively. The configuration of the frontal recess should be thoroughly characterized, particularly the anatomic dimensions in the anterior-posterior and lateral directions (Fig. 23.2). A number of anatomic variations can alter the anatomy of the frontal recess and are described elsewhere in detail in this textbook. The frontal recess is bordered laterally by the lamina papyracea, which may be dehiscent or eroded in more advanced disease states. Violation of this structure may result in orbital injury. The depth of the cribriform plate, often graded using the Keros classification [4] (Fig. 23.3), is another important safety consideration. Patients with particularly deep cribriform plates are generally at a greater risk for skull base injury and iatrogenic cerebrospinal fluid (CSF) leak. Finally, it is important to note

vascular structures that may run in or near the surgical field. In frontal sinus surgery, the vessel most at risk is the anterior ethmoid artery (AEA), which normally courses anteriorly along the border of the bony skull base and lamina papyracea. In some patients, the artery may travel instead through a mesentery and is thus at greater risk of injury (Fig. 23.4) [5]. Careful review of the above anatomic variations, especially when carried out in a systematic approach, is a critical component of complication prevention (Table 23.1).

Complications of the Endoscopic Approach

This section will focus on some of the more common complications encountered in endoscopic frontal sinus surgery. Given that the endoscopic approach to the frontal sinus has only become widely utilized relatively recently [6], there is a paucity of literature examining frontal sinus-specific complications. A single

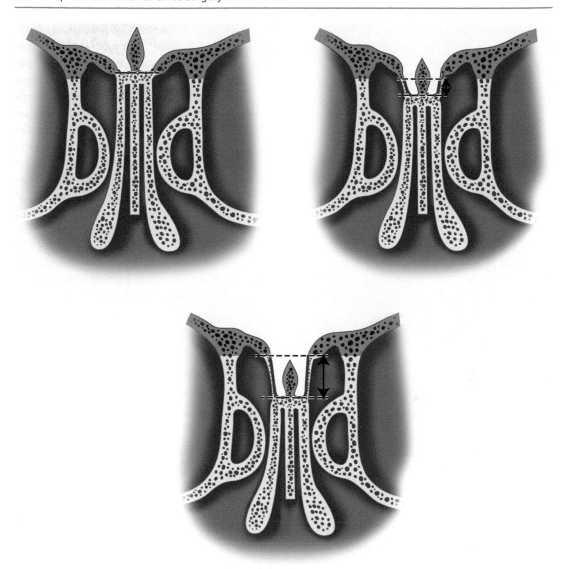

Fig. 23.3 Keros classification of cribriform depth (Class I, 0–3 mm; Class II. 4–7 mm; Class III, >7 mm). This is only one of several features that need to be evaluated when examining the relationship of the sinuses to the anterior skull base

institutional experience documenting 298 frontal sinus approaches found an overall complication rate of roughly 10%, with 2.7% of these consisting of major complications [7]. The authors documented an increased rate of complications with revision procedures and with extended techniques.

Despite careful patient selection and preoperative planning, complications may arise, even in the most experienced hands. After a brief discussion of critical technical points, this chapter will cover the prevention and management of impor-

tant complications encountered during endoscopic frontal sinus surgery, including:

- Scarring and restenosis
- Mucocele formation
- Hemorrhage and vascular injury
- Orbital injury
- CSF leak and intracranial injury

These complications, and others associated with endoscopic frontal sinus surgery, are summarized in Table 23.2.

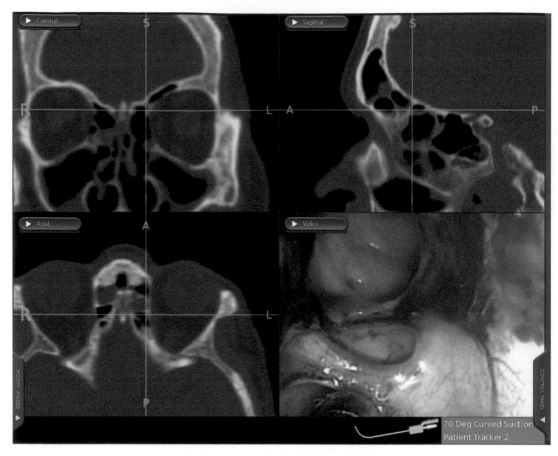

Fig. 23.4 Intraoperative image-guidance snapshot of the left dehiscent anterior ethmoid artery, using a 45-degree endoscope during frontal recess dissection. The artery is just outside of the skull base in a thin bony canal, coursing anteriorly as it traverses across the skull base

Table 23.1 CT scan checklist for frontal sinus surgery

Integrity of lamina papyracea
Integrity of skull base
Keros classification
Skull base height, slope, asymmetry
Course of anterior ethmoid artery
Insertion of uncinate process
Pneumatization pattern of agger nasi and accessory frontal cells
Patency of frontal sinus outflow tract
Anterior-posterior and lateral dimensions of frontal sinus ostia
Extent of pneumatization of frontal sinus
Posterior table erosion

Basic Technical Considerations

As with any surgery, prevention of complications is achieved in part with complete comprehension of anatomy, careful surgical planning, and meticulous surgical technique. For frontal sinus surgery, a thorough understanding of the agger nasi cell and its relation to surrounding structures, which should be ascertained during the review of preoperative imaging, is essential for safe dissection of the frontal recess [8]. Once identified, the bony septations that comprise the agger nasi cell and suprabullar cells must be removed in a sequential fashion to open the frontal sinus outflow tract. Failure to open these cells may result in recurrence or persistence of frontal sinus disease and also predisposes to incomplete dissection resulting in scarring and stenosis. Careful mucosal sparing technique during surgical dissection in this area is needed to prevent scarring and synechiae and delayed neo-osteogenesis [9].

Table 23.2 Complications of endoscopic surgery

Complication	Risk factors	Prevention	Management
Scarring and ostial stenosis	Smaller ostium Nasal polyps, asthma, heavy disease burden Middle turbinate lateralization Neo-osteogenesis	Mucosal sparing technique Frontal sinus stents not generally recommended Mucosal-free grafting techniques for extended procedures Meticulous postoperative care	In clinical revision, possible balloon dilation Revision with extended frontal sinusotomy (Draf IIB, III) when indicated
Mucocele formation	Sinus outflow tract obstruction Neo-osteogenesis History of frontal sinus obliteration procedure	Mucosal sparing technique Maintenance of ostial patency	Endoscopic marsupialization
Hemorrhage and vascular injury	Bleeding diathesis Anticoagulant therapy Hypertension Dehiscent AEA	Reverse Trendelenburg position Total intravenous anesthesia Preoperative corticosteroids Topical/injectable vasoconstrictors Routine use of nasal packing is *not* indicated	Bipolar cautery Nasal packing for postoperative bleeding Avoid pro-inflammatory hemostatic agents (e.g., thrombin)
Orbital complications	Dehiscent AEA Dehiscent lamina papyracea Use of powered instrumentation Drilling/cautery near trochlea	Preoperative imaging review	Bipolar cautery Ophthalmology consult Lateral canthotomy/cantholysis Medial orbital wall decompression
Skull base injury and intracranial complications	Low ethmoidal skull base height Keros 3 classification Sloped skull base Posterior table erosion	Preoperative imaging review	Intraoperative CSF leak: repair Suspected CSF leak postoperatively: β2-transferrin testing, imaging Intracranial infections: neurosurgical consult Intracranial hemorrhage: emergent neurosurgical consult

Utilization of extended approaches to the frontal sinus, such as the Draf type IIA/B and III sinusotomies, may be indicated in patients who have failed primary frontal sinusotomy. While the proper surgical technique for these extended approaches will be discussed elsewhere in this book, it should be noted that these techniques can carry an increased risk of skull base injury, CSF leak, and orbital complications.

Scarring and Frontal Ostial Stenosis

Maintaining ostial patency of the frontal sinus is critical for the long-term success of frontal sinus surgery. Patients who experience stenosis of the frontal ostium following surgery are at risk of disease recurrence and return of symptoms. For primary frontal sinusotomy (Draf IIA), retrospective studies have demonstrated long-term patency rates of 92% [10]. Risk factors for failure of primary frontal sinusotomy are primarily related to frontal ostium size [11], but other contributing factors have been identified, such as nasal polyposis, asthma, and heavy disease burden and presence of osteitis or neo-osteogenesis [12, 13].

Extended frontal surgery, such as Draf IIB or Draf III sinusotomy, can be used to create the largest ostium possible. Despite the aggressive nature of these techniques, symptomatic restenosis is still often encountered. The failure rate of the Draf III in which a revision procedure is encountered is estimated to be 13.9% [14]. The unexpectedly high failure rate may be related to the severity of the underlying disease process, the amount of exposed bone resulting from this technique, and the expected stenosis seen postoperatively [15]. Utilization of mucosal grafting techniques may facilitate rapid wound healing while minimizing stenosis [16].

A number of nasal biomaterials have been developed with the goal of preventing frontal ostial stenosis, albeit to varying degrees of success. Nonabsorbable frontal sinus stents have been designed to prevent restenosis of the neo-ostium, although their efficacy appears to be mixed. While shorter periods of stenting (e.g., 2 months) of the frontal sinus have not been shown to be effective in the long term [17], maintenance of a frontal stent over an extended period (e.g., 6 months minimum) seems to be well tolerated [18]. However, this is rarely required or recommended due to the risk of chronic stent infection and inflammation which may increase the likelihood of neo-osteogenesis (Fig. 23.5).

Chitosan gel is a newer bioabsorbable material derived from chitinous crustacean exoskel-

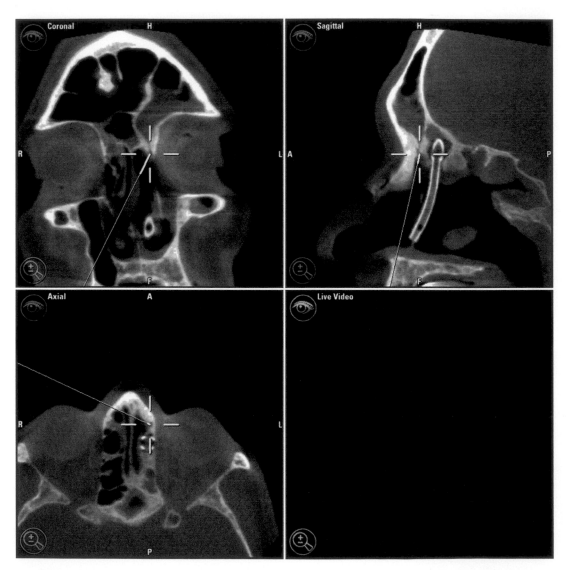

Fig. 23.5 Intraoperative triplanar CT scan imaging on a patient who has undergone prior frontal sinus surgery frontal sinus stent was attempted. Note the significant neo-osteogenesis around the stent indicative of ongoing chronic inflammation. Removal of the stent from the frontal recess in this scenario will likely result in rapid restenosis

etons that have been developed as a hemostatic agent and middle meatal spacer. When applied to neo-ostia, the product appears to improve frontal ostial patency at 12 weeks when compared to control, although long-term follow-up has not been documented [19]. While bioabsorbable steroid-releasing stents have been shown to be effective in preventing adhesion formation when used for ethmoid applications, these stents have only recently been FDA approved for use in frontal sinus applications. More study is needed to gauge the efficacy of these stents in the long term.

Mucocele Formation

Mucoceles are cyst-like, expansile growths lined by sinonasal mucoperiosteum that contain inspissated mucus. They tend to form when the sinus outflow tract is obstructed, leading to the accumulation of mucus within a confined space. Mucoceles must be surgically addressed when they expand or erode into nearby structures, including the orbit and anterior cranial fossa. When infected, they are termed mucopyoceles

and demand more urgent attention due to the risk of intracranial or intraorbital spread of infection. Patients with frontal sinus mucoceles may often present with orbital symptoms, including proptosis, diplopia, ophthalmoplegia, as well as cardinal symptoms of chronic rhinosinusitis, i.e., nasal congestion, facial pressure and pain, and rhinorrhea (Fig. 23.6). Retrospective analyses have determined that mucoceles are most often diagnosed 5 years following endoscopic sinus surgery [20].

In endoscopic frontal sinus surgery, the most critical factor in the prevention of frontal sinus mucoceles is mucosal preservation and maintenance of sinus ostial patency postoperatively. Careless disruption of mucosa around the frontal sinus outflow tract increases the risk of restenosis and obstruction, as mentioned previously.

In the past, definitive treatment for frontal sinus mucoceles consisted of complete excision of the cyst with obliteration of the surrounding sinus mucoperiosteum via an external approach. However, endoscopic marsupialization of these lesions is now regarded as the preferred treatment modality for the vast majority of cases.

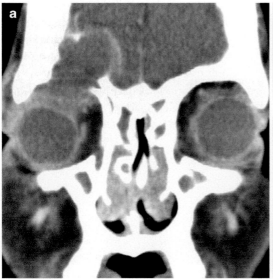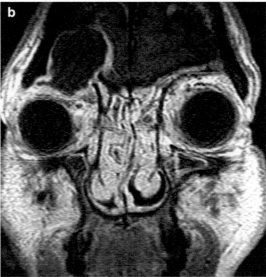

Fig. 23.6 Corresponding noncontrast coronal sinus CT (**a**) and postcontrast T1 coronal MR (**b**) demonstrating a fronto-orbital mucopyocele. Destruction of the orbital roof and right globe dystopia is noted, with intracranial extension of the rim-enhancing fluid collection

The endoscopic approach is preferred over external sinus obliteration as normal frontal sinus physiology is retained. Monitoring for mucocele recurrence is also more readily facilitated when endoscopic techniques are used. Even for so-called "giant" mucoceles that have significant intracranial or intraorbital extension, surgical outcomes for endoscopic and external approaches are roughly equivalent [21]. A minimum of a Draf IIA sinusotomy is suggested for endoscopic management of iatrogenic mucoceles.

Hemorrhage and Vascular Injury

Maintaining excellent hemostasis intraoperatively is necessary for optimizing visibility of the surgical field and consequently the safety and efficiency of the operation. A number of different factors must be considered in the prevention of hemorrhage. Aside from the aforementioned patient factors (e.g., anticoagulation status), variables at play include the type of anesthesia, preoperative steroids, use of local anesthetics, and patient positioning. While reverse Trendelenburg position has been confirmed to reduce intraoperative blood loss during FESS [22], some debate exists with regard to optimizing the other factors. A recent meta-analysis demonstrated significantly less blood loss when using total intravenous anesthesia as opposed to balanced anesthesia. The same study also demonstrated less bleeding when preoperative steroids were used [23]. The benefits of using topical or injectable vasoconstrictors like epinephrine are clear but must be weighed against the potential cardiovascular side effects [24].

Postoperative hemorrhage is estimated to occur in less than 1% of cases [1, 2]. Interestingly, the use of nasal packing has not been shown to decrease this risk [25]. The use of topical hemostatic agents at the end of surgery should only be used when absolutely necessary given their association with postoperative scarring [26]. While postoperative IV NSAIDs like ketorolac are generally contraindicated in other common head and neck procedures, they have not been shown to increase the risk of postoperative hemorrhage [27].

Aside from these general preventative measures, a thorough knowledge of vulnerable vascular structures is necessary. For surgery of the frontal sinus, the vessel most at risk during surgical dissection is the AEA, as previously mentioned. If damaged, this vessel will bleed briskly and is at risk of retracting into the orbit, which may lead to orbital hematoma formation. Prompt recognition and treatment, ideally with bipolar cautery, is the preferred method of addressing this problem before further complications can arise.

Orbital Complications

In surgical dissection of the frontal recess, the orbit remains particularly at risk for iatrogenic injury given its close proximity to the surgical field and the relative ease with which the lamina papyracea may be penetrated. The risk of injury increases when powered instrumentation is used [28]. The gravity of orbital complications can vary considerably, ranging from the relatively inconsequential herniation of periorbital fat, to more serious events such as extraocular muscle disruption and orbital hematoma, the latter of which may cause blindness if not appropriately addressed (Fig. 23.7).

With thoughtful preoperative planning, injury to the orbit may be prevented. The surgeon should

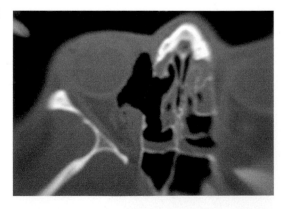

Fig. 23.7 Axial CT image demonstrates a dramatic microdebrider injury that occurred during endoscopic sinus surgery. Removal of the medial orbital contents to the level of the globe is observed

carefully review CT scan to gauge for the integrity of the lamina papyracea, as well as the course of the AEA. The AEA may be dehiscent in 6–66% of cases [29]. Damage to this vessel can result in orbital hematoma, a serious complication that requires emergent action. Intraoperatively, it is important that the eye not be covered or draped. Transparent tape should be used instead so that the surgeon may periodically inspect and palpate the globe. Orbital hematoma may be suspected if the eye becomes tense and proptotic or if there is chemosis or ecchymosis. Blindness may result when the orbital pressure exceeds the perfusion pressure of the optic nerve, which can occur in less than 30 min for arterial bleeds [30]. Examination should include ballottement of the orbit, checking for afferent pupillary defect, and tonometry. Once suspected, immediate ophthalmology consultation should be requested in order to obtain objective measurements of intraocular

pressure. Should an ophthalmologist not be readily available, the sinus surgeon should be prepared to decompress the orbit.

The most effective method for orbital decompression is lateral canthotomy and inferior cantholysis (Fig. 23.8). The procedure begins by making a small horizontal incision in the lateral canthus using scissors and then directing a second cut inferiorly until reaching the orbital rim, so that the inferior lateral canthal tendon is completely transected. It is important to understand that orbital decompression is not achieved until this tendon is severed. Attempts to decompress the orbit via transection of the superior crus of canthal tendon should be avoided, as damage to the lacrimal gland and levator muscle may occur.

Should the orbit continue to feel tense after canthotomy and cantholysis, intraocular pressure may be further reduced with medial orbital wall

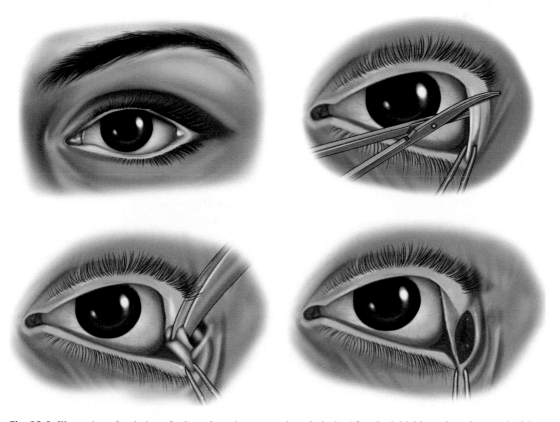

Fig. 23.8 Illustration of technique for lateral canthotomy and cantholysis. After the initial lateral canthotomy incision, division of the lower crus of the tendon (inferior cantholysis) is the key part of the left eye procedure for optimal orbital pressure release

decompression. This method is less effective at reducing intraocular pressure and should only be pursued after lateral canthotomy has been performed. In medial orbital decompression, the lamina papyracea is identified and removed along the length of the anterior and posterior ethmoidectomy cavity. Powered instrumentation should not be used so as to avoid damage to orbital fat or the extraocular muscles. Once the periorbita is exposed, multiple parallel periorbital incisions are made with a sickle knife in a posterior to anterior direction, allowing periorbital fat to extrude into the ethmoidectomy cavity and thus decompressing the tense orbit.

Once the orbit has been decompressed, attention should be directed toward resolving continued AEA hemorrhage if necessary. While rarely required, this is best achieved with ligation of the artery via clips or bipolar cautery. Monopolar cautery within the confines of the orbit should be avoided due to the potential of thermal injury to this delicate area. Nasal packing should not be used so as to prevent placing additional pressure on the orbit.

Diplopia is another potential orbital complication that may result if one of the extraocular muscles is injured. Drilling or cautery around the trochlea places the medial rectus and superior oblique muscles at risk (Fig. 23.9). Patients will present with double vision and an inability to either adduct or internally rotate the affected eye. Patients who sustain extraocular muscle injury should be referred to ophthalmology for further care.

Skull Base Injury and Intracranial Complications

Sequelae that may arise from violation of the bony skull base during sinus surgery include CSF rhinorrhea, the presentation of which may either be immediate or delayed, and the complications stemming from this event, such as meningitis and other intracranial infections. Limited case series exist documenting the incidence of this complication with regard to frontal sinus surgery specifically. Certain variations in anatomy, such as lower ethmoidal skull base height [31], increase the risk of iatrogenic injury and should be carefully reviewed during preoperative planning as previously discussed. In cases with bony erosion of the posterior table of the frontal sinus, either from expansile mucoceles or long-standing sinusitis, CSF leak may be more likely to occur. Once intracranial penetration occurs, the use of powered instrumentation may be associated with the creation of larger defects or more substantial injury [32].

Recognition of skull base injury with CSF leak may occur intraoperatively or in a delayed fash-

Fig. 23.9
Representation of the relationship of the trochlea and superior oblique muscle and its proximity to the frontal sinus outflow tract. While rare, aggressive drilling or cautery in this region can cause temporary or permanent diplopia

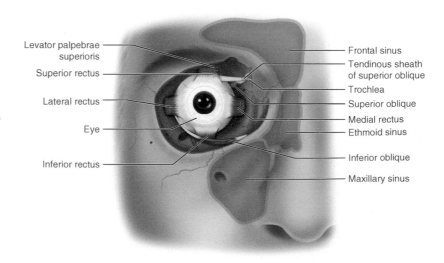

ion. Intraoperatively, injury to the skull base may often initially present with significant hemorrhage, after which the surgeon may visualize streaming clear fluid or pulsations of the dura. A delayed presentation is estimated to occur about 50% of the time [33]. Patients may endorse clear thin rhinorrhea that is positional, a salty postnasal drip, or headache, or they may present with evidence of intracranial infection, including meningitis or intracranial abscess (Fig. 23.10).

When a diagnosis of CSF leak is made intraoperatively, the defect should be repaired before the end of the case. When a delayed CSF leak is suspected, further workup may be required to make the diagnosis, including nasal endoscopy, β2-transferrin testing, and CT imaging of the bony skull base to assess for defects. In the delayed setting, a persistent CSF leak should be repaired once identified given the risk of intracranial infection.

Iatrogenic CSF leaks may be repaired in a single- or multilayered fashion using a variety of materials and techniques. Differences in these methods are often based on surgeon preference, as well as the size and location of the skull base defect. The technical aspects of skull base reconstruction and CSF leak repair are discussed in detail else-

where in this book. Skull base defects localized to the frontal recess will often require the surgeon to perform an extended frontal sinusotomy for exposure, so that the frontal sinus outflow tract is not obstructed after graft placement. The literature does not support the routine use of prophylactic antibiotics or postoperative lumbar drain placement [34]. For patients who develop more serious sequelae of skull base injury, such as meningitis, intracranial abscess, vascular injury, or stroke, emergent neurosurgical evaluation is required.

Skull base injury and CSF leak are rare and potentially serious complications of endoscopic frontal sinus surgery. Preoperative imaging review is the most important component of preventing this complication. Except for very low flow leaks, these injuries should be repaired to prevent intracranial infection.

Complications of External Approaches

While external approaches to the frontal sinus are less often used today than they were in the past, they still remain useful in cases where the endoscopic approach has failed. Open

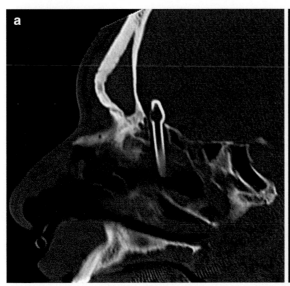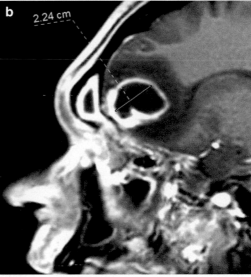

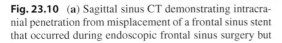

Fig. 23.10 (a) Sagittal sinus CT demonstrating intracranial penetration from misplacement of a frontal sinus stent that occurred during endoscopic frontal sinus surgery but was detected in a delayed postoperative setting. (b) Corresponding post-gadolinium MR shows an associated brain abscess

Table 23.3 Complications specific to external procedures

Procedure	Complications
Open (transfacial) frontoethmoidectomy	Telecanthus (medial canthal tendon disruption)
	Epiphora (nasolacrimal system disruption)
	Poor cosmesis: scarring
Frontal sinus trephination	Supratrochlear nerve injury
	Poor cosmesis: scarring, alopecia
Osteoplastic flap	Poor cosmesis: scarring, frontal bossing/depression, alopecia
	Facial nerve (temporal branch) weakness
	Mucocele formation

approaches relevant to frontal sinus surgery include external frontoethmoidectomy, trephination, and the osteoplastic flap technique. General complications are summarized in Table 23.3, and those specific to particular procedures are outlined below.

External Frontoethmoidectomy

External frontoethmoidectomy is rarely indicated today over conventional endoscopic technique due to a number of significant drawbacks, although it may still be used in cases of complex fronto-orbital neoplasms. In many respects, the complications that arise from this procedure are similar to the endoscopic approach to the frontal recess, including hemorrhage and orbital hematoma secondary to AEA transection, CSF leak, and frontal outflow tract obstruction. However, due to the inferior visualization of the surgical field that is offered by this approach, these complications may be more severe and less easily managed.

The modified Lynch incision that is used in this technique may scar and lead to poor cosmesis. Aggressive dissection near the anterior orbit may cause damage to the medial canthus, resulting in telecanthus. Injury to the nasolacrimal system is also possible during dissection down to the sinus. Mastery of the anatomy in this region is

necessary to avoid complications. For patients who sustain either of these latter two complications, referral to an oculoplastic surgeon for further management should be considered.

Frontal Sinus Trephination

Frontal sinus trephination is an adjunctive technique that may be indicated for difficult to access frontal sinus lesions that otherwise cannot be reached endoscopically. In this approach, a small incision is made just superior to the medial brow, through which a burr can be introduced for drilling through the anterior table and into the frontal sinus.

When performed correctly, complications for this procedure are generally minor. As with any incision made on the face, scar formation with poor cosmetic result is a possibility. The surgeon should be careful not to take the incision through the brow hair follicles, as noticeable alopecia may result after healing. Injury to the supratrochlear nerve, resulting in anesthesia of the forehead, may be temporary or permanent. Many of the other potential serious complications, such as orbital injury and inadvertent craniotomy, are generally avoided with the use of image-guidance systems or detailed anatomic planning.

Osteoplastic Flap

The osteoplastic flap procedure, once considered the gold standard treatment for frontal sinus disease, has fallen out of favor since the development extended endoscopic techniques that achieve similar results but still maintain normal frontal sinus drainage. Revision rates for this external technique have been estimated to be around 17% and possibly higher in patients who have inflammatory disease [35]. However, even in today's era where the endoscopic approach dominates, the osteoplastic flap may be indicated for neoplasms, meningoencephaloceles, disease in the lateral aspects of the sinus, or in cases where repeated attempts at endoscopic management have failed.

Briefly, the osteoplastic flap technique is performed through a coronal incision, and a skin flap is raised inferiorly. Using image guidance, the frontal sinus contours are outlined, and cuts are made through the bony anterior table with a powered saw (Fig. 23.11). Disease management is dictated by the pathology and preoperative plan. The procedure may be performed in an obliterative fashion, which is achieved by meticulously stripping away all sinus mucosa, plugging the sinus outflow tract, and then filling the sinus cavity with fat. The bone and skin layers are then replaced.

Complications that may arise with the osteoplastic flap procedure can be grouped into one of three categories:

- Cosmetic
- Intracranial or orbital injury
- Mucocele formation

There are many aspects of this procedure that may lead to cosmetically undesirable results. The coronal incision is generally well disguised when properly carried out through the hair-bearing scalp, although patients with significant alopecia may find the resulting scar unacceptable. Raising the skin flap also places the temporal branch of the facial nerve at risk, which, if damaged, may result in brow and forehead asymmetry. Dissection should be carried deep to the temporoparietal fascia so that the frontal division of the facial nerve is preserved superficially within the flap. If the bone flap does not sit properly when replaced, deformity of the forehead can be observed, such as frontal bossing or depression of the frontal table. Modifications to the classical technique have been devised to overcome this issue [36].

Dissection outside the confines of the frontal sinus, especially when raising the bone flap, may result in orbital or intracranial injury. This is prevented by carefully demarcating the borders of the frontal sinus. Historically, this was achieved with overlaying a 6-foot Caldwell radiograph, although this has been almost entirely replaced with computerized image-guidance systems. Intracranial penetration can result in CSF leak if frontal bone cuts are misdirected, leading to violation of the dura. If encountered, dural tears can be repaired in a multilayered fashion as previously described. Neurosurgical consultation is advised in these situations. Damage to the supe-

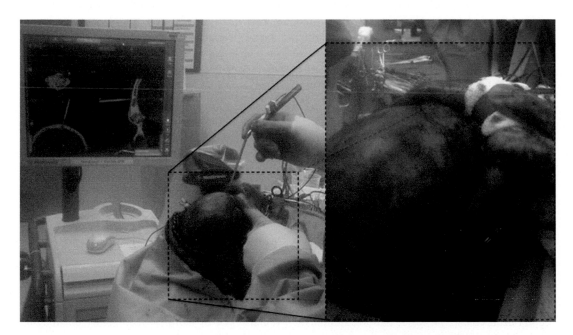

Fig. 23.11 Image guidance can be used to help outline the frontal sinus boundary in preparation for an osteoplastic flap approach, in this case for a large frontal osteoma

rior orbit is also possible, resulting in the exposure of periorbital fat or damage to the extraocular
muscles. Ophthalmologic evaluation is suggested
if the latter complication has occurred.

Finally, patients who undergo the osteoplastic
flap procedure are at risk of forming mucoceles
postoperatively. This is best prevented by ensuring that all mucosa is stripped during the obliteration part of the procedure, which may be achieved
with polishing the sinus cavity with powered
drills. Alternatively, if obliteration is not required,
the mucosa of the frontal sinus outflow can be left
completely intact to preserve normal sinus physiology. The use of bone cement in the obliterated
cavity should be avoided due to the propensity
for infection [35]. For patients who undergo
obliteration, monitoring for disease recurrence
with CT and/or MRI may be more difficult. When
mucoceles do occur following the procedure, surgical revision, either with a repeat osteoplastic
flap or endoscopic "unobliteration" procedure
[37, 38], may be needed.

The osteoplastic flap technique, while used
less often in today's paradigm of extended endoscopic approaches, may still be performed in
select cases of frontal sinus disease. The various
complications inherent to this procedure, namely,
issues with cosmesis and the potential for recurrence and postoperative mucocele formation,
may be difficult to prevent. As such, the procedure is generally considered only for select cases
not amenable to endoscopic or minimally invasive combined approaches.

Complications with Frontal Balloon Sinuplasty

Balloon sinuplasty has become a popular alternative to conventional endoscopic surgery for the
management of patients with mild to moderate
frontal sinus inflammatory disease due to its relative ease of use and the fact that it may be performed in a clinic setting. While discussion of the
efficacy of this surgical modality is out of the
scope of this chapter, in-office balloon sinuplasty
appears to have a low complication rate, with retrospective analyses demonstrating a postopera-

tive hemorrhage rate of 1.1% and orbital
complications in 0.3% of patients [39].
Unfortunately, no data specific to the frontal
sinus exist.

Complications of frontal balloon sinuplasty
may stem from the dilation of the wrong area.
False cannulation and incorrect dilation may
result in failure to resolve symptoms, or potentially worsening frontal sinus drainage if an
accessory frontal recess cell is dilated, or a narrow frontal outflow is traumatized. Patients with
variations in anatomy of the frontal recess, which
can be further exacerbated by prior ethmoidectomy, may be at increased risk of false passage
and procedural failure [40]. More serious complications, such as CSF leak, are extremely rare,
although those have been documented in the case
report literature [41].

As with conventional endoscopic sinus surgery, all patients should have preoperative CT,
which will alert the surgeon to anatomic variations in the frontal recess that may make balloon
dilation difficult (e.g., neo-osteogenesis), as well
as demonstrate instances in which this treatment
would be inappropriate, such as heavy disease
burden. During the procedure itself, care should
be taken to confirm correct placement; this can be
done with direct visualization of passage into the
frontal sinus, transillumination of the sinus with a
lighted guide wire, or use of computer-assisted
navigation associated with the balloon
instrumentation.

Balloon sinuplasty of the frontal sinuses carries a low complication rate when performed correctly. Complications and poor surgical outcomes
stem from false cannulation and can generally be
avoided by reviewing the anatomy of the frontal
sinus outflow tract and confirming correct
placement.

Summary

Despite continued advances in surgical technique
and technologies, surgery of the frontal sinus
remains one of the most technically challenging
areas in rhinology. Complications of frontal sinus
surgery may impact successful outcomes and can

be morbid or even life-threatening. Careful review of the preoperative CT scan, along with other patient factors, remains one of the most important aspects in preventing serious complications. This holds true regardless of the surgical approach used. Even in the most experienced hands, complications can and do occur. Although serious complications are rare, surgeons must be prepared to address these issues in an expeditious manner. Finally, recognition of one's own limitations in skill and experience are critical to performing safe surgery. Patients with extensive frontal disease or complex anatomy should be cared for by those with appropriate expertise and training in this area.

References

1. Ramakrishnan VR, Kingdom TT, Nayak JV, Hwang PH, Orlandi RR. Nationwide incidence of major complications in endoscopic sinus surgery. Int Forum Allergy Rhinol. 2012;2(1):34–9.
2. Krings JG, Kallogjeri D, Wineland A, Nepple KG, Piccirillo JF, Getz AE. Complications of primary and revision functional endoscopic sinus surgery for chronic rhinosinusitis. Laryngoscope. 2014;124(4):838–45.
3. Hahn S, Palmer JN, Purkey MT, Kennedy DW, Chiu AG. Indications for external frontal sinus procedures for inflammatory sinus disease. Am J Rhinol Allergy. 2009;23(3):342–7.
4. Keros P. On the practical value of differences in the level of the lamina cribrosa of the ethmoid. Z Für Laryngol Rhinol Otol Ihre Grenzgeb. 1962;41:809–13.
5. Hoang JK, Eastwood JD, Tebbit CL, Glastonbury CM. Multiplanar sinus CT: a systematic approach to imaging before functional endoscopic sinus surgery. AJR Am J Roentgenol. 2010;194(6):W527–36.
6. Psaltis AJ, Soler ZM, Nguyen SA, Schlosser RJ. Changing trends in sinus and septal surgery, 2007 to 2009. Int Forum Allergy Rhinol. 2012;2(5):357–61.
7. Hoskison E, Daniel M, Daudia A, Jones N, Sama A. Complications of endoscopic frontal sinus surgery. Otolaryngol Head Neck Surg. 2010;143(2 Suppl):P272–P272.
8. Wormald PJ. The agger nasi cell: the key to understanding the anatomy of the frontal recess. Otolaryngol Head Neck Surg. 2003;129(5):497–507.
9. Moriyama H, Yanagi K, Ohtori N, Asai K, Fukami M. Healing process of sinus mucosa after endoscopic sinus surgery. Am J Rhinol. 1996;10(2):61–6.
10. Naidoo Y, Wen D, Bassiouni A, Keen M, Wormald PJ. Long-term results after primary frontal sinus surgery. Int Forum Allergy Rhinol. 2012;2(3):185–90.
11. Hosemann W, Kühnel T, Held P, Wagner W, Felderhoff A. Endonasal frontal sinusotomy in surgical management of chronic sinusitis: a critical evaluation. Am J Rhinol. 1997;11(1):1–9.
12. Chandra RK, Palmer JN, Tangsujarittham T, Kennedy DW. Factors associated with failure of frontal sinusotomy in the early follow-up period. Otolaryngol Head Neck Surg. 2004;131(4):514–8.
13. Naidoo Y, Bassiouni A, Keen M, Wormald P-J. Risk factors and outcomes for primary, revision, and modified Lothrop (Draf III) frontal sinus surgery. Int Forum Allergy Rhinol. 2013;3(5):412–7.
14. Anderson P, Sindwani R. Safety and efficacy of the endoscopic modified Lothrop procedure: a systematic review and meta-analysis. Laryngoscope. 2009;119(9):1828–33.
15. Tran KN, Beule AG, Singal D, Wormald P-J. Frontal ostium restenosis after the endoscopic modified Lothrop procedure. Laryngoscope. 2007;117(8):1457–62.
16. Conger BT, Riley K, Woodworth BA. The Draf III mucosal grafting technique: a prospective study. Otolaryngol Head Neck Surg. 2012;146(4):664–8.
17. Banhiran W, Sargi Z, Collins W, Kaza S, Casiano R. Long-term effect of stenting after an endoscopic modified Lothrop procedure. Am J Rhinol. 2006;20(6):595–9.
18. Orlandi RR, Knight J. Prolonged stenting of the frontal sinus. Laryngoscope. 2009;119(1):190–2.
19. Ngoc Ha T, Valentine R, Moratti S, Robinson S, Hanton L, Wormald P-J. A blinded randomized controlled trial evaluating the efficacy of chitosan gel on ostial stenosis following endoscopic sinus surgery. Int Forum Allergy Rhinol. 2013;3(7):573–80.
20. Scangas GA, Gudis DA, Kennedy DW. The natural history and clinical characteristics of paranasal sinus mucoceles: a clinical review. Int Forum Allergy Rhinol. 2013;3(9):712–7.
21. Stokken J, Wali E, Woodard T, Recinos PF, Sindwani R. Considerations in the management of giant frontal mucoceles with significant intracranial extension: a systematic review. Am J Rhinol Allergy. 2016;30(4):301–5.
22. Hathorn IF, A-RR H, Manji J, Javer AR. Comparing the reverse Trendelenburg and horizontal position for endoscopic sinus surgery: a randomized controlled trial. Otolaryngol Head Neck Surg. 2013;148(2):308–13.
23. Khosla AJ, Pernas FG, Maeso PA. Meta-analysis and literature review of techniques to achieve hemostasis in endoscopic sinus surgery. Int Forum Allergy Rhinol. 2013;3(6):482–7.
24. Higgins TS, Hwang PH, Kingdom TT, Orlandi RR, Stammberger H, Han JK. Systematic review of topical vasoconstrictors in endoscopic sinus surgery. Laryngoscope. 2011;121(2):422–32.
25. Eliashar R, Gross M, Wohlgelernter J, Sichel J-Y. Packing in endoscopic sinus surgery: is it really required? Otolaryngol Head Neck Surg. 2006;134(2):276–9.

26. Chandra RK, Conley DB, Haines GK, Kern RC. Long-term effects of FloSeal packing after endoscopic sinus surgery. Am J Rhinol. 2005;19(3):240–3.

27. Moeller C, Pawlowski J, Pappas AL, Fargo K, Welch K. The safety and efficacy of intravenous ketorolac in patients undergoing primary endoscopic sinus surgery: a randomized, double-blinded clinical trial. Int Forum Allergy Rhinol. 2012;2(4):342–7.

28. Bhatti MT, Giannoni CM, Raynor E, Monshizadeh R, Levine LM. Ocular motility complications after endoscopic sinus surgery with powered cutting instruments. Otolaryngol Head Neck Surg. 2001;125(5):501–9.

29. Jang DW, Lachanas VA, White LC, Kountakis SE. Supraorbital ethmoid cell: a consistent landmark for endoscopic identification of the anterior ethmoidal artery. Otolaryngol Head Neck Surg. 2014;151(6):1073–7.

30. Stankiewicz JA. Blindness and intranasal endoscopic ethmoidectomy: prevention and management. Otolaryngol Head Neck Surg. 1989;101(3):320–9.

31. Ramakrishnan VR, Suh JD, Kennedy DW. Ethmoid skull-base height: a clinically relevant method of evaluation. Int Forum Allergy Rhinol. 2011;1(5):396–400.

32. Church CA, Chiu AG, Vaughan WC. Endoscopic repair of large skull base defects after powered sinus surgery. Otolaryngol Head Neck Surg. 2003;129(3):204–9.

33. Bedrosian JC, Anand VK, Schwartz TH. The endoscopic endonasal approach to repair of iatrogenic and noniatrogenic cerebrospinal fluid leaks and encepha-loceles of the anterior cranial fossa. World Neurosurg. 2014;82(6 Suppl):S86–94.

34. Oakley GM, Orlandi RR, Woodworth BA, Batra PS, Alt JA. Management of cerebrospinal fluid rhinorrhea: an evidence-based review with recommendations. Int Forum Allergy Rhinol. 2016;6(1):17–24.

35. Ochsner MC, DelGaudio JM. The place of the osteoplastic flap in the endoscopic era: indications and pitfalls. Laryngoscope. 2015;125(4):801–6.

36. Healy DY, Leopold DA, Gray ST, Holbrook EH. The perforation technique: a modification to the frontal sinus osteoplastic flap. Laryngoscope. 2014;124(6):1314–7.

37. Javer AR, Sillers MJ, Kuhn FA. The frontal sinus unobliteration procedure. Otolaryngol Clin N Am. 2001;34(1):193–210.

38. Hwang PH, Han JK, Bilstrom EJ, Kingdom TT, Fong KJ. Surgical revision of the failed obliterated frontal sinus. Am J Rhinol. 2005;19(5):425–9.

39. Sillers MJ, Lay KF. Balloon catheter dilation of the frontal sinus Ostium. Otolaryngol Clin N Am. 2016;49(4):965–74.

40. Heimgartner S, Eckardt J, Simmen D, Briner HR, Leunig A, Caversaccio MD. Limitations of balloon sinuplasty in frontal sinus surgery. Eur Arch Oto-Rhino-Laryngol Off J Eur Fed Oto-Rhino-Laryngol Soc EUFOS Affil Ger Soc Oto-Rhino-Laryngol – Head Neck Surg. 2011;268(10):1463–7.

41. Tomazic PV, Stammberger H, Koele W, Gerstenberger C. Ethmoid roof CSF-leak following frontal sinus balloon sinuplasty. Rhinology. 2010;48(2):247–50.

Management of Frontal Headaches

Andrew Thamboo, John M. DelGaudio,
and Zara M. Patel

Introduction

Frontal headaches, commonly called "sinus headaches" by patients, primary care physicians, and general media, are an imprecise term that often leads to improper management. Given the commonality of this term, it is important that otolaryngologists have a good understanding of the possible causes of "sinus headaches" and the different management options available. The International Headache Society (IHS) provides a number of conditions with diagnostic criteria that otolaryngologists should be aware of to help manage patients who are referred for "sinus headache."

Diagnostic Criteria of Acute and Chronic Rhinosinusitis

The American Academy of Otolaryngology–Head and Neck Surgery Foundation (AAO-HNSF) provides evidence-based recommendations regarding the management of acute and chronic rhinosinusitis. The criteria were first established in 1997 but have evolved with an updated document elaborating on the condition in 2014 [1]. Facial pain is described as a cardinal symptom in the setting acute rhinosinusitis (ARS) if associated with purulent nasal discharge. In the setting of chronic rhinosinusitis (CRS), facial pain is a cardinal symptom of CRS as long as it is found in combination with one more cardinal nasal symptom and confirmed by objective findings seen either on nasal endoscopy or sinus CT scan or both (Table 24.1).

The international community, including Canada and Europe, has also established their guidelines for diagnosing ARS and CRS. In similar fashion to AAO-HNSF, the Canadian guidelines state facial pain in the setting of an acute sinus infection must be associated with purulence, but may also be associated with nasal obstruction [2]. The Canadian guidelines view facial pain in the setting of CRS similarly to the AAO-HNSF. The European guidelines on CRS patients also state that patients must have facial pain in the presence of either purulence or nasal

A. Thamboo · Z. M. Patel (✉)
Department of Otolaryngology – Head and Neck Surgery, Stanford University School of Medicine, Stanford, CA, USA

J. M. DelGaudio
Department of Otolaryngology – Head and Neck Surgery, Emory University School of Medicine, Atlanta, GA, USA

© Springer Nature Switzerland AG 2019
D. Lal, P. H. Hwang (eds.), *Frontal Sinus Surgery*, https://doi.org/10.1007/978-3-319-97022-6_24

Table 24.1 AAO-HSNSF diagnostic criteria for acute and chronic rhinosinusitis [1]

Acute rhinosinusitis

Up to 4 weeks of *purulent nasal drainage* (anterior, posterior, or both) accompanied by *nasal obstruction, facial pain pressure fullness,* or both:[a]

    Purulent nasal discharge cloudy or colored, in contrast to the clear secretions that typically accompany viral upper respiratory infection, and may be reported by the patient or observed on physical examination

    Nasal obstruction may be reported by the patient as nasal obstruction, congestion, blockage, or stuffiness or may be diagnosed by physical examination

    Facial pain pressure fullness may involve the anterior face and periorbital region or manifest with headache that is localized or diffuse

Chronic rhinosinusitis

12 weeks or longer of two or more of the following signs and symptoms:

    Mucopurulent drainage (anterior, posterior, or both)

    Nasal obstruction (congestion)

    Facial pain pressure fullness

    Decreased sense of smell

and inflammation is documented by one or more of the following findings:

    Purulent (not clear) mucus or edema in the middle meatus or anterior ethmoid region

    Polyps in nasal cavity or the middle meatus

    Radiographic imaging showing inflammation of the paranasal sinuses

[a]Facial pain pressure fullness in the absence of purulent nasal discharge is insufficient to establish diagnosis of acute rhinosinusitis

Table 24.2 IHS diagnostic criteria for headaches associated with rhinosinusitis [4]

1. Frontal headaches accompanied by pain in one or more regions of the face, ear, or teeth and fulfilling criteria 3 and 4

2. Clinical, nasal endoscopic, CT and/or MRI, and/or laboratory evidence of acute or acute-on-chronic rhinosinusitis[a]

3. Headache and facial pain develop simultaneously with onset or acute exacerbation of rhinosinusitis

4. Headache and facial pain resolve within 7 days after remission or successful treatment of acute or acute-on-chronic rhinosinusitis

[a]Clinical evidence: purulence, nasal obstruction, hyposmia, anosmia, and/or fever

obstruction to be considered a valid symptom in the setting of a sinus disorder [3]. While all guidelines convey that facial pain is a valid symptom as long as it is associated with other nasal symptoms, the IHS has further removed the association of facial pain from CRS. They describe CRS as "not a validated cause of headache or facial pain unless relapsing into an acute state" [4] (Table 24.2).

Diagnostic Approach to Frontal Headaches

Otolaryngologists seeing a patient for frontal headaches need to perform a thorough head and neck history and physical exam to determine if the sinuses are contributing to their symptoms. Asking appropriate questions regarding sinus-related symptoms is common practice for many otolaryngologists, and history alone may be able rule out sinus disease. Sinus-related pain is usually described as pressure-like and dull as well as bilateral, unless an isolated sinus is infected, and will most often have accompanying signs and symptoms directing the practitioner to a diagnosis of sinusitis [5]. Sinus pain usually lasts for days and is not associated with nausea, vomiting, visual disturbance, phonophobia, or photophobia [5]. If patients have confirmation on physical exam of sinusitis such as purulence draining from the sinuses on endoscopy, or findings of disease within the frontal sinuses on imaging, then certainly treatment for sinusitis should be initiated. The appropriate treatment choices for acute and chronic sinusitis have been well documented elsewhere and are beyond the scope of this chapter. Our purpose here is to help elucidate other diagnoses that are important to recognize and treat appropriately. Instead of simply informing patients their symptoms are unrelated to sinus problems, it is important to also have a grasp of common neurological causes of frontal headaches in order to better counsel, educate, and guide these patients. Otolaryngologists should be familiar with basic history taking for neurologic and other causes of frontal pressure. Providing patients with a good understanding of other causes of frontal headaches will help them understand the reason they may require a referral to another specialist and can avoid delay in the treatment of their symptoms.

The timing of nasal endoscopy or CT scan at a time that the patient is symptomatic with "sinus headache/pain" is helpful in confirming or ruling out the role of sinonasal infection or inflammation in their symptoms. Nasal endoscopy, especially when patients are able to see the findings real time on a monitor, as well as going over a negative CT scan in detail, can provide reassurance to patients. On the other hand, positive CT scans can be more difficult to reassure a patient there may be other causes to their frontal pain. It is important to educate the patient that there is poor correlation between location and magnitude of radiographic findings with facial pain location and severity and that other causes of pain should potentially be explored [6–8].

There is substantial evidence that frontal headaches often do not have a rhinologic etiology. As illustrated in Fig. 24.1, there are a number of conditions that can mimic frontal sinusitis. The upcoming sections describe neurologic causes of frontal headaches that will help guide otolaryngologists regarding pertinent history taking to ascertain the correct diagnosis and also

possible management options as they wait for their referral to another specialist.

Diagnostic Criteria of Neurogenic Causes of Frontal Headaches

The *International Classification of Headache Disorders, 2nd edition* [4], is an extensive publication and by no means is an otolaryngologist expected to know the exact details of each diagnostic criteria, but one should have a general idea of each of the following conditions and an article to reference if further information is required.

Migraines

Migraines are one of the most common causes of frontal headaches. There are a high number of patients suffering from migraines who have unfortunately not been diagnosed based on the IHS criteria [9]. Therefore, it is not surprising to find patients referred to our clinics mislabeled as individuals having sinus headaches. A summary of studies misdiagnosing migraines as sinus headaches is illustrated in Table 24.3. The Sinus, Allergy, and Migraine Study

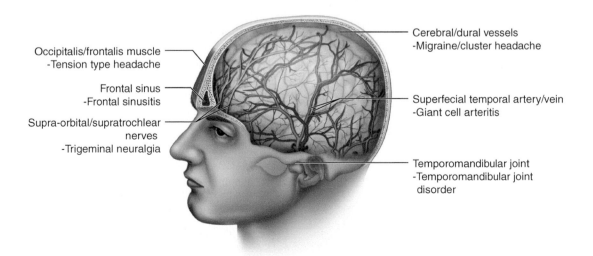

Fig. 24.1 Conditions that mimic frontal sinus headaches

(SAMS) recruited 100 consecutive adults who self-diagnosed themselves with sinus headaches and found out that 63% of patients had a diagnosis of migraine based on the IHS criteria [10]. Moreover, 58% of patients in a tertiary rhinology practice with no evidence of sinus disease or mucosal contact points and normal CT scan were later diagnosed with migraines following a neurology referral [11]. Patients who are eventually treated for the underlying migraine attribute their misdiagnosis of sinus headaches to misunderstanding of their cranial autonomic symptoms during headaches which can include nasal congestion, eyelid edema, rhinorrhea, conjunctival injection, and lacrimation [10]. Consequently, if nasal endoscopy and CT scan is negative, migraine is most likely the correct diagnosis and a trial of medical therapy, and referral to a neurologist should be undertaken (Table 24.4, IHS diagnostic criteria of migraines).

The initial treatment of migraine management is easy for an otolaryngologist to begin, but preventative and long-term therapy should be managed by a neurologist or primary care physician who is well versed in migraine management. Otolaryngologists should feel comfortable initiating treatment following a negative endoscopy and CT scan findings for patients presenting with frontal headaches while patients await their neurology referral. If patients have failed nonspecific medications such as NSAIDs, triptans are the best headache abortive drug to manage acute migraines [12]. Triptans are a class of selective serotonin receptor agonists that result in vasoconstriction of cranial vessels leading to inhibition of pro-inflammatory neuropeptide release. There is growing evidence that triptans also act on peripheral nerves, specifically inhibiting the trigeminal nerve [13]. Triptans have shown to be effective in the management of mild to severe forms of migraine and specifically in relieving symptoms such as nausea, vomiting, phonophobia, and photophobia [14, 15]. Besides being contraindicated in patients with cardiovascular disease [16], the medication is quite tolerable. There are a number of studies that show successful empirical management of "sinus headaches" with triptans [17–19].

Trigeminal Neuralgia

Trigeminal neuralgia (TN), previously known as tic douloureux, is a unilateral disorder that may encompass one or more divisions of the trigeminal nerve. Patients feel brief electric shock-like pains, which is abrupt in onset and termination. While the pain is usually triggered spontane-

Table 24.3 Studies illustrating misdiagnosis of "sinus headaches" in the setting of migraines

Study	Design	Level of evidence	Number of subjects	Conclusion
Barbanti et al. [46]	Prospective cohort	2b	177	Approximately 1/2 of migraine patients have unilateral cranial autonomic symptoms
Perry et al. [11]	Prospective cohort	2b	36	Majority of patients in tertiary rhinology practice have migraines
Schreiber et al. [47]	Prospective cohort	2b	2991	Majority of patients diagnosed with sinus headaches have migraines
Eross et al. [10]	Prospective cohort	1b	100	Most common reasons for misdiagnosis were triggers, provocation, and location
Mehle and Kremer [48]	Prospective cohort	2b	35	Majority of patients with sinus headache are diagnosed with migraine. Positive migraine history still requires ENT workup
Foroughipour et al. [49]	Prospective cohort	2b	58	Majority of patients with sinus headache are diagnosed with migraine

ously, it can be evoked by such actions as face washing, shaving, and talking. Frontal headaches can be elicited by irritation of V1 [4]. Close attention to the history will facilitate a clinician in making the diagnosis of TN (Table 24.5) as the pain experienced in TN is much different from sinus pain. However, illustrating to patients a negative endoscopy and CT scan may help educate and convince patients regarding the source of their pain.

V1 is affected in less than 5% of patients suffering from TN [4]. When a branch of the trigeminal nerve is affected, it either can be from a structural cause compressing the nerve (symptomatic) or from the nerve itself (classical). Patients suffering from classical TN have a refractory period between episodes while symptomatic TN may have a persistent aching between paroxysms. While standard nomenclature differentiates classical and symptomatic TN by absence or presence of a structural cause, MRI and posterior fossa exploration surgery have shown that a number of classical TN is due to tortuous or aberrant vessels compressing the trigeminal root [4].

First-line medical therapy is carbamazepine, which can also serve as a diagnostic tool. Patients with TN tend to have a good response to carbamazepine [20]. There are a number of other options which include oxcarbazepine, baclofen, lamotrigine, and gabapentin [21]. There are also a number of ablative procedural options, which include radiofrequency ablation, gamma knife surgery, and balloon compression. Radiofrequency is arguably the most common procedure performed after medical therapy. Surgical microvascular decompression (MVD) is performed on those who are debilitated from the pain and have failed all other forms of medical and ablative procedures. Patients must undergo a craniotomy, and therefore the morbidity is higher than other forms of management. However, the outcome of surgery is quite successful with approximately 71% reporting complete resolution [22]. Otolaryngologists should be comfortable in prescribing first-line therapy medications for TN while patients are waiting for their referral to a neurologist.

Giant Cell Arteritis

Giant cell arteritis (GCA) commonly presents as a unilateral headache, most commonly in the temporal region, but can certainly involve the frontal region as well. While the headache is considered to be more persistent than conditions like TN, the pain worsens with chewing from jaw claudication. However, the most

Table 24.4 IHS diagnostic criteria for migraine [4]

Migraine with aura
1. At least two attacks fulfilling criteria 2–4 if aura is present
2. Headache lasts 4–72 h
3. Headache that has two of the following: unilateral, pulsating quality, moderate or severe pain intensity, aggravated by or causing avoidance of routing physical activity
4. One of the following occurs during the headache: nausea, vomiting, photophobia, phonophobia
5. Headache cannot be attributed to another disorder
Migraine without aura
1. At least five attacks fulfilling criteria 2–4 when aura is not present
2. Headache lasts 4–72 h
3. Headache that has two of the following: unilateral, pulsating quality, moderate or severe pain intensity, aggravated by or causing avoidance of routine physical activity
4. One of the following occurs during the headache: nausea, vomiting, photophobia, phonophobia
5. Headache cannot be attributed to another disorder

Table 24.5 IHS diagnostic criteria for classic trigeminal, neuralgia [4]

1. Paroxysmal attacks of pain lasting from a fraction of a second to 2 min, affecting one or more divisions of the trigeminal nerve and fulfilling criteria 2 and 3
2. Pain has at least one of the following characteristics:
(a) Intense, sharp, superficial, or stabbing
(b) Precipitated from trigger areas or trigger factors
3. Attacks are stereotyped in the individual patient
4. There is no clinically evident neurologic deficit
5. Not attributed to another disorder

important symptom that should prompt a physician to do an urgent workup for GCA is repeated attacks of amaurosis fugax associated with the headaches. Physicians should have high suspicion for GCA, especially when a female older than 60 years old presents with such symptoms (Table 24.6, diagnostic criteria of GCA). The major risk of GCA is blindness due to anterior ischemic optic neuropathy, which can occur in both eyes. The time interval between visual loss in one eye and the other is about 1 week. Fortunately, this can be prevented by immediate treatment with steroids. Patients who have GCA are also at risk for cerebral ischemic attacks and dementia.

Initial workup for GCA usually begins with blood work showing elevated erythrocyte sedimentation rate (ESR) and C-reactive protein (CRP); however, the gold standard investigation is a temporal artery biopsy. Histologically, there is variability in the location of the GCA as they present as skip lesions; consequently, it is important to either obtain a large piece of the temporal artery or to use a duplex study to direct the biopsy to regions of high suspicion.

Primary management of GCA is steroids but the optimal dose and length of treatment is

unclear. Consensus-based recommendations suggest 40–60 mg/day followed by individualized length and tapering of dose [23]. While any further management should be managed by a rheumatologist, other adjuvant therapies include methotrexate, which has been shown to decrease the cumulative dose of steroids, and tocilizumab, which has been shown to decrease remission rate [24, 25].

Temporomandibular Joint Disorder

Temporomandibular joint disorder (TMD) is a common problem many otolaryngologists see; therefore, it is important to be able to differentiate this condition from a rhinogenic problem. The initial source of the pain originates at the temporomandibular joint but can often radiate over the frontal sinus/temple due to the muscles overlying these regions that attach to the joint. TMD can be divided into three subtypes: intra-articular, muscular (myofascial), and arthritic. Patients presenting with history of clicking and popping with jaw opening suffer from intra-articular TMD. On physical exam, crepitus can be felt on palpation. It is more difficult to diagnose muscular subtype as the pain is associated with a misaligned jaw resulting in persistently strained muscles of mastication. Arthritic subtype is best appreciated through history, especially those with history of osteoarthritis, as this is the most common cause of TMD [26]. Obtaining a history of jaw clenching; bruxism; pain with eating, talking, or yawning; limited range of motion; or looking for signs of flattened cuspid ridges should direct a physician to consider TMD as the likely cause of frontal headaches (Table 24.7, diagnostic criteria of TMD).

The initial treatment of TMD should be conservative. Educating the patient regarding the anatomy of the temporomandibular joint and muscle attachments can improve patient compliance with respect to conservative treatment. When TMD is mild to moderate in nature,

Table 24.6 IHS diagnostic criteria for giant cell arteritis [4]

1. Any new persisting headache fulfilling criteria 3 and 4
2. At least one of the following:
(a) Swollen tender scalp artery with elevated ESR or CRP
(b) Temporal artery biopsy demonstrating GCA
3. Headache develops in close temporal relation to other symptoms and signs of GCA (these may include jaw claudication, polymyalgia rheumatic, recent repeated attacks of amaurosis fugax)[a]
4. Headache resolves within 3 days of high-dose steroid treatment

[a]Signs and symptoms may be so variable that any recent persisting headache in a patient over 60 years old should suggest this diagnosis. There is a major risk of blindness that is preventable by immediate steroid treatment and the time interval between visual loss in one eye and in the other is usually less than a week

Table 24.7 IHS diagnostic criteria for headaches associated to temporomandibular joint disorder [4]

1. Recurrent pain in one or more regions of the head and/or face, fulfilling criteria 3 and 4
2. Radiographic, MRI, or bone scintigraphy demonstrates temporomandibular joint (TMD) disorder
3. Evidence that pain can be attributed to TMD, based on at least one of the following:
(a) Pain is precipitated by jaw movements and/or chewing of hard or tough food
(b) Reduced range of or irregular jaw opening
(c) Noise from one or both TMDs during jaw movements
(d) Tenderness of the joint capsules(s) of one or both TMDs
4. Headache resolves within 3 months and does not recur after successful treatment of the TMD

Table 24.8 IHS diagnostic criteria for tension-type headaches [4]

1. Headache lasting from 30 min to 7 days (or even more persistent if diagnosing chronic TTH)
2. Headache has at least two of the following characteristics:
(a) Bilateral location
(b) Pressing/tightening (nonpulsating) quality
(c) Mild or moderate intensity
(d) Not aggravated by routine physical activity, such as walking or climbing stairs
3. Both of the following:
(a) No nausea or vomiting (anorexia may occur)
(b) No more than one of phonophobia or photophobia
4. Not attributed to another disorder

NSAIDS such as ibuprofen or naproxen can help address the acute pain. Oral steroids are also an option if the pain is worse or the pain is not managed well with NSAIDS. Heat or ice to painful areas, massage, and range of motion exercises have shown to reduce pain [27]. Physiotherapists who specialize in TMD are great resources for patients who require long-term management. Intra-oral appliances and surgery are also options, and appropriate referrals to local dentists or oral surgeons should also be considered.

Tension-Type Headaches

Tension-type headache (TTH) is the most common type of headache experienced by individuals. Most commonly they are episodic so management is not pursued, but patients with chronic TTH tend to present to the clinic. The prevalence of frequent and chronic TTH is 21.6–34% and 0.9–2%, respectively [28, 29]. Patients who have TTH describe the pain as being bilateral, band-like squeezing headache from the frontal or temporal region and can extend to the parietal and occipital region (Table 24.8, diagnostic criteria of TTH). TTH can often be mistaken as frontal sinus headaches, migraines, and cervicogenic headaches given the location of the pain. However, migraines can often be differentiated from TTH, as TTH does not have the same throbbing character that migraines tend to have. Patients with cervicogenic headaches tend to have a history of neck problems. Patient with TTH can have underlying anxiety or depression disorder [30].

Primary treatment of TTH is with NSAIDS to address acute attacks. Care must be taken to limit the use of NSAIDS as they may cause medication overuse headaches (discussed later). For those with chronic TTH, lifestyle changes which include addressing underlying stress, proper sleep, and regular exercise will improve the severity and frequency of the TTH. Tricyclic antidepressants and muscle relaxants have been shown to work, but if patients are requiring this degree of management, they should already be in the care of a neurologist [31, 32].

Cluster Headaches

Cluster headaches (CH), nicknamed "suicidal headaches," can be episodic or chronic in nature. Approximately 85% of CH are episodic [33]. Episodic CH occur at least once every 24 h for weeks at a time and then be in remission for weeks to years (Table 24.9, diagnostic criteria of CH). The attacks are unilateral and rarely switch sides. The pain comes on without warning and patients have described the feeling as if "the eye is being pushed out" [33]. When the pain presents, patients are restless and are unwilling to lie down as most prefer to rock back and forth. The pain is located around the eye and orbit radiating to the temple, forehead, and cheek [33]. Patients also experience autonomic symptoms which include lacrimation and conjunctival injection [34]. Only 3% of patients do not have autonomic symptoms [35].

Otolaryngologists can provide basic patient education and management. Successful cluster headache treatment requires prophylactic and symptomatic medication. Due to the rapid onset of symptoms, fast-acting therapy is needed. Oxygen and subcutaneous sumatriptan provide the most effective relief. Oxygen given via a face mask at 7–10 L/min for approximately 15 min will help patients achieve relief within 15 min [36]. Subcutaneous sumatriptan can be self-administered by patients. A 6 mg dose has been found to relieve up to 74% of patients within 15 min [37]. Patients also may present to the emergency department to receive intravenous dihydroergotamine to achieve quick relief of their symptoms [33].

Medication Overuse Headaches

The indiscriminate management of primary headache disorders can lead to an unintended secondary headache disorder known as medication overuse headaches (MOH) (Table 24.10, diagnostic criteria of MOH). The overall prevalence of MOH is 0.5–2.6% in the general population [38]. In about 80% of patients with MOH, they have an underlying migraine headache, while the remaining patients either have TTH or post-traumatic headaches [39, 40]. Most commonly, MOH is due to overuse of opioids but it is also seen in those overusing triptans [41]. The pathophysiology of MOH is unclear but believed to be due to an underlying susceptibility and/or presence of genetic risk factors [42].

Management of MOH can be complex as the primary treatment involves withdrawing the MOH-inducing medication. Sometimes the withdrawal needs to done as an in-patient as intravenous medications can be used to manage the pain as the primary underlying drug is being weaned. However, as otolaryngologists, patient education can dramatically improve patients with MOH. A prospective cohort study in Norway showed a dramatic decrease in medication overuse with patient education alone [43]. Patient education regarding MOH can be beneficial as patients await their neurology appointment.

Table 24.9 IHS diagnostic criteria for cluster headache [4]

1. At least five attacks fulfilling criteria 2–4
2. Severe or very severe unilateral orbital, supraorbital, and/or temporal pain lasting 15–180 min if untreated
3. Headache is accompanied by at least one of the following:
(a) Ipsilateral conjunctival injection and/or lacrimation
(b) Ipsilateral nasal congestion and/or rhinorrhea
(c) Ipsilateral eyelid edema
(d) Ipsilateral forehead and facial sweating
(e) Ipsilateral miosis and/or ptosis
(f) A sense of restlessness or agitation
4. Attacks have a frequency from one every other day to eight per day
5. Not attributed to another disorder

Table 24.10 IHS diagnostic criteria for medication overuse headache [4]

1. Headache present on ≥15 days/months fulfilling criteria 3 and 4
2. Regular overuse for ≥3 months of one or more drugs that can be taken for acute and/or symptomatic treatment of headache
3. Headache has developed or markedly worsened during medication overuse
4. Headache resolves or reverts to its previous pattern within 2 months of discontinuation of overused medication

Mucosal Contact Points

A controversial cause of focal headaches are rhinogenic mucosal contact points. There is very poor evidence for this condition as many of the studies lack a sham group, omit information regarding abortive medications used postoperatively, and demonstrate unclear patient selection. However, this condition should not be dismissed. While the pathophysiology is unclear, as a number of patients have contact points incidentally found on endoscopy or imaging and have no focal pain, there is belief that some patients may experience localized nerve irritation as particular contact points produce excess substance P and calcitonin gene-related peptide release [44]. Patients can present with focal frontal headaches from radiation to the cutaneous distribution of ophthalmic (V1) division of the trigeminal nerve as the anterior aspect of the middle turbinate is innervated by the anterior ethmoid nerve, which is a branch of V1. Potential triggers include sharp septal spur, concha bullosa of the middle turbinate, pneumatized uncinate process, or other anatomic alterations causing mucosa on mucosa contact.

Management involves a multidisciplinary team. Given that 50% of patients with contact points have one in the contralateral nasal cavity [45], immediately moving to surgical intervention is not recommended. Medical options include starting topical nasal steroid as well as an antihistamine sprays to reduce the inflammation between the contact points. Patients should also be thoroughly worked up for a primary headache disorder; the patient can undergo an in-office procedure to anesthetize the mucosa containing the irritated nerves at points of contact. This is best done topically with a mix of phenylephrine and topical lidocaine placed on a small cotton applicated directly placed between the contact points. The cotton applicator is then removed after 5 min. Often patients with this disorder will experience a dramatic decrease or even resolution of their headache with this maneuver. If a patient has this positive result, the senior author will have them come back on a different day to ensure this improvement can be replicated. If a patient does not find any improvement from topical nasal therapy and potential management of a primary headache disorder, and the patient appreciates a marked decrease in their facial pain with repeat pinpoint application of anesthetic to the contact point, surgical removal is then considered. Patients should always be aware and properly informed during the consent process that although having a positive result from the application of local anesthetic is a good prognostic indicator that surgery may be helpful to their symptoms, the procedure may still produce minimal or no improvement of their symptoms.

Summary

Frontal headaches can be from a variety of rhinogenic and non-rhinogenic causes. Appropriate history taking and physical exam, with imaging when indicated, are always the key in making the correct diagnosis [50]. If a non-rhinogenic cause is found to be the etiology of the frontal headache, otolaryngologists should be knowledgeable and equipped to begin the first appropriate step in management while referring the patient to another specialist.

References

1. Rosenfeld RM, Piccirillo JF, Chandrasekhar SS, et al. Clinical practice guideline (update): adult sinusitis. Otolaryngol Head Neck Surg. 2015;152(2 Suppl):S1–S39.
2. Desrosiers M, Evans GA, Keith PK, et al. Canadian clinical practice guidelines for acute and chronic rhinosinusitis. J Otolaryngol Head Neck Surg. 2011;40(Suppl 2):S99–193.
3. Fokkens WJ, Lund VJ, Mullol J, et al. EPOS 2012: European position paper on rhinosinusitis and nasal polyps 2012. A summary for otorhinolaryngologists. Rhinology. 2012;50(1):1–12.
4. Headache Classification Subcommittee of the International Headache S. The international classification of headache disorders: 2nd edition. Cephalalgia. 2004;24 Suppl 1:9–160.

5. Tarabichi M. Characteristics of sinus-related pain. Otolaryngol Head Neck Surg. 2000;122(6):842–7.

6. Falco JJ, Thomas AJ, Quin X, et al. Lack of correlation between patient reported location and severity of facial pain and radiographic burden of disease in chronic rhinosinusitis. Int Forum Allergy Rhinol. 2016;6(11):1173–81.

7. Hansen AG, Stovner LJ, Hagen K, et al. Paranasal sinus opacification in headache sufferers: a population-based imaging study (the HUNT study-MRI). Cephalalgia. 2016;37(6):509–16.

8. DelGaudio JM, Wise SK, Wise JC. Association of radiological evidence of frontal sinus disease with the presence of frontal pain. Am J Rhinol. 2005;19(2):167–73.

9. Lipton RB, Diamond S, Reed M, Diamond ML, Stewart WF. Migraine diagnosis and treatment: results from the American migraine study II. Headache. 2001;41(7):638–45.

10. Eross E, Dodick D, Eross M. The sinus, allergy and migraine study (SAMS). Headache. 2007;47(2):213–24.

11. Perry BF, Login IS, Kountakis SE. Nonrhinologic headache in a tertiary rhinology practice. Otolaryngol Head Neck Surg. 2004;130(4):449–52.

12. Bigal ME, Bordini CA, Antoniazzi AL, Speciali JG. The triptan formulations: a critical evaluation. Arq Neuropsiquiatr. 2003;61(2A):313–20.

13. Goadsby PJ. The pharmacology of headache. Prog Neurobiol. 2000;62(5):509–25.

14. Silberstein SD. Practice parameter: evidence-based guidelines for migraine headache (an evidence-based review): report of the quality standards subcommittee of the American academy of neurology. Neurology. 2000;55(6):754–62.

15. Diener HC, Limmroth V. Advances in pharmacological treatment of migraine. Expert Opin Investig Drugs. 2001;10(10):1831–45.

16. Welch KM, Mathew NT, Stone P, Rosamond W, Saiers J, Gutterman D. Tolerability of sumatriptan: clinical trials and post-marketing experience. Cephalalgia. 2000;20(8):687–95.

17. Cady RK, Schreiber CP. Sinus headache or migraine? Considerations in making a differential diagnosis. Neurology. 2002;58(9 Suppl 6):S10–4.

18. Kari E, DelGaudio JM. Treatment of sinus headache as migraine: the diagnostic utility of triptans. Laryngoscope. 2008;118(12):2235–9.

19. Dadgarnia MH, Atighechi S, Baradaranfar MH. The response to sodium valproate of patients with sinus headaches with normal endoscopic and CT findings. Eur Arch Otorhinolaryngol. 2010;267(3):375–9.

20. Bagheri SC, Farhidvash F, Perciaccante VJ. Diagnosis and treatment of patients with trigeminal neuralgia. J Am Dent Assoc. 2004;135(12):1713–7.

21. Cruccu G, Gronseth G, Alksne J, et al. AAN-EFNS guidelines on trigeminal neuralgia management. Eur J Neurol. 2008;15(10):1013–28.

22. Sarsam Z, Garcia-Finana M, Nurmikko TJ, Varma TR, Eldridge P. The long-term outcome of microvascular decompression for trigeminal neuralgia. Br J Neurosurg. 2010;24(1):18–25.

23. Waldman CW, Waldman SD, Waldman RA. Giant cell arteritis. Med Clin North Am. 2013;97(2):329–35.

24. Carbonella A, Berardi G, Petricca L, et al. Immunosuppressive therapy (Methotrexate or Cyclophosphamide) in combination with corticosteroids in the treatment of Giant cell arteritis: comparison with corticosteroids alone. J Am Geriatr Soc. 2016;64(3):672–374.

25. Regent A, Redeker S, Deroux A, et al. Tocilizumab in Giant cell arteritis: a multicenter retrospective study of 34 patients. J Rheumatol. 2016;43(8):1547–52.

26. Stegenga B, de Bont LG, Boering G. Osteoarthrosis as the cause of craniomandibular pain and dysfunction: a unifying concept. J Oral Maxillofac Surg. 1989;47(3):249–56.

27. Ager JW. Discussion: statistical analysis in treatment and prevention program evaluation. NIDA Res Monogr. 1992;117:31–40.

28. Russell MB. Tension-type headache in 40-year-olds: a Danish population-based sample of 4000. J Headache Pain. 2005;6(6):441–7.

29. Russell MB, Levi N, Saltyte-Benth J, Fenger K. Tension-type headache in adolescents and adults: a population based study of 33,764 twins. Eur J Epidemiol. 2006;21(2):153–60.

30. Puca F, Genco S, Prudenzano MP, et al. Psychiatric comorbidity and psychosocial stress in patients with tension-type headache from headache centers in Italy. The Italian collaborative group for the study of psychopathological factors in primary headaches. Cephalalgia. 1999;19(3):159–64.

31. Cerbo R, Barbanti P, Fabbrini G, Pascali MP, Catarci T. Amitriptyline is effective in chronic but not in episodic tension-type headache: pathogenetic implications. Headache. 1998;38(6):453–7.

32. Bettucci D, Testa L, Calzoni S, Mantegazza P, Viana M, Monaco F. Combination of tizanidine and amitriptyline in the prophylaxis of chronic tension-type headache: evaluation of efficacy and impact on quality of life. J Headache Pain. 2006;7(1):34–6.

33. Dodick DW, Rozen TD, Goadsby PJ, Silberstein SD. Cluster headache. Cephalalgia. 2000;20(9):787–803.

34. Lance JW, Anthony M. Migrainous neuralgia or cluster headache? J Neurol Sci. 1971;13(4):401–14.

35. Nappi G, Micieli G, Cavallini A, Zanferrari C, Sandrini G, Manzoni GC. Accompanying symptoms of cluster attacks: their relevance to the diagnostic criteria. Cephalalgia. 1992;12(3):165–8.

36. Fogan L. Treatment of cluster headache. A double-blind comparison of oxygen v air inhalation. Arch Neurol. 1985;42(4):362–3.

37. Treatment of Acute Cluster Headache with Sumatriptan. The sumatriptan cluster headache study group. N Engl J Med. 1991;325(5):322–6.

38. Westergaard ML, Hansen EH, Glumer C, Olesen J, Jensen RH. Definitions of medication-overuse headache in population-based studies and their implica-

tions on prevalence estimates: a systematic review. Cephalalgia. 2014;34(6):409–25.

39. Shand B, Goicochea MT, Valenzuela R, et al. Clinical and demographical characteristics of patients with medication overuse headache in Argentina and Chile: analysis of the Latin American section of COMOESTAS project. J Headache Pain. 2015;16:83.

40. Heyer GL, Idris SA. Does analgesic overuse contribute to chronic post-traumatic headaches in adolescent concussion patients? Pediatr Neurol. 2014;50(5):464–8.

41. Radat F, Creac'h C, Guegan-Massardier E, et al. Behavioral dependence in patients with medication overuse headache: a cross-sectional study in consulting patients using the DSM-IV criteria. Headache. 2008;48(7):1026–36.

42. Diener HC, Holle D, Solbach K, Gaul C. Medication-overuse headache: risk factors, pathophysiology and management. Nat Rev Neurol. 2016;12:575.

43. Grande RB, Aaseth K, Benth JS, Lundqvist C, Russell MB. Reduction in medication-overuse headache after short information. The Akershus study of chronic headache. Eur J Neurol. 2011;18(1):129–37.

44. Stammberger H, Wolf G. Headaches and sinus disease: the endoscopic approach. Ann Otol Rhinol Laryngol Suppl. 1988;134:3–23.

45. Baroody FM, Brown D, Gavanescu L, DeTineo M, Naclerio RM. Oxymetazoline adds to the effectiveness of fluticasone furoate in the treatment of perennial allergic rhinitis. J Allergy Clin Immunol. 2011;127(4):927–34.

46. Barbanti P, Fabbrini G, Pesare M, Vanacore N, Cerbo R. Unilateral cranial autonomic symptoms in migraine. Cephalalgia. 2002;22(4):256–9.

47. Schreiber CP, Hutchinson S, Webster CJ, Ames M, Richardson MS, Powers C. Prevalence of migraine in patients with a history of self-reported or physician-diagnosed "sinus" headache. Arch Intern Med. 2004;164(16):1769–72.

48. Mehle ME, Kremer PS. Sinus CT scan findings in "sinus headache" migraineurs. Headache. 2008;48(1):67–71.

49. Foroughipour M, Sharifian SM, Shoeibi A, Ebdali Barabad N, Bakhshaee M. Causes of headache in patients with a primary diagnosis of sinus headache. Eur Arch Otorhinolaryngol. 2011;268(11):1593–6.

50. Lal D, Rounds AM, Dodick DW. Comprehensive management of patients presenting to the otolaryngologist for Sinus pressure, pain, or headache. Laryngoscope. 2015;125(2):303–10.

Outcomes and Quality of Life from Frontal Sinus Surgery

Jessica E. Southwood, Todd A. Loehrl, and David M. Poetker

Introduction

The goal of surgical treatment of medically refractory frontal sinusitis is to improve the quality of life (QOL) of patients that have failed medical therapy. The decision to operate should include an understanding of the underlying pathology whether inflammatory vs neoplastic, the fundamental limits of dissection inherent in the narrow boundaries of the frontal sinus, and the need for adequate exposure for long-term postoperative follow-up. Given the complex anatomic region of the frontal sinus and its outflow tract, surgical interventions of the frontal sinus are not without risks, particularly scarring.

Historical approaches to management of frontal sinus disease such as the Lynch and Lothrop procedures provided short-term patency rates with failures of 30% on a long-term basis [1]. The propensity for high failure rates led to the popularity of the osteoplastic flap with frontal sinus obliteration; however the associated morbidity of this procedure including supraorbital neuralgia, frontal bossing, and inability to monitor the frontal sinus with surveillance has caused this surgery to fall out of favor [2]. Innovation and technology have significantly increased the armamentarium of surgical options, specifically with the advent of endoscopic sinus surgery (ESS) as an alternative to the open approaches. The unique features of surgical instrumentation for the frontal sinus have popularized the more standard endoscopic approaches described by Draf [3] which range from a total ethmoidectomy without instrumentation of the frontal recess (Draf I), mucosal-sparing removal of tissue from the frontal recess (Draf IIA), and removal of the superior anterior attachment of the middle turbinate and the floor of the frontal sinus (Draf IIB) to an extensive drill-out procedure with removal of the superior septum, the frontal beak, and the frontal intersinus septum (Draf III) (Table 25.1). In addition to endoscopic dissection, balloon catheter dilation (BCD) offers another instrument for increasing ostial patency of the frontal sinus; however unlike endoscopic sinus surgery, BCD does not remove tissue. BCD is typically not recommended for chronic rhinosinusitis (CRS) with polyps or eosinophilic disease, where tissue removal and maximal widening of the outflow tract by removal of frontal recess cells is

J. E. Southwood
Department of Otolaryngology, Medical College of Wisconsin, Milwaukee, WI, USA

T. A. Loehrl · D. M. Poetker (✉)
Department of Otolaryngology, Medical College of Wisconsin, Milwaukee, WI, USA

Division of Surgery, Zablocki VA Medical Center, Milwaukee, WI, USA

© Springer Nature Switzerland AG 2019
D. Lal, P. H. Hwang (eds.), *Frontal Sinus Surgery*, https://doi.org/10.1007/978-3-319-97022-6_25

Table 25.1 Description of frontal sinusotomies

Draf I	Total ethmoidectomy without instrumentation of the frontal recess
Draf IIA	Mucosal-sparing removal of tissue of the frontal recess
Draf IIB	Removal of the superior anterior attachment of the middle turbinate to the septum and removal of the floor of the frontal sinus
Draf III	Drill-out procedure which includes a bilateral Draf IIB with removal of the superior septum, frontal beak, and intersinus septum of the frontal sinus

necessary for efficacious topical drug delivery [4]. BCD is contraindicated if there is suspicion or documentation of neoplastic disease [5]. In addition to the variety of instrumentation and techniques for frontal sinusotomies, frontal sinus stents may be considered for patients with aggressive disease when recurrent restenosis occurs or in unique primary cases for which patients are at high risk of recurrence or who have other comorbidities where multiple procedures are ill-advised [6].

The purpose of this chapter is to summarize the evidence for surgical intervention of the frontal sinus specifically focusing on the outcomes and QOL related to such procedures. Special attention will be paid to evaluation of the research to date that discusses outcomes in frontal sinus surgery which focus on patient-focused QOL measures, the effectiveness of surgical interventions in creating a patent frontal sinusotomy, and the safety profile of various techniques.

Comparative effectiveness studies comparing ESS with medical therapy support the indication for ESS in patients with medically recalcitrant CRS [7–9]. A study to determine the efficacy of frontal sinusotomy on the basis of QOL, in the absence of the total effect of ESS on CRS, is difficult to construct. The QOL measures associated with addressing the other sinuses at the time of frontal sinusotomy may obscure the differential impact of frontal sinus surgery [10]. The outcome measurements taken into account include not only subjective measures of QOL but also frequency of frontal recess patency on endoscopic or imaging studies and incidence of revision surgery.

Draf IIA Frontal Sinusotomy

Endoscopic frontal sinus surgery for medically recalcitrant frontal sinus disease is generally very successful when performed by an experienced sinus surgeon [11]. DeConde and Smith recently reviewed the data examining outcomes of Draf IIA frontal sinusotomy and discussed certain limitations of studies in the literature, such as the lack of patient baseline characteristics and the rare use of validated disease-specific measures, even in more recent studies when such tools were available [12]. With these caveats in mind, the literature in the last 10 years found that most patients do experience symptomatic improvement (68.5–92%) after frontal sinusotomy with most studies reporting endoscopic patency in the mid-80% (range 67.6–92%) [12–15]. Naidoo et al. performed a retrospective review on 109 patients undergoing primary frontal sinus sinusotomy (Draf IIA) and measured the success rate with technical and subjective measures including sinus patency and resolution of symptoms [11]. The frontal ostium patency rate measured 92%, revision surgery was less than 9%, and complete resolution of symptoms with long-term benefit was noted in 78%. Interestingly, there was no significant correlation between patient factors such as the presence of eosinophilic mucin, asthma, polyposis, or smoking on patency or resolution of symptoms. Frontal ostium size correlated with a higher risk of stenosis. The intraoperative frontal ostium dimensions of the group which developed stenosis were statistically smaller ($p < 0.0068$), with a minimum dimension of >4.8 mm the critical measurement for maintaining long-term patency. The sinusotomy threshold dimension by Naidoo et al. [11] is similar to a study by Chandra et al. [16] which postulated that a diameter of 4–5 mm increases the likelihood of maintaining patency of the frontal sinus. In a study by Hosemann et al., the stenosis rate of the frontal sinus increased from 16% to 30% when the diameter of the ostium dropped below 5 mm [17].

Although achieving a maximal opening of the frontal sinus is a critical goal within the confines of the restricted anatomy, this should not come at the expense of poor technique and mucosal stripping.

Such iatrogenic trauma may lead to cicatricial scarring and increased failure rates. Such dogma is supported not by large evidence-based studies but by historical experience with mucosal trauma associated with external approaches [1], as well as early Draf IIA procedures performed with a diamond drill [18], both leading to high frontal sinus failure rates. Assessing the anatomic limits of the frontal recess using preoperative imaging may differentiate those patients with intrinsic narrowness who may be at risk for failure [12]. Patients with relatively narrow outflow tracts, whether in anterior-to-posterior and/or medial-to-lateral dimensions, are more likely to require revision surgery or salvage Draf III surgery. Patients who have persistent inflammatory disease burden of the frontal sinus are more likely to have persistent sinonasal symptoms [11], and those with retained frontal sinus cells and/or middle turbinate lateralization are more likely to require revision sinus surgery [19].

Draf IIB Frontal Sinusotomy

Despite optimized surgical technique with meticulous frontal recess dissection using mucosal-sparing techniques, stenosis of the frontal sinus can be a cumbersome complication of ESS. Synechiae formation, intrinsic narrowed anatomy, and the underlying disease process itself can predispose patients to frontal sinus stenosis. Extended frontal sinus surgery approaches can often improve long-term frontal sinus patency and surgical outcomes [20, 21]. The Draf IIB extends the Draf IIA by removing the ipsilateral floor of the frontal sinus to widen the frontal ostium. This can also include removal of the frontal beak which results in exposed bone. Some authors, who believe that the exposed bone and underlying inflammation of chronic rhinosinusitis lead to scarring and stenosis postoperatively, feel that Draf IIB surgery should be reserved for isolated frontal sinus disease without pansinusitis, or for improving access to remove small frontal sinus tumors [22, 23]. Other authors have supported the Draf IIB as a viable option in patients with recalcitrant disease [24].

The Draf IIB procedure incorporates resection of the middle turbinate thereby decreasing the potential for middle turbinate recurrent lateralization and synechia formation. Turner et al. performed a retrospective review of patients who underwent a Draf IIB frontal sinusotomy as part of their ESS after failing medical treatment [24]. All procedures were performed by a single surgeon at a single institution. Primary outcomes included SNOT-20 and sinus patency with width ≥ 3 mm which was diagnosed on the ability to pass a standard curved suction during postoperative endoscopy. In their series, 18 patients underwent the Draf IIB procedure, 5 of which had undergone previous surgery on the frontal sinus. The most common indications for the extended procedure were lateralized middle turbinate or middle turbinate remnant (8 patients), mucocele or mucopyocele [6], and postoperative synechiae [5]. Patients were followed for a mean of 16.2 months (range 1–64 months), and frontal sinus patency measured with endoscopy was achieved in >90% cases, including 5 of 6 primary cases and 15 of 16 revision procedures. Patients who underwent primary frontal sinus Draf IIB had a significant improvement in SNOT-20 scores (2.64 to 1.15, $p = 0.02$), whereas those who underwent revision surgery did not (1.89 to 1.46, $p = 0.46$). Although Turner et al. [24] demonstrated patency over a mean follow-up period of 16 months using the Draf IIB technique, some authors [22] advocate for Draf III over the Draf IIB due to the risk of intensive inflammatory fibrosis leading to scarring and stenosis if the frontal beak is drilled exposing bone in CRS cases.

Draf III Frontal Sinusotomy

Although the Draf IIA and Draf IIB procedures have shown high rates of frontal sinus patency, there are certain clinical scenarios that may make these techniques infeasible or prone to restenosis. Frontal ostium size has previously been reported as a risk factor for failure of the Draf IIA and IIB procedure [11, 16, 17]. The smaller the ostia, the greater the risk of adhesion formation or risk of polyp recurrence leading to complete occlusion of the frontal sinus ostium.

The smaller ostium is also less likely to function as an adequate conduit for saline irrigations or other topical therapies. For patients unresponsive to medical therapy, a graduated surgical approach has been recommended [25]. The final tier, frontal sinus obliteration, is performed through an osteoplastic flap and obliterates the sinus with fat or other material. The osteoplastic flap showed a significant success rate of 93% at 8 years [26]; however the 20% major complication rate of this procedure has rendered it a less favorable surgical option [27]. The complications of dural exposure, dural laceration with cerebrospinal fluid leak (CSF), and orbital injury were related to misdirected osteotomies that extended beyond the frontal sinus [27, 28]. An endoscopic alternative to frontal obliteration, was described by Draf [3], Close [29], and Gross [21], using an approach modified from Lothrop's technique described in 1914, in which a combined external and internal approach was used to resect the frontal sinus floor and septum, with the goal of restoring normal ventilation and drainage of the frontal sinuses. The endoscopic modified Lothrop procedure (EMLP), otherwise known as a Draf III frontal sinusotomy or frontal drill-out, is considered a salvage procedure for failed frontal sinusotomy or Draf IIB in which a large combined frontal sinus allows for the drainage through a common central pathway. The surgical borders of the endoscopic Lothrop cavity are well characterized. The orbital plates of the frontal bone and the periosteum of the skin overlying the frontal process of the maxilla are the lateral borders. The first olfactory fascicle of the olfactory bulb marks the posterior border. The anterior table of the frontal sinus demarcates the anterior limit of dissection.

A systematic review and meta-analysis of the safety and efficacy of the EMLP procedure was performed by Anderson and Sindwani [30] which included 18 studies containing data from 612 patients. Major complications which included CSF leak, tension pneumocephalus, and posterior table dehiscence were less than 1%, and minor complications such as increased crusting, epistaxis, anosmia/hyposmia, nasal bone dehiscence, philtral pressure ulcer, and transient blurry vision were 4% combined. The endoscopic frontal patency was reported in 81% of 394 reported cases, and there was symptomatic improvement with 82% of 430 patients. The overall surgical success rates as measured by single vs revision surgery were 86% and 14% of 612 patients, respectively. Of the 85 of 612 (14%) patients who underwent revision surgery, 80% had revision EMLP, and 20% underwent osteoplastic frontal sinus obliteration. Comorbidities have been studied as a potentiating factors in restenosis after EMLP such as aspirin sensitivity, gastroesophageal reflux disease, allergy, asthma, nasal polyposis, and eosinophilic mucin chronic rhinosinusitis; however only the diagnosis of eosinophilic mucin chronic rhinosinusitis was associated with higher rate of ostial restenosis in a study by Tran et al. [31].

Naidoo et al. reviewed the long-term outcomes of EMLP in 229 patients over a 10-year time period who had previously failed FESS and maximal medical therapy [32]. Prior to EMLP, patients had undergone on average 3.8 standard ESS procedures, and over half of the patients (135/229) had a diagnosis of CRS with nasal polyposis (CRSwNP). All patients reported an improvement in overall postoperative symptom score which included nasal obstruction, facial pain, anosmia, anterior rhinorrhea, and post nasal drip. The frontal neo-ostium remained patent in 221/229 patients over an average follow-up period of 45 months. Only 12 patients developed disease recurrence and persistence of symptoms requiring revision EMLP. Allergic fungal sinusitis (AFRS) was stated as significant risk factors for failure of the EMLP with recurrence of fungal debris and polyposis occluding the frontal sinus occurring in 7/12 patients. Other factors such as persistent colonization of the sinuses with recalcitrant S. aureus which is influenced by antibiotic sensitivity, environmental, and immune factors were thought to lead to scar tissue or osteogenesis and consequently narrowing of the frontal neo-ostium.

The EMLP has been shown to decrease the risk of revision sinus surgery especially in asthma and aspirin intolerant CRSwNP patients compared to standard ESS [33]. In a retrospective cohort study by Bassiouni and Wormald, the revision rate in ESS group was 37% versus a revision rate of 7% in the EMLP ($p < 0.001$). Survival analysis showed that the EMLP significantly reduced the risk of revision surgery (hazard ratio = 0.258, $p = 0.0026$).

Balloon Catheter Dilation

Balloon catheter dilation in the frontal sinus outflow tract fractures and laterally displaces the medial and superior wall of obstructing frontal cells, medially displaces the intersinus septal cell wall, and dilates soft tissue stenosis in revision cases [4]. Balloon dilation may be used in the office setting and eliminates the risks associated with general anesthesia. Its use is contraindicated in cases of questionable underlying histology, dense neo-osteogenesis of the frontal bones in which the walls are unlikely to be fractured and displaced adequately, and in patients with extensive polyposis [5]. Balloon dilation of the frontal sinus is generally considered safe with no cases of CSF leak, orbital injury, or severe epistaxis reported in a multi-centered trial in 115 patients [34]; and only 1 adverse event – transient periorbital swelling – reported in a similarly designed multi-institutional prospective study involving 203 patients [35]. Unlike clinical trials which exclude patients with a history of extensive polyps, extensive sinus surgery, severe osteoneogenesis, sinonasal malignancy, or history of facial trauma, the OpenFDA database reports adverse events associated with balloon dilation in "real-world" patient settings, including cases of distorted sinus anatomy and severe inflammatory conditions such as cystic fibrosis. In the 114 adverse events reported in the OpenFDA database over an 8-year time period in a study by Prince and Bhattacharyya, there were 17 skull base injuries, 15 of which had a CSF leak [36]. Balloon dilation of the frontal sinuses was found to be significantly associated with these injuries. The difference between the observed degree of adverse events in the OpenFDA database and prior studies underscores the importance of patient selection and the surgeon's experience to mitigate the potential for complications using balloon dilation.

A nonrandomized prospective trial of 107 patients undergoing BCD indicated that 98% of sinus ostia remained patent at 24 weeks with positive 1- and 2-year results [34, 37, 38]. Plaza et al. evaluated frontal sinus ostium balloon dilation versus Draf I in patients with CRS and found that patients who underwent dilation had significant improvement on Lund-Mackay stage with resolution of frontal sinus disease confirmed by computed tomographic scan as well as equivalent outcomes on endoscopy during 12-month follow-up period [39]. Hathorn et al. evaluated frontal sinus ostial patency, surgical time, and mean blood loss in 30 patients with CRS using a hybrid approach combining standard instrumentation to expose the frontal recess followed by balloon dilation compared with traditional Draf IIA on the opposite side of the same patient [40]. Patients acted as their own controls, and ostial patency and size were assessed 5 weeks, 3 months, and 1 year postoperatively using endoscopy. All frontal sinus ostia that were assessed at 1 year remained patent, and no patients required revision frontal surgery. The surgical times and blood loss were lower in the hybrid approach vs standard ESS ($p = 0.03$ and $p = 0.008$, respectively) [40]. The largest study to date which included in-office BCD of the frontal sinuses in a multi-institutional trial reported that 251 of 268 frontal sinuses were successfully dilated (93.7%) with 5 frontal sinuses requiring revision procedures (2%) [35]. SNOT-20 and Lund-Mackay computed tomography scoring showed significant improvement at 24 weeks ($p < 0.0001$) and clinically significant improvement in QOL, which included all study subjects that received not only frontal sinus dilation but also maxillary and sphenoid dilation.

In addition to primary frontal sinusotomy and dilation, balloons have been studied in revision frontal cases. Small case series have shown benefit with sustained frontal sinus patency in patients treated with balloon dilation after frontal sinusotomy in limited follow-up periods [41]. Wycherly et al. reported patency in 21 of 24 frontal sinus ostia after an average of 12 months in 13 patients who underwent balloon dilation in revision frontal sinus surgery [42]. Although shorter follow-up periods limit the conclusions that can be made for long-term outcomes, Weiss et al. showed that QOL following balloon sinus dilation are stable from 6 months out to at least 2 years [34].

The majority of studies show equivocal patency results of balloon dilation compared to standard ESS in the cohorts studied; however the efficacy and feasibility of frontal balloon dilation are not necessarily the same across the wide range of severities and rhinosinusitis subtypes [22]. The use of the balloon for frontal sinusitis remains controversial among rhinologists and otolaryngologists performing frontal sinus surgery; however in mild to moderately severe disease and in select revision cases, the balloon appears to be a safe and effective instrument and does not preclude endoscopic surgery in the future.

Frontal Sinus Stenting

The role of stenting the frontal sinus is controversial. The potential benefits of stenting include separation of the mucosal edges to prevent synechia and subsequent stenosis, filling in a potential dead space to prevent occlusive clots and debris from occluding the frontal recess, and creating a scaffold for mucosal reepithelization [22]. These positive features must be weighed against the concerns of placing a foreign body into the frontal sinus. Formation of biofilms has been shown to form on stents after only 1–6 weeks [43]. The role of CRS and biofilms is established [44–46], and it is postulated that stents may potentiate chronic infection [22]. In the most severe infectious scenario, Chadwell et al. discuss a case report of a patient who underwent placement of a frontal sinus stent and developed toxic shock syndrome 18 days after ESS despite concurrent antibiotic use [47]. Additionally, if the stent is too short, granulation tissue can form around the stent and embed the stent in scar tissue. If the stent is too long, persistent crusting of the nasal end may occur and lead to an unpleasant odor.

There is no agreed upon consensus on the indications for frontal sinus stenting. Rather the surgeon must assess the need for frontal sinus stenting based on the risk of restenosis which may include the following factors: (1) size of the neo-ostium frontal sinus outflow tract diameter (<5 mm diameter doubles the rate of restenosis, <2 mm diameter increases rate of stenosis to 50%), (2) extensive severe polyposis, (3) demucosalization with exposed bone, (4) revision frontal sinus surgery with extensive scar, (5) osteitic bone in the frontal recess, (6) flail middle turbinate, and (7) history of traumatic frontal sinus fracture [6, 17]. Several studies of uncontrolled case series exist. Weber et al. retrospectively reviewed the cases of 12 patients who received 21 frontal nasal stents, which were left in place for 6 months [48]. Eight patients had a history of recurrent polypoid frontal sinus disease with scarred off outflow tracts, two patients had an osteoma of the frontal sinus with denuded bone, and the remaining two patients had mucopyoceles after previous sinus surgery for major scarring. In nine patients, a successful outcome was ascertained by visualization of either an open frontal recess on nasal endoscopy or an aerated frontal sinus on imaging, suggesting that stenting prevented restenosis by scar tissue in the majority of very difficult revision cases. Use of a Silastic stent in patients with a Draf III sinusotomy did not show a significant difference in outcomes in patency or symptomatic improvement [49].

Several studies have shown decreased inflammation and scarring of the sinuses with use of a mometasone-eluting bioabsorbable stent compared to placebo stent [50–52], with recent FDA approval for use in the frontal sinus outflow tract. Other biomaterials, such as dissolvable steroid-impregnated nasal dressings and a novel chitosan gel with hemostatic and wound healing properties [53–55], have been employed in ESS studies.

Chitosan is prepared from chitin, a polymer that is found in crustaceans, fungi, insects, annelids, mollusks, and coelenterata [56]. Chitosan is a biodegradable substance manufactured in various physical forms including solutions, filaments, powder, film, and hydrogels [55] that has shown not only improved hemostasis but also potential for improved post-ESS sinus patency. Ha et al. performed a prospective, blinded, randomized controlled trial to quantify the effect of chitosan gel on circumferential scarring of sinus ostia following ESS [54]. All 26 patients underwent bilateral complete functional ESS, with a total of 10 primary and 16 revision procedures performed for CRS. Patients acted as their own control with one side receiving chitosan gel and the other receiving no nasal gel or packing. Intraoperative frontal ostial areas were comparable for chitosan gel and control sides ($p > 0.05$). Postoperative measurements showed that chitosan gel significantly improved frontal sinus ostial patency at 12 weeks, compared to their baseline frontal areas ($p < 0.001$). The underlying mechanisms by which chitosan exerts its favorable wound healing effects are incompletely understood; however it is theorized that chitosan inhibits fibroblast migration and proliferation with enough time to allow reepithelization and reciliation to occur without collagen deposition and subsequent adhesion formation [57].

Summary

ESS improves QOL for patients with medically refractory sinus disease. Despite this, surgical management of frontal sinus disease remains challenging due to the close anatomic proximity of the orbit and skull base. In addition, individual anatomic patient factors may put patients at high risk for stenosis. Draf IIA studies show very high patency rates for mucosally preserved openings of at least 4.5 mm in diameter. A graded approach, reserving the Draf III procedure as salvage surgery in recalcitrant disease shows high rates of subjective improvement and neo-ostium patency. BCD has shown favorable safety and efficacy in clinical trials. Stenting serves as an adjunct to help decrease the risk of stenosis. As with all techniques and indications for surgical intervention, patient selection remains of the utmost importance.

References

1. Chiu AG. Frontal sinus surgery: its evolution, present standard of care, and recommendations for current use. Ann Otol Rhinol Laryngol Suppl. 2006;196:13–9.
2. Wormald PJ. Salvage frontal sinus surgery: the endoscopic modified lothrop procedure. Laryngoscope. 2003;113(2):276–83.
3. Draf W. Endonasal micro-endoscopic frontal sinus surgery: the fulda concept. Oper Tech Otolaryngol Head Neck Surg. 1991;2(4):234–40.
4. Sillers MJ, Lay KF. Balloon catheter dilation of the frontal sinus ostium. Otolaryngol Clin N Am. 2016;49(4):965–74.
5. Heimgartner S, Eckardt J, Simmen D, Briner HR, Leunig A, Caversaccio MD. Limitations of balloon sinuplasty in frontal sinus surgery. Eur Arch Otorhinolaryngol. 2011;268(10):1463–7.
6. Hunter B, Silva S, Youngs R, Saeed A, Varadarajan V. Long-term stenting for chronic frontal sinus disease: case series and literature review. J Laryngol Otol. 2010;124:1216–22.
7. Smith TL, Kern R, Palmer JN, et al. Medical therapy vs surgery for chronic rhinosinusitis: a prospective, multi-institutional study with 1-year follow-up. Int Forum Allergy Rhinol. 2013;3(1):4–9.
8. DeConde AS, Mace JC, Alt JA, Soler ZM, Orlandi RR, Smith TL. Investigation of change in cardinal symptoms of chronic rhinosinusitis after surgical or ongoing medical management. Int Forum Allergy Rhinol. 2015;5(1):36–45.
9. DeConde AS, Mace JC, Alt JA, Schlosser RJ, Smith TL, Soler ZM. Comparative effectiveness of medical and surgical therapy on olfaction in chronic rhinosinusitis: a prospective, multi-institutional study. Int Forum Allergy Rhinol. 2014;4:725–33.
10. DeConde AS, Suh JD, Mace JC, Alt JA, Smith TL. Outcomes of complete vs targeted approaches to endoscopic sinus surgery. Int Forum Allergy Rhinol. 2015;5(8):691–700.
11. Naidoo Y, Wen D, Bassiouni A, Keen M, Wormald PJ. Long-term results after primary frontal sinus surgery. Int Forum Allergy Rhinol. 2012;2(3):185–90.
12. DeConde AS, Smith TL. Outcomes after frontal sinus surgery: an evidence-based review. Otolaryngol Clin N Am. 2016;49(4):1019–33.
13. Friedman M, Bliznikas D, Vidyasagar R, Joseph NJ, Landsberg R. Long-term results after endoscopic sinus surgery involving frontal recess dissection. Laryngoscope. 2006;116(4):573–9.
14. Chan Y, Melroy CT, Kuhn CA, Kuhn FL, Daniel WT, Kuhn FA. Long-term frontal sinus patency after endoscopic frontal sinusotomy. Laryngoscope. 2009;119(6):1229–32.
15. Askar MH, Gamea A, Tomoum MO, Elsherif HS, Ebert C, Senior BA. Endoscopic management of chronic frontal sinusitis: prospective quality of life analysis. Ann Otol Rhinol Laryngol. 2015;124(8):638–48.

16. Chandra RK, Palmer JN, Tanqsujarittham T, Kennedy DW. Factors associated with failure of frontal sinusotomy in the early follow-up period. Otolaryngol Head Neck Surg. 2004;131(4):514–8.

17. Hosemann W, Kuhnel T, Held P, Wagner W, Felderhoff A. Endonasal frontal sinusotomy in surgical management of chronic sinusitis: a critical evaluation. Am J Rhinol. 1997;11(1):1–9.

18. Wigand ME, Hosemann WG. Endoscopic surgery for frontal sinusitis and its complications. Am J Rhinol. 1991;5(3):85–9.

19. Valdes CJ, Bogado M, Samaha M. Causes of failure in endoscopic frontal sinus surgery in chronic rhinosinusitis patients. Int Forum Allergy Rhinol. 2014;4(6):502–6.

20. Weber R, Draf W, Kratzsch B, Hosemann W, Schaefer SD. Modern concepts of frontal sinus surgery. Laryngoscope. 2001;111(1):137–46.

21. Gross WE, Gross CW, Becker D, Moore D, Phillips D. Modified transnasal endoscopic lothrop procedure as an alternative to frontal sinus obliteration. Otolaryngol Head Neck Surg. 1995;113(4):427–34.

22. Chen PG, Wormald PJ, Payne SC, Gross WE, Gross CW. A golden experience: fifty years of experience managing the frontal sinus. Laryngoscope. 2016;126:802–7.

23. Eloy JA, Friedel ME, Kuperan AB, Govindaraj S, Folbe AJ, Liu JK. Modified mini-lothrop/extended draf IIB procedure for contralateral frontal sinus disease: a case series. Int Forum Allergy Rhinol. 2012;2:321–4.

24. Turner JH, Vaezeafshar R, Hwang PH. Indications and outcomes for draf IIB frontal sinus surgery. Am J Rhinol Allergy. 2016;30(1):70–3.

25. Metson R, Sindwani R. Endoscopic surgery for frontal sinusitis–a graduated approach. Otolaryngol Clin North Am. 2004;37:411–22.

26. Hardy JM, Montgomery WW. Osteoplastic frontal sinusotomy: an analysis of 250 operations. Ann Otol Rhinol Laryngol. 1976;85(4 pt 1):523–32.

27. Weber R, Draf W, Keerl R, et al. Osteoplastic frontal sinus surgery with fat obliteration: techniques and long term results using MRI in 82 operations. Laryngoscope. 2000;110:1037–44.

28. Sindwani R, Metson R. The impact of image-guidance on osteoplastic frontal sinus obliteration surgery. Otolaryngol Head Neck Surg. 2004;131:150–5.

29. Close LG, Lee NK, Leach JL, Manning SC. Endoscopic resection of the intranasal frontal sinus floor. Ann Otol Rhinol Laryngol. 1994;103:952–8.

30. Anderson P, Sindwani R. Safety and efficacy of the endoscopic modified lothrop procedure: a systematic review and meta-analysis. Laryngoscope. 2009;119:1828–33.

31. Tran KN, Beule AG, Singal D, Wormald PJ. Frontal ostium restenosis after the endoscopic modified lothrop procedure. Laryngoscope. 2007;117:1457–62.

32. Naidoo Y, Bassiouni A, Keen M, Wormald PJ. Long-term outcomes for the endoscopic modified lothrop/draf III procedure: a 10-year review. Laryngoscope. 2014;124(1):43–9.

33. Bassiouni A, Wormald PJ. Role of frontal sinus surgery in nasal polyp recurrence. Laryngoscope. 2013;123(1):36–41.

34. Weiss RL, Church CA, Kuhn FA. Long-term outcome analysis of balloon catheter sinusotomy: two year follow up. Otolaryngol Head Neck Surg. 2008;139:S38–46.

35. Karanfilov B, Silvers S, Pasha R, et al. Office-based balloon sinus dilation: a prospective, multicenter study of 203 patients. Int Forum Allergy Rhinol. 2013;3(5):404–11.

36. Prince A, Bhattacharyya N. An analysis of adverse event reporting in balloon sinus procedures. Otolaryngol Head Neck Surg. 2016;154(4):748–53.

37. Bolger WE, Brown CL, Church AC, et al. Safety and outcomes of balloon catheter sinusotomy: a multicenter 24-week analysis in 115 patients. Otolaryngol Head Neck Surg. 2007;137:10–20.

38. Kuhn FA, Church CA, Goldberg AN, et al. Balloon catheter sinusotomy: one-year follow-up – outcomes and role in functional endoscopic sinus surgery. Otolaryngol Head Neck Surg. 2008;139:S27–37.

39. Plaza G, Eisenberg G, Montojo J, Onrubia T, Urbasos M, O'Connor C. Balloon dilation of the frontal recess: a randomized clinical trial. Ann Otol Rhinol Laryngol. 2011;120:511–8.

40. Hathorn IF, Pace-Asciak P, Habib AR, Sunkaraneni V, Javer AR. Randomized controlled trial: hybrid technique using balloon dilation of the frontal sinus drainage pathway. Int Forum Allergy Rhinol. 2015;5(2):167–73.

41. Eloy JA, Friedel ME, Eloy JD, Govindaraj S, Folbe AJ. In-office balloon dilation of the failed frontal sinusotomy. Otolaryngol Head Neck Surg. 2012;146(2):320–2.

42. Wycherly BJ, Manes RP, Mikula SK. Initial clinical experience with balloon dilation in revision frontal sinus surgery. Ann Otol Rhinol Laryngol. 2010;119(7):468–71.

43. Perloff J, Palmer J. Evidence of bacterial biofilms on frontal recess stem in patients with chronic rhinosinusitis. Am J Rhinol. 2004;18:377–80.

44. Bendouah Z, Barbeau J, Hamad WA, Desrosiers M. Biofilm formation by staphylococcus aureus and pseudomonas aeruginosa is associated with an unfavorable evolution after surgery for chronic sinusitis and ansal polyposis. Otolaryngol Head Neck Surg. 2006;134(991):996.

45. Foreman A, Wormald PJ. Different biofilms, different disease? A clinical outcomes study. Laryngoscope. 2010;120:1701–6.

46. Psaltis AJ, Weitzel EK, Ha KR, Wormald PJ. The effect of bacterial biofilms on post-sinus surgical outcomes. Am J Rhinol. 2008;22:1–6.

47. Chadwell JS, Gustafson LM, Tami TA. Toxic shock syndrome associated with frontal sinus stents. Otolaryngol Head Neck Surg. 2001;124(5):573–4.

48. Weber R, Mai R, Hosemann W, Draf W, Toffel P. The success of 6-month stenting in endonasal frontal sinus surgery. Ear Nose Throat J. 2000;79(12):930–2.

49. Banhiran W, Sargi Z, Collins W, Kaza S, Casiano R. Long term effect of stenting after an endoscopic modified lothrop procedure. Am J Rhinol. 2006;20(6):595–9.

50. Murr AH, Smith TL, Hwang PH, et al. Safety and efficacy of a novel bioabsorbable, steroid-eluting sinus stent. Int Forum Allergy Rhinol. 2011;1(1):23–32.

51. Marple BF, Smith TL, Han JK, et al. Advance II: a prospective, randomized study assessing safety and efficacy of bioabsorbable steroid-releasing sinus implants. Otolaryngol Head Neck Surg. 2012;146(6):1004–11.

52. Han JK, Marple BF, Smith TL, et al. Effect of steroid-releasing sinus implants on postoperative medical and surgical interventions: an efficacy meta-analysis. Int Forum Allergy Rhinol. 2012;2(4):271–9.

53. Valentine R, Athanasiadis T, Moratti S, Robinson S, Wormald PJ. The efficacy of a novel chitosan gel on hemostasis after endoscopic sinus surgery in a sheep model of chronic rhinosinusitis. Am J Rhinol Allergy. 2009;23(1):71–5.

54. Ngoc Ha T, Valentine R, Moratti S, Robinson S, Hanton L, Wormald PJ. A blinded randomized controlled trial evaluating the efficacy of chitosan gel on ostial stenosis following endoscopic sinus surgery. Int Forum Allergy Rhinol. 2013;3(7):573–80.

55. Valentine R, Athanasiadis T, Moratti S, Hanton L, Robinson S, Wormald PJ. The efficacy of a novel chitosan gel on hemostasis and wound healing after endoscopic sinus surgery. Am J Rhinol Allergy. 2010;24(1):70–5.

56. Muzzarelli A. Chitin and chitosan: unique cationic polysaccharides. In: Mark H, Bikales N, Overberger CG, Menges G, Kroschwitz J, editors. In encyclopedia of polymer science and engineering, vol. 430. Hoboken: Wiley Interscience; 1990.

57. Athanasiadis T, Beule AG, Robinson BH, Robinson SR, Shi Z, Wormald PJ. Effects of a novel chitosan gel on mucosal wound healing following endoscopic sinus surgery in a sheep model of chronic rhinosinusitis. Laryngoscope. 2008;118:1088–94.

Pediatric Frontal Sinus Surgery

Brian D'Anza, Janalee K. Stokken, and Samantha Anne

Introduction

Surgical intervention to the frontal sinus is rarely pursued in the pediatric population, as the sinus does not begin to pneumatize until around the age of 8, and there is variability in the rate of development. Additionally, chronic frontal rhinosinusitis is often resolved by management of the adenoids and/or maxillary and ethmoid sinuses. Though pediatric frontal sinus surgery is uncommon, a thorough understanding of frontal sinus anatomy, pathology, and management is important for all otolaryngologists as complications of acute sinusitis can result from frontal sinusitis and should be treated expediently.

Embryology

The frontal sinus begins to develop around the fourth to fifth week of gestation and continues to develop well into adolescence. Around 4 weeks gestation, when the embryo begins to develop of branchial arches and pouches, the frontonasal prominence derives from the cranial neural crest mesenchyme. Inferiorly, the frontonasal prominence develops nasal placodes, thickened areas of ectoderm, which develop on both sides. The nasal placodes invade the mesenchyme and further differentiate into the medial and lateral nasal processes. The two medial nasal processes form the primary nasal septum, middle part of the upper lip, and premaxilla. The nasal processes together eventually contribute to development of the nasal cavity and choanae. The frontonasal prominence extends caudally and involves the mesoderm to form the septum [1, 2].

Around the 25th to 28th week of development, there are three medial projections from lateral wall of the nose. The anterior and inferior projections give rise to the agger nasi cell, inferior turbinate, and maxillary sinus. The superior projection forms the middle and superior turbinate and ethmoidal cells. The meatus begins to form as lateral diverticula between the turbinates. The middle meatus forms between the inferior and middle turbinates and expands laterally giving rise to the infundibulum. The infundibulum continues to expand superiorly which eventually

B. D'Anza
Division of Rhinology, Allergy, and Skull Base Surgery, Department of Otolaryngology, University Hospitals – Case Western Reserve University, Cleveland, OH, USA

J. K. Stokken (✉)
Department of Otorhinolaryngology, Mayo Clinic, Rochester, MN, USA

S. Anne
Pediatric Otolaryngology, Head and Neck Institute, Cleveland Clinic, Cleveland, OH, USA

© Springer Nature Switzerland AG 2019
D. Lal, P. H. Hwang (eds.), *Frontal Sinus Surgery*, https://doi.org/10.1007/978-3-319-97022-6_26

gives rise to the frontonasal recess, and this continues to elongate to form the frontal sinus. At onset of the elongation, the frontal recess contains thickened regions of cartilage. By term, this is replaced with complex folds and furrows and includes ethmoidal cells. Around 2 years of age, pneumatization of the frontal bone begins. The frontal sinus continues to grow well into adolescence, when it becomes fully pneumatized [1, 2].

Acute Rhinosinusitis

Upper respiratory illness (URI) is very common in children, and the symptoms can be difficult to differentiate from acute sinusitis. Symptoms of acute sinusitis in a child include purulent nasal drainage, day and nighttime cough, nasal obstruction, fever, postnasal drainage, and/or headache. The American Academy of Pediatrics' (AAP) clinical practice guideline for diagnosis and management of sinusitis in children defines acute sinusitis when the URI symptoms last more than 10 days without improvement, worsening of symptoms after initial improvement (double sickening), or severe symptoms such as high fevers and purulent nasal drainage for 3 consecutive days [3].

A diagnosis of sinusitis is primarily based on history and physical exam findings. Signs of infection include nasal mucosal edema, discolored nasal drainage, and inferior eyelid or maxilla swelling [3]. Nasal endoscopy can be used to evaluate for purulent drainage and polyps; however, this may be poorly tolerated in young children [4]. Computed tomography (CT) of sinuses offers a highly accurate assessment of the sinuses. However, due to concern for radiation exposure and risk for childhood malignancies, CT scans should be reserved for cases that absolutely require imaging (such as surgical preoperative scanning). The AAP guidelines advise against the use of sinus CT for diagnosis of acute sinusitis [3]. Lastly, magnetic resonance imaging (MRI) can be used when there is concern for intraorbital or intracranial extension.

Initial medical treatment of acute pediatric sinusitis is with antibiotic therapy directed to the most common pathogens. These organisms are the same pathogens that affect the upper respiratory tract: *Streptococcus pneumoniae*, *Haemophilus influenzae*, and *Moraxella catarrhalis* [5]. As such, the recommended antibiotic is amoxicillin (45 mg/kg in two divided doses) in uncomplicated acute bacterial sinusitis in ages 2 and older, with no recent antibiotic use in the month prior. When there is concern for high prevalence of resistance in the community, then high-dose amoxicillin is warranted at 90 mg/kg/day in two divided doses. When there is moderate to severe illness, if there is prior recent antibiotic use, or if the child is less than 2 years of age, then amoxicillin-clavulanate is recommended. Additional recommended therapy includes nasal saline, although there is reported poor compliance in children [6].

Frontal sinusitis, if present, is often treated appropriately in the context of treating acute maxillary or ethmoid sinusitis. However, it is important to recognize that frontal sinusitis does have the risk of complications with spread to the orbit and brain. Common intracranial complications from frontal sinusitis are meningitis, epidural abscess, subdural empyema, brain abscess, and venous sinus thrombosis [7]. Infections affecting the orbit can progress along the widely accepted Chandler's classification: preseptal cellulitis, orbital cellulitis, subperiosteal abscess, orbital abscess, and cavernous sinus thrombosis [8]. When complications arise from frontal sinusitis, pediatric frontal sinus surgery becomes critical to control the disease process and sequelae.

Chronic Rhinosinusitis

Chronic rhinosinusitis (CRS) is defined in the pediatric population in a similar fashion as it is for adults. However, it has been noted that CRS is indistinguishable from adenoiditis, and there is considerable overlap in the symptoms of these with viral upper respiratory tract infections and allergic rhinitis. A diagnosis of CRS is made by the presence of two or more symptoms, for at least 12 weeks, in addition to either endoscopic findings or CT changes consistent with the

CRS. The symptoms of CRS include nasal obstruction or congestion, nasal drainage, facial pain or pressure, and cough, and one of the patient's symptoms must be obstruction or drainage.

An endoscopic exam can be difficult to obtain in younger patients but is crucial in older children. Findings of nasal polyps should warrant an evaluation for cystic fibrosis. The adenoids should be evaluated for hypertrophy and purulent drainage. Other endoscopic findings can be mucopurulent discharge primarily from the middle meatus, mucosal edema, or obstruction of the middle meatus (EPOS 2012). Plain X-rays do not have a role in the diagnosis of pediatric CRS. CT imaging should be obtained only when surgical interventions are planned.

Frontal Sinus Anatomy

Pediatric sinonasal anatomy can be difficult to navigate via endoscopy simply because of the often immature and constricted nature of the nose. This challenge can be magnified in the pediatric frontal sinus due to the varied and changing pneumatization patterns. In adults, image guidance has become commonplace within many sinus practices, and the same can be said for pediatrics. However, relying on surgical navigation can be difficult to follow in pediatric patients due to the smaller head and desire to keep radiation dosage low leading to less detailed imaging capture. In light of the smaller volume of the sinuses and difficult visualization due to limited nasal corridors, pediatric sinus surgery can be fraught with risk of complications if the surgeon's knowledge is not rooted in basic anatomy.

Normal Anatomy

The frontal sinuses are bounded by an anterior and posterior table, the frontal bone superiorly and laterally, and usually an intersinus septum medially [1, 2, 9]. The intersinus septum separates the two frontal sinuses and at its most infe-

rior extent is continuous with the crista galli posteriorly, the frontal bone and nasal spine anteriorly, and the perpendicular plate of the ethmoid inferiorly. The inferior boundary is more complex but commonly involves the orbital roof and frontal sinus ostium more medially. The ostium flows into the much more complex frontal sinus infundibulum or frontal sinus outflow tract and drainage pathway. The location of these basic anatomical structures is highly variable depending on the degree of sinus pneumatization and age of the child [1, 2, 9].

The size of the frontal sinus will vary as the child ages and pneumatization progresses. Starting at age 1–4 years, secondary pneumatization will occur [1, 9]. And, while the sinus will be embryologically present at birth, it is not until after ages 3–8 that the frontal sinus will be more obviously seen in radiologic scans [1, 9]. Usually at about 6 years of age, the superior extent of the frontal sinus is at the superior orbital rim [10]. Secondary pneumatization will continue through adolescence at variable rates, finally completing around 18 years of age [1, 7].

The degree of pneumatization has been hypothesized to be influenced by multiple factors including mucociliary clearance, comorbidities, climate, and geography [11, 12]. Cystic fibrosis patients are a perfect case study for the importance of mucociliary clearance impacting eventual sinus formation, as nearly 50% of patients have aplastic frontal sinuses [13]. This is thought to be due to the genetic deficiencies in the CFTR transmembrane receptor negatively impacting mucociliary function, thereby resulting in a lack of pneumatization of the frontal sinuses [7]. Additionally, patients may have small sphenoid sinuses and a congested ethmoid sinus cavity resulting in a low-lying ethmoid skull base. All of these facts are extremely important to the pediatric sinus surgeon.

The boundaries of the frontal sinus drainage pathway are complex in the adult and can be even more varied in the pediatric population. The outflow tract or "infundibulum" can be thought of as a funnel, which typically angles posteromedially toward the ethmoid cells, but can be highly variable in its caliber, location, and eventual drainage path. In prepubescent children, this drainage pathway is typically shorter secondary to the limited pneumatization of frontal sinus [13, 14]. Thus, the chances of anatomic obstruction are somewhat lower than seen in the adult population [13, 14]. There are a multitude of anatomic variations that can be present in the pediatric population, such as the site of uncinate process attachment, size and presence of agger nasi cells, or presence of suprabullar ethmoid cells.

Anatomic Variations

There are multiple variations to normal anatomy in the area of the frontal sinus that are described well in the adult literature and elsewhere. This includes the Kuhn classification of frontal sinus cells (I–IV) as well as the Keros classification for the depth of the olfactory fossa [15, 16]. While these anatomic variations are certainly important to know and applicable to frontal sinus surgery in children, we will not be defining these in great detail here. Instead we will be commenting on literature reviewing those variations applicable to pediatric frontal sinus surgery.

In 2015, a radiologic case series study evaluated the anatomy of the frontal recess in patients 5–14 years of age [17]. The purpose was to review the frequency of frontoethmoidal cells in the pediatric population. They found that 97% of patients had a well-formed agger nasi cell, while 86% had at least 1 frontal cell [17]. The authors felt this indicated a high frequency of frontoethmoidal cells in children and is likely a result of changing anatomy during development. It must be noted that this was purely a radiologic review, and none of the patients had documented sinus disease or surgery.

Kim et al. performed a retrospective study of 113 pediatric patients (mean age 11.2 years) with persistent chronic sinusitis not responsive to medical management [14]. They documented the sinonasal anatomic variations as seen on CT scans. They found that among the most common was the presence of an agger nasi cell as an early

pneumatization pattern (69.1%) [14]. Also, they found the frontal sinus to be the least likely disease location, with an incidence of 47.6% [14]. They concluded that there was no association between an agger nasi cell and the frequency or location of frontal sinus disease. The authors contended pediatric chronic sinusitis in their population was caused primarily by a functional mucosal issue due to various environmental, systemic, or local factors.

This idea was also supported by a study completed by Silvasli et al. that looked at anatomic variations in the lateral sinonasal wall [18]. They reported on 47 patients ranging in age from 2 to 16 years, with an average age of 10 years [18]. Among the most common were concha bullosa and agger nasi cells. They found the ethmoid bulla to be underdeveloped and less prominent than in the adult [18]. The authors concluded the data did not support a relationship between anatomic variations and chronic sinus disease in children. The authors recommended against aggressive surgical management in pediatric populations due to the lack of this significant relationship [18].

Indications and Contraindications to Surgical Management

Indications

Surgery for frontal sinusitis in pediatric patients has been shown to be effective with recent American Academy of Otolaryngology (AAO) clinical consensus statements supporting its use. Surgery for pediatric CRS can take many forms from adenoidectomy to limited endoscopic sinus surgery (ESS) to maxillary antral irrigation to frontal sinusotomy. The specific procedures employed and their indications are a source of controversy, with a wide range of opinions as to what constitutes appropriate surgical intervention. These topics will be covered in greater detail later in this chapter. Briefly, there is a general consensus in the literature that surgery should be reserved for

Table 26.1 Indications for surgery related to pediatric frontal sinusitis

Indication	Details
Acute orbital complications of frontal sinus disease: subperiosteal abscess, orbital abscess	Endoscopic surgery to address anatomic issue unresponsive to medical therapy
Acute neurologic complications: epidural abscess, subdural abscess, meningitis, venous sinus thrombosis, brain abscess	Anterior ethmoidectomy, uninectomy, or maxillary antrostomy usually suffice
Chronic frontal sinusitis with or without polyposis and symptomatic sequelae unresponsive to maximal medical management	Maxillary antrostomy with anterior ethmoidectomy advocated as initial surgery. Frontal sinusotomy can be considered for recalcitrant disease
Frontal bone osteomyelitis, subperiosteal abscess. also known as Pott's puffy tumor	May require trephination or incision and drainage. Anterior ethmoidectomy and maxillary antrostomy may be sufficient endonasally
Mucopyocele of frontal sinus	Requires endoscopic frontal sinusotomy to drain fluid
Benign tumors of frontal sinus	Fibrous dysplasia, ossifying fibroma, osteoma, teratoma, inverted papilloma
CSF leak repair	May be related to congenital encephalocele, meningocele, nasal dermoid tract, etc.

acute sinusitis complications and intractable cases of chronic sinus disease with severe symptomatology [3, 7, 9, 19]. Table 26.1 presents generally accepted indications for pediatric endoscopic surgery involving the frontal sinus or frontal sinus drainage pathway. Pediatric patients with tumors within and around the frontal sinus may be candidates indications for endoscopic procedures based on the anatomic favorability for complete resection of tumor. Frontal CSF leaks are generally rare, but are more commonly seen in the pediatric population associated with a congenital encephalocele, prior trauma or nasal dermoid tract.

Contraindications

The primary contraindications to undergoing a frontal sinus surgical procedure revolve around medical comorbidities or the inability to tolerate a general anesthetic. Patients with bleeding disorders or critically sick children fit under this category. As well, in some children undergoing surgery for relative indications such as CRS, the surgeon must be cognizant of the family situation, as the child will need good postoperative care, regular follow-up, and possibly repeat surgical debridements under general anesthesia. The family should be apprised of these necessities at

the outset, and if their expectations are unreasonable, surgical planning should be delayed until appropriate understanding is demonstrated.

Of note, one of the early concerns regarding ESS was for disturbing the growth of the pediatric facial skeleton. Early reports in piglet models had revealed some facial growth disturbances [20]. However, since then several studies have looked at anthropomorphic measurements over time for pediatric patients and failed to show growth disturbances associated with sinus surgery [21, 22].

Surgical Techniques and Strategy

Various surgical methods have been employed and can vary widely from surgeon to surgeon. Acute sinus-related complications including subperiosteal orbital abscess formation or frontal bone osteomyelitis were historically treated with a trephination via an exterior medial brow incision. Today, many of the complications associated with acute frontal sinusitis can be treated with directed endoscopic sinus surgery. The goal of this surgery is to provide source control of the infection. If appropriate access to the frontal sinus cannot be obtained, a "minitrephine" can be included to allow for the passage of instruments or irrigations directly into the frontal sinus from above. Literature in this realm is sparse beyond case reports; thus, we will focus most of the discussion on surgery for chronic sinusitis.

The data supports different types of approaches for chronic sinusitis in the pediatric patient who is not responsive to medical therapy. This includes conservative management via adenoidectomy to more aggressive first-line ESS [1, 3, 9, 19, 23]. There is also a suggested difference between the treatments of adolescent versus younger children [19, 23]. Studies have shown that children between 6 and 12 years of age gain the most long-term benefit from adenoidectomy, while there is little data regarding patients 13–18 years of age [19, 23].

Unfortunately, there are no large-scale randomized, controlled studies in the literature that specifically address pediatric frontal CRS. Part of this is due to the fact that surgical management for frontal sinus disease in children is extremely rare [7, 14]. There are often technical issues with accessing the frontal sinus as the space is narrow and often underdeveloped depending on the age. This can prevent adequate visualization and requires smaller endoscopes that limit the field of view. There are also concerns for scarring when operating in a small space. Therefore, we are left to glean results from those studies that include frontal sinus disease in the data.

In 2014, the AAO released a series of clinical consensus statements regarding pediatric CRS [19]. Among other subjects, they addressed the effectiveness of adenoidectomy and functional ESS based on a literature review and panel of experts. Below we list the recommended options for surgical management and the AAO consensus statements. We also review other literature pertaining to the subject of surgical management.

Adenoidectomy

One of the stated purposes of the AAO consensus statement on pediatric CRS was to get a sense of the benefits of adenoidectomy [19]. No frontal sinus-specific statements were made as there was no literature to support such. Regardless, they

reported the literature showed a strong clinical consensus in recommending adenoidectomy as a first-line surgical treatment for CRS in children 12 years of age and younger [19]. This is supported by microbiologic studies showing adenoidectomy, regardless of adenoid hypertrophy, resulted in a dramatic decrease in nasopharyngeal pathogens associated with pediatric CRS [24, 25]. Based on this reasoning, it would make sense that pediatric frontal sinus disease refractory to medical management could be equally improved with adenoidectomy. There is a benefit to adenoidectomy with respect to improved symptom outcomes compared to medical management in up to 70% of patients [26]. There are no prospective studies looking specifically at clinical improvements for frontal sinus disease. Further study in this area is needed.

Endoscopic Sinus Surgery

ESS for pediatric sinus disease is an often debated topic regarding its indications in pediatric populations. Included in this is the extent of ESS involving uncinectomy, maxillary antrostomy, anterior ethmoidectomy, and/or frontal sinusotomy. It is clear, however, that ESS plays a role in surgical management of pediatric frontal CRS that has failed maximal medical therapy. The AAO consensus statement on pediatric CRS discussed a systematic database review reporting success rates of 82–100% for ESS in pediatric patients [19, 27]. Similarly, a meta-analysis of 15 studies involving 1301 patients concluded that ESS improved sinus-related symptoms and quality of life [28].

A study by Ramadan looked at the efficacy of adenoidectomy versus ESS [23]. This was a prospective non-randomized study over 10 years involving 202 patients, of which 183 had follow-up of at least 1 year [23]. Patients were split into one of three groups: adenoidectomy alone, ESS alone, or adenoidectomy plus ESS. They found that the lowest revision rate for surgery was found in the adenoidectomy plus ESS group at 7.6% [23]. The other two groups showed revision surgical rates for controlling symptoms of 12.5%

(ESS) and 25% (adenoidectomy) [23]. The results also showed a higher number of asthma patients, and older children required ESS after adenoidectomy. Thus, the authors believed children 6 years and younger without asthma benefitted from adenoidectomy alone as a primary surgery. Meanwhile, children older than 6 years with asthma and exposure to cigarette smoke were recommended to have concurrent ESS with adenoidectomy. All ESS in this sample was defined as an anterior ethmoidectomy and maxillary antrostomy. Approximately 28% of the patients had a posterior ethmoidectomy. None of the patients was reported to have a frontal sinusotomy.

Rarely, a pediatric patient will undergo an endoscopic frontal sinusotomy or frontal sinus exploration. It has been reported in adolescents and cystic fibrosis patients but is often avoided due to the delayed pneumatization of the frontal sinus and technical difficulties previously outlined [7]. As can be seen from the above cited literature, there is no adequate prospective data investigating the use of frontal sinusotomy in children, including its effect on outcomes versus more conservative approaches.

Balloon Catheter Technology

The use of balloon catheter technology (BCT) for dilation of sinuses has been investigated in recent years as an alternative to ESS in the operating room setting. The use of this technology in pediatric patients is intuitive as it lends itself to narrow sinonasal outflow tracts, reduces damage to surrounding tissue, and is based on the idea of minimally invasive treatment. As well, it has been shown to have an excellent safety profile in adults [29–31].

Studies have evaluated BCT for sinus outflow dilation on pediatric patients. There is evidence for feasibility and efficacy among all sinuses, but unfortunately the trials have not offered much data regarding frontal sinus balloon dilation. A recent study by Ramadan et al. in 2010 compared the results of 30 children who had balloon dilation of their sinuses versus adenoidectomy [32].

The mean age of the children was significantly less in the BCT dilation group (7.7 years) versus the adenoidectomy group (4.8 years) [32]. Only two of the dilations were performed on frontal sinuses. Nevertheless, they reported improved outcomes on multivariate analysis in the usage of BCT when compared to adenoidectomy alone [32]. They reported that age was not a significant confounder.

A cross-sectional analysis by Ference et al. reviewed state surgical databases comparing average OR time and cost between traditional functional ESS techniques and procedures utilizing BCT [33]. They found that charges were higher and operating room time did not change with using BCT. This raises a question of the benefits of routine use of BCT in pediatric patients. Clearly, further study is needed to determine the appropriate patients and indications for use in the pediatric population.

Complications

Endoscopic sinus surgery in the pediatric population has been shown to be safe with a reported complication rate of 1.4%. Makary and Ramadan reviewed 11 articles published between 1990 and 2012 and found 6 complications in 440 pediatric patients undergoing ESS for CRS. Patients with nasal polyposis, cystic fibrosis, primary ciliary dysmotility, and primary immunodeficiency were excluded [27]. Three of the reported complications were violation of the orbit, two were periorbital ecchymosis, and the last was epistaxis requiring transfusion. There were no reports of CSF rhinorrhea or major orbital injury resulting in vision changes or loss. They did not report the minor complication rates of nasal synechiae or mild epistaxis, and recalcitrant disease was not reported. Ference et al. did not report any orbital complications or deaths in their analysis of 537 endoscopic approaches to the frontal sinus and 72 frontal balloon dilations.

When comparing the overall complication rates in the pediatric population to adults, Krings et al. reported no difference in major complication rates, with no skull base complications in just under 3000 cases. In the same study, they did show that at all age groups, cases involving the sphenoid (0.45%), frontal (0.53%), or all sinuses (0.44%) were more likely to have a complication as compared to cases involving only the maxillary and/or ethmoid sinuses (0.28%). The use of image guidance was not associated with a lower complication rate [34].

Understanding the patient's frontal sinus anatomy in conjunction with choosing an appropriate management intervention is the best way to avoid complications in pediatric frontal sinus surgery. Parasagittal CT images are the best preoperative modality when preparing for surgery involving the frontal recess. In patients with a pneumatized frontal sinus and obstructing frontal or suprabullar cells, balloon dilation may be appropriate; future research will help clarify the role of balloon catheter technology in this population. Avoiding destabilization to middle turbinate and mucosal stripping injury to the axilla in addition to placement of a dissolvable middle meatal spacer can help to prevent middle turbinate lateralization and adhesions. Image guidance navigation should be utilized if endoscopic dissection of the frontal recess is warranted to ensure all obstructing anterior ethmoid cells are addressed as retained agger nasi cells and retained ethmoids have been noted to be the cause of failure in 13% and 53% of revision frontal sinus surgeries, respectively [35].

Summary

Frontal sinus surgery is rarely indicated in the pediatric population. However, rare indications, including life-threatening complications may necessitate surgery in this patient population. Clinicians therefore must be familiar with the indications for undertaking frontal surgery, anatomical considerations in this age group as well as the techniques necessary for managing recalcitrant frontal sinusitis in the pediatric population.

References

1. Duque CS, Casiano RS. Surgical anatomy and embryology of the frontal sinus. In: Kountakis SE, Senior BA, Draf W, editors. The frontal sinus. Berlin\Heidelberg: Springer; 2005. p. 21–32.
2. Rontal M, Anon JB, Zinreich SJ. Embryology and anatomy of the paranasal sinuses. In: Bluestone CD, Stool SE, Alper CM, editors. Pediatric otolaryngology, vol. 2. 4th ed. Philadelphia: Saunders; 2003. p. 861.
3. Wald ER, Applegate KE, Bordley C, et al. Clinical practice guideline for the diagnosis and management of acute bacterial sinusitis in children aged 1 to 18 years. Pediatrics. 2013;132(1):e262–80.
4. Lusk RP. Pediatric rhinosinusitis. In: Johnson JT, Rosen CA, Bailey BJ, editors. Bailey's head and neck surgery—otolaryngology. Philadelphia: Wolters Kluwer Health/Lippincott Williams & Wilkins. p. 1456–66.
5. Wald ER, Milmoe GJ, Bowen A, Ledesma-Medina J, Salamon N, Bluestone CD. Acute maxillary sinusitis in children. N Engl J Med. 1981;304(13):749–54.
6. Kassel JC, King D, Spurling GK. Saline nasal irrigation for acute upper respiratory tract infection. Cochrane Database Syst Rev. 2010;3:CD006821.
7. Gross CW, Han JK. Pediatric frontal sinusitis. In: Kountakis SE, Senior BA, Draf W, editors. The frontal sinus. Berlin\Heidelberg: Springer. p. 127–32.
8. Chandler JR. The pathogenesis of orbital complications in acute sinusitis. Laryngoscope. 1970;80:1414–28.
9. Wise SK, Orlandi RR, Delgaudio JM. Sinonasal development and anatomy. In: Kennedy DW, Hwang PH, editors. Rhinology: diseases of the nose, sinuses, and skull base. New York: Thieme Medical Publishers; 2012. p. 1–20.
10. Ahmed A. Imaging of the paediatric paranasal sinuses. S Afr J Rad. 2013;17(3):91–7.
11. Aydinhoglu A, Kavakli A, Erdem S. Absence of frontal sinus in Turkish individuals. Yonsei Med J. 2003;44(2):215–8.
12. Lang J. Clinical anatomy of the nose, nasal cavity and paranasal sinuses. New York: Thieme Medical Publishers; 1989. p. 1–3.
13. Eggesbo HB, Sovik S, Dolvik S, et al. CT characterization of developmental variations of the paranasal sinuses in cystic fibrosis. Acta Radiol. 2001;42:482–93.
14. Kim HJ, Jung Cho M, Lee JW, Tae Kim Y, Kahng H, Sung Kim H, Hahm KH. The relationship between anatomic variations of paranasal sinuses and chronic sinusitis in children. Acta Otolaryngol. 2006;126(10):1067–72.
15. Bent J, Kuhn FA, Cuilty C. The frontal cell in frontal recess obstruction. Am J Rhinol. 1994;8:185–91.
16. Stammberger HR, Kennedy DW, Anatomic Terminology Group, et al. Paranasal sinuses: ana-

tomic terminology and nomenclature. Ann Otol Rhinol Laryngol Suppl. 1995;177:7–16.

17. Al-Qudah M, Mardini D. Computed tomographic analysis of frontal recess cells in pediatric patients. Am J Rhinol Allergy. 2015;29(6):425–9.

18. Sivasli E, Sirikçi A, Bayazýt YA, et al. Anatomic variations of the paranasal sinus area in pediatric patients with chronic sinusitis. Surg Radiol Anat. 2003;24:400–5.

19. Brietzke SE, Shin JJ, Choi S, et al. Clinical consensus statement: pediatric chronic rhinosinusitis. Otolaryngol Head Neck Surg. 2014;151(4):542–53.

20. Mair EA, Bolger WE, Breisch EA. Sinus and facial growth after pediatric endoscopic sinus surgery. Arch Otolaryngol Head Neck Surg. 1995;121(5):547–52.

21. Senior B, Wirtschafter A, Mai C, Becker C, Belenky W. Quantitative impact of pediatric sinus surgery on facial growth. Laryngoscope. 2000;110:1866–70.

22. Bothwell MR, Piccirillo JF, Lusk RP, Ridenour BD. Long-term outcome of facial growth after functional endoscopic sinus surgery. Otolaryngol Head Neck Surg. 2002;126:628–34.

23. Ramadan HH. Surgical management of chronic sinusitis in children. Laryngoscope. 2004;114:2103–9.

24. Tallat AM, Baghat YS, El-Ghazzawy E, et al. Nasopahryngeal bacterial flora before and after adenoidectomy. J Laryngol Otol. 1989;103:372–4.

25. Lee D, Rosenfeld RM. Adenoid bacteriology and sinonasal symptoms in children. Otolaryngol Head Neck Surg. 1997;116:301–7.

26. Brietzke SE, Brigger MT. Adenoidectomy outcomes in pediatric rhinosinusitis: a meta-analysis. Int J Pediatr Otorhinolaryngol. 2008;72:1541–5.

27. Makary CA, Ramadan HH. The role of sinus surgery in children. Laryngoscope. 2013;123:1348–52.

28. Vlastarakos PV, Fetta M, Segas JV, et al. Functional endoscopic sinus surgery improves sinus-related symptoms and quality of life in children with chronic rhinosinusitis: a systematic analysis and meta-analysis of published interventional studies. Clin Pediatr. 2013;52:1091–7.

29. Bolger WE, Vaughan WC. Catheter-based dilation of the sinus ostia: initial safety and feasibility analysis in a cadaver model. Am J Rhinol. 2006;20:290–4.

30. Brodner D, Nachlas N, Mock P, et al. Safety and outcomes following hybrid balloon and balloon-only procedures using a multifunction, multisinus balloon dilation tool. Int Forum Allergy Rhinol. 2013;3(8):652–8.

31. Batra PS, Ryan MW, Sindwani R, Marple BF. Balloon catheter technology in rhinology: reviewing the evidence. Laryngoscope. 2011;121(1):226–32.

32. Ramadan HH, Terrell AM. Balloon catheter sinuplasty ad adenoidectomy in children with chronic rhinosinusitis. Ann Oto Rhinol Laryngol. 2010;119(9):578–82.

33. Ference EH, Schroeder JW, Qureshi H. Current utilization of balloon dilation versus endoscopic techniques in pediatric sinus surgery. Otolaryngol Head Neck Surg. 2014;151(5):852–60.

34. Krings JG, Kallogjeri D, Wineland A, Nepple KG, Piccirillo JF, Getz AE. Complications of primary and revision functional endoscopic sinus surgery for chronic rhinosinusitis. Laryngoscope. 2014;124:838–45.

35. Otto KJ, DelGaudio JM. Operative findings in the frontal recess at time of revision surgery. Am J Otolaryngol. 2010;31(3):175–80.

Congenital and Pediatric Frontal Pathology

Joseph S. Schwartz and Nithin D. Adappa

Introduction

Congenital nasal and paranasal sinus anomalies may arise from either an error in embryogenesis or an intrauterine interruption in fetal growth. Congenital midline nasal masses (nasal dermoids, gliomas, and encephaloceles) share a common embryologic origin and are the product of a developmental error of the anterior neuropore, which contributes to the development of the anterior skull base. The frontal sinus develops anterior to the anterior neuropore, with developmental errors of the latter presenting as masses that are intimately related anatomically to frontal structures.

Pediatric rhinosinusitis is a disease entity commonly encountered by pediatric otolaryngologists with rare instances of associated complications. Though rare, the sequelae of sinusitis-related complications can be devastating, necessitating prompt recognition and management. Frontal sinusitis in the pediatric population represents an important risk factor for intracranial spread of infection given its close relationship to the cranial vault.

The goal of this chapter is to provide a comprehensive review of both congenital midline nasal masses and complications of pediatric frontal sinusitis with particular attention given to the underlying pathophysiology, clinical approach, and treatment strategies of these disease entities.

Congenital Midline Nasal Masses

Overview of the Embryology of the Anterior Neuropore

An understanding of the underlying pathophysiology of congenital midline nasal masses necessitates knowledge of the normal embryologic development of the anterior neuropore. The embryologic precursor to the central nervous system is an ectodermally derived neural tube that forms in the midline by the third week of gestation along the dorsal surface of the embryo. Closure of the neural tube occurs during the fourth week of gestation, commencing initially in the midportion of the neural tube with neuropores at the cranial (anterior neuropore) and caudal (posterior neuropore) limits of the neural tube closing last. Neural tube closure is accompanied by neural crest migration along the neural tube into the mesenchyme, which once organized forms crucial skeletal structures and spaces of the anterior skull base. These spaces include:

J. S. Schwartz
Department of Otolaryngology – Head and Neck Surgery, McGill University, Montreal, QC, Canada

N. D. Adappa (✉)
Department of Otorhinolaryngology – Head and Neck Surgery, University of Pennsylvania, Perelman School of Medicine, Philadelphia, PA, USA

© Springer Nature Switzerland AG 2019
D. Lal, P. H. Hwang (eds.), *Frontal Sinus Surgery*, https://doi.org/10.1007/978-3-319-97022-6_27

- Fonticulus nasofrontalis – gap between the frontal and nasal bones
- Foramen cecum – gap between the frontal and ethmoid bones which is continuous with the prenasal space
- Nasal capsule – precursor to the nasal septum and cartilages which is continuous with the ethmoid sinuses
- Prenasal space – located between the nasal bones and nasal capsule

Under normal circumstances, these spaces are obliterated by progressive growth of neighboring bones. Persistence or faulty closure of these spaces can give rise to a congenital midline nasal mass.

At the anterior limit of neural crest migration and neural tube closes, the anterior neuropore is predisposed to embryologic defects given its comparative deficiency in neural crest cells and belated neural tube closure. Frontal, nasal, and ethmoid structures form immediately anterior to the anterior neuropore, with errors in development of the latter manifesting in close proximity with these structures [1, 2].

Nasal Dermoids

Epidemiology

Midline congenital nasal masses are rare overall (1:20,000–40,000 births) with the majority (over 60%) of such cases comprising nasal dermoids [3]. Moreover, nasal dermoids make up a minority of all dermoids in the head and neck region (up to 12%) as well as throughout the body (up to 3%) [3–5]. A slight male predominance has been observed in addition to suggestions of a potential hereditary basis [6]. While most nasal dermoids occur in isolation, an association with a variety of craniofacial abnormalities has been described [7].

Pathophysiology

Three principal theories have prevailed in the literature to account for the development of nasal dermoids: the prenasal theory, the trilaminar theory, and the superficial sequestration theory. Among these, the prenasal theory first proposed

by Grunwald in the early 1900s has garnered the greatest support [3]. This theory states that at approximately 8 weeks' gestation, a dural diverticulum projects from the anterior cranial fossa through the foramen cecum, traversing the prenasal space to eventually contact the skin of the caudal surface of the nasal bones (eventual site of the rhinion). As the prenasal space involutes, the dural diverticulum detaches from the overlying skin and retracts intracranially thereby severing any neuroectodermal connection. Faulty regression of the dural diverticulum can result in the persistence of a midline tract [6, 8]. If a cutaneous-dural connection persists, cutaneous elements may be drawn anywhere along the course of the diverticulum from the nasal tip to the anterior cranial fossa though the majority are confined to the superficial nasal region. Proliferation of entrapped cutaneous elements (ectoderm and mesoderm) results in the formation of a nasal dermoid cyst, an epithelial-lined sac comprised of adnexal structures such as glands and hair [2, 4]. Often, a sinus tract communicates the cyst with the overlying skin surface anywhere in the midline between the glabella and columella. In instances of intracranial extension (up to 20% in a recent meta-analysis [9] though this figure varies widely in the literature), communication often occurs via an unobliterated foramen cecum with the potential for extradural adherence to the falx cerebri [9].

Clinical Presentation

Nasal dermoids are most often diagnosed in childhood though delayed presentations have been described in several instances. The pathognomonic presentation of a nasal dermoid, present in less than half of patients [10], is that of a midline cutaneous pit with a protruding hair [9]. When presenting as a nasal mass, several features distinguish a nasal dermoid from that of an encephalocele. Nasal dermoids are noncompressible masses which do not transilluminate and fail to enlarge when the child cries (Valsalva maneuver) or with compression of the internal jugular veins (Furstenberg's sign) [11]. The majority of nasal dermoids manifest along the nasal dorsum (60%), with 30% occurring intranasally and 10% having a combined presentation [12]. With endonasal presentations, nasal dermoids typically manifest endoscopically as a bilaterally protruding submucosal mass along the nasal septum [4]. Commonly, sebaceous material can be expressed from the sinus tract and recurrent infections are likewise commonplace. Intracranial communication predisposes to intracranial spread of infection resulting in meningitis, cavernous sinus thrombosis, or brain abscess [11]. If left in place, distortion in nasal development may arise thereby dictating the need for prompt surgical removal [13].

Imaging

Radiologic imaging is an essential component in the clinical workup of a congenital midline nasal mass for the purposes of diagnostic confirmation, evaluation of intracranial extension, and operative planning. Both MRI and thin-section high-resolution CT are valuable imaging modalities for diagnosing and delimiting the extent of nasal dermoids, providing complimentary information. Historically, imaging algorithms dictated the need for both CT and MRI in the workup of nasal dermoids. Recent literature has increasingly advocated in favor of MRI as a first-line imaging modality due to concerns of ionizing radiation associated with CT in the pediatric population and demonstration of a higher sensitivity of MRI in the detection of intracranial extension [9, 14]. The latter observation is particularly relevant in the neonate and infant presenting with a midline nasal mass due to normal anatomic variations present in the nasofrontal region of this age group that may be mistaken for radiologic evidence of intracranial extension. These normal variations include the presence of a midline gap between the nasal bones which may be confused for a dermal sinus tract, non-ossification of the cribriform plate which can be mistaken for a communication between the anterior cranial fossa and nasal cavity, and fatty replacement of the crista galli which ordinarily occurs by age 5 and may be confused with the presence of a dermoid cyst [6]. Fat may also be normally distributed within the nasal bones and nasal process of the frontal bone con-

tributing further to diagnostic pitfalls in the radiologic identification of nasal dermoids [15].

While the literature may suggest a more judicious application of CT in the diagnostic workup of nasal dermoids, the superior bony detail it provides is of considerable value in guiding preoperative decision-making and may also supplement ambiguous MRI findings. CT findings consistent with intracranial extension include a widened foramen cecum (which can be as wide as 10 mm normally) and a bifid crista galli (Fig. 27.1) [11]. While these findings raise suspicion of intracranial extension, they are by no means pathognomonic. Both may manifest in the absence of intracranial extension, brought about by the presence of fibrous tissue connecting the dermoid cyst to adjacent dura [16]. Conversely, an absent foramen cecum and normal crista galli render the presence of intracranial extension unlikely [8]. The addition of contrast may be of benefit in visualizing the immature cartilaginous anterior cranial fossa [14] and in cases of suspected infection [6]. Multiplanar high-resolution MRI provides superior soft tissue detail

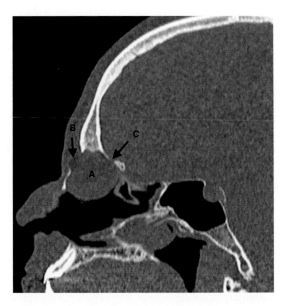

Fig. 27.1 Preoperative CT scan of a nasal dermoid. Preoperative CT scan, bone window, sagittal view of a nasal dermoid. The lesion (**A**) is relatively isodense to adjacent brain matter and soft tissues of the nose. The expansile nature of the lesion has eroded portions of the nasal bones (**B**) and anterior skull base (**C**)

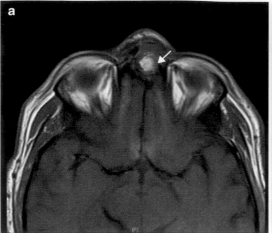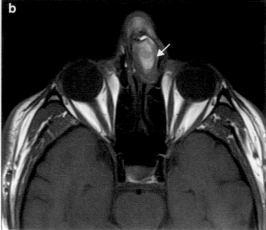

Fig. 27.2 Preoperative MRI of a nasal dermoid. Preoperative MRI, T1-weighted, non-infused axial view of a nasal dermoid at the level of the orbits. An intrinsic hyperintense T1-weighted intralesional signal (arrows in **a**, **b**) is seen indicative of fatty internal contents, an important radiologic feature differentiating nasal dermoids from other midline nasal masses such as nasal glioma

compared to CT and best delimits local disease extension both extracranially and intracranially (Fig. 27.2). The addition of gadolinium contrast facilitates the differentiation of non-enhancing nasal dermoids with other enhancing lesions such as hemangiomas and teratomas as well as normally enhancing nasal mucosa [4]. An additional important radiologic feature of nasal dermoids on MRI is an intrinsic hyperintense T1-weighted intralesional signal indicative of fatty internal contents. This finding serves to differentiate nasal dermoids from other midline nasal masses such as nasal gliomas which are typically hypointense on T1 compared to cerebral gray matter [17].

Histology

Histologically, nasal dermoids are defined as a keratinizing squamous epithelium-lined cyst containing mesodermal adnexal structures. The presence of adnexal structures (hair follicles, glandular structures) serves to histologically differentiate nasal dermoids from epidermoid cysts which do not contain the latter. Similarly, presence of all three embryonic layers (endoderm, mesoderm, and ectoderm) distinguishes teratomas from dermoids, the latter lacking endodermal elements [6].

Surgical Management

Definitive management of nasal dermoids includes complete surgical resection of both the cyst and associated sinus tract. Failure to do so has been demonstrated to confer a rate of recurrence of up to 100% in some series [11, 18]. Early intervention is advocated to minimize potential distortions in nasal cosmesis as well as potentially devastating infectious complications [9]. The ideal surgical approach should adhere to the following four basic tenets first described by Pollock et al. [19]: (1) provide exposure to all midline lesions and readily permit medial and lateral osteotomies, (2) provide exposure to the skull base and permit rapid repair of a defect and control of a cerebrospinal fluid (CSF) leak, (3) permit reconstruction of the nasal dorsum, and (4) allow for cosmetically acceptable scar formation. Both open and endoscopic approaches have been described, the former being more commonplace, with the lesion's extent and location dictating the preferred surgical approach. Presence of an external punctum requires an external incision, with a midline vertical incision incorporating the punctum most often employed which permits adequate exposure for resection of small sinus tracts. Open rhinoplasty approaches permit the resection of longer tracts or subcutaneous lesions within the lower soft tissue vault of the nose. Nasal osteotomies may be performed to correct an open roof deformity subsequent to diastasis of the nasal bones or to optimize exposure of the sinus tract [14]. Traditionally, a bifrontal craniotomy was employed to address nasal dermoids tracking intracranially with this approach increasingly falling out of favor due to the associated risks of brain edema and olfactory impairment secondary to brain retraction. More recently, a subcranial approach has been described which provides excellent exposure of the anterior cranial fossa without the need for brain retraction and minimal impact on long-term growth of the facial skeleton [20–22]. Descriptions of endoscopic endonasal approaches for the resection of endonasal and/or intracranial components are comparatively few, with a recent evidence-based review listing five studies totaling eight patients wherein complete surgical resection was accomplished in all instances [4]. Accruing surgical experience with expanded endonasal approaches for the management of intracranial pathology in both adult and pediatric patient populations suggests that midline nasal masses are likewise amenable to such minimally invasive approaches as an alternative to traditional open approaches [23]. In cases of skin involvement, an endoscopic approach may be combined with a limited midline vertical excision allowing for resection of the punctum and sinus tract up to the endonasal portion of the resection (Figs. 27.3 and 27.4) [4].

Nasal Gliomas and Encephaloceles

Epidemiology

Nasal gliomas and congenital encephaloceles are both relatively rare midline nasal masses. Only 250 cases of nasal glioma have been reported in the English literature, with a 3:2 male to female ratio observed and no known familial predisposition [24]. An increased incidence of encephaloceles has been observed in Southeast Asia (1:5000 live births) compared to Western countries (1:40,000) though the exact explanation for this geographic distribution has yet to be clearly defined [25]. The distribution of encephaloceles based on location is also known to vary geo-

graphically, with the occipital type predominating in Western countries and the sincipital/nasal type predominating in Southeast Asia [26].

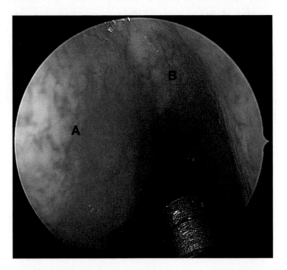

Fig. 27.3 Preoperative endoscopic view of nasal dermoid. Preoperative endoscopic view of the left nasal cavity demonstrating fullness in the region of the superior septum (**A**) and roof of the nasal vault (**B**) corresponding to the location of a nasal dermoid

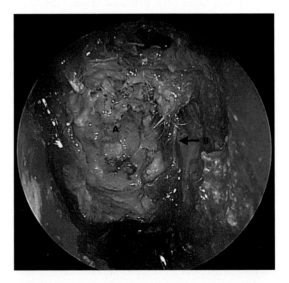

Fig. 27.4 Intraoperative endoscopic view of nasal dermoid contents. Intraoperative endoscopic view of a nasal dermoid as seen through the left nasal cavity. The anterior face of the lesion has been unroofed revealing its internal contents (**A**) comprised of hair follicles and glandular secretions. A squamous epithelium lining (**B**) is clearly visualized surrounding the cyst contents

Pathophysiology

Several mechanisms for the pathogenesis of nasal gliomas and encephaloceles have been described with the encephalocele theory being the most widely accepted view. This theory attributes the formation of nasal gliomas and encephaloceles to faulty closure of the anterior neuropore and failed regression of the dural diverticulum, which ordinarily protrudes through the foramen cecum or fonticulus nasofrontalis during development in utero. In the case of encephaloceles, intracranial tissue herniates into the extracranial dural projection through a patent foramen cecum or fonticulus nasofrontalis thereby maintaining a direct central nervous system (CNS) communication. Conversely, nasal gliomas are sequestered encephaloceles, wherein brain parenchyma is heterotopically situated extracranially due to prior closure of the cranial vault during gestation [24, 27]. In up to 20%, a fibrous stalk remains allowing for a communication between the glioma and the intracranial space (Fig. 27.5) [27]. Extranasal gliomas arise via herniation through the fonticulus nasofrontalis, whereas intranasal gliomas herniate through the foramen cecum and become sequestered within the prenasal space. The term glioma is in fact a misnomer as it implies a true neoplasm. It is now more widely termed nasal neuroglial/cerebral heterotopia given the absence of neoplastic features and its developmental origin as a sequestered mass of neuroglial tissue [2].

Classification

Congenital encephaloceles are classified based on their contents and the site of the cranial defect. Encephalocele is an umbrella term that refers to the herniation of intracranial contents through a defect in the skull base. A meningocele implies a herniation of the meninges with CSF; a meningoencephalocele refers to the herniation of meninges, brain parenchyma, and CSF; and a meningoencephalocystocele designates the herniation of meninges, brain parenchyma, CSF, and ventricles (Fig. 27.6). The most widely employed site-based classification organizes encephaloceles into occipital, sincipital/nasal (also termed frontoethmoidal), or basal encephaloceles. In Western countries, occipital encephaloceles comprise the majority of cases (75%), whereas sin-

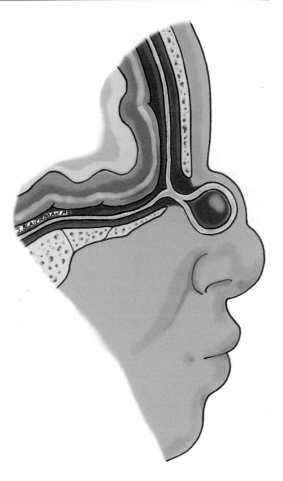

Fig. 27.5 Nasal glioma. Illustration demonstrating a nasal glioma with a persistent fibrous stalk communicating intracranially via an anterior skull base defect

cipital (15%) and basal (10%) are far less frequent. Sincipital encephaloceles manifest externally in the midface and are subdivided into nasofrontal (herniation through both foramen cecum and fonticulus nasofrontalis), nasoethmoidal (herniation into the prenasal space via the foramen cecum), and naso-orbital encephaloceles, of which the nasofrontal subtype is the most common (up to 60%) [28]. Basal encephaloceles most often manifest intranasally and are subdivided into transethmoidal (through the cribriform plate), sphenoethmoidal (through the sphenoethmoidal junction), transsphenoidal (through the sphenoid body), sphenomaxillary (through the junction of the sphenoid body and wing into the pterygopalatine fossa), or sphenoorbital (through the superior orbital fissure) vari-

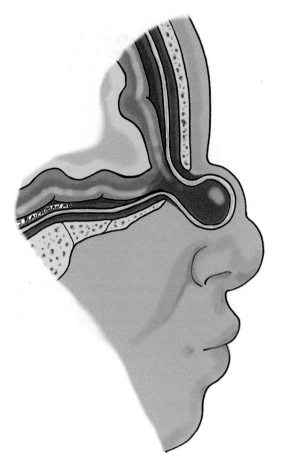

Fig. 27.6 Nasal encephalocele (red shaded area). Illustration demonstrating herniation of a cerebrospinal fluid-filled sac corresponding to an encephalocele with an associated anterior skull base defect

ations [25]. Nasal gliomas may be classified into extranasal (60%), intranasal (30%), or a combination of the two (10%) [2].

Clinical Presentation
Nasal gliomas, when present extranasally, appear as a firm, noncompressible, smooth, skin-covered mass most commonly located in the glabellar region [28]. Its bluish hue and telangiectatic surface may be mistaken for a hemangioma or vascular malformation [27]. Intranasal gliomas appear as a pale, polyp-like mass within the nasal cavity arising most commonly from the lateral nasal wall at the axilla of the middle turbinate [24]. Nasal gliomas may be distinguished clinically from encephaloceles, as

the former fails to enlarge with maneuvers that may elevate intracranial pressure (Valsalva maneuver, coughing, crying, Furstenberg sign) due to their lack of communication with the intracranial compartment [27].

The presentation of encephaloceles may likewise vary based on the site of the cranial defect. Sincipital encephaloceles typically present as a midfacial mass at the nasofrontal suture (nasofrontal), along the nasal sidewall at the junction between the nasal bone and cartilage (nasoethmoidal) or at the medial canthal region (naso-orbital). A broad nasal root and hypertelorism may also be present [15]. Basal encephaloceles, like intranasal gliomas, may mimic a nasal polyp though they typically originate medial to the middle turbinate. Basal encephaloceles or intranasal gliomas may present with upper airway obstruction and respiratory distress owing to the obligate nasal breathing that characterizes the neonatal period [25].

Imaging
MRI is the imaging modality of choice for the initial evaluation of both nasal gliomas and encephaloceles. In so far as encephaloceles, MRI is better able to ascertain the extent and nature of the herniated contents in addition to screening for any associated intracranial anomalies [28]. Herniated brain parenchyma is typically isointense to normal brain tissue though hyperintensity on T2-weighted sequences may be seen due to gliosis and surrounding CSF [2]. Communication of the herniated contents with the intracranial compartment is critical for diagnosis [15]. Nasal gliomas display similar MR characteristics save for the lack of an intracranial communication.

High-resolution CT imaging provides complementary information in so far as detailing the bony anatomy and morphology of the skull base defect [29]. The limitations of this imaging modality in the infant have been previously outlined, with the potential for erroneous interpretations of skull base defects attributed to incomplete ossification of the skull base seen in this age group. Three-dimensional CT reconstructions may also be of value for surgical planning and preoperative family counseling [30].

Finally, Doppler ultrasound may be valuable in differentiating extranasal gliomas, which display a low diastolic flow velocity, from vascular anomalies such as hemangiomas which display a high diastolic flow velocity, particularly during the proliferative phase [15, 31].

Histology

It is often challenging to histologically distinguish nasal glioma and encephalocele as both may be comprised either exclusively or predominantly of glial tissue [29]. Histologic features that strongly favor the diagnosis of glioma include the presence of leptomeninges, ependyma, or choroid plexus [27]. Should these features be absent, the diagnosis is made on the grounds of both clinical and radiologic information [24, 29].

Surgical Management

Overriding Surgical Principles

Surgical intervention is the mainstay of treatment for both nasal gliomas and encephaloceles. While the ideal timing for surgery for nasal gliomas or encephaloceles has yet to be clearly defined, circumstances that dictate urgent operative intervention include complete nasal airway obstruction, active CSF leak, apparent skin defect and/or ulceration, and infectious complications including intracranial spread [25]. While the literature to date lacks high-grade evidence quantifying the long-term risk of meningitis in patients with congenital encephalocele, anecdotal evidence from a small case series suggests that the risk is quite low in the absence of a CSF leak [32]. This is often the situation with both sincipital and basal encephaloceles given that both more often present with intact skin or an epidermal lining thereby allowing for an adequate barrier between the intracranial space and the external non-sterile environment. Additional considerations for early intervention exist for lesions that distort the facial skeleton, with concerns that delaying surgery may further exacerbate any existing facial deformity [25]. There exists some debate in the literature as to which types of lesions this encompasses with some authors arguing that even certain basal encephaloceles, if sufficiently large and/or anterior, have

the potential to create craniofacial distortion (e.g. telecanthus) if surgical intervention is delayed [32].

The remainder of cases should be addressed in a timely manner sometime during the course of early childhood though discrepancy exists in the literature as to the exact age this entails, ranging from the age of 3 months to age 5 [26, 32, 33]. The rationale given for this delay, particularly when an endoscopic approach is planned, includes allowing for sufficient facial growth to transpire. This augments both the nasal aperture and distal surgical corridor thereby rendering an endoscopic approach more feasible. It also ensures the child is better suited to tolerate intraoperative blood loss and the physiologic changes associated with general anesthesia [26, 32].

The extensive nature of these lesions frequently dictates a two-team approach with our neurosurgical colleagues, not unlike the existing relationship between otolaryngologists and neurosurgeons widely practiced in the vast majority of skull base centers worldwide. Close communication with a neuroradiologist is also invaluable in characterizing the nature of the lesion and associated skull-based defect in view of establishing the most appropriate surgical plan for the pathology in question. Intrathecal fluorescein injection may be considered to supplement deficiencies intrinsic to pediatric neuroimaging by improving the likelihood of identifying multiple and/or occult CSF leaks. Safety of this technique has been well demonstrated in both adult and pediatric populations when employed with the correct dosage [34].

The overriding surgical aim is to create a surgical corridor that permits optimal exposure for complete resection of the lesion while taking into consideration the postoperative cosmetic result, which invariably includes the correction of any existing facial deformity. Resection of the herniated or sequestered brain matter does not predispose to an increased risk of neurologic deficit given that it is devoid of normally functioning brain parenchyma. An exception to this would be in the case of a transsphenoidal encephalocele that may contain vital structures (hypothalamus, optic nerve, or portions of the circle of Willis), which must be reduced and not resected [35].

Surgical Approaches

The approach-based algorithm for the surgical management of nasal gliomas and encephaloceles mirrors that of nasal dermoids in that both external and endoscopic approaches are described, with the location and extent of the pathology ultimately dictating the preferred approach. Extranasal gliomas are preferentially excised via an open rhinoplasty approach that provides adequate exposure and a favorable cosmetic outcome due to discrete scar placement. Vertical midline or bicoronal incisions may be required in particularly large lesions or those with a significant rostral extent. Nasal osteotomies can facilitate exposure of components deep to the nasal bones with extension toward and through the anterior skull base such as in the case of a fibrous stalk [24]. Intranasal gliomas are increasingly approached with a purely endoscopic approach, including any intracranial component, applying the same principles that govern expanded endoscopic approaches for other skull base pathologies. The advantage of this approach includes scar avoidance and preservation of normal facial anatomy without comprising completeness of resection [29]. The surgical approach for congenital encephaloceles is quite analogous, with the extranasal portion seen in sincipital encephaloceles approached via a bicoronal incision and the intranasal component seen in either basal or sincipital encephaloceles resected via an endoscopic approach. A shift in the literature can be observed as of late with an increasing acceptance and promotion of endonasal approaches for both intracranial resection and repair of the skull base defect associated with congenital encephalocele. A variety of endoscopic reconstructive methods have been reported, with both free grafts (e.g., fascia lata) and pedicled vascularized flaps (e.g., nasoseptal flap, inferior turbinate flap) described [24, 25, 32, 34, 36].

Intracranial Complications of Pediatric Frontal Sinusitis

Epidemiology

Intracranial spread of infection secondary to paranasal sinusitis is a rare complication most commonly associated with acute involvement of the frontal sinus [37–39]. The reported incidence of sinogenic intracranial complications ranges from 3% to 17% [40–42], whereas the largest pediatric series of patients admitted for acute sinusitis reported a 3% intracranial complication rate [43]. Adolescent males between the ages of 11 and 15 appear to be the most frequently affected group, though the exact reason for this association remains to be clearly elucidated [38, 40, 44, 45]. Some authors have postulated a predisposition for intracranial spread in this age group due to a peak in vascularity of the diploic veins of the frontal sinus resulting in hematogenous intracranial spread of infection [46]. When individuals within this demographic group present with significant frontal sinus involvement, an accrued incidence of simultaneous intracranial and orbital complications of acute sinusitis is seen particularly in the context of a superior or superolaterally situated subperiosteal orbital abscess [42].

Pathophysiology

Intracranial spread of infection originating in the paranasal sinuses has been theorized to occur via one of two mechanisms: direct extension or hematogenously (retrograde thrombophlebitis). Direct extension of infection may occur via preformed pathways such as a dehiscence in the skull base (congenital or traumatic) or existing foramina or alternatively via erosions in the posterior frontal table due to osteomyelitis-induced necrosis [44]. Direct extension of infection is more commonly observed in otologic sources of intracranial infection than in sinusitis [47].

Hematogenous intracranial spread of frontal sinusitis is facilitated by the rich network of valveless diploic veins (also known as Bechet's plexus) that interconnects the vasculature of the sinus mucosa with the intracranial venous system. Owing to this communication, thrombophlebitis originating in the mucosal veins of the frontal sinus can progress in a retrograde fashion through this valveless venous network to the emissary skull veins, dural venous sinuses, and subdural and cerebral veins [44, 47].

Microbiology

The microbiology of sinusitis-induced intracranial infection has been studied extensively with an overall consensus described regarding the polymicrobial nature of this complication [47]. Anaerobic, aerobic, and microaerophilic bacteria are commonly isolated with streptococcal species, *Haemophilus influenzae*, and anaerobes identified as the most common causative organisms [44]. *Streptococcus milleri*, a common commensal organism of the oral, oropharyngeal, and nasopharyngeal flora, has drawn considerable attention by multiple publications in recent years citing it as the most common causative organism responsible for sinogenic intracranial complications [48–50]. In studies where both the sinus and associated intracranial infectious process were cultured, an overall concordance was seen in the microbiological organisms recovered [51].

Clinical Workup and Treatment Strategies

Sinusitis is often overlooked as the origin of an intracranial infection due in part to the rarity of this complication, absence of classic sinonasal symptoms, nonspecific clinical presentation, and possible masking of symptoms due to prior antibiotic exposure [40]. When present, neurological signs often portend a poor prognosis [48]. As such, radiologic imaging represents an important tool in the diagnosis and workup of sinogenic intracranial complications. Computed tomography (CT) scan of the brain has been advocated by some authors as the diagnostic modality of choice for intracranial complications with simultaneous acquisition of the sinuses to identify a potential infectious source [40]. Others have expressed caution with this imaging modality due to its reportedly poor sensitivity and poor correlation with intraoperative findings. In up to 50% of cases, an initial CT evaluation may overlook the presence of an intracranial infectious process [42]. Serial CT imaging is therefore recommended should a high index of suspicion remain in addition to assessing treatment response should an intracranial infection be identified initially. Some studies have demonstrated improved sensitivity of magnetic resonance imaging (MRI)

compared to CT, with the former demonstrating improved delineation of intracranial suppuration [42, 52, 53]. However, the need for sedation in young children, additional cost, and accessibility limitations associated with MRI have been cited as potential drawbacks [42].

Sinogenic intracranial complications necessitate the implementation of a concerted multidisciplinary management strategy comprised of microbiologists, otolaryngologists, neurosurgeons, and neuroradiologists. Surgical intervention strategies have evolved considerably in recent years with the advent of endoscopic sinus and skull base surgical approaches. While infectious complications of this nature were historically addressed exclusively via transcranial open neurosurgical approaches, endoscopic transnasal approaches are increasingly employed solely or in conjunction with traditional neurosurgical approaches. In a recent systematic review by Patel et al., subgroup analysis of the reviewed literature based on year of publication revealed that an increased proportion of patients with sinogenic intracranial complications underwent functional endoscopic sinus surgery (FESS) in recent studies compared to older publications [39].

Despite the attractiveness of a minimally invasive approach in the surgical management of pediatric sinogenic intracranial complications, there exists some debate in the literature as to the exact role and relevance of endoscopic sinus surgery in this disease entity's surgical algorithm. In a single-center retrospective cohort of pediatric sinogenic empyema, Garin et al. reviewed their surgical treatment outcomes over a 2-year period. Once again in this series, the frontal sinus was most frequently implicated as the anatomical origin for the intracranial infection based on radiologic imaging. Despite a relatively small sample size ($n = 17$), the authors highlighted vastly distinct treatment outcomes of neurosurgical versus sinus surgery treatment modalities based on the location of the empyema (subdural vs. epidural). In cases of subdural empyema, craniotomy was deemed vastly superior compared to sinus surgery. As an initial surgical procedure, its success rate was 100% compared to 14% when other techniques were employed. When all surgical procedures were considered, the success rate of craniotomy was 88% compared to 25% using other techniques. Limited success of ESS was observed in the setting of subdural empyema even in cases of limited extension. Based on this data, the authors discouraged the employment of ESS alone in the setting of subdural empyema, with craniotomy advised as the treatment modality of choice. Nonetheless, the authors did attribute some merit to FESS as an adjunctive procedure in cases of subdural empyema for the purposes of harvesting a bacteriological sample. In so far as epidural empyema, FESS was deemed as an appropriate alternative to craniotomy particularly in instances where direct endoscopic drainage of the collection is feasible through a Draf III approach. Wherein this is not feasible, an open craniotomy approach is preferred. Interestingly, no influence in surgical outcome was observed with drainage or obliteration of the frontal sinus [54].

A retrospective review by DelGaudio et al. likewise downplayed the relevance of FESS in the initial surgical management of sinogenic intracranial complications. In a cohort of 23 patients comprised of pediatric patients in majority (median age = 14), an acute frontal sinusitis was once again deemed to be the most important predisposing factor for intracranial infection. In patients with small (<1 cm) intracranial abscesses, the addition of FESS in conjunction with intravenous medical therapy as the initial management strategy did not appear to alter the subsequent need for an open neurosurgical intervention. Over 80% of these patients later underwent craniotomy for persistent or progressive intracranial disease despite resolution of their sinus disease. The author's rationale for this observation relates to the hematogenous intracranial spread of infection in sinogenic intracranial complications thereby precluding any immediate benefit with interventions aimed at establishing surgical drainage of the sinuses. Given the underwhelming data and challenges associated with FESS in the acute setting due to significant inflammation and bleeding, the authors ascribed a limited number of contexts in which FESS would be indicated in the management of intracranial complications of sinusitis. In cases where a direct extension of infection from the sinus to the intracranial space is clearly established, FESS, as per the authors, is indicated. Other indications for FESS listed by the authors include persistence or recurrence of intracranial infection despite adequate prior neurosurgical intervention or intracranial resolution of infection with persistent chronic rhinosinusitis despite maximal medical therapy. For small intracranial abscess (<1 cm) with no bony defect of the skull base identified and no neurological signs, conservative medical therapy alone (intravenous antibiotics and topical decongestants) is deemed as an appropriate initial treatment strategy by the authors with the addition of FESS yielding no additional benefit based on their reported experience [55]. One apparent limitation of this study was the absence of any subgroup analysis of treatment outcomes based on the nature and location of the intracranial infection. Subdural empyema comprised the most common complication of this cohort (43%) for which FESS has previously demonstrated limited benefit [54]. Whether this may have contributed to the underwhelming evidence in favor of FESS for the management of intracranial infection is unclear.

Other authors advocate in favor of an aggressive initial surgical management approach that entails a combination of FESS and open neurosurgical interventions. This strategy, argue the authors, allows for evacuation of the intracranial collection while providing infectious source control and microbiologic sampling via a rhinologic route. In a pediatric cohort of 27 children collected over a 5-year period, a variety of surgical approaches were employed based on surgeon preference with a combined FESS-craniotomy strategy performed in the majority of instances at initial presentation. The extensiveness of FESS likewise varied from minimal clearance of the ostiomeatal complex in conjunction with frontal sinus trephination to a more comprehensive endoscopic intervention comprising a complete dissection of the offending sinus and associated drainage pathway, the frontal sinus being the most commonly implicated. Interestingly, patients who underwent a more comprehensive versus a limited endoscopic approach demonstrated faster recovery with shorter length of stay, thereby supporting an aggressive rhinologic

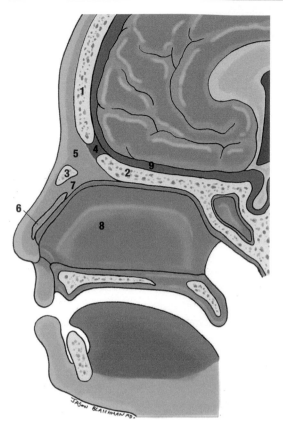

Fig. 27.7 Embryologic anatomy of the nose and anterior skull base. 1, frontal bone; 2, ethmoid bone; 3, nasal bone; 4, foramen cecum; 5, fonticulus nasofrontalis; 6, nasal cartilage;7, prenasal space; 8, nasal capsule; 9, dura

approach. Compared to this combined approach, both rhinologic and neurosurgical interventions employed in isolation demonstrated an increased likelihood of requiring further neurosurgical procedures. Altogether, this study's findings reinforce prior support for neurosurgical drainage procedures as a mainstay in the treatment of sinogenic intracranial infection with accrued benefit derived from the addition of a comprehensive endoscopic rhinologic procedure. Figure 27.7 summarizes the embryologic and anatomical underpinnings of congenital frontal pathology.

Summary

Congenital midline nasal masses represent a rare group of lesions that arise from faulty development of the anterior neuropore. An understanding of the embryologic underpinnings of this category of disorders provides critical insight into its clinical presentation and definitive management. The otolaryngologist and skull base surgeon comprise an essential role in the multidisciplinary effort responsible for the diagnosis, clinical workup, and definitive management of these conditions. A transition in the surgical management of these disease processes is observed in recent literature, with an endoscopic approach increasingly favored for the extirpation of both intranasal and intracranial portions in addition to the reconstruction of any associated skull base defect.

Acute frontal sinusitis is among the most important predisposing factors for intracranial spread of infection with adolescent males most frequently affected. The potential for neurological sequelae and death arising from this complication dictates prompt recognition and management with varying treatment strategies described in the literature. While neurosurgical drainage remains critical in the initial surgical approach of this infectious complication, a comprehensive endoscopic rhinologic approach has proven to be complementary in some instances. Nonetheless, further clarification is required to determine when and in whom would FESS be optimally beneficial.

Disclosure None for either author.

References

1. Krakovitz PR, Koltai PJ. Neonatal nasal obstruction. NeoReviews. 2007;8:e199–205.
2. Baxter DJ, Shroff M. Congenital midface abnormalities. Neuroimaging Clin N Am. 2011;21(3):563–84. vii-viii
3. Rohrich RJ, Lowe JB, Schwartz MR. The role of open rhinoplasty in the management of nasal dermoid cysts. Plast Reconstr Surg. 1999;104(5):1459–66; quiz 67; discussion 68
4. Pinheiro-Neto CD, Snyderman CH, Fernandez-Miranda J, Gardner PA. Endoscopic endonasal surgery for nasal dermoids. Otolaryngol Clin N Am. 2011;44(4):981–7, ix
5. Denoyelle F, Ducroz V, Roger G, Garabedian EN. Nasal dermoid sinus cysts in children. Laryngoscope. 1997;107(6):795–800.

6. Zapata S, Kearns DB. Nasal dermoids. Curr Opin Otolaryngol Head Neck Surg. 2006;14(6):406–11.
7. Wardinsky TD, Pagon RA, Kropp RJ, Hayden PW, Clarren SK. Nasal dermoid sinus cysts: association with intracranial extension and multiple malformations. Cleft Palate Craniofac J. 1991;28(1):87–95.
8. Paradis J, Koltai PJ. Pediatric teratoma and dermoid cysts. Otolaryngol Clin N Am. 2015;48(1):121–36.
9. Hanikeri M, Waterhouse N, Kirkpatrick N, Peterson D, Macleod I. The management of midline transcranial nasal dermoid sinus cysts. Br J Plast Surg. 2005;58(8):1043–50.
10. Sreetharan V, Kangesu L, Sommerlad BC. Atypical congenital dermoids of the face: a 25-year experience. J Plast Reconstr Aesthet Surg. 2007;60(9):1025–9.
11. Bloom DC, Carvalho DS, Dory C, Brewster DF, Wickersham JK, Kearns DB. Imaging and surgical approach of nasal dermoids. Int J Pediatr Otorhinolaryngol. 2002;62(2):111–22.
12. Szeremeta W, Parikh TD, Widelitz JS. Congenital nasal malformations. Otolaryngol Clin N Am. 2007;40(1):97–112, vi–vii
13. Heywood RL, Lyons MJ, Cochrane LA, Hayward R, Hartley BE. Excision of nasal dermoids with intracranial extension – anterior small window craniotomy approach. Int J Pediatr Otorhinolaryngol. 2007;71(8):1193–6.
14. Herrington H, Adil E, Moritz E, Robson C, Perez-Atayde A, Proctor M, et al. Update on current evaluation and management of pediatric nasal dermoid. Laryngoscope. 2016;126(9):2151–60.
15. Hedlund G. Congenital frontonasal masses: developmental anatomy, malformations, and MR imaging. Pediatr Radiol. 2006;36(7):647–62; quiz 726–7
16. Pensler JM, Bauer BS, Naidich TP. Craniofacial dermoids. Plast Reconstr Surg. 1988;82(6):953–8.
17. Huisman TA, Schneider JF, Kellenberger CJ, Martin-Fiori E, Willi UV, Holzmann D. Developmental nasal midline masses in children: neuroradiological evaluation. Eur Radiol. 2004;14(2):243–9.
18. Posnick JC, Bortoluzzi P, Armstrong DC, Drake JM. Intracranial nasal dermoid sinus cysts: computed tomographic scan findings and surgical results. Plast Reconstr Surg. 1994;93(4):745–54; discussion 55–6
19. Pollock RA. Surgical approaches to the nasal dermoid cyst. Ann Plast Surg. 1983;10(6):498–501.
20. Kellman RM, Goyal P, Rodziewicz GS. The transglabellar subcranial approach for nasal dermoids with intracranial extension. Laryngoscope. 2004;114(8):1368–72.
21. Goyal P, Kellman RM, Tatum SA 3rd. Transglabellar subcranial approach for the management of nasal masses with intracranial extension in pediatric patients. Arch Facial Plast Surg. 2007;9(5):314–7.
22. Shlomi B, Chaushu S, Gil Z, Chaushu G, Fliss DM. Effects of the subcranial approach on facial growth and development. Otolaryngol Head Neck Surg. 2007;136(1):27–32.
23. Khalili S, Palmer JN, Adappa ND. The expanded endonasal approach for the treatment of intracranial skull base disease in the pediatric population. Curr Opin Otolaryngol Head Neck Surg. 2015;23(1):65–70.
24. Rahbar R, Resto VA, Robson CD, Perez-Atayde AR, Goumnerova LC, McGill TJ, et al. Nasal glioma and encephalocele: diagnosis and management. Laryngoscope. 2003;113(12):2069–77.
25. Tirumandas M, Sharma A, Gbenimacho I, Shoja MM, Tubbs RS, Oakes WJ, et al. Nasal encephaloceles: a review of etiology, pathophysiology, clinical presentations, diagnosis, treatment, and complications. Childs Nerv Syst. 2013;29(5):739–44.
26. Singh AK, Upadhyaya DN. Sincipital encephaloceles. J Craniofac Surg. 2009;20(Suppl 2):1851–5.
27. Ajose-Popoola O, Lin HW, Silvera VM, Teot LA, Madsen JR, Meara JG, et al. Nasal glioma: prenatal diagnosis and multidisciplinary surgical approach. Skull Base Rep. 2011;1(2):83–8.
28. Lowe LH, Booth TN, Joglar JM, Rollins NK. Midface anomalies in children. Radiographics. 2000;20(4):907–22; quiz 1106–7, 12
29. Adil E, Robson C, Perez-Atayde A, Heffernan C, Moritz E, Goumnerova L, et al. Congenital nasal neuroglial heterotopia and encephaloceles: an update on current evaluation and management. Laryngoscope. 2016;126(9):2161–7.
30. Schlosser RJ, Faust RA, Phillips CD, Gross CW. Three-dimensional computed tomography of congenital nasal anomalies. Int J Pediatr Otorhinolaryngol. 2002;65(2):125–31.
31. Dasgupta NR, Bentz ML. Nasal gliomas: identification and differentiation from hemangiomas. J Craniofac Surg. 2003;14(5):736–8.
32. Woodworth BA, Schlosser RJ, Faust RA, Bolger WE. Evolutions in the management of congenital intranasal skull base defects. Arch Otolaryngol Head Neck Surg. 2004;130(11):1283–8.
33. Keshri A, Shah S, Patadia S, Sahu R, Behari S. Transnasal endoscopic repair of pediatric meningoencephalocele. J Pediatr Neurosci. 2016;11(1):42–5. https://doi.org/10.4103/1817-745.181249.
34. Castelnuovo P, Bignami M, Pistochini A, Battaglia P, Locatelli D, Dallan I. Endoscopic endonasal management of encephaloceles in children: an eight-year experience. Int J Pediatr Otorhinolaryngol. 2009;73(8): 1132–6.
35. Hoving EW. Nasal encephaloceles. Childs Nerv Syst. 2000;16(10–11):702–6.
36. Nogueira JF Jr, Stamm AC, Vellutini E, Santos FP. Endoscopic management of congenital meningoencephalocele with nasal flaps. Int J Pediatr Otorhinolaryngol. 2009;73(1):133–7.
37. Lang EE, Curran AJ, Patil N, Walsh RM, Rawluk D, Walsh MA. Intracranial complications of acute frontal sinusitis. Clin Otolaryngol Allied Sci. 2001;26(6):452–7.
38. Oxford LE, McClay J. Complications of acute sinusitis in children. Otolaryngol Head Neck Surg. 2005;133(1):32–7.
39. Patel NA, Garber D, Hu S, Kamat A. Systematic review and case report: intracranial complications

of pediatric sinusitis. Int J Pediatr Otorhinolaryngol. 2016;86:200–12.

40. Ong YK, Tan HK. Suppurative intracranial complications of sinusitis in children. Int J Pediatr Otorhinolaryngol. 2002;66(1):49.

41. Reid JR. Complications of pediatric paranasal sinusitis. Pediatr Radiol. 2004;34(12):933–42.

42. Herrmann BW, Forsen JW Jr. Simultaneous intracranial and orbital complications of acute rhinosinusitis in children. Int J Pediatr Otorhinolaryngol. 2004;68(5):619–25.

43. Lerner DN, Choi SS, Zalzal GH, Johnson DL. Intracranial complications of sinusitis in childhood. Ann Otol Rhinol Laryngol. 1995;104(4 Pt 1):288–93.

44. Kombogiorgas D, Seth R, Athwal R, Modha J, Singh J. Suppurative intracranial complications of sinusitis in adolescence. Single institute experience and review of literature. Br J Neurosurg. 2007;21(6):603–9.

45. Glickstein JS, Chandra RK, Thompson JW. Intracranial complications of pediatric sinusitis. Otolaryngol Head Neck Surg. 2006;134(5):733–6.

46. Quraishi H, Zevallos JP. Subdural empyema as a complication of sinusitis in the pediatric population. Int J Pediatr Otorhinolaryngol. 2006;70(9):1581–6.

47. Brook I. Microbiology and antimicrobial treatment of orbital and intracranial complications of sinusitis in children and their management. Int J Pediatr Otorhinolaryngol. 2009;73(9):1183–6.

48. Patel AP, Masterson L, Deutsch CJ, Scoffings DJ, Fish BM. Management and outcomes in children

with sinogenic intracranial abscesses. Int J Pediatr Otorhinolaryngol. 2015;79(6):868–73.

49. Jones RL, Violaris NS, Chavda SV, Pahor AL. Intracranial complications of sinusitis: the need for aggressive management. J Laryngol Otol. 1995;109(11):1061–2.

50. Fenton JE, Smyth DA, Viani LG, Walsh MA. Sinogenic brain abscess. Am J Rhinol. 1999;13(4):299–302.

51. Brook I, Frazier EH. Microbiology of subperiosteal orbital abscess and associated maxillary sinusitis. Laryngoscope. 1996;106(8):1010–3.

52. Germiller JA, Monin DL, Sparano AM, Tom LW. Intracranial complications of sinusitis in children and adolescents and their outcomes. Arch Otolaryngol Head Neck Surg. 2006;132(9):969–76.

53. Felsenstein S, Williams B, Shingadia D, Coxon L, Riordan A, Demetriades AK, et al. Clinical and microbiologic features guiding treatment recommendations for brain abscesses in children. Pediatr Infect Dis J. 2013;32(2):129–35.

54. Garin A, Thierry B, Leboulanger N, Blauwblomme T, Grevent D, Blanot S, et al. Pediatric sinogenic epidural and subdural empyema: the role of endoscopic sinus surgery. Int J Pediatr Otorhinolaryngol. 2015;79(10):1752–60.

55. DelGaudio JM, Evans SH, Sobol SE, Parikh SL. Intracranial complications of sinusitis: what is the role of endoscopic sinus surgery in the acute setting. Am J Otolaryngol. 2010;31(1):25–8.

Optimal Strategies in Medical Management of Frontal Sinusitis

28

Kristine A. Smith, Jeremiah A. Alt,
and Richard R. Orlandi

Introduction

Chronic rhinosinusitis (CRS) is an inflammatory condition of the sinonasal passages [1]. Medical therapy is an essential component in the management of CRS and is often necessary for successful long-term symptom control and the prevention of disease recurrence [2]. The primary goal of medical therapy is to reduce sinonasal mucosal inflammation [2]. The frontal sinus is the most complex sinus to manage in patients with CRS, in part due to its challenging anatomy. Delivery of topical medications to the frontal recess is limited by its anterosuperior position as well as the presence of variable and complex frontal cells, which may partially or completely obstruct the frontal recess [3, 4]. While endoscopic sinus surgery (ESS) may improve the delivery of medication to the frontal recess, stenosis and disease recurrence are common, and prolonged medical therapy is often required [2, 5].

There is increasing evidence to suggest that different endotypes and phenotypes of CRS exist and may influence which therapies are effective [6, 7]. Currently, CRS is divided into two main phenotypic groups: CRS with nasal polyposis (CRSwNP) and without nasal polyposis (CRSsNP) [1, 4]. While there is overlap between the management of these two groups, it diverges in some areas, and not all therapies are equally effective between or within these two groups [8]. As the pathogenesis of CRS becomes more defined, medications targeting specific processes are being developed in hopes of providing more effective patient-specific treatment processes.

A variety of medical therapies are currently available for the management of CRS and many innovative therapies are being investigated. Understanding the different types of therapies available, as well as the evidence and role for these therapies, is essential to aid clinicians in managing frontal sinusitis. The objective of this chapter is to review the available medical therapies, the most up-to-date evidence for these therapies, and their role in the management of frontal sinusitis.

Medical Management of Chronic Rhinosinusitis

The mainstay of the management of CRS includes saline irrigations and topical intranasal corticosteroids [2, 4]. In addition, systemic therapies

K. A. Smith
Division of Otolaryngology – Head and Neck Surgery, Department of Surgery, University of Calgary, Calgary, AB, USA

J. A. Alt · R. R. Orlandi (✉)
Division of Otolaryngology – Head and Neck Surgery, University of Utah School of Medicine, Salt Lake City, UT, USA

© Springer Nature Switzerland AG 2019
D. Lal, P. H. Hwang (eds.), *Frontal Sinus Surgery*, https://doi.org/10.1007/978-3-319-97022-6_28

such as corticosteroids and antibiotics are often utilized for patients with severe symptoms or disease flares. The role of additional therapies such as allergy treatment has also been investigated. As the pathophysiology of CRS is better understand, innovative biologic treatments have been developed and are currently under investigation. This section will review these medical therapies. However, many of these therapies have not been evaluated for their specific impact on frontal sinusitis. Where possible, their role in the specific management of frontal sinusitis will be discussed. Table 28.1 details the available medical therapies for CRS.

Table 28.1 Medical therapies for chronic rhinosinusitis

	Recommendation		Consideration for frontal sinusitis
	CRSwNP	CRSsNP	
Topical intranasal therapies			
Saline irrigations	Recommendation for[a]	Recommendation for[a]	High-volume or nasal drops for improved penetration to frontal recess
Topical intranasal Corticosteroids	Recommendation for[a]	Recommendation for[a]	
Topical antibiotics	Recommendation against	Recommendation against	–
Topical antifungals	Recommendation against	Recommendation against	–
Manuka honey	*No recommendation*	*No recommendation*	–
Surfactants	*No recommendation*	*No recommendation*	–
Xylitol	*No recommendation*	*No recommendation*	–
Drug-eluting stents	Treatment option	Treatment option	May improve frontal recess patency and short term outcomes
Systemic therapies			
Systemic corticosteroids	Recommendation for[a]	Treatment option	May improve patency of frontal recess to improve delivery of topical therapies
Systemic antibiotics			
Short-term antibiotics	Treatment option	Recommendation for[a]	–
Long-term antibiotics	Treatment option	Recommendation for[a]	–
Leukotriene receptor antagonist	Treatment option	*No recommendation*	–
Allergy therapy[b]			
Antihistamines	Treatment option[b]	Treatment option[b]	–
Allergy immunotherapy	Treatment option[b]	Treatment option[b]	–
Aspirin desensitization	Treatment option[b]	*No recommendation*	–
Biologic therapies			
Anti-immunoglobulin E therapy	Treatment option	*No recommendation*	–
Anti-interleukin-5 therapy	Treatment option	*No recommendation*	–
Anti-interleukin-4 therapy	Treatment option	*No recommendation*	–

Adapted from the International Consensus Statement on Allergy and Rhinology: Rhinosinusitis [4]
Recommendation for: therapy is recommended in routine CRS management
Recommendation against: therapy is not recommended for routine CRS management
Treatment option: may be considered on a case-by-case basis
No recommendation: inadequate evidence available to make a recommendation for or against therapy
CRSwNP chronic rhinosinusitis with nasal polyposis, *CRSsNP* chronic rhinosinusitis without nasal polyposis
[a]As a part of appropriate medical therapy recommendations
[b]May be considered in patients with comorbid allergic disease

Topical Intranasal Therapies

Saline Irrigations

Saline irrigations are one of the most common treatment modalities for CRS, and their clinical effectiveness has been well established [2, 9]. Sinonasal irrigations decrease inflammation by removing mucus and environmental irritants while aiding in mucociliary clearance [2]. Irrigations have been shown to improve disease-specific quality of life (QoL) and have a synergistic benefit when combined with topical intranasal corticosteroids [9, 10]. High-volume saline irrigations (>50 ml) can also be used to deliver topical medications to the sinonasal cavity, such as budesonide. High-volume techniques have also been shown to have better penetration in the frontal recess and frontal sinus [11]. High-volume sinonasal saline irrigations are currently recommended as part of appropriate medical therapy (AMT) for all CRS patients [4, 12].

Topical Intranasal Corticosteroids

Topical intranasal corticosteroids are a staple in the management of CRS. They reduce sinonasal inflammation by decreasing vascular permeability, reducing glycoprotein release from submucosal glands, and reducing mucus viscosity [2, 10]. Intranasal corticosteroids have the highest grade of evidence supporting their use in CRS patients [2]. They have been associated with improvements in overall symptom scores, improvements in QoL and reduction in polyp size in CRSwNP [10]. Corticosteroid sprays are the most common form of intranasal corticosteroids used, and multiple formulations are available; no one formulation has been shown to be superior to the others [2]. The off-label use of budesonide respules has become increasingly common, due to its proven clinical effectiveness and improved distribution to the paranasal sinuses utilizing high-volume saline irrigations as a delivery method [13, 14]. While the safety profile for this method of delivery has not been fully evaluated, recent investigations suggest the risks of long-term use are low [13]. Intranasal drops are another method of delivering corticosteroids to the nasal cavity and may provide better penetration to the frontal recess compared to nasal sprays [11, 15]. High-volume irrigations and nasal drops may be particularly useful in the management of frontal sinusitis due to the improved penetration into the frontal recess [15]. The use of topical intranasal corticosteroids is strongly recommended as part of the appropriate medical therapy for CRSwNP and CRSsNP.

Topical Antibiotics

Topical antibiotics are thought to provide higher concentration of medication to the sinonasal cavity without subjecting patients to the systemic risks [2]. However, there is little evidence to support the use of topical antibiotics in the management of routine CRS [2, 4]. However, the use of topical antibiotics may be useful in select patients with CRS. Mupirocin irrigations have been shown to improve CRS symptoms in patients with CRSsNP with positive *Staphylococcus aureus* cultures [2]. Recalcitrant cases of CRS including patients with cystic fibrosis or immunodeficiency may also benefit from topical antibiotics [2]. Currently, the evidence *recommends against* the "routine" use of topical antibiotics in the management of CRS; however, topical antibiotics may be effective in select cases of recalcitrant CRS [1, 2, 4].

Topical Antifungals

Fungal colonization of the paranasal sinuses is ubiquitous [16]. The role that fungal colonization plays in the pathophysiology of CRS is unclear and is an area of ongoing investigation [4, 16]. Topical antifungals, such as amphotericin B, have been trialed to eradicate fungal elements with the idea that these elements are causing inflammation and clearing them may improve the control of CRS. However, these trials did not demonstrate any clinical benefit in the majority of CRSsNP and CRSwNP patients [2, 4]. A small subset of patients with allergic fungal rhinosinusitis may receive some benefit, but the evidence is limited [4]. Currently, the routine use of topical antifungals in the management of CRS is not recommended [1, 2, 4].

Alternative Topical Therapies

Several alternative medical therapies, such as Manuka honey, surfactants, and xylitol have been evaluated in CRS management [17]. Surfactants are amphipathic molecules that act as mucolytics, by decreasing mucus viscosity. They may also have antibacterial or anti-biofilm properties [18]. Baby shampoo is a surfactant that is sometimes used in sinonasal irrigations and may decrease postnasal drip symptoms. However, these rinses can cause local irritation [17]. Manuka honey is a naturally occurring honey with antibacterial properties, specifically toward *Staphylococcus* and *Pseudomonas* biofilms [17]. While in vitro studies suggest Manuka honey has anti-biofilm characteristics, this data has not been reproduced in rigorous clinical trials [17]. Xylitol is a sugar alcohol with antimicrobial properties that has limited evidence to suggest that in sinonasal irrigations it may decrease bacterial loads and improve disease-specific QoL in CRS [17]. The data regarding the potential clinical benefit of these therapies is limited. However, they may be beneficial in select CRS patients. Further study is required to determine their role in management of CRS.

Delivery of Topical Intranasal Medication

Impact of Delivery Method

Delivery methods for topical intranasal medications can be divided into high-volume (>50 ml) and low-volume (<50 ml) techniques [15]. Table 28.2 describes the available methods as well as their associated sinonasal distributions and the optimal head position for best delivery to the paranasal sinuses [11, 15]. The distribution of low-volume techniques is generally limited to the nasal cavity, with little to no penetration into the paranasal sinuses [15]. High-volume techniques provide significantly improved delivery to the paranasal sinuses and are more effective at larger volumes (i.e., 240 ml sinus irrigations) [15]. As such, high-volume techniques are recommended as the optimal delivery method [11].

Impact of Head Position

Head position is commonly cited as an important factor affecting delivery of topical medications to

Table 28.2 Common topical delivery methods

Device	Examples	Sinonasal delivery sites	Optimal head position
Low volume[a]	Nasal drops	Nasal cavity Olfactory cleft Middle meatus	Lying head back Lying head low Nose upward
	Nasal spray	Nasal cavity Middle meatus	
High volume[b]	NeilMed Sinus Rinse Neti pot	Nasal cavity sinus Ethmoid sinus Maxillary sinus Frontal sinus Sphenoid sinus	Head down forward

[a]Less than 50 ml
[b]Greater than 50 ml

the paranasal sinuses [15]. Head position has the greatest impact on sinus distribution in low-volume delivery methods [11]. With these devices, the lying head low/lying head back/nose upward position provides the greatest distribution, as well as improved distribution to the olfactory cleft and possibly the frontal recess [11]. The head down forward position has the most optimal delivery to all of the paranasal sinuses, including the frontal sinus [11, 15]. As such, high-volume delivery methods combined with the head down forward position are recommended as the optimal delivery head position. When low-volume techniques are utilized, the nose upward position may improve delivery for this method [11, 15].

Impact of Endoscopic Sinus Surgery

One of the goals of ESS is to open the paranasal sinuses to facilitate the delivery of topical intranasal medications. ESS is the most significant factor influencing the distribution and penetration of medications into the paranasal sinuses [11]. In unoperated sinuses, distribution to the paranasal sinuses is inconsistent and limited. Following ESS, distribution to all of paranasal sinuses is significantly improved, especially to the frontal sinus [11]. The extent of ESS also influences the distribution of medication; for example, a Draf III provides significantly better penetration of topical medication into the frontal recess compared to a Draf IIA [15, 19]. In general, as the degree of frontal recess dissection increases (i.e., Draf I to Draf III), the penetration of topical intranasal medications into the frontal sinus increases [11, 20]. In patients where delivery of medication to the frontal sinus is one of the primary therapeutic goals, clinicians may consider these factors when determining the extent of frontal recess dissection to perform in ESS.

Systemic Therapies

Systemic Corticosteroids

Systemic corticosteroids are typically used for acute exacerbations of CRS and severe recalcitrant CRS and to help reduce the size of polyps in patients with CRSwNP [2]. Short courses of systemic corticosteroids (<3 weeks) have been shown to reduce polyp size in CRSwNP, improve disease-specific QoL and improve sinonasal symptoms [2]. However, these improvements are not sustained longer than 3–6 months after the course [21]. In addition, the potential benefit in CRSsNP is controversial [2]. Systemic corticosteroids are associated with a significant risk for adverse events with short courses, repeated use, and prolonged use [2, 4]. Balancing the risks and benefits of systemic corticosteroids is an ongoing challenge in the management of CRS. The best available evidence suggests that they do improve symptom severity and QoL in CRSwNP patients for a short duration [21, 22]. Their routine use in CRSsNP remains controversial partially because of a lack of studies examining this specific population [4]. The use of systemic corticosteroids may be considered on a case-by-case basis, carefully weighing the risks and benefits and involving patients in the shared decisionmaking process.

Systemic Antibiotics

Systemic antibiotics historically made up a significant proportion of medical therapy for CRS. As understanding of the underlying pathophysiology has clarified that CRS is primarily an inflammatory, not infectious, condition, the use of systemic antibiotics in the management of CRS has decreased [17]. Systemic antibiotics may be divided into two therapeutic options: short-term antibiotics and long-term anti-inflammatory antibiotics [2]. Short-term antibiotics are generally comprised of culture-directed or broad-spectrum antibiotics for less than 4 weeks. The evidence for short-term antibiotics is conflicting but tends to support their use in CRS patients with active mucopurulence [2, 4]. Long-term antibiotics involve prolonged courses (great than 12 weeks) of antibiotics with anti-inflammatory properties such as macrolides. The evidence supporting their use is limited to CRSsNP patients. Their use has been associated with improved symptom scores and QoL, which are sustained for up to 3 months after completing treatment [2, 4]. As with systemic corticosteroids, there are significant risks of both short- and long-term courses of antibiotics, and their use should be carefully considered on a case-by-case basis.

Leukotriene Pathway Antagonists

Leukotrienes are inflammatory mediators that play a role in the pathophysiology of CRS by increasing vasodilation, increasing mucosal edema, and increasing eosinophilic infiltration and inflammation [17]. They may play a more significant role in the development of CRSwNP versus CRSsNP. Leukotriene pathway antagonists (LTA) are a class of medication that either block leukotrienes from binding to their respective receptors (montelukast), or inhibit the production of leukotrienes (zileuton), thereby decreasing the resulting inflammation [2, 4]. They are primarily used in patients with severe, uncontrolled asthma. The use of LTAs in CRSwNP is associated with improved sinonasal symptoms and may be considered for select CRSwNP patients [2, 4].

Allergy Therapy

Approximately 20–60% of CRS patients suffer from concurrent allergic rhinitis [17]. Whether allergy plays a causal role in the pathogenesis of CRS remains unclear [4]. However, patients with a significant allergic component receive some improvement in their disease-specific QoL with treatment of concurrent allergies. As such, the investigation and treatment of comorbid allergy are an option in CRS patients [4].

Antihistamines

Topical and systemic antihistamines reduce inflammation by reducing histamine release [17]. This results in improved sinonasal symptoms by decreasing vascular permeability, vasodilation, and mucus production [2]. They are recommended in patients with concurrent allergic symptoms [2]. They are not recommended for the treatment of CRS without comorbid allergy.

Allergy Immunotherapy

Immunotherapy has been well established as a beneficial therapeutic option for allergic disease. Allergy immunotherapy is recommended for patients with moderate to severe allergic rhinitis with persistent symptoms despite allergy avoidance and antihistamines. In addition these patients must have demonstrable evidence of specific immunoglobulin E (IgE)-mediated response to clinically relevant allergens. Subcutaneous immunotherapy (SCIT) and sublingual immunotherapy (SLIT) expose the patient to progressively larger doses of the respective allergen(s) in order to downregulate the immune reaction to the allergen [17]. As a component of the management of concurrent allergy, immunotherapy may be useful in select CRS patients with severe, refractory allergic disease [2, 4].

Aspirin Desensitization

A subset of patients with CRSwNP suffer from aspirin (ASA)-exacerbated respiratory disease (AERD). There is evidence to suggest that desensitizing these patients to ASA improves associated pulmonary and sinonasal disease, reduces polyp recurrence, and decreases the revision rates for ESS [4, 17]. A thorough pulmonary assessment is necessary prior to desensitization, as patients with a FEV1 (expected functional expiratory volume within 1 s) of less than 75% should not be desensitized [4]. ASA desensitization is ideally performed 4–6 weeks after surgical removal of polyps with the goal of reducing the ongoing inflammation in the postoperative period as well as the potential for the most significant impact on polyp recurrence and QoL improvements [4]. ASA desensitization should be considered in patients with AERD, especially those refractory to both medical and surgical therapies.

Biologic Therapies

As the pathophysiology of CRS is further defined, various inflammatory pathways have been identified as possible targets for biologic therapies. Some of these have led to the development of therapies that have shown some promise in the management of CRS. These therapies will be discussed below. Of note, all of these therapies are meant to target pathways in CRSwNP and have not been tested in CRSsNP. As these are innovative therapies with only a few studies examining each, there is no evidence examining their role in treating the frontal sinus specifically.

Anti-immunoglobulin E Therapy

IgE is a potent inflammatory mediator responsible for mast cell activation that has been implicated in the pathophysiology of CRS [2, 23]. High levels of serum IgE are also associated with the presence of asthma and a history of asthma in CRS patients [23–25]. Monoclonal anti-IgE antibodies function by binding free serum IgE as well as decreasing availability of IgE receptors located on mast cells, basophils and dendritic cells. This results in a degree of antigen "insensitivity" [23, 24]. Two limited randomized control trials have examined the efficacy of omalizumab, an anti-IgE therapy, in CRSwNP [23, 24, 26]. A clinical benefit was only demonstrated in one of the trials and was limited to mild improvements in objective measures (radiologic imaging and polyp size) and patient-reported outcomes (total symptoms and QoL) [2]. Anti-IgE therapy remains a promising potential medical therapy for a specific subgroup of patients with CRSwNP, with more research needed to better define those who would most benefit from it.

Anti-interleukin-5 Therapy

Over 80% of CRSwNP is associated with significant eosinophilia, particularly in patients with a history of aspirin sensitivity and asthma [25, 27]. Interleukin-5 (IL-5) is thought to play a significant role in the pathophysiology of CRSwNP, since it mediates eosinophil growth, recruitment, and activation [25]. Anti-IL-5 antibodies bind free IL-5, impair eosinophil-mediated inflammation, and have been shown to induce eosinophil apoptosis and reduce tissue eosinophilia in nasal polyps [2, 28]. Anti-IL-5 therapy has been investigated in two small, randomized control trials (RCT) in CRSwNP and resulted in mild improvements in serum eosinophil levels and polyp scores [27, 28]. However, there were no improvements in symptoms scores or QoL. While anti-IL-5 therapy may provide some benefit in CRSwNP, further studies are needed before it can be recommended as a routine therapeutic option for CRSwNP.

Anti-interleukin-4 Therapy

Interleukin-4 (IL-4) plays a role in type 2 helper T-cell-mediated inflammation, which is associated with CRSwNP [29]. IL-4 also potentiates the immune response of fibroblasts in CRS [30–32]. Dupilumab is a monoclonal anti-IL-4 antibody that targets the α subunit of the IL-4 receptor (Rα), which inhibits signaling of IL-4 and IL-13 [33]. A RCT investigated the impact of subcutaneous dupilumab in patients with CRSwNP who continued to have symptoms despite topical intranasal corticosteroids [33]. Results demonstrated significant improvements in radiographic imaging and polyp size. Additionally, patients received significant improvements in QoL. These effects were more pronounced in patients with concurrent asthma [33]. Dupilumab appears to be a promising medical therapy; however, larger trials with longer duration of follow-up are required to better determine its role in CRSwNP treatment.

Appropriate Medical Therapy

The above section details the available options for the medical management of CRS. However, not all of these interventions are appropriate for all CRS patients. Appropriate medical therapy (AMT) is a recent concept in the management of CRS that is meant to replace the concepts of maximal medical therapy (MMT) [4, 12, 34]. MMT referred to the process of exhausting medical treatment options before surgical interventions were offered. AMT aims to balance a reasonable trial of medical therapy without delaying patients' access to ESS [4]. AMT has been described by the International Consensus Statement on Allergy and Rhinology: Rhinosinusitis as well as Rudmik et al. [4, 12, 34]. These suggest that AMT should consist of high-volume sinonasal irrigations and topical intranasal corticosteroids, for a minimum of 3–4 weeks for all CRS patients [4]. Specific CRS phenotypes (CRSwNP and CRSwNP) should receive additional directed therapy as well as a component of AMT. CRSsNP patient should also receive a short course of systemic [12, 34]. CRSwNP patients should receive a short course of systemic corticosteroids (1–3 weeks) [12, 34]. Patients with persistent symptoms and objective evidence of inflammation following a trial of these therapies may be appropriate candidates for ESS [35]. Of note, the recommendations regarding AMT do not address specific sites of sinusitis, such as frontal sinusitis. Currently there is no evidence to suggest that AMT for frontal sinusitis should deviate from these recommendations [35].

Considerations for Medical Management of the Frontal Sinus

Currently there are no recommendations for medical strategies specific to frontal sinusitis [4, 12, 34, 35]. Short courses (<3 weeks) of systemic corticosteroids may be considered on an individual basis considering the associated therapeutic risks [2]. They may be beneficial in patients with frontal sinusitis to decrease edema and inflammation in the frontal recess and reduce the resulting obstruction of the frontal recess. This strategy may also improve delivery of medication to the frontal recess by decreasing obstruction and facilitating the penetration of topical intranasal medications. Delivery methods with improved penetration into the frontal recess, such as high-volume saline irrigations in the head down forward position or nasal drops in the nose upward position, may be considered in the management of frontal sinusitis specifically [11, 15]. The delivery of intranasal medications is also proportionally related to the dissection of the frontal recess [21]. In patients where facilitating delivery to the frontal sinus is a goal of ESS, clinicians may consider a more extensive frontal recess dissection. Drug-eluting stents have shown promising initial data suggesting that their placement at the time of surgery may improve short-term postoperative outcomes [36]. The accepted, evidenced-based medical management for frontal sinusitis in CRS remains AMT, as described above [12, 34]. However, further investigation is required to determine whether any of the specific therapies outlined may play a unique role in the management of frontal sinusitis.

Summary

Frontal sinusitis in CRS represents a unique challenge. Medical therapy is an essential component of initial and maintenance therapy for successful patient outcomes. High-volume saline irrigations and topical intranasal steroids are necessary components of medical management, with CRSsNP and CRSwNP requiring different additional therapies for complete AMT. A variety of other therapeutic options are available, which may be considered on a case-by-case basis to optimize the management of CRS. Balancing the risks and benefits of these treatments can be difficult; however, the majority of patients receive significant symptomatic improvement with medical therapy in conjunction with ESS and adjunctive therapies.

Potential Conflict(s) of Interest Kristine A. Smith: None.

Jeremiah A. Alt: Consultant for Medtronic, Spirox, and GlycoMira Therapeutics.

Richard R. Orlandi: Consultant for Medtronic, Intersect, 480 Biomedical, and BioInspire.

References

1. Fokkens WJ, Lund VJ, Mullol J, Bachert C, Alobid I, Baroody F, et al. EPOS 2012: European position paper on rhinosinusitis and nasal polyps 2012. A summary for otorhinolaryngologists. Rhinology. 2012;50(1):1–12.
2. Rudmik L, Soler ZM. Medical therapies for adult chronic sinusitis: a systematic review. JAMA. 2015;314(9):926–39.
3. Lee WT, Kuhn FA, Citardi MJ. 3D computed tomographic analysis of frontal recess anatomy in patients without frontal sinusitis. Otolaryngol Head Neck Surg. 2004;131(3):164–73.
4. Orlandi RR, Kingdom TT, Hwang PH, Smith TL, Alt JA, Baroody FM, et al. International consensus statement on allergy and rhinology: rhinosinusitis. Int Forum Allergy Rhinol. 2016;6(Suppl 1):S22–209.
5. DeConde AS, Smith TL. Outcomes after frontal sinus surgery: an evidence-based review. Otolaryngol Clin N Am. 2016;49(4):1019–33.
6. Kalish L, Snidvongs K, Sivasubramaniam R, Cope D, Harvey RJ. Topical steroids for nasal polyps. Cochrane Database Syst Rev. 2012;12:CD006549.
7. Snidvongs K, Kalish L, Sacks R, Craig JC, Harvey RJ. Topical steroid for chronic rhinosinusitis without polyps. Cochrane Database Syst Rev. 2011(8):CD009274.
8. Kerr EA, Hayward RA. Patient-centered performance management: enhancing value for patients and health care systems. JAMA. 2013;310(2):137–8.
9. Chong LY, Head K, Hopkins C, Philpott C, Glew S, Scadding G, et al. Saline irrigation for chronic rhinosinusitis. Cochrane Database Syst Rev. 2016;4:CD011995.
10. Chong LY, Head K, Hopkins C, Philpott C, Schilder AG, Burton MJ. Intranasal steroids versus placebo or no intervention for chronic rhinosinusitis. Cochrane Database Syst Rev. 2016;4:CD011996.
11. Thomas WW 3rd, Harvey RJ, Rudmik L, Hwang PH, Schlosser RJ. Distribution of topical agents to the paranasal sinuses: an evidence-based review with recommendations. Int Forum Allergy Rhinol. 2013;3(9):691–703.
12. Rudmik L, Soler ZM, Hopkins C, Schlosser RJ, Peters A, White AA, et al. Defining appropriateness criteria for endoscopic sinus surgery during management of uncomplicated adult chronic rhinosinusitis: a RAND/UCLA appropriateness study. Int Forum Allergy Rhinol. 2016;6(6):557–67.

13. Smith KA, French G, Mechor B, Rudmik L. Safety of long-term high-volume sinonasal budesonide irrigations for chronic rhinosinusitis. Int Forum Allergy Rhinol. 2016;6(3):228–32.
14. Harvey RJ, Snidvongs K, Kalish LH, Oakley GM, Sacks R. Corticosteroid nasal irrigations are more effective than simple sprays in a randomized double-blinded placebo-controlled trial for chronic rhinosinusitis after sinus surgery. Int Forum Allergy Rhinol. 2018;8(4):461–70.
15. Smith KA, Rudmik L. Delivery of topical therapies. In: Woodworth BA, Poetker DM, Reh DD, editors. Advances in oto-rhino-laryngology – Rhinosinusitis with nasal polyposis. Basel/New York: Karger; 2016.
16. Fokkens WJ, Ebbens F, van Drunen CM. Fungus: a role in pathophysiology of chronic rhinosinusitis, disease modifier, a treatment target, or no role at all? Immunol Allergy Clin N Am. 2009;29(4):677–88.
17. Schwartz JS, Tajudeen BA, Cohen NA. Medical management of chronic rhinosinusitis – an update. Expert Rev Clin Pharmacol. 2016;9(5):695–704.
18. Lee JT, Chiu AG. Topical anti-infective sinonasal irrigations: update and literature review. Am J Rhinol Allergy. 2014;28(1):29–38.
19. Barham HP, Ramakrishnan VR, Knisely A, Do TQ, Chan LS, Gunaratne DA, et al. Frontal sinus surgery and sinus distribution of nasal irrigation. Int Forum Allergy Rhinol. 2016;6(3):238–42.
20. Singhal D, Weitzel EK, Lin E, Feldt B, Kriete B, McMains KC, et al. Effect of head position and surgical dissection on sinus irrigant penetration in cadavers. Laryngoscope. 2010;120(12):2528–31.
21. Vaidyanathan S, Barnes M, Williamson P, Hopkinson P, Donnan PT, Lipworth B. Treatment of chronic rhinosinusitis with nasal polyposis with oral steroids followed by topical steroids: a randomized trial. Ann Intern Med. 2011;154(5):293–302.
22. Head K, Chong LY, Hopkins C, Philpott C, Burton MJ, Schilder AG. Short-course oral steroids alone for chronic rhinosinusitis. Cochrane Database Syst Rev. 2016;4:CD011991.
23. Hong CJ, Tsang AC, Quinn JG, Bonaparte JP, Stevens A, Kilty SJ. Anti-IgE monoclonal antibody therapy for the treatment of chronic rhinosinusitis: a systematic review. Syst Rev. 2015;4:166.
24. Chang TW, Shiung YY. Anti-IgE as a mast cell-stabilizing therapeutic agent. J Allergy Clin Immunol. 2006;117(6):1203–12; quiz 13
25. Para AJ, Clayton E, Peters AT. Management of rhinosinusitis: an evidence based approach. Curr Opin Allergy Clin Immunol. 2016;16(4):383–9.
26. Pinto JM, Mehta N, DiTineo M, Wang J, Baroody FM, Naclerio RM. A randomized, double-blind, placebo-controlled trial of anti-IgE for chronic rhinosinusitis. Rhinology. 2010;48(3):318–24.
27. Gevaert P, Lang-Loidolt D, Lackner A, Stammberger H, Staudinger H, Van Zele T, et al. Nasal IL-5 levels determine the response to anti-IL-5 treatment in patients with nasal polyps. J Allergy Clin Immunol. 2006;118(5):1133–41.
28. Gevaert P, Van Bruaene N, Cattaert T, Van Steen K, Van Zele T, Acke F, et al. Mepolizumab, a humanized anti-IL-5 mAb, as a treatment option for severe nasal polyposis. J Allergy Clin Immunol. 2011;128(5):989–95, e1–8
29. Gandhi NA, Bennett BL, Graham NM, Pirozzi G, Stahl N, Yancopoulos GD. Targeting key proximal drivers of type 2 inflammation in disease. Nat Rev Drug Discov. 2016;15(1):35–50.
30. Akdis CA, Bachert C, Cingi C, Dykewicz MS, Hellings PW, Naclerio RM, et al. Endotypes and phenotypes of chronic rhinosinusitis: a PRACTALL document of the European academy of allergy and clinical immunology and the American academy of allergy, asthma & immunology. J Allergy Clin Immunol. 2013;131(6):1479–90.
31. Bachert C, Zhang N, Holtappels G, De Lobel L, van Cauwenberge P, Liu S, et al. Presence of IL-5 protein and IgE antibodies to staphylococcal enterotoxins in nasal polyps is associated with comorbid asthma. J Allergy Clin Immunol. 2010;126(5):962–8, 8.e1–6
32. Bachert C, van Steen K, Zhang N, Holtappels G, Cattaert T, Maus B, et al. Specific IgE against Staphylococcus aureus enterotoxins: an independent risk factor for asthma. J Allergy Clin Immunol. 2012;130(2):376–81.e8.
33. Bachert C, Mannent L, Naclerio RM, Mullol J, Ferguson BJ, Gevaert P, et al. Effect of subcutaneous dupilumab on nasal polyp burden in patients with chronic sinusitis and nasal polyposis: a randomized clinical trial. JAMA. 2016;315(5):469–79.
34. Rudmik L, Soler ZM, Hopkins C, Schlosser RJ, Peters A, White AA, et al. Defining appropriateness criteria for endoscopic sinus surgery during management of uncomplicated adult chronic rhinosinusitis: a RAND/UCLA appropriateness study. Rhinology. 2016;54(2):117–28.
35. Sohal M, Tessema B, Brown SM. Medical management of frontal sinusitis. Otolaryngol Clin N Am. 2016;49(4):927–34.
36. Santarelli GD, Han JK. Evaluation of the PROPEL(R) mini sinus implant for the treatment of frontal sinus disease. Expert Opin Drug Deliv. 2016;13(12):1789–93.

Frontal Barotrauma and Aerosinusitis

Adrienne M. Laury and Kevin C. McMains

Introduction

Sinus barotrauma, also known as aerosinusitis or barosinusitis, is defined as sinus damage induced by a pressure differential which occurs between the air trapped in the sinuses and the surrounding environment. This condition most frequently occurs as a result of flying or diving but can occur in any situation where the environmental pressure changes while the intrasinus pressure cannot. If this pressure variation supercedes what the body's compensatory mechanisms can accommodate, sinus discomfort or physical mucosal damage can occur. In severe cases, sinus barotrauma can even result in blurred vision, difficulties in oxygenation from a mask, extreme pain, and shock [1, 2].

Sinus barotrauma is a relatively common disease for pilots with an incidence of 1.5–44% in hypobaric chamber simulations [3]. In a retrospective survey of Danish civilian aviation pilots, 12% were found to have had aerosinusitis, with approximately 70–80% of cases involving the frontal sinuses [4]. In turn, military pilots, who are typically exposed to even greater physiologic extremes, are at an even greater risk for significant barotrauma sequelae [5]. This explains why aerosinusitis is the fourth most common otolaryngologic disease to result in the hospitalization of fighter pilots [6]. Additionally, skydivers and military personnel who participate in high altitude-low opening (HALO) jumps are also at an increased risk for aerosinusitis.

Barosinusitis is also a significant and frequent complication for deep-sea divers. Scuba divers who descend to 10 m will double their ambient pressure compared with sea level, and an additional atmosphere of pressure will be added for every subsequent 10 m. This rapid change in pressure over a relatively short distance significantly increases a diver's risk for sinus barotrauma. One group from Germany found the lifetime incidence of barosinusitis in experienced divers to reach up to 11% [7].

Sinus barotrauma has a unique pathophysiology, and subsequently its diagnosis and treatment algorithm are distinctive from acute or chronic rhinosinusitis.

Pathophysiology

The mechanism behind sinus barotrauma is inherent upon the body's adherence to the laws of physics. Typically, gas naturally flows through the sinus ostia to equilibrate the air in the sinuses with that of the environment. Upon ascent or descent and diving or flying, these pressure changes can occur much more rapidly, necessitat-

A. M. Laury · K. C. McMains (✉)
Otolaryngology, South Texas Veterans Health Care
System, San Antonio, TX, USA

© Springer Nature Switzerland AG 2019
D. Lal, P. H. Hwang (eds.), *Frontal Sinus Surgery*, https://doi.org/10.1007/978-3-319-97022-6_29

ing an even quicker gas exchange. However, if the sinus ostium is blocked secondary to edema, polyps, etc., this gas exchange is prohibited. Additionally, Boyle's law states that, at a constant temperature, the volume of a gas is inversely proportional to the pressure ($C_T = V/P$). Therefore, if a pressure differential occurs between the sinuses and ambient air, the volume of gas in the sinus will also be altered inversely to the pressure. In turn, within the incompressible bony walls of the sinuses, this pressure/volume alteration can result in significant mucosal damage including edema, hemorrhage, and even soft tissue avulsion.

When flying, differences in the severity and frequency of aerosinusitis have been shown to be related to the timing of the injury, specifically in ascent versus descent. As a plane descends, barometric pressure increases, creating a negative pressure differential within a sinus, which, in turn, can cause collapse of the mucosal pathway/sinus ostia [8]. Subsequently, this prevents air from entering the sinus, creating an even greater negative intrasinus pressure and resulting in a condition known as sinus "squeeze." Alternatively, on ascent, pressure increases within a sinus compared to the environment, and in the face of blocked ostia, air will be forced out along the path of least resistance – physiologically or nonphysiologically. This is referred to as "reverse squeeze." Sinus barotrauma during descent is at least twice as frequent as ascent; however, barotrauma suffered during ascent is associated with more severe sequelae [5]. For example, "reverse squeeze" injuries can include subcutaneous or orbital emphysema, blindness, pneumocephalus, and trigeminal nerve dysfunction, almost always secondary to the nonphysiological escape of trapped air from a sinus [9].

Sinus barotrauma's propensity toward the frontal sinus is also based upon physical laws, specifically Poiseuille's equation which states that flow is directly proportional to the radius (r) by a power of four and inversely proportional to the length (L) ($Q = \Delta P \, \pi r4/8\mu L$, where Q is the flow rate, P is the pressure, and μ is the fluid viscosity). The frontal sinus outflow tract is significantly longer and narrower than any of the other

sinus ostia. Therefore, in the frontal sinuses, there will be more obstruction from smaller amounts of mucosal edema, resulting in barotrauma occurring most frequently in the frontal sinuses.

Overall, the pathophysiology behind sinus barotrauma can occur in any environment where a pressure differential occurs, including commercial airline flights or weather-related barometric pressure changes. However, the frequency and severity of the injury are often directly related to the rapidity and magnitude of the pressure differential between the ambient atmosphere and the intrasinus environment.

Diagnosis

History and Physical

Patients typically present with the report of significant facial or dental pain during rapid changes in atmospheric pressure. This symptom is then relieved as the pressure differential is eliminated. The pain is usually localized over the frontal or maxillary sinuses but may also be retro-orbital or even diffuse in nature [8]. Case series in military pilots confirms the predominant symptom of frontal pain (97%), followed by premolar pain (27%), and bloody rhinorrhea (13–58%) [10, 11]. It is important to note the differences in symptom localization as it may significantly impact one's treatment plan if surgery is required. Additionally, ascent barotrauma will more commonly result in the symptom of epistaxis, as the expansion of enclosed air is more likely to expel blood mixed with mucus from the pressurized sinus/es [12].

The frequency and severity of symptoms can also vary based on any underlying sinonasal comorbidity which may predispose the patient to barosinusitis, i.e., chronic rhinosinusitis, allergies, upper respiratory infection, etc. Additionally, the timing of the symptoms – ascent vs descent – should be sought out and documented, as it may suggest a different underlying cause or comorbidity and may predispose patients to different sequelae.

In 1972, the Weissman classification system was proposed as a means to correlate the clinical symptoms of sinus barotrauma with its intrasinus pathology and radiographic findings (Table 29.1) [13]. Negative intrasinus pressures of less than 100 mmHg are typically associated with Weissman Class I, 100–250 mmHg with Class II, and > 250 mmHg with Class III. To put this in perspective, typical commercial flights descend at roughly 300 ft./min *with* cabin pressurization resulting in a pressure differential of <200 mmHg and therefore, a lower Weissman classification (I or II). Alternatively, a military combat flight can descend at speeds greater than 10,000 ft./min *without* cabin pressurization resulting in significantly higher pressure changes almost always resulting in a Weissman Class III injury.

Physical examination findings may greatly vary. Typically, the large majority of patients will appear completely unremarkable on nasal endoscopy without evidence of hemorrhage, mucosal edema, or mucosal avulsions. This may be because of a prolonged time between injury and evaluation by an otolaryngologist, allowing for the resolution of physical findings. Alternatively, the physical signs may be completely localized within the sinus cavity and therefore not visible in a surgery-naïve patient. However, some patients may present with obvious mucosal edema or hemorrhage acutely or possibly polyps or even sinonasal tumors which predisposed them to barosinusitis. In patients with descent barotrauma, extrasinus pathology such as polyps or mucosal edema are not uncommon, while in

ascent barotrauma, intrasinus tumors or skull base or cranial nerve dehiscences may be identified [14–16]. Additionally, relatively common findings such as septal deviation, concha bullosa, and turbinate hypertrophy may place patients at an increased risk for barotrauma either by direct mass effect or altered nasal airflow, although this has not been investigated in a prospective clinical trial [5].

Imaging

Computerized tomography (CT) scans can provide useful information in the patient with suspected sinus barotrauma. This allows for the evaluation of any intrasinus pathology which may not be visible on physical exam or nasal endoscopy. If a CT is obtained immediately following the barotrauma, an opacification can sometimes be seen in the involved sinus representing acute submucosal hemorrhage or polypoid edema (Fig. 29.1). Additionally, a repeat CT obtained a few weeks later will often show reso-

Table 29.1 Weissman classification of frontal sinus barotrauma [13]

	Symptoms	Plain films	Pathology
Class I	Transient frontal discomfort	Normal	Minimal edema of sinonasal mucosa
Class II	Frontal sinus pain <24 h	Thickening of frontal sinus mucosa	Blood tinged fluid in the sinus
Class III	Severe pain over the frontal sinus (squeeze only)	Air-fluid level or polypoid mass	Hematoma, edema, avulsed mucosa, and serosanguinous fluid

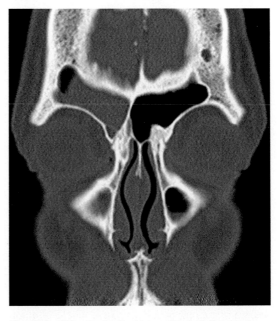

Fig. 29.1 CT scan obtained immediately following barotrauma showing an opacification in the involved sinus representing acute submucosal hemorrhage or polypoid edema

lution of the opacification/hemorrhage further supporting the diagnosis of barosinusitis (Fig. 29.2). Additional radiographic findings suggestive of barotrauma can include mucosal thickening along the sinus outflow tract/s as well as diffuse mucosal edema within the sinus.

Oftentimes, imaging may be unremarkable, owing to the resolution of the mucosal trauma associated with the inciting event. In these cases, the only radiologic clues may be narrow sinus outflow tracts (that ideally correlate with the patient's symptomatic sinus/sinuses) or minimal mucosal inflammation. Alternatively, some patients may present without direct evidence of barosinusitis but with anatomic variants that alter the nasal airflow or potentially block the sinus where the symptoms exist. In these cases, consideration should be given to ensure that the patient's symptoms and history correlate with the observed anatomic variant.

Magnetic resonance imaging (MRI) is rarely necessary for diagnosis; however, if obtained, one might expect to see an unenhanced mass lesion in the paranasal sinuses that is hyperin-

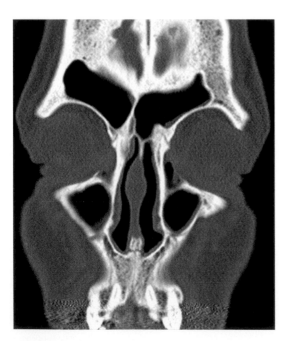

Fig. 29.2 A repeat CT obtained a few weeks later for the same patient showing the resolution of the opacification/hemorrhage, further supporting the diagnosis of barosinusitis

tense both on T1- and T2-weighted images [17]. Other pathologies that may be consistent with this MRI appearance include a mucocele or sinus cholesterol granuloma; however, sinus hemorrhage secondary to barotrauma is unique in that it would likely decrease in size or resolve on repeat imaging.

Treatment

Medical

Medical management is typically the first-line treatment for sinus barotrauma. This can include a variety of options such as both topical and oral decongestants, intranasal steroid sprays, nasal saline irrigations, oral steroids, and analgesics [5, 7]. The use of antibiotics is typically reserved for those cases initiated by bacterial sinusitis and antihistamines for those related to allergies [18, 19].

Medical treatment of acute sinus barotrauma is predominantly focused on nasal decongestion [14]. A typical regimen utilized by the authors consists of 5–7 days of intranasal decongestants (such as oxymetazoline nasal spray), a 5-day oral steroid taper, oral decongestants (such as pseudoephedrine), and analgesia as needed depending on the severity of symptoms. One study from Germany identified 40 divers with sinus barotrauma, of which 19 were successfully treated with the initiation of 6 weeks of nasal saline irrigations and mometasone spray bid as well as 5 days of PO steroids [7]. Additionally, patients should be restricted from repeat flying or diving for at least 1 week or until the evidence of barotrauma and its inciting risk factors have resolved [8, 19]. CT imaging and nasal endoscopy can be repeated at that time, and if evidence of barosinusitis persists, continued activity limitations should be considered. Since baseline mucosal thickening can exist in asymptomatic individuals, this should not be the sole criterion for continued restriction [20, 21]. Rather, the entire clinical picture including history, symptoms, and endoscopic and radiographic changes during recovery should be considered. For professional divers and pilots with Weissman Class III injuries, a hypobaric chamber simulation dive may be useful prior to medical release to help predict the likelihood of imminent repeat injury [8].

Once barotrauma has occurred and resolved, patients should be counseled and offered prophylactic treatment. This typically involves an oral decongestant 1 h prior to flying or diving and a nasal decongestant spray approximately 20 min before flight descent. Underwater application of intranasal decongestants has even been described for special operation divers in order to prevent barotrauma upon resurfacing [22]. Additionally, utilization of an intranasal steroid spray is an alternate prophylactic treatment option that can be considered, but this does require consistent daily use which may be less appealing to the intermittent recreational flier or diver.

Surgical

Surgical management of sinus barotrauma should be considered in all patients who do not respond to medical management or who experience repeat symptoms despite prophylactic treatment. Additionally, patients identified with an underlying inciting pathology such as diffuse nasal polyposis or sinonasal mass should undergo surgical intervention as a first-line treatment.

For those who fail medical management, consideration should first be given to understand the anatomic area responsible for the patients' symptoms – whether it is an isolated blocked frontal sinus outflow tract or diffuse mucosal edema throughout all paranasal sinuses [5]. This information is essential and should be used to guide any surgical intervention. For the isolated sinus barotrauma, a direct surgical approach opening only the affected sinus is often all that is required to alleviate symptoms. Specifically, for mucosal edema in the frontal sinus outflow tract, balloon sinuplasty has been proposed as a possibly less invasive, in-office treatment option to obtain ostial patency. However, only one case report currently exists describing this technique, and unfortunately, it was unsuccessful in relieving the patient's symptoms [23]. Therefore, more investigation into the utility of balloon dilation of

sinus ostia for the treatment of frontal sinus barotrauma is necessary. Additionally, directed surgery may also be of utility in patients with specific anatomic variants that can lead to ostiomeatal complex obstruction when coupled with mucosal edema. For example, patients with concha bullosa, septal deviations, paradoxical middle turbinates, etc. and correlative barotrauma symptoms often will obtain relief from correction of the inciting anatomy in addition to opening the symptomatic sinus.

For patients with diffuse mucosal edema or bilateral, diffuse sinus pain, a more extensive surgical intervention is often required. Currently, the standard of care management of these patients is a full-house functional endoscopic sinus surgery (FESS) with a Draf IIA [21, 24, 25]. In pilot cohorts, this intervention strategy has repeatedly been shown to result in a 92–100% resolution of symptoms and return to flying status [24, 25]. Additionally, in professional divers, surgical management results in significantly improved SNOT-20 scores [7]. Unfortunately, failure does still occasionally occur and is typically most often due to stenosis of a frontal sinus ostium [25]. Frontal stenting may have some benefit in preventing these sequelae and should be considered during initial surgical intervention [26]. However, in the rare case where stenosis does occur, a Draf III or endoscopic modified Lothrop procedure should be considered as a definitive management option [27].

Postoperative management consists of typical postsurgical sinus irrigations and in-office debridements for several weeks. For professional divers and pilots, returning to work after surgery is dependent upon mucosal healing and can usually be accomplished within 6–8 weeks. A repeat trial in a hypobaric chamber is a reasonable option to confirm resolution of symptoms in a simulated environment prior to return to duty.

Summary

Sinus barotrauma is a unique pathophysiology which most often occurs in divers and pilots. The frontal sinus because of its long and narrow sinus outflow tract is most frequently affected. The diagnosis of barosinusitis is based upon a history of frontal, maxillary, or retro-orbital pain that occurs with significant changes in barometric pressure. This may or may not be accompanied by physical evidence of mucosal damage on nasal endoscopy or CT imaging. Treatment should begin with medical management including topical and oral decongestants, oral steroids, and possibly analgesia. Surgery should be reserved for those patients with recurrent barotrauma or those with significant sinonasal pathology which may predispose them to frequent episodes. The extent of surgical intervention should be based upon the patient's symptoms, physical exam, and radiographic findings and may vary between a unilateral Draf IIA and a full-house FESS with Draf III.

References

1. Larsen AS, Buchwald C, Besterhauge S. Sinus barotraumas – late diagnosis and treatment with computer-aided endoscopic surgery. Aviat Space Environ Med. 2003;74(2):180–3.
2. Lewis ST. Barotrauma in United States Air Force: accidents-incidents. Aerosp Med. 1973;44(9):1059–61.
3. Dickson ED, King PF. Results of treatment of otitic and sinus barotrauma. J Aviat Med. 1956;27(2):92–9.
4. Rosenkvist L, Klokker M, Katholm M. Upper respiratory infections and barotrauma in commercial pilots: a retrospective survey. Aviat Space Environ Med. 2008;79(10):960–3.
5. Weitzel EK, McMains KC, Wormald PJ. Comprehensive surgical management of the aerosinusitis patient. Curr Opin Otolaryngol Head Neck Surg. 2009;17:11–7.
6. Wang Y, Xu XR. Contrastive analysis on disease spectrum of otorhinolaryngology in 230 pilots of three generation fighters. J Clin Otorhinolaryngol (China). 2006;20(1):13–5.
7. Skevas T, Baumann I, Bruckner T, et al. Medical and surgical treatment in divers with chronic rhinosinusitis and paranasal sinus barotrauma. Eur Arch Otorhiniolaryngol. 2012;269:853–60.
8. Weitzel EK, McMains KC, Rajapaksa S, Wormald PJ. Aerosinusitis: pathophysiology, prophylaxis, and management in passengers and aircrew. Aviat Space Environ Med. 2008;79(1):50–3.
9. Becker GD, Parell GJ. Barotrauma of the ears and sinuses after scuba diving. Eur Arch Otorhinolaryngol. 2001;258:159–63.
10. Singletary EM, Reilly JF Jr. Acute frontal sinus barotrauma. Am J Emerg Med. 1990;8:329–31.
11. Wolf CR. Aerotitis in air travel. Calif Med. 1972;117:10–2.
12. Fagan P, McKenzie B, Edmonds C. Sinus barotrauma in divers. Ann Otol Rhinol Laryngol. 1976;85(1 Pt 1):61–4.
13. Weissman B, Green RS, Roberts PT. Frontal sinus barotrauma. Laryngoscope. 1972;82:2160–8.
14. Stewart TW Jr. Common otolaryngologic problems of flying. Am Fam Physician. 1979;19:113–9.
15. Tryggvason G, Briem B, Guomundsson O, et al. Sphenoid sinus barotrauma with intracranial air in sella turcica after diving. Acta Radiol. 2006;47:872–4.
16. Sharma N, DE M, Pracy P. Recurrent facial patesthesis secondary to maxillary antral cyst and dehiscent infraorbital canal: case report. J Laryngol Otol. 2007;121:e6.
17. Segev Y, Landsberg R, Fliss DM. MR imaging appearance of frontal sinus barotrauma. AJNR Am J Neuroradiol. 2003;24:346–7.
18. Kraus RN. Treatment of sinus barotrauma. Ann Otol Rhinol Laryngol. 1959;68:80–9.
19. Smith JP, Furry DE. Aeromedical considerations in the management of paranasal sinus barotrauma. Aerosp Med. 1972;43:1031–3.
20. Brandt MT. Oral and maxillofacial aspects of diving medicine. Mil Med. 2004;169:137–41.
21. O'Reilly BJ, Lupa H, Mcrae A. The application of endoscopic sinus surgery to the treatment of recurrent sinus barotrauma. Clin Otolaryngol Allied Sci. 1996;21:528–32.
22. Mutzbauer TS, Mueller PH, Sigg O, Tetzlaff K, Neubauer B. Underwater application of nasal decongestants: method for special operations. Mil Med. 2000;165(11):849–51.
23. Andrews JN, Weitzel EK, Eller R, McMains CK. Unsuccessful frontal balloon sinuplasty for recurrent sinus barotrauma. Aviat Space Environ Med. 2010;81(5):514–6.
24. Bolger WE, Parsons DE, Matson RE. Functional endoscopic sinus surgery in aviators with recurrent sinus barotrauma. Aviat Space Environ Med. 1990;61:148–56.
25. Parsons DS, Chambers DW, Boyd EM. Long-term follow-up of aviators after functional endoscopic sinus surgery for sinus barotrauma. Aviat Space Environ Med. 1997;69:1029–34.
26. Rains BM 3rd. Frontal sinus stenting. Otolaryngol Clin N Am. 2001;34:101–10.
27. Boston AG, McMains KC, Chen PG, Weitzel EK. Management of the refractive aerosinusitis patient: an algorithm used in the US military experience. Unpublished data.

Frontal Sinus Surgery: Selection of Technique

30

Devyani Lal and Peter H. Hwang

Introduction

The goal of any frontal sinus procedure is to address disease effectively while minimizing complications and the need for a revision procedure. In the contemporary era, the selection of surgical approaches to the frontal sinus should be personalized. Patient factors that determine the choice of approach include the location of the disease, the extent and type of pathology, variants in frontal sinus anatomy, as well as patient preference. The technical expertise and experience of the surgeon is a determinant of great import that should be honestly self-evaluated. The surgeon must be technically proficient and masterful of both the anatomy

and necessary instrumentation. Frontal sinus surgery demands meticulous intraoperative dissection and postoperative care. Inadequate frontal surgery may not only leave the disease untreated but also create complications of scarring and stenosis that can worsen prognosis and symptoms in addition to making revision surgery more challenging [1–5]. Through continual study of the three-dimensional frontal recess anatomy and through cadaveric dissection exercises, the frontal surgeon can acquire the expertise to address simpler cases and build experience for more complex surgery [6–8]. Lastly, modern endoscopic sinus surgery requires the availability of specific instrumentation and endoscopes not only in the operating suite but also in the office. Additional equipment such as navigation systems (image guidance) are useful for frontal sinus surgery and can be invaluable for addressing complex pathology and anatomy effectively.

The advancement of technology and navigation systems has enhanced the safety of both endoscopic and external frontal sinus surgery. Modern endoscopes offer superior optics and diverse angles of visualization. CT imaging can be now conducted routinely in sub-millimeter cuts, offering greater detail of anatomical features. Magnetic resonance imaging technology offers the ability to study frontal sinus pathologies with much greater sophistication, defining both the type of pathology and location and

Electronic Supplementary Material The online version of this chapter (https://doi.org/10.1007/978-3-319-97022-6_30) contains supplementary material, which is available to authorized users.

D. Lal (✉)
Department of Otolaryngology – Head and Neck Surgery, Mayo Clinic College of Medicine and Science, Mayo Clinic, Phoenix, AZ, USA

P. H. Hwang
Department of Otolaryngology – Head and Neck Surgery, Stanford University School of Medicine, Stanford, CA, USA

extent. Modern navigation systems have not only facilitated the development of endoscopic techniques but have also made external techniques such as the osteoplastic approach and frontal trephination more precise and safe.

The frontal sinus can be surgically addressed through transnasal endoscopic and external approaches or a combination thereof. In the modern era, endoscopic techniques have supplanted most indications for external procedures on the frontal sinus. However, external techniques can be invaluable for specific indications, where they can be indeed more effective and less morbid than the modern endoscopic approach. For example, external frontal trephination may provide an effective, safe, and efficient supplement to endoscopic transnasal surgery when frontal disease is far lateral or high. The modern frontal sinus surgeon therefore must have expertise in both endoscopic and external techniques.

Historically, external fronto-ethmoidectomy was a mainstay of surgical drainage options for the frontal sinus. However, long-term success was elusive due to recurrent stenosis and scarring of the ostium. This led to the development of salvage external procedures to "obliterate" or externalize the frontal sinuses, sacrificing the functionality of the frontal sinus. Obliteration and cranialization of the frontal sinus remain valuable techniques but are necessary only for rare indications. In the contemporary era, external techniques do not necessarily have to be used with an obliterative philosophy. Approaches such as the bicoronal osteoplastic approach can also be performed to restore mucociliary function ("functional external sinus surgery"). In select cases, these external procedures may less be morbid and shorter in duration than an endoscopic technique used for the same purpose [9, 10].

This chapter will detail the editors' philosophical approach to the selection of technique and the extent of frontal sinus surgery. This chapter will highlight anatomical and pathological considerations that dictate choices using illustrative cases and videos. Select cases presented in the chapters on endoscopic and external frontal techniques are further detailed here to discuss the thought process employed to choose the surgical approach.

The Evolution of Surgical Philosophy

While technology has contributed to the evolution of techniques in frontal surgery, continued growth in the understanding of paranasal sinus physiology and disease pathophysiology has directed the migration from the philosophy of obliterating sinuses toward one of restoring function [6, 11]. All frontal endoscopic techniques for inflammatory disease respect the fundamental tenets of mucosal preservation and functional restoration. For instance, we now understand that mucoceles are lined by normal sinus mucosa. Therefore marsupialization of the mucocele is a not only the safer alternative to extirpation, but it is also a function-restoring choice [7]. Modern frontal sinus surgery should be personalized and patient-specific, and the surgeon thus should employ a variety of surgical strategies to address different indications such as recurrent acute sinusitis, recurrent barotrauma, or recurrent nasal polyposis. Referral to subspecialist surgeons may be considered for recalcitrant and complex pathology.

Choice of Techniques in Frontal Sinus Surgery: Pros vs. Cons

The contemporary literature has established that endoscopic techniques are at least as efficacious as external approaches (if not more so) but with potentially reduced morbidity. Recent studies have also addressed the challenges associated with choosing the right endoscopic technique. Philosophically, the frontal sinus may be approached with a broad array of surgical options, ranging from the least aggressive to the most aggressive approaches. While a more minimal approach may minimize the risk of complications, it may be inadequate to manage disease in the immediate or the long term. On the other hand, more extensive procedures such as the Draf III require technical expertise and potentially increase the length of surgery and the risk of complications. Debate between those who favor more conservative approaches over more aggressive approaches continues. We favor

Table 30.1 Common indications for frontal sinus surgery

A. Chronic inflammatory disease
(a) Chronic rhinosinusitis (with [CRSwNP] or without nasal polyposis [CRSsNP])
(b) Complications of chronic rhinosinusitis
(c) Noninvasive fungal ball
B. Acute inflammatory disease
(a) Acute frontal sinusitis unresponsive to medical therapy
(b) Recurrent acute frontal rhinosinusitis
(c) Acute frontal sinusitis with (impending) complications
(d) Acute invasive fungal rhinosinusitis
C. Mucocele
D. Frontal barosinusitis
E. Tumors of the fronto-ethmoidal region
(a) Benign tumors: osteoma, inverted papilloma, etc.
(b) Malignant tumors: primary and metastatic lesions
F. Cerebrospinal fluid leak and meningoencephalocele of the fronto-ethmoidal region
G. Frontal sinus trauma requiring surgical repair
H. Foreign body removal
I. Transfrontal approaches to pathology in other areas
(a) Anterior cranial base pathology
(b) Pathology of the medial and superior orbit
J. Pneumatocele of the frontal sinus

tailoring the approach to the specific patient, choosing an option that is effective long-term, efficient, and the least morbid. The choice of technique is dictated by the indication of surgery (Table 30.1), the general health status of the patient, and patient preference. The decision to surgically address the frontal sinus should be made thoughtfully, and similar diligence must be exercised in selecting the technique.

The indications, pros, and cons of frontal sinus techniques are detailed in Table 30.2 (modern endoscopic techniques) and Table 30.3 (external techniques). Contemporary endoscopic techniques for frontal sinus surgery include ethmoidectomy and formal frontal ostioplasty via the endoscopic Draf I, Draf II, and Draf III (EMLP) approaches. These techniques are further discussed in detail in the relevant sections (Chaps. 6 and 7). In certain circumstances, these techniques may be supplemented by external approaches such as the frontal trephination approach [2, 8, 12, 13].

Clinical Indications and Their Impact on Technique Selection

Table 30.1 lists common indications for frontal sinus surgery. These indications include chronic and acute inflammatory pathology of the frontal sinus that is unresponsive to medical therapy, as well as their complications. Other indications for surgery include mucoceles, tumors, fractures, cerebrospinal fluid leak, recurrent barosinusitis, etc. which have been discussed earlier in the book. The technical details of surgical procedures have also been presented in the earlier chapters. Here we elaborate our approach to the selection of the frontal technique based on surgical indication.

Inflammatory Frontal Sinus Disease

The authors' approach uses a tiered, personalized approach that is based on the severity and recalcitrance of inflammatory disease, as well as the associated anatomy (Fig. 30.1). In our experience, the vast majority of frontal sinus inflammatory disease chronic rhinosinusitis (CRS) can be addressed by a Draf I or a Draf IIA approach. Most CRS patients presenting to us for revision frontal sinus surgery can also be addressed by these approaches. The Draf IIB and Draf III approaches are not utilized uncommonly in our practices but are reserved for special circumstances as outlined by Table 30.2. External approaches such as the frontal trephination technique are used as needed to assist with transnasal endoscopic surgery. External surgeries such as the osteoplastic flap and cranialization procedures are used on rare occasions in our practice. Finally, balloon-assisted frontal sinusotomy is utilized in our practices for managing the stenosing frontal sinus, as well as in the management of acute frontal sinusitis as a stand-alone tool. Additionally, the balloon is used selectively along with formal frontal recess dissection ("hybrid" technique).

Acute Rhinosinusitis (ARS)

Immunocompromised and intubated patients may develop severe symptoms and can be at risk for developing complications from ARS unre-

Table 30.2 Contemporary indications for endoscopic frontal sinus surgery

Procedure	Description	Applications
Draf I	Removal of ethmoidal cells in the frontal recess without formal instrumentation of the frontal ostium	1. CRSsNP with minimal frontal recess disease 2. Acute frontal sinusitis 3. Recurrent acute frontal sinusitis
Draf II	Complete removal of all anterior ethmoidal cells in the frontal recess with widening of the frontal ostium area	1. Primary surgery for CRSsNP and CRSwNP 2. Revision surgery for CRSsNP and CRSwNP 3. Frontal mucoceles 4. Acute frontal sinusitis 5. Frontal barotrauma 6. Benign tumors 7. Recurrent acute frontal sinusitis
Draf IIA	Medial extent of frontal ostioplasty limited to the vertical attachment of the middle turbinate into the frontal sinus floor	1. Primary surgery for CRSsNP and CRSwNP 2. Revision surgery for CRSsNP and CRSwNP 3. Frontal mucoceles 4. Acute frontal sinusitis 5. Frontal barotrauma 6. Small fronto-ethmoidal osteoma 7. Recurrent acute frontal sinusitis 8. Pneumatocele of the frontal sinus
Draf II B	Widening of the frontal ostium with removal of the floor of the frontal sinus medial to the attachment of the middle turbinate, extending the frontal ostioplasty to the nasal septum or interfrontal sinus septum	1. Revision surgery for CRSsNP and CRSwNP 2. Address a lateralized middle turbinate causing persistent frontal disease 3. Address middle turbinate remnants from prior resection that have scarred or lateralized, causing frontal sinusitis or mucocele 4. Osteoneogenesis 5. Resection of fronto-ethmoidal osteoma 6. Resection of inverted papilloma 7. Endoscopic repair of frontal sinus trauma 8. Endoscopic repair of posterior frontal table CSF leak and meningoencephaloceles 9. As a unilateral approach to the anterior cranial base 10. As a unilateral approach to the medial and superior orbit
Draf III (endoscopic modified Lothrop procedure)	Converting bilateral frontal sinuses into a common cavity by removal of the interfrontal sinus septum and associated fronto-ethmoidal cells; a common drainage path into the nose is achieved by removal of the frontal sinus floor and superior nasal septum	1. Revision surgery for CRSsNP associated with extensive scarring or neo-osteogenesis 2. Revision surgery for CRSwNP with recalcitrant disease subtype 3. Endoscopic repair of frontal sinus trauma 4. Endoscopic repair of posterior frontal table CSF leak and meningoencephalocele 5. Endoscopic resection of benign and malignant tumors involving the frontal sinus 6. As an approach to the anterior cranial base 7. As an approach to the medial and superior orbit

sponsive to appropriate surgery. Odontogenic sinusitis that does not resolve with appropriate therapy directed to the root cause can also cause acute on CRS. In such patients, anterior ethmoidectomy or Draf I or Draf IIA procedure may be effective to manage these conditions (Fig. 30.2). However, if the frontal mucosa is extremely inflamed and friable, stenting may be necessary to inhibit granulation and scar tissue formation.

In those with severe inflammation, mucosal stripping, and narrow, osteitic frontal recess, a Draf IIB with drill out and stenting may be occasionally warranted (Video 30.1).

Other indications for surgery on the frontal sinus include recurrent acute frontal sinusitis. Balloon-assisted frontal recess dilatation in these patients may have advantageous applications in the office-based setting or bedside in the critical

Table 30.3 Contemporary indications for external techniques in frontal sinus surgery

Procedure	Description	Applications
Frontal mini-trephination	Trephining the anterior frontal sinus table by means of a small cannula	1. Acute frontal sinusitis (severe or with complications) to evacuate pus 2. Irrigate frontal sinus 3. Identify frontal recess drainage endoscopically by indentifying colored dye that has been flushed through a mini-trephination
Frontal trephination	Formal incision through brow or lid crease with removal of the anterior frontal table bone	1. In combination with a transnasal endoscopic technique for removal of high fronto-ethmoidal cells 2. Removal of disease (polyp, tumor, mucocele, etc.) in the lateral frontal sinus with or without endoscopic approach 3. Repair of frontal trauma 4. Repair of CSF leak 5. Obliteration of a hypoplastic frontal sinus 6. Approach to the supraorbital area
Osteoplastic flap without obliteration	Utilized to address frontal sinus disease with a goal to restoring frontal sinus function	1. Removal of disease (polyp, tumor, mucocele, etc.) in the lateral or superior frontal sinus with or without endoscopic approach 2. Repair of frontal trauma 3. Repair of CSF leak 4. Approach to the supraorbital area
Osteoplastic flap with obliteration	Utilized to address situations where restoring frontal sinus function is deemed to be not feasible	1. Irreversible, recurrent, unsalvageable scarring of the frontal recess 2. Small hypoplastic frontal sinus with repeated failure of functional approaches 3. Removal of the anterior table for malignancy or extensive trauma that cannot be functionally reconstructed
Cranialization	Removal of the entire posterior table and frontal sinus mucosa, allowing the frontal lobe to fall forward into the frontal sinus. This is not a procedure used for inflammatory sinus disease or mucoceles	1. Malignancy requiring removal of the posterior frontal table 2. Extensive comminuted posterior table fracture that cannot be reconstructed
Riedel's approach	Removal of anterior frontal table with exteriorization of the sinus	1. Rarely performed due to crippling cosmetic deformity. In most instances, the anterior table is reconstructed and frontal sinus obliterated after Riedel's approach

care unit. It is helpful to confirm a diagnosis of recurrent acute sinusitis by endoscopic examination or a computerized tomography (CT) scan at the time of an infection.

Chronic Frontal Sinusitis

The most common indication for performing frontal sinus surgery is symptomatic chronic frontal sinusitis unresponsive to appropriate medical therapy [14]. This includes patients with chronic rhinosinusitis with nasal polyps (CRSwNP) as well as those without nasal polyps (CRSsNP). Within this broad categorization, the disease being addressed may have been relatively responsive to medical or surgical intervention or have exhibited a recalcitrant course [15–17]. Post-traumatic or iatrogenic frontal sinusitis may either be relatively responsive to surgical intervention or be recalcitrant, based on the location and extent of injury. Subtypes of CRS with greater predilection for recalcitrance include nasal polyposis, allergic fungal rhinosinusitis (AFRS), aspirin-exacerbated respiratory disease (AERD), cystic fibrosis (CF), eosinophilic granulomatous polyangiitis (EGPA, formerly

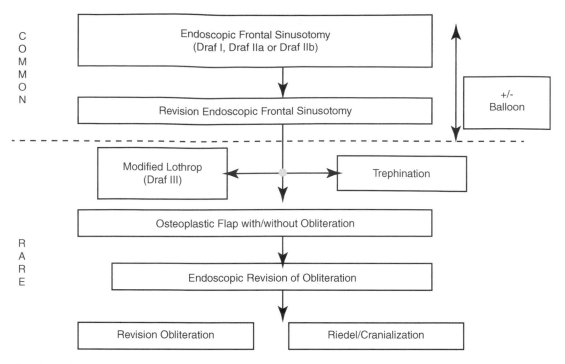

Fig. 30.1 Figure one outlines the editors' approach and use of techniques for frontal sinus surgery

known as Churg-Strauss vasculitis), granulomatosis with polyangiitis (GPA), and immunodeficiency. This group of conditions may require multiple revision procedures. Our group recently published revision endoscopic sinus surgery rates by subtypes of CRS. In a retrospective review of 424 CRS patients [18], our overall revision ESS rate was 4% (3.5% in CRSwNP and 5.1% for CRSsNP). AFS, AERD, and EGPA groups demonstrated low revision rates, while immunodeficiency and GPA patients required more revision surgery. Revision ESS rates for subtypes were AERD, 2%; AFS, 2%; immunodeficiency, 14%; GPA, 40%; EGPA, 0%; and "all other CRS," 4% at median follow-up duration of 36, 28, 41, 37, 44, and 26 months, respectively. Growth in contemporary understanding of CRSwNP subtypes has facilitated the development of surgical and medical strategies that have improved outcomes for AERD, AFS, and EGPA patients. Each of these pathologies requires specific considerations in the preparation for surgery, selection of surgical technique and the extent of surgery, as well as postoperative care. For CRSsNP, Draf I and Draf IIA are the most commonly selected procedures for primary surgery

(Fig. 30.1, Video 30.2). CRSsNP patients with mild disease that do not wish to undergo formal frontal sinusotomy or may be poor surgical candidates (hypoplastic sinuses, etc.) may be managed by anterior ethmoidectomy (Fig. 30.2d). Abuzeid and Hwang et al. reported that anterior ethmoidectomy in these cases may suffice [8]. In revision frontal sinus surgery, Draf IIB may be especially suitable for specific indications such as a lateralized and unsalvageable middle turbinate remnant (Video 30.2). The Draf III procedure is usually used to salvage persistent, recalcitrant sinusitis. In rare cases, the Draf III procedure may be necessary as a primary procedure (Video 30.3), such as in patients with extensive neo-osteogenesis of the frontal recess (Fig. 30.3). The Draf III procedure may also be indicated in patients with severe immunodeficiency, recurrent florid polyposis, or those who have poor mucociliary function; these patients continue to accumulate debris and pus despite adequate frontal ostioplasty (Fig. 30.4). In these patients the Draf III cavity affords gravitational drainage, improves access for delivery of sinonasal lavage and medications, and facilitates in-office debridement.

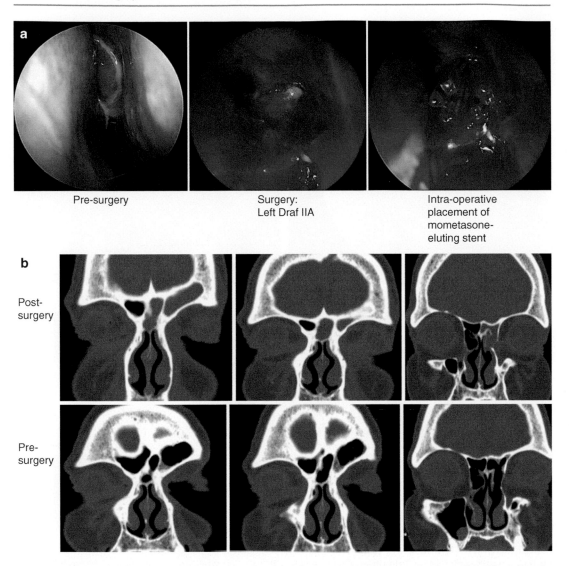

Fig. 30.2 Anterior ethmoidectomy and Draf 1 and Draf IIA procedures can be effective for acute and chronic rhinosinusitis (**a–d**). (**a**) Endoscopic images of a 76-year-old patient with left odontogenic sinusitis unresponsive to dental and medical treatment. The first picture shows pus in the left middle meatus. The patient underwent a left Draf IIA procedure. We placed a mometasone-eluting stent since the left frontal sinus mucosa was extremely inflamed, and the sinus had osteitic changes and was hypoplastic. (second image). The third image shows the stent in position. Placement of a silastic stent or a larger stent would have been difficult and resulted in mucosal stripping. (**b**) Coronal CT images done 15 months after surgery show complete resolution of opacification of the left frontal sinus with persistent osteitis. Note that the postoperative imaging confirms the performance of a Draf IIB procedure. (**c**) Thirty-degree endoscopy images of the left frontal sinus show mild scarring in the medial aspect of an otherwise well-healed ostioplasty. MT: middle turbinate; FS: frontal sinus: SB: Skull base. (**d**) CT scans of a 60-year-old patient with chronic rhinosinusitis without nasal polyps recalcitrant to appropriate medical therapy. The patient has hypoplastic frontal sinuses bilaterally. He underwent anterior ethmoidectomy and maxillary antrostomy. Postoperative imaging performed for new headache after 1 year shows resolution of opacification in the frontal sinuses and demonstrates the performance of anterior ethmoidectomy.

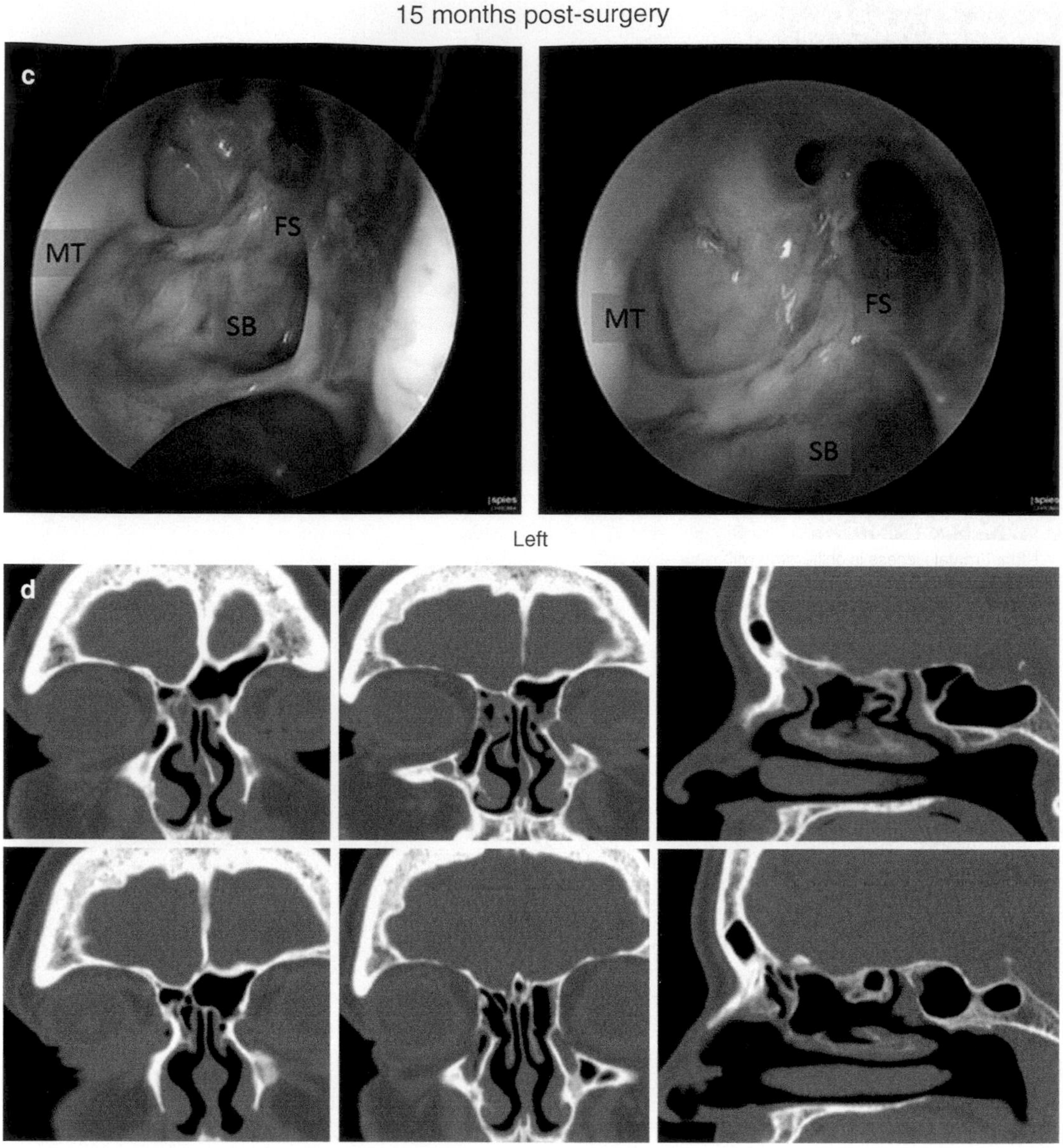

15 months post-surgery

Left

Fig. 30.2 (continued)

For CRSwNP patients, complete and meticulous dissection of all ethmoidal cells in the frontal sinus drainage pathway is essential. Our approach for CRSwNP is usually a Draf IIA procedure, but the choice of technique is personalized based on the anatomy and pathology. It is rare for us to perform more extensive procedures such as Draf IIB or Draf III for primary surgery for CRSwNP patients, unless anatomical considerations warrant those. During surgery, the goal is to perform a thorough ethmoidectomy by skeletonizing the lamina papyracea and skull base and creating a wide ethmoidal corridor. The widest Draf IIA procedure possible is aimed for. This philosophy also encompasses CRSwNP subtypes such as AFS, AERD, or EGPA. Targeted surgery on the ostiomeatal complex may be inadequate to address frontal disease in these CRSwNP subtypes (Fig. 30.5). The creation of wide frontal sinusotomy helps with mucociliary clearance and is a conduit to evacuate all allergic/eosinophilic mucin and nasal polyps intraoperatively; these maneu-

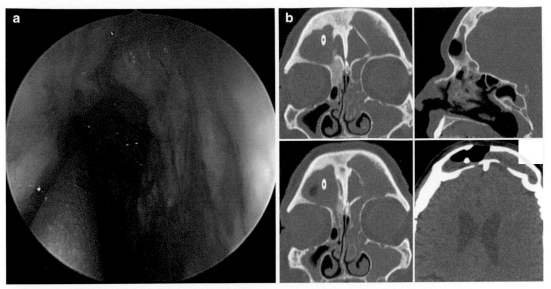

Right Frontal Recess is obliterated with Neo-osteogenesis

Fig. 30.3 In the rare patient with extensive neo-osteogenesis of the frontal recess, the Draf III procedure may be necessary as a primary procedure. Note the extensive neo-osteogenesis in the right frontal recess on the endoscopic image (**a**) and CT images (**b**) of an 80-year-old female that presents with pre-septal orbital cellulitis. An urgent frontal trephination with placement of a drain was performed, as seen on the CT images

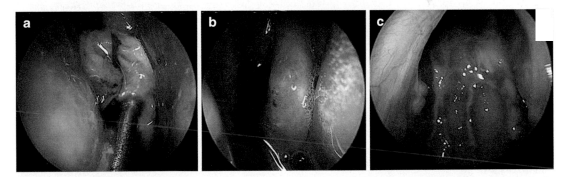

Fig. 30.4 More extensive procedures such as a Draf III surgery may be necessary in "crippled" frontal sinuses that fail to regain function and continue to collect debris and purulence as shown in **a** and **b** panels. Panel **c** shows purulence accumulating in the modified Lothrop cavity, but this large cavity is much more amenable to office debridement and toilet, as well as gravitational drainage

vers are critical to optimizing outcomes for patients with eosinophilic chronic rhinosinusitis [19]. Studies also show that larger ostia size also facilitates topical drug delivery through sinonasal irrigations [20]. Topical corticosteroid sinonasal irrigations after endoscopic sinus surgery have been shown to be more effective than nasal steroid sprays in the management of patients with CRS [14, 21]. Wider frontal sinusotomy can also facilitate office-based debridement and polypectomy.

Figure 30.5 shows CT images of a patient with allergic fungal sinusitis treated with bilateral Draf IIA procedures, maxillary antrostomy, and sphenoethmoidectomy. Her 6-month postoperative examination, shown in Video 30.4, demonstrates an excellent response to the combination of meticulous surgery and diligent maintenance medical therapy. Cystic fibrosis patients may also form nasal polyps but usually have hypoplastic or absent frontal sinuses. However, when disease is present

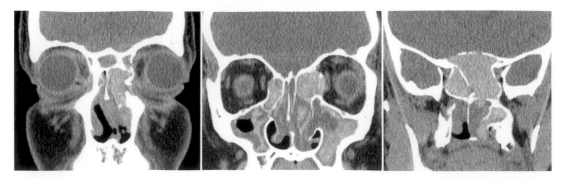

Fig. 30.5 Sinus CT of a patient with CRS with nasal polyposis (CRSwNP) and allergic fungal sinusitis. Targeted surgery on the ostiomeatal complex may be inadequate to address frontal disease in eosinophilic CRSwNP subtypes. Our selection for CRSwNP is usually a Draf IIA procedure in these patients

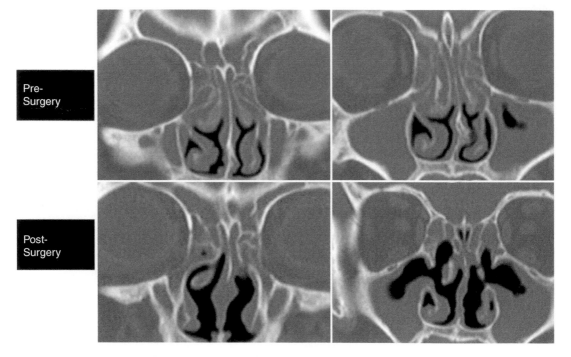

Pre-Surgery

Post-Surgery

Fig. 30.6 Sinus CT scans before and after frontal sinusotomy in two patients requiring revision frontal surgery. The imaging reveals incomplete ethmoidectomy and frontal sinusotomy; these are likely contributors to surgical recalcitrance. Many of these patients can still be effectively managed by revision Draf I or Draf IIA procedures

in pneumatized frontal sinuses, these patients are likely to require the facilitation of gravitational drainage and toilet via large openings to the frontal sinuses as well. In patients of CRSwNP with early recurrent nasal polyposis, or those with diffuse recurrence, we may still consider a revision Draf IIA procedure. In CRSwNP, we typically choose the Draf IIB procedure to address lateralized or scarred middle turbinates, or when middle turbi-

nates resection is necessitated due to extensive polypoid degeneration or instability. The decision to perform a Draf III procedure is made if the sinus CT scan shows the previous procedures to have been thoroughly executed. In some instances, endoscopy and imaging reveal incomplete ethmoidectomy and frontal sinusotomy; these are likely contributors to disease recalcitrance despite surgery (Fig. 30.6). Many of these patients can still

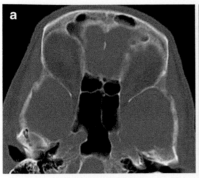 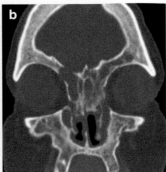 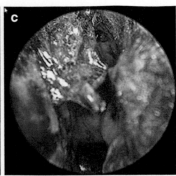

Fig. 30.7 CT and endoscopy images from a patient with granulomatosis with polyangiitis (GPA; formerly known as Wegener's granulomatosis) showing extensive neo- osteogenesis and loculated mucoceles. In such patients, it may be prudent to avoid surgery and follow the patient closely

be effectively managed by revision Draf I or Draf IIA procedures, but some may require Draf IIB or Draf III procedures.

Systemic pathology such as GPA, EGPA, immunodeficiency, etc. also requires multidisciplinary management with rheumatologists, pulmonologists, and immunologists. Input from these specialists on the advisability of surgery as well as postoperative medical management is essential. Patients with GPA may have extensive osteoneogenesis and loculated mucoceles. In these patients, it may be prudent to avoid surgery and follow the patient closely to monitor for disease control and impending complications (Fig. 30.7).

Mucoceles
Mucoceles of the frontal sinus result from scarring of the frontal recess secondary to prior trauma or surgery, sometimes years after the primary insult [22, 23]. In most instances, these are relatively simple to address by endoscopic techniques [7, 24–26]. However, frontal mucoceles that occur in the setting of prior frontal sinus obliteration can be difficult to manage [27, 28]. In these situations, multiple and loculated mucoceles may be present far laterally and superiorly (Fig. 30.8). These may require being addressed by larger endoscopic techniques or external approaches [7, 27]. Functional approaches are preferred, as a repeat obliteration or cranialization procedure is not only associated with increased risk of immedi-

ate complications but also delayed complications such as mucocele recurrence, frontal anesthesia, and neuralgia.

Tumors

Most benign tumors can be managed by transnasal endoscopic techniques. Endoscopic techniques supplemented by a trephination or a purely external technique may be needed for tumors that extend far lateral or cranial in the frontal sinus. In these situations, external techniques may be more efficient and effective.

Osseous Tumors
Benign fibro-osseous neoplasms such as osteoma frequently affect the fronto-ethmoid area. These can cause obstruction of the frontal sinus drainage and may require surgery (detailed in Chap. 16) [29]. Small and large osteomas that are nonobstructive can be observed, especially if they do not cause symptoms or problems with cosmesis (Fig. 30.9). Depending on the size and location of bony neoplasms, a purely endoscopic or external technique or a combined approach may be necessary to be most effective and least morbid (Fig. 30.9).

Inverted Papilloma
Inverted papilloma is likely the most common benign sinonasal tumor of the frontal sinus for which surgery is undertaken (detailed in Chap.

17). Special considerations in the choice of technique are dictated by tumor location, access for visualization and instrumentation, extent of surgical resection, and need for reconstruction [30–33]. The selected approach should give the surgeon adequate room to

pass instrumentation, visualize tumor, and achieve negative resection margins. The intent is to resect the tumor completely, along with margins as deemed necessary. When endoscopic resection is performed, preserving the interfrontal sinus septum is advantageous in

Above and Below Approach:
Trephination with Bilateral Draf IIB

Dissect through Trephination

Fig. 30.8 Images from a patient who has undergone previous frontal sinus obliteration. (**a**) Bicoronal incision scar is visible, along with proptosis secondary to bilateral mucoceles. CT and MRI show that multiple and loculated mucoceles may be far laterally and superiorly in the frontal sinuses and supraorbital cells. There is extensive erosion of the skull base and orbital bone, which would make another obliteration procedure difficult. Distinguishing mucocele from fat may be difficult even with MRI scans when the mucocele content becomes inspissated with the passage of time. (**b–d**) "Above and below" approach employed with a combination of Draf IIB and bilateral frontal trephination procedures to marsupialize all the mucoceles. (**d**) Postoperative MRI showing complete evacuation of the mucoceles; the axial images show the space between the compressed left frontal lobe and the dura has filled up with CSF

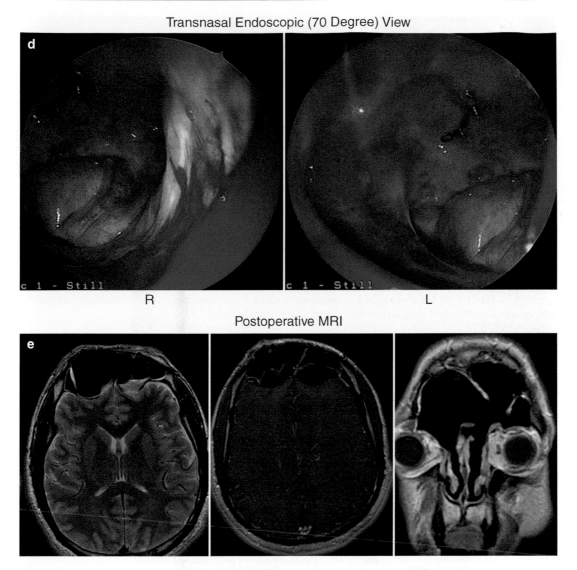

Fig. 30.8   (continued)

minimizing the spread of disease to the contralateral sinus (Video 30.5). External approaches such as a trephination or an osteoplastic flap may be necessary for very large and far lateral tumors or tumors that are located very high in the frontal sinus (Figs. 30.10 and 30.11). For certain inverted papilloma tumors, a purely external technique may be quicker and less morbid (Fig. 30.11).

Malignant Tumors

Malignant tumors of the fronto-ethmoid area include primary sinonasal tumors (adenocarcinoma, olfactory neuroblastoma, squamous cell carcinoma, undifferentiated carcinoma, melanoma, etc.) or metastatic disease (renal cell carcinoma is the most frequent source). These malignancies may be managed endoscopically or in conjunction with external approaches. The primary concern is the ability to

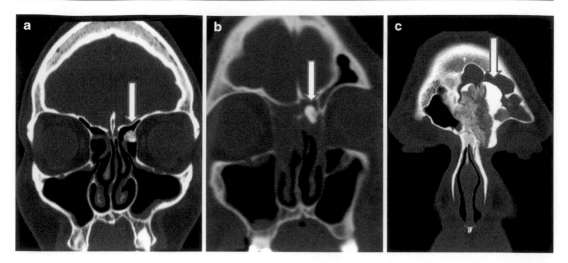

Fig. 30.9 Fronto-ethmoidal osteoma. (**a**) Small (and large) osteomas that are nonobstructive can be observed, especially if they do not cause symptoms or problems with cosmesis. (**b**) Small fronto-ethmoidal osteoma, which can be addressed via a Draf IIA or IIB approach. (**c**) Large osteoma affecting the orbit and skull base, for which a combined endoscopic-external approach may be most effective

Pre-surgery

Post-surgery

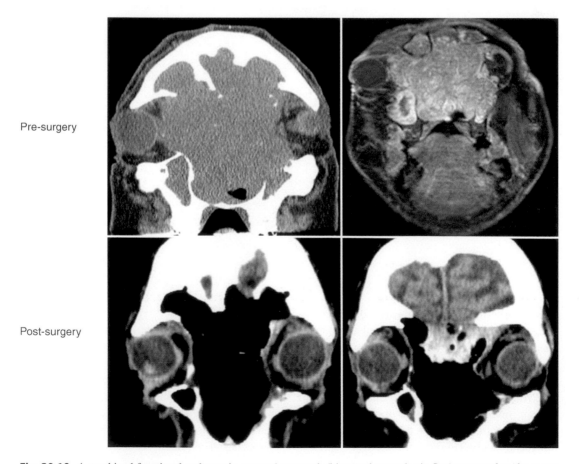

Fig. 30.10 A combined functional endoscopic-external approach (bicoronal osteoplastic flap) was used as the tumor here is very bulky, high, and far lateral in the frontal sinus. CT imaging before and after surgery is shown

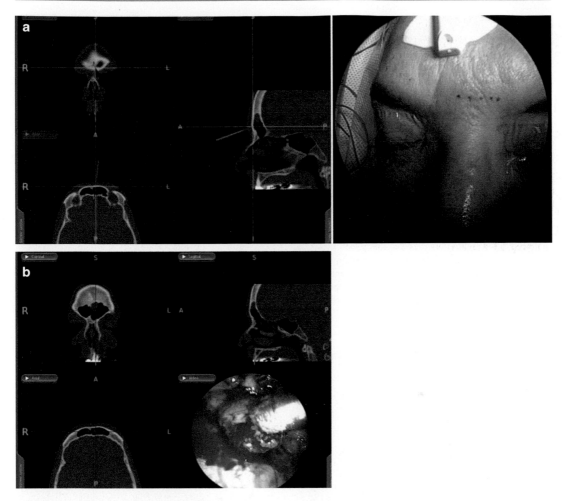

Fig. 30.11 (**a**) Triplanar linked CT Images showing a mass in the left frontal sinus to be high and medial. Based on the location, an external frontal trephination approach was chosen versus an endoscopic approach. The image guidance probe was used to map the trajectory of approach, and plan the incision on the left forehead incision. (**b**) Resection of the mass shown in figure a using a trephination approach only; the pathology was reported to be inverted papilloma

resect the tumor with negative margins. Therefore the approach is dictated by the tumor location, histopathology, soft tissue or bone involvement, as well as extent of required resection and the need for reconstruction [34, 35]. Orbital and soft tissue invasion and high and lateral intracranial involvement are likely to require external approaches or combined endoscopic-external approaches (Fig. 30.12). While endoscopic resection for malignancy is feasible (Fig. 30.13), the full discussion of the choice of treatment for malignancy is beyond the scope of this chapter and is addressed in Chap. 21.

Trauma

The algorithm for managing frontal sinus trauma has been refined in the contemporary era. The vast majority of frontal trauma requiring repair can be managed endoscopically or combined with trephination technique (Fig. 30.13) [36, 37]. Cosmetic deformities, frontal recess obstruction, or cerebrospinal fluid leak are indications for which surgical repair may be required for frontal sinus trauma. These are detailed further in Chap. 15.

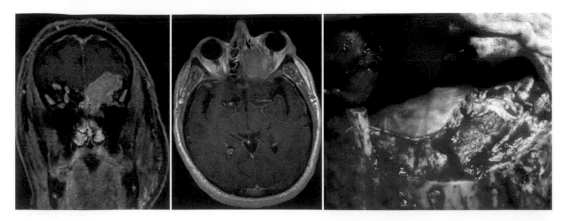

Fig. 30.12 The coronal (**a**) and axial (**b**) gadolinium enhanced T1-weighted images on the panel show the extent of a biopsy proven squamous cell carcinoma of the left fronto-ethmoid area. The tumor has intracranial extension which is very high and lateral; transnasal endoscopic techniques are unlikely to successfully access the lateral extent of the tumor. Addtionally, there is invasion into the orbital soft tissue and orbital apex which will require orbital exenteration. An external approach with bicoronal incision was therefore used for tumor resection and orbital exenteration; repair of the dural defect was performed with fascia lata graft (**c**)

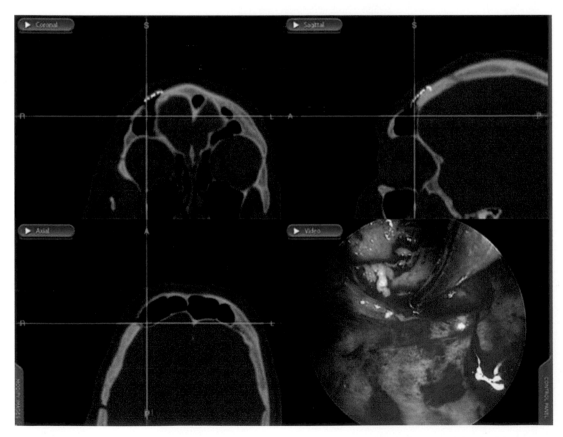

Fig. 30.13 An isolated right frontal trephination approach was used to close a frontal roof fracture that was causing subcutaneous emphysema. This was from a persistent post-surgical fistula caused inadvertently at a previous subfrontal craniotomy where the roof of the frontal sinus was breached

Anterior Skull Base Surgery

The frontal sinus is frequently used as an approach to the anterior cranial base or the orbital for the management of skull base pathology [34, 38, 39]. Procedures such as the endoscopic modified Lothrop procedure or external frontal techniques are utilized for access, resection, and reconstruction [35, 40]. Rarer indications for frontal sinus surgery include frontal sinus barotrauma, aerosinusitis, and pneumatoceles [41]. These are discussed further in Chap. 29.

Caveats

Surgery for Headaches

Surgery for frontal headaches must be undertaken after a thorough evaluation. If the sinus appears to be healthy on CT scan during episodes of pain, the pain is unlikely from inflammatory frontal sinus disease [42]. Other causes of frontal headache such as primary headache disorders (migraine, tension headaches, cluster headaches, etc.) and tumors should be ruled out [42–44]. Surgery on such patients can not only result in unsatisfactory outcomes but mislead the surgeon into performing more extensive revision surgery. The rhinologic surgeon should become familiar with diagnosing and managing patients with frontal headaches, and this is discussed further in Chap. 25.

Osteoplastic Approach with and Without Obliteration

Historically, the osteoplastic approach has been used concomitantly with frontal obliteration [10]. However, the osteoplastic approach can be utilized without subsequent obliteration; by preserving the mucosa and following principles employed in functional endoscopic sinus surgery, the functional status of the frontal sinus can be preserved or restored [45–47]. Contemporary indications for osteoplastic approaches include frontal pathologies that cannot be addressed via an endoscopic approach. Indications for osteoplastic approach without obliteration include inflammatory or neoplastic disease that is high and far lateral that cannot be addressed endoscopically or with a frontal trephination. In this situation, the osteoplastic approach can be used with preservation of frontal mucosa. The frontal sinus drainage pathway is not manipulated if drainage is adequate (Fig. 30.14) or formally enlarged if necessary. The goal of function restoration is philosophically similar to functional endoscopic approaches. Indications for osteoplastic approach with obliteration are limited; this approach is used when restoration of frontal sinus function is deemed impossible. Obliteration may be indicated for CRS with extensive scarring or neo-osteogenesis causing irreversible, unsalvageable scarring of the frontal recess; small hypoplastic frontal sinus with repeated failure of functional approaches; or extensive frontal trauma that cannot be functionally reconstructed or endoscopically addressed.

Cranialization

Cranialization of the frontal sinus consists of meticulous removal of the sinus mucosa and the posterior wall of the frontal sinus, causing the frontal lobe to occupy the frontal sinus, abutting the anterior table and floor of the frontal sinus [48]. It is usually not indicated for inflammatory frontal disease in the contemporary era, but used in cases where there is unsalvageable destruction of the posterior table by trauma or tumor (Fig. 30.15).

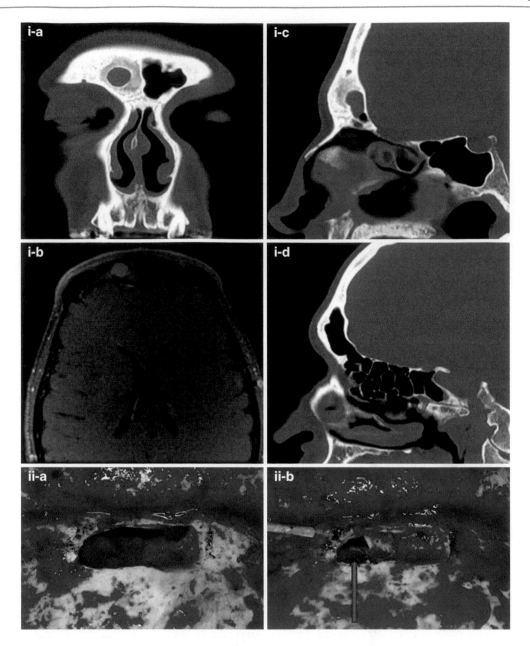

Fig. 30.14 (**i-a**) Coronal section CT scan of patient demonstrating complete opacification of a hypoplastic right frontal sinus. (**i-b**) Axial section MRI T1-weighted sequence with contrast shows a discrete cyst or mass in the right frontal sinus. (**i-c**) Sagittal section CT scan demonstrating opacified and hypoplastic right frontal sinus. CT images of the right frontal sinus show dense, thick bone that will need to be drilled via an endoscopic transnasal approach to the sinus. (**i-d**) Sagittal section CT scan demonstrating a well-pneumatized and healthy left frontal sinus with a wide frontal sinus drainage pathway. (**ii-a**) An osteoplastic flap with a bicoronal approach was used for the patient shown in Figure (**i-iii**). Mucoid material was found and evacuated from the right frontal sinus, and the underlying mucosa was found to be healthy. (**iii-b**) The left frontal sinus was completely healthy with a wide frontal sinus drainage pathway; its ostium and recess can also be visualized (arrow). We therefore elected not to drill the right frontal recess but instead marsupialize the right frontal sinus into the left frontal sinus. (**iii**) Three-month follow-up CT imaging shows the osteoplastic flap to be well healed (**iii-a**) and the "modified external Lothrop" common cavity to be adequately ventilated by the left frontal sinus drainage pathway (**iii-b**). A 66-year-old male with a history of renal cell carcinoma presented with a frontal forehead bulge and headache

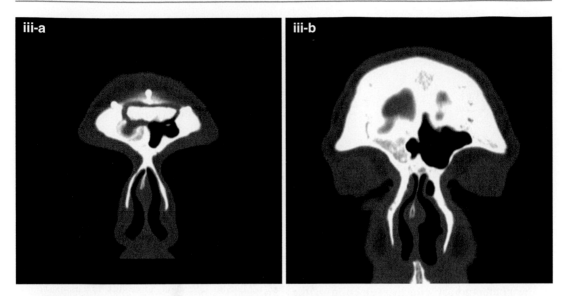

Fig. 30.14 (continued)

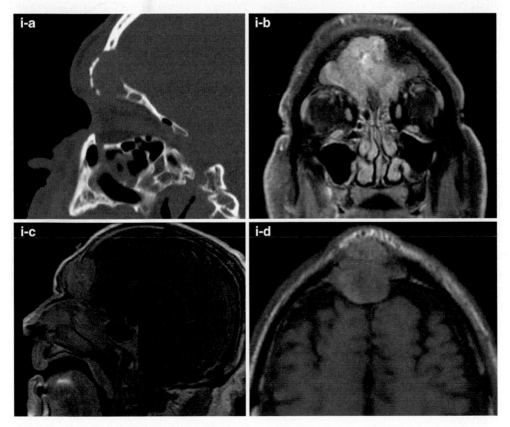

Fig. 30.15 (**i-a**) Sinus CT scan demonstrating an expansile mass of the frontal sinus eroding the anterior, posterior, and inferior (orbital) walls on sagittal view in a patient with metastatic renal cell carcinoma. (**i-b, c, d**) T1-weighted MRI sequence with gadolinium contrast shows a large contrast-enhancing mass in the bilateral frontal sinus with extension into adjacent structures in the coronal (**i-b**), axial (**i-c**), and sagittal (**i-d**) sections; the contrast-enhancing mass to infiltrate the soft tissue anteriorly and the dura posteriorly. (**ii**) The patient subsequently underwent resection of the mass with a cranialization procedure and reconstruction using mesh and a free flap

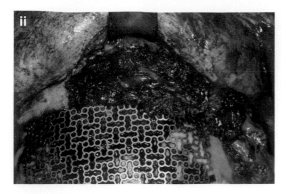

Fig. 30.15 (continued)

Summary

In the contemporary era, the selection of the surgical approach to the frontal sinus surgery should be personalized. The selected technique should address the disease effectively while minimizing the risks of complications and postoperative sequelae. Factors that determine the choice of approach include the location, extent, and pathology of the disease, the frontal sinus anatomy, the surgeon's expertise, and the availability of instrumentation. In our experience, the vast majority of frontal sinus inflammatory disease [chronic rhinosinusitis (CRS)] can be addressed by a Draf I or a Draf IIA approach. Most CRS patients presenting for revision frontal sinus surgery can also be addressed by these approaches. The Draf IIB and Draf III approaches are not infrequently employed in our practice, but reserved for select cases. External approaches such as the frontal trephination technique are used to assist with transnasal endoscopic surgery as needed. External surgery such as the osteoplastic flap and cranialization procedures are applied only on rare occasions.

References

1. Tomazic PV, Stammberger H, Koele W, Gerstenberger C. Ethmoid roof CSF-leak following frontal sinus balloon sinuplasty. Rhinology. 2010;48(2):247–50.
2. Valdes CJ, Bogado M, Samaha M. Causes of failure in endoscopic frontal sinus surgery in chronic rhinosinusitis patients. Int Forum Allergy Rhinol. 2014;4(6):502–6.
3. Graham SM, Nerad JA. Orbital complications in endoscopic sinus surgery using powered instrumentation. Laryngoscope. 2003;113(5):874–8.
4. Bartley J, Eagleton N, Rosser P, Al-Ali S. Superior oblique muscle palsy after frontal sinus minitrephine. Am J Otolaryngol Head Neck Med Surg. 2012;33(1):181–3.
5. Stankiewicz JA, Lal D, Connor M, Welch K. Complications in endoscopic sinus surgery for chronic rhinosinusitis: a 25-year experience. Laryngoscope. 2011;121(12):2684–701.
6. Weber W, Kratzsch B, Hosemann W, Schaefer SD. Modern concepts of frontal sinus surgery. Laryngoscope. 2001;111(1):137–46.
7. Courson AM, Stankiewicz JA, Lal D. Contemporary management of frontal sinus mucoceles: a meta-analysis. Laryngoscope. 2014;124(2):378–86.
8. Abuzeid WM, Mace JC, Costa ML, Rudmik L, Soler ZM, Kim GS, et al. Outcomes of chronic frontal sinusitis treated with ethmoidectomy: a prospective study. Int Forum Allergy Rhinol. 2016;6(6):597–604.
9. Hahn S, Palmer JN, Purkey MT, Kennedy DW, Chiu AG. Indications for external frontal sinus procedures for inflammatory sinus disease. Am J Rhinol Allergy. 2009;23(3):342–7.
10. Ramadan HH. History of frontal sinus surgery. Arch Otolaryngol Head Neck Surg. 2000;126(1):98–9.
11. Draf W, Weber R. Draf microendoscopic sinus procedures Am J Oto 1999.pdf. Am J Otolaryngol. 1993;14(6):394–8.
12. Becker SS, Han JK, Nguyen TA, Gross CW. Initial surgical treatment for chronic frontal sinusitis: a pilot study. Ann Otol Rhinol Laryngol. 2007;116(4 I):286–9.
13. Kennedy DW, Josephson JS, Zinreich SJ, Mattox DE, Goldsmith MM. Endoscopic sinus surgery for mucoceles: A viable alternative. Laryngoscope. 1989;99(9):885–95
14. Orlandi RR, Kingdom TT, Hwang PH, Smith TL, Alt JA, Baroody FM, et al. International consensus statement on allergy and rhinology: rhinosinusitis. Int Forum Allergy Rhinol. 2016;6(November 2015):S22–209.
15. Han JK. Subclassification of chronic rhinosinusitis. Laryngoscope. 2013;123(SUPPL. 2):15–27.
16. Akdis CA, Bachert C, Cingi C, Dykewicz MS, Hellings PW, Naclerio RM, et al. Endotypes and phenotypes of chronic rhinosinusitis: a PRACTALL document of the European Academy of Allergy and Clinical Immunology and the American Academy of Allergy, Asthma & Immunology. J Allergy Clin Immunol. 2013 Jun;131(6):1479–90.
17. López-Chacón M, Mullol J, Pujols L. Clinical and biological markers of difficult-to-treat severe chronic rhinosinusitis. Curr Allergy Asthma Rep. 2015;15(5):19.
18. Miglani A, Divekar RD, Azar A, Rank MA, Lal D. Revision endoscopic sinus surgery rates by chronic rhinosinusitis subtype. Int Forum Allergy Rhinol. 2018;(0):1–5. https://doi.org/10.1002/alr.22146.

19. Snidvongs K, Chin D, Sacks R, Earls P, Harvey RJ. Eosinophilic rhinosinusitis is not a disease of ostiomeatal occlusion. Laryngoscope. 2013;123(5): 1070–4.

20. Snidvongs K, Pratt E, Chin D, Sacks R, Earls P, Harvey RJ. Corticosteroid nasal irrigations after endoscopic sinus surgery in the management of chronic rhinosinusitis. Int Forum Allergy Rhinol. 2012;2(5): 415–21.

21. Harvey RJ, Snidvongs K, Kalish LH, Oakley GM, Sacks R. Corticosteroid nasal irrigations are more effective than simple sprays in a randomized double-blinded placebo-controlled trial for chronic rhinosinusitis after sinus surgery. Int Forum Allergy Rhinol. 2018;8(4):461–70.

22. Herndon M, McMains KC, Kountakis SE. Presentation and management of extensive fronto-orbital-ethmoid mucoceles. Am J Otolaryngol Head Neck Med Surg. 2007;28(3):145–7.

23. Mourouzis C, Evans BT, Shenouda E. Late presentation of a mucocele of the frontal sinus: 50 years postinjury. J Oral Maxillofac Surg. 2008;66(7):1510–3.

24. Bockmühl U, Kratzsch B, Benda K, Draf W. Surgery for paranasal sinus mucocoeles: efficacy of endonasal microendoscopic management and long-term results of 185 patients. Rhinology. 2006 Mar;44(1):62–7.

25. Cervantes SS, Lal D. Crista galli mucocele: endoscopic marsupialization via frontoethmoid approach. Int Forum Allergy Rhinol. 2014;4(7):598–602.

26. Serrano E, Klossek JM, Percodani J, Yardeni E, Dufour X. Surgical management of paranasal sinus mucoceles: a long-term study of 60 cases. Otolaryngol Head Neck Surg. 2004;131(1):133–40.

27. Wormald PJ, Ananda A, Nair S. Modified endoscopic lothrop as a salvage for the failed osteoplastic flap with obliteration. Laryngoscope. 2003;113(11): 1988–92.

28. Weber R, Draf W, Keerl R, Kahle G, Schinzel S, Thomann S, et al. Osteoplastic frontal sinus surgery with fat obliteration: technique and long-term results using magnetic resonance imaging in 82 operations. Laryngoscope. 2000;110(June):1037–44.

29. Ooi EH, Glicksman JT, Vescan AD, Witterick IJ. An alternative management approach to paranasal sinus fibro-osseous lesions. Int Forum Allergy Rhinol. 2011;1(1):55–63.

30. Lawson W, Patel ZM. The evolution of management for inverted papilloma: an analysis of 200 cases. Otolaryngol Head Neck Surg. 2009;140(3):330–5.

31. Chiu AG, Jackman AH, Antunes MB, Feldman MD, Palmer JN. Radiographic and histologic analysis of the bone underlying inverted papillomas. Laryngoscope. 2006;116(9):1617–20.

32. Cannady SB, Batra PS, Sautter NB, Roh H-J, Citardi MJ. New staging system for sinonasal inverted papilloma in the endoscopic era. Laryngoscope. 2007;117(7):1283–7.

33. Wormald PJ, Ooi E, van Hasselt CA, Nair S. Endoscopic removal of sinonasal inverted papil-

loma including endoscopic medial maxillectomy. Laryngoscope. 2003;113(5):867–73.

34. Eloy JA, Vivero RJ, Hoang K, Civantos FJ, Weed DT, Morcos JJ, et al. Comparison of transnasal endoscopic and open craniofacial resection for malignant tumors of the anterior skull base. Laryngoscope. 2009;119(5):834–40.

35. Har-El G, Casiano RR. Endoscopic management of anterior skull base tumors. Otolaryngol Clin N Am. 2005;38(1):133–44.

36. Chaaban MR, Conger B, Riley KO, Woodworth BA. Transnasal endoscopic repair of posterior table fractures. Otolaryngol Head Neck Surg. 2012;147(6):1142–7.

37. Koento T. Current advances in sinus preservation for the management of frontal sinus fractures. Curr Opin Otolaryngol Head Neck Surg. 2012;20(4):274–9.

38. Lee JM, Ransom E, Lee JYK, Palmer JN, Chiu AG. Endoscopic anterior skull base surgery: intraoperative considerations of the crista galli. Skull Base. 2011;21(2):83–6.

39. Kabil MS, Shahinian HK. The endoscopic supraorbital approach to tumors of the middle cranial base. Surg Neurol. 2006;66(4):396–401.

40. Lal D, Cain RBB. Updates in reconstruction of skull base defects. Curr Opin Otolaryngol Head Neck Surg. 2014;22(5):419–28.

41. Weitzel EK, McMains KC, Wormald PJ. Comprehensive surgical management of the aerosinusitis patient. Curr Opin Otolaryngol Head Neck Surg. 2009;17(1):11–7.

42. Lal D, Rounds A, Dodick DW. Comprehensive management of patients presenting to the otolaryngologist for sinus pressure, pain, or headache. Laryngoscope. 2015;125(2):303–10.

43. Patel ZM, Kennedy DW, Setzen M, Poetker DM, Delgaudio JM. "Sinus headache": Rhinogenic headache or migraine? An evidence-based guide to diagnosis and treatment. Int Forum Allergy Rhinol. 2013;3(3):221–30.

44. Lal D, Rounds AB, Rank MA, Divekar R. Clinical and 22-item Sino-Nasal Outcome Test symptom patterns in primary headache disorder patients presenting to otolaryngologists with "sinus" headaches, pain or pressure. Int Forum Allergy Rhinol. 2015;5(5):408–16.

45. Rivera T, Rodríguez M, Pulido N, García-Alcántara F, Sanz L. Current indications for the osteoplastic flap. Acta Otorrinolaringol (English Ed). 2016;67(1):33–9.

46. Ochsner MC, Delgaudio JM. The place of the osteoplastic flap in the endoscopic era: indications and pitfalls. Laryngoscope. 2015;125(4):801–6.

47. Healy DY, Leopold DA, Gray ST, Holbrook EH. The perforation technique: a modification to the frontal sinus osteoplastic flap. Laryngoscope. 2014;124(6):1314–7.

48. Donath A, Sindwani R. Frontal sinus cranialization using the pericranial flap: an added layer of protection. Laryngoscope. 2006;116(9):1585–8.

Index

Printed by Printforce, the Netherlands